Java 22 for Healthcare and Medical Applications

This comprehensive book delves into the key features introduced in Java 22, providing insights and practical examples to help readers understand and implement these enhancements within the context of medical applications with the goal of enhancing medical practices, streamlining processes, and improving patient care.

Java 22 for Healthcare and Medical Applications explores the latest Java 22 and features the newest advancements in Java programming, including unnamed variables, launch multi-file source-code programs, and foreign function and memory APIs. From implementing advanced algorithms for medical image analysis to developing efficient healthcare management systems, this book shows how this tool can revolutionize the medical field. With its focus on accessibility, interoperability, and data security, this book empowers healthcare professionals to leverage technology in innovative ways, ultimately leading to better patient outcomes and improved healthcare delivery. Whether it's optimizing electronic health record systems, developing telemedicine platforms, or advancing medical research through data analysis, the author equips medical professionals with the knowledge and skills needed to harness the full potential of Java programming in the healthcare industry. With clear explanations and 300+ hands-on examples, readers will learn how to leverage Java 22's cutting-edge features to build powerful and efficient applications.

The book caters to a diverse audience ranging from students to professionals and provides valuable insights into the latest advancements in Java programming and its applications within healthcare and medical technology.

Usharani Bhimavarapu is an Assistant Professor at Koneru Lakshmaiah Education Foundation in Andhra Pradesh, India, where she teaches Computer Science and Engineering. With a career spanning 17 years, she has become a respected authority in Data Mining, Machine Learning, and Data Structure. Dr. Bhimavarapu's research prowess is evidenced by her publication of over 100 papers and 50 books on programming languages like CPP, Java, Fullstack, Databases, R, Node.js, Python, HTML, and CSS.

Biomedical and Robotics Healthcare
Series Editors: Utku Kose, Jude Hemanth, and **Omer Deperlioglu**

Artificial Intelligence for the Internet of Health Things
Deepak Gupta, Eswaran Perumal and K. Shankar

Biomedical Signal and Image Examination with Entropy-Based Techniques
V. Rajinikanth, K. Kamalanand, C. Emmanuel and B. Thayumanavan

Robotic Technologies in Biomedical and Healthcare Engineering
Edited by Deepak Gupta, Moolchand Sharma, Vikas Chaudhary, and Ashish Khanna

Mechano-Electric Correlations in the Human Physiological System
A. Bakiya, K. Kamalanand and R. L. J. De Britto

Machine Learning and Deep Learning in Medical Data Analytics and Healthcare Applications
Edited by Om Prakash Jena, Bharat Bhushan, and Utku Kose

Applied Artificial Intelligence: A Biomedical Perspective
Edited by Swati V. Shinde, Varsha Bendre, D. Jude Hemanth, and MA Balafar

Combating Women's Health Issues with Machine Learning: Challenges and Solutions
Edited by Jude Hemanth and Meenu Gupta

Soft Computing Techniques in Connected Healthcare Systems
Edited by Moolchand Sharma, Suman Deswal, Umesh Gupta, Mujahid Tabassum, and Isah A. Lawal

Explainable Artificial Intelligence (XAI) in Healthcare
Edited by Utku Kose, Nilgun Sengoz, Xi Chen, and Jose Antonio Marmolejo Saucedo

Java 22 for Healthcare and Medical Applications
Usharani Bhimavarapu

For more information about this series, please visit: www.routledge.com/Biomedical-and-Robotics-Healthcare/book-series/BRHC

Java 22 for Healthcare and Medical Applications

Usharani Bhimavarapu

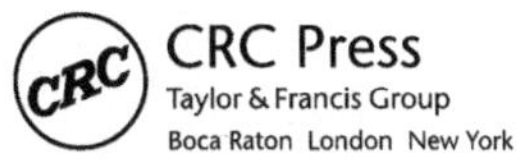

CRC Press is an imprint of the
Taylor & Francis Group, an informa business

Designed cover image: Shutterstock ©

First edition published 2025
by CRC Press
2385 NW Executive Center Drive, Suite 320, Boca Raton FL 33431

and by CRC Press
4 Park Square, Milton Park, Abingdon, Oxon, OX14 4RN

CRC Press is an imprint of Taylor & Francis Group, LLC

ISBN: 978-1-032-89726-4 (hbk)
ISBN: 978-1-032-89719-6 (pbk)
ISBN: 978-1-003-54431-9 (ebk)

DOI: 10.1201/9781003544319

Typeset in Times
by Newgen Publishing UK

Contents

Preface

Java has been a cornerstone of enterprise and application development for decades, and with the release of Java 22, it continues to evolve, offering new features and enhancements that boost productivity, performance, and security. This book is designed for developers who are already familiar with the fundamentals of Java and are eager to expand their knowledge to the latest features and their applications.

Java 22 introduces several enhancements to improve code flexibility, readability, and maintainability. JEP 456 introduces unnamed variables and patterns for improved readability in variable declarations and nested patterns (Chapters 3 and 9). JEP 459 simplifies string handling with runtime-computed values within strings, enhancing security and readability (Chapter 4). Additionally, JEP 463 makes it easier for beginners to write single-class programs, facilitating a smoother transition to complex programming (Chapter 6). JEP 461 enriches the Stream API with custom intermediate operations, enhancing the expressiveness of stream pipelines (Chapter 11). JEP 447 allows developers to place statements before explicit constructor invocations, offering more flexibility in constructor behavior (Chapter 7). Structured concurrency (JEP 462) and scoped values (JEP 464) streamline concurrent programming by enhancing error handling, cancellation, and data sharing across threads (Chapter 10).

To bring these features to life, this book emphasizes real-time examples, particularly in the medical field. By working through these practical examples, you'll not only learn the new features but also understand how they can be applied to solve complex, real-world problems. We will explore how to manage and process large sets of medical data using Java 22's enhanced APIs and performance improvements, develop diagnostic tools that utilize Java's pattern matching and new APIs, and create secure medical applications that protect sensitive data. Additionally, you will learn how to interface with medical devices using the Foreign Function & Memory API, capturing and processing data directly from various medical instruments.

This book is ideal for Java developers who want to upgrade their skills to Java 22, software engineers looking for practical examples of Java in the medical field, medical application developers who need to build efficient, secure, and high-performance applications, and students and educators in computer science and software engineering who are interested in the latest Java features and their applications. Each chapter introduces new features and demonstrates their use with practical, real-world examples, with code samples provided to illustrate concepts and exercises included to reinforce learning. We hope this book will serve as a valuable resource in your journey to mastering advanced Java programming and building impactful medical applications.

About the Author

Usharani Bhimavarapu is an Assistant Professor at Koneru Lakshmaiah Education Foundation in Andhra Pradesh, India, where she teaches Computer Science and Engineering. With a career spanning 17 years, she has become a respected authority in Data Mining, Machine Learning, and Data Structure. Dr. Bhimavarapu's research prowess is evidenced by her publication of over 100 papers and 50 books on programming languages like CPP, Java, Fullstack, Databases, R, Node.js, Python, HTML, and CSS.

1 Java Introduction

1.1 INTRODUCTION

OOPs stands for object-oriented programming, which is a programming paradigm that organizes software design around objects rather than functions and logic. In OOP, objects are instances of classes, which encapsulate data (attributes) and behaviors (methods). This paradigm promotes modularity, reusability, and extensibility in software development by allowing developers to model real-world entities and their interactions more effectively. Key principles of OOP include encapsulation, inheritance, polymorphism, and abstraction.

1.1.1 Fundamental OOP Concepts in Java

These concepts form the foundation of object-oriented programming in Java and are essential for building modular, maintainable, and scalable software systems.

1.1.1.1 Abstraction

Abstraction is the process of hiding the implementation details and showing only the essential features of an object. It helps in reducing programming complexity and effort by focusing on the high-level functionalities. Abstraction is achieved using abstract classes and methods, where the implementation details are hidden, and only the essential features are provided.

1.1.1.2 Encapsulation

Encapsulation refers to the bundling of data (variables) and methods that operate on that data into a single unit or class. It helps in data hiding and protects the data from unauthorized access. Encapsulation is achieved using access modifiers to restrict access to certain components of a class, thus protecting data from unauthorized access.

1.1.1.3 Inheritance

Inheritance allows a class (subclass or derived class) to inherit properties and behaviors from another class (superclass or base class). It promotes code reusability and establishes a hierarchical relationship between classes. Inheritance allows a subclass to inherit properties and behaviors from a superclass, promoting code reuse and establishing a hierarchical relationship between classes.

1.1.1.4 Polymorphism

Polymorphism allows objects of different classes to be treated as objects of a common superclass. It enables methods to be written that can work with objects of various types and classes at runtime.

DOI: 10.1201/9781003544319-1

Polymorphism allows objects of different types to be treated as objects of a common superclass, enabling flexibility and code reuse.

1.1.2 Impact of OOP Concepts on Performance

The implementation of object-oriented programming (OOP) concepts, such as encapsulation and inheritance, can enhance code reusability and maintainability, leading to more efficient development processes.

1. Memory Usage:
    a. Objects and Classes: Each object in Java occupies memory. Excessive use of objects, especially large ones, can lead to increased memory consumption and reduced application performance.
    b. Inheritance and Polymorphism: Deep inheritance hierarchies and extensive use of polymorphism can lead to increased memory usage and slower runtime performance due to dynamic method dispatch.
2. CPU Overhead:
    a. Method Calls: Frequent method calls, especially in deep inheritance structures or complex polymorphic scenarios, can introduce CPU overhead.
    b. Encapsulation and Accessor Methods: Overuse of getters and setters for encapsulation can result in additional method calls, impacting CPU performance.
3. Optimizing Java Code for Performance
4. Efficient Use of Objects:
    a. Minimize object creation, especially in performance-critical sections of the code. Use object pooling for frequently used objects.
5. Optimizing Inheritance and Polymorphism:
    a. Prefer composition over inheritance where appropriate to reduce complexity and memory footprint.
    b. Use interfaces wisely and avoid deep inheritance trees to reduce the overhead of dynamic method dispatch.
6. Effective Memory Management:
    a. Monitor and manage memory usage actively. Utilize Java profiling tools to identify and fix memory leaks.
    b. Optimize data structures, preferring efficient collections like ArrayList over LinkedList when random access is frequent.
7. Code Refactoring for Performance:
    a. Refactor code to eliminate unnecessary method calls, especially in loops or frequently called methods.
    b. Use inline code for trivial methods where appropriate.
8. Lazy Initialization and Eager Loading:
    a. Use lazy initialization for heavy resources when their immediate loading might impact startup performance.
    b. Conversely, use eager loading to pre-load resources and reduce latency in critical sections of the application.
9. Leveraging Modern JVM Features:
    a. Stay updated with the latest Java versions, which often include performance enhancements in the JVM.
    b. Utilize JIT compilation and understand how Java's HotSpot VM optimizes code at runtime.

10. Concurrency and Multithreading:
    a. Use multithreading judiciously to improve application performance, especially for I/O bound or computationally intensive operations.
    b. Ensure thread safety and avoid common pitfalls like deadlock or race conditions.

1.2 CONCEPTS OF OOPS IN JAVA

In Java, object-oriented programming (OOP) is based on several key concepts:

1.2.1 Classes and Objects

Classes are blueprints for objects, defining their attributes (fields) and behaviors (methods). Objects are instances of classes.

Syntax

```
// Abstract class Student
abstract class Student {
  // Abstract method (no implementation)
  abstract void registerCourse();

  // Abstract method (no implementation)
  abstract void attendClass();

  // Concrete method (optional to include in abstract class)
    static void getDetails() {
    // Method can have implementation
  }

}
// Concrete class Course extends Student
class Course extends Student {
  //constructor
public Course(String courseName, Student student)
{
this.courseName = courseName;
this.student = student;
// A course is composed of a student
}
// Main method in Course class
  void main(String[] args) {
    System.out.println("Main method in Course class.");
  Student s=new Course();
Course c= new Course();
  }

  // Method implementations would go here
}
```

In the above syntax, the `Student` class is defined as an abstract class, which means it cannot be instantiated directly and serves as a blueprint for other classes. It contains abstract methods (`registerCourse` and `attendClass`) that do not have implementations, requiring any subclass to provide specific behavior for these methods. The `Course` class, which extends `Student`, is a concrete implementation that inherits the structure of the `Student` class and is responsible for implementing the abstract methods, thereby showcasing the relationship between abstract and concrete classes in object-oriented programming.

1.2.1.1 Objects

In Java, an object is a fundamental concept that represents a real-world entity or concept within a program's runtime environment. Objects are instances of classes, which serve as blueprints or templates defining their structure and behavior. An object is created using the new keyword followed by a constructor invocation. It is an instance of a class and holds its own set of data (attributes or fields) and methods (functions or behaviors).

The line `Course c = new Course();` in the syntax given in (A)(i.e. classes) creates an instance of the `Course` class, allowing you to work directly with a concrete object that inherits from the abstract `Student` class. By doing so, you can implement and access the specific behaviors defined by the `Course` class, including any methods that were declared as abstract in `Student`. This enables you to utilize the functionality associated with a student enrolled in a course, such as registering for classes or attending lectures. Moreover, since `Course` extends `Student`, it can also leverage any concrete methods defined in the `Student` class, promoting code reuse. This instantiation showcases the use of concrete objects in object-oriented programming, allowing for the practical implementation of the abstract class's template.

1.2.2 Inheritance

Inheritance allows a class (subclass) to inherit properties and behaviors from another class (superclass). This promotes code reuse and establishes a hierarchical relationship between classes.

In the syntax given in (A)(i.e. classes), the `Student` class serves as an abstract base class, defining two abstract methods (`registerCourse` and `attendClass`) that must be implemented by any subclass. The `Course` class inherits from `Student`, allowing it to leverage the defined structure while implementing specific behavior for the abstract methods.

1.2.3 Polymorphism

Polymorphism allows objects of different types to be treated as objects of a common superclass. It enables methods to be overridden in subclasses to provide different implementations.

In the syntax given in (A)(i.e. classes), the line `Student s = new Course();` exemplifies the concept of polymorphism in object-oriented programming. By declaring `s` as a `Student` type and initializing it with an instance of the `Course` class, we achieve upcasting, allowing the `Course` object to be treated as a `Student`. This enables the use of `s` to call methods defined in the `Student` class, while the actual method implementations executed will be those from the `Course` class. This design encapsulates behavior, allowing for flexibility in managing different types of students while adhering to a common interface. It promotes code reusability and adaptability, showcasing how objects can interact with one another through their defined relationships, ultimately enhancing the overall functionality of the program.

1.2.4 Abstraction

Abstraction involves hiding the implementation details and exposing only the essential features of an object. Abstract classes and interfaces are used to achieve abstraction in Java.

In the syntax given in (A)(i.e. classes), the `Student` class is defined as an abstract class with two abstract methods: `registerCourse()` and `attendClass()`, which must be implemented by any subclass. The `getDetails()` method is a concrete method that can provide common functionality.

The `Course` class extends `Student`, indicating that it will provide specific implementations for the abstract methods, although they are not defined in this outline.

1.2.5 Encapsulation

Encapsulation refers to bundling the data (attributes) and methods that operate on the data within a single unit (class). Access modifiers like private, protected, and public are used to control access to class members.

In the syntax given in (A)(i.e. classes), encapsulation is demonstrated through the use of the abstract class `Student`, which contains abstract methods that define essential behaviors without exposing their implementations. By encapsulating the behavior of registering for courses and attending classes, the `Student` class establishes a blueprint that can be inherited by concrete classes like `Course`. This ensures that the internal workings of how these methods are executed are hidden from the user, promoting a clear separation between the interface and the implementation.

When a `Course` object is created with `Course c = new Course();`, it encapsulates the specific details of course management, allowing the class to define its own implementations of the abstract methods. The encapsulated nature of the `Student` class ensures that the core functionalities are protected and can only be modified through defined interfaces, enhancing data integrity and reducing the risk of unintended interactions. This encapsulation fosters a robust design that facilitates maintainability and scalability in object-oriented programming.

1.2.6 Methods

Methods are functions defined within classes to perform specific tasks. They encapsulate behavior and can accept parameters and return values.

In the syntax given in (A)(i.e. classes), the Student class declares abstract methods, registerCourse() and attendClass(), which serve as contracts that must be fulfilled by any subclass, ensuring that specific behaviors are implemented while keeping the method implementations hidden. This means that the details of how these operations are carried out are encapsulated within the subclass. When the Course class extends Student, it can provide concrete implementations for these abstract methods, thereby encapsulating the specific logic related to course registration and attendance. The encapsulated methods allow for controlled access and modification of functionality, ensuring that the internal workings of the Course class are not exposed to the outside world. This separation of method declaration in the abstract class and implementation in the concrete class promotes a clean interface, enabling code reuse and reducing complexity while maintaining the integrity of the methods defined in the Student class.

1.2.7 Packages

Packages are used to organize classes and interfaces into namespaces, providing a way to manage and control access to classes and interfaces. For example, to create a simple package named `com.java22`, you would start your Java file with:

```
package com.java22;
```

This declaration must be the first line of your Java source file and indicates that the classes defined in that file belong to the `com. java22` package.

1.2.8 Constructors and Destructors

Constructors are special methods used for initializing objects when they are created. Java doesn't have destructors, but it has finalizers that are called before an object is garbage collected.

These components form the foundation of OOP in Java and are essential for building robust, modular, and maintainable software systems.

```
public Course(String courseName, Student student)
{
this.courseName = courseName;
this.student = student;
// A course is composed of a student
}
```

This constructor initializes a `Course` object by setting its `courseName` and associating it with a `Student` object, establishing a composition relationship where the course contains a student.

1.2.9 Access Modifiers

Keywords that set the access level for classes, variables, methods, and constructors. Common modifiers include public, protected, private, and default (no modifier).

1. public: The member is accessible from any other class.
2. protected: The member is accessible within its own package and by subclasses.
3. default (no modifier): The member is accessible only within its own package.
4. private: The member is accessible only within its own class.

These modifiers help encapsulate data and restrict access to class members, promoting better data management and security in object-oriented programming.

1.2.10 Association

A relationship between two objects that shows how they are related to each other, is often represented by the use of instance variables that reference other objects.

Association is a relationship where one class references another, indicating a "has-a" relationship, such as a `Student` having a `Course`.

1.2.11 Aggregation

A form of association with a whole-part relationship where the part can exist independently of the whole. It represents a "has-a" relationship.

In the context of the `Student` and `Course` classes, aggregation can be illustrated by a `Student` object that contains references to multiple `Course` objects, indicating that a student can enroll in various courses independently of the courses themselves.

1.2.12 Composition

A stronger form of aggregation where the part cannot exist independently of the whole, implying a "contains-a" relationship.

In the context of Student and Course classes, composition can be represented by a Course class that contains a Student object, indicating that a course is made up of students, and if the course is deleted, the associated students are also no longer relevant.

1.2.13 Static Binding

The process of linking a method call to its method body at compile time, is used in method overloading.

In the context of `Student` and `Course` classes, static binding occurs when a static method, such as ` getDetails()`, is called on a `Student` reference, resolving to the method in the `Student` class at compile time, regardless of the actual object type.

1.2.14 Dynamic Binding

The process of linking a method call to its method body at runtime, used in method overriding.

In the context of `Student` and `Course` classes, dynamic binding occurs when a method, such as `registerCourse()`, is invoked on a `Student` reference, allowing the specific implementation in the subclass (e.g., `Course`) to be executed at runtime based on the actual object type.

1.2.15 Superclass

A class from which other classes inherit properties and behavior.

1.2.16 Subclass

A class that inherits properties and behavior from another class, known as the superclass.

In the context of `Student` and `Course`, the `Student` class serves as a superclass that defines common attributes and behaviors, while the `Course` class can extend `Student` as a subclass, inheriting its properties and methods.

1.2.17 Overloading

The ability to define multiple methods with the same name but different parameters within the same class.

1.2.18 Overriding

The ability of a subclass to provide a specific implementation for a method that is already defined in its superclass.

In the context of `Student` class, overriding allows a subclass to implement its own version of a method like `registerCourse()` that is defined in the `Student` superclass, enabling specialized behavior.

1.3 JAVA IS NOT PURE OOPS

Java is often considered not to be a pure object-oriented programming (OOP) language because it supports primitive data types, such as `int`, `float`, `boolean`, etc., which are not objects. This deviation from pure OOP principles is mainly due to performance considerations and historical reasons. The reasons for Java not considered a pure OOP language:

1.3.1 Primitive Data Types

Java includes primitive data types like `int`, `float`, `boolean`, etc., which are not objects. These types do not have associated methods or properties, unlike objects.

1.3.2 Static Methods and Fields

Java allows the declaration of static methods and fields within classes. Static methods and fields are associated with the class itself rather than with instances of the class, which is not strictly in line with the instance-based nature of OOP.

1.3.3 Procedural Programming Features

Java supports procedural programming features such as static methods, which can be called without creating an instance of a class. This approach is more aligned with procedural programming paradigms than with pure OOP.

1.3.4 Primitive Wrappers

Although Java includes primitive data types, it also provides wrapper classes (e.g., `Integer`, `Float`, `Boolean`, etc.) that encapsulate primitive values within objects. While this allows primitive types to be treated as objects, it introduces complexity and is not inherently pure OOP.

Despite these deviations, Java remains predominantly object-oriented in its design and approach. It emphasizes the use of classes and objects for modeling real-world entities, inheritance, polymorphism, encapsulation, and other OOP principles. However, the presence of primitive types and static elements makes it less strictly adherent to the principles of pure object-oriented programming.

1.4 OOPS VS PROCEDURAL ORIENTED APPROACH

Object-Oriented Programming (OOP) is a programming paradigm that focuses on organizing code around objects, which are instances of classes. OOP emphasizes concepts such as encapsulation, inheritance, polymorphism, and abstraction to structure and manage complex systems efficiently.

Procedural Oriented Approach (POA), also known as procedural programming, is a programming paradigm where the program structure revolves around procedures or functions. It emphasizes the sequential execution of instructions, with a primary focus on procedures that perform tasks and manipulate data using functions and control structures like loops and conditionals. Table 1.1 summarizes differences between object-oriented programming (OOP) and procedural programming:

1.5 COMPARISON OF JAVA WITH OTHER PROGRAMMING LANGUAGES

Java, Python, and C++ are high-level programming languages used for developing software applications across various platforms. Java is a strongly-typed, object-oriented programming language known for its platform independence, achieved through the Java Virtual Machine (JVM). It emphasizes security, robustness, and portability in application development. Table 1.2 shows the comparison of programming languages Java, Python and CPP.

This table provides a high-level overview of how Java, Python, and C++ differ in their approach to OOP, highlighting key aspects like inheritance, memory management, and ease of use. Each language has its unique strengths and is suited to different types of applications and developer preferences.

While Java, Python, and C++ all support OOP, their approaches and capabilities differ significantly, catering to different programming needs and scenarios. Java offers an OOP experience with a strong emphasis on safety and portability. Python provides a more flexible but less structured OOP approach, making it ideal for rapid development. C++, on the other hand, offers a powerful but complex OOP experience with its close-to-hardware capabilities.

TABLE 1.1
OOPs vs procedure oriented programming

Aspect	Object-Oriented Programming (OOP)	Procedural Programming
Main Focus	Focuses on objects and their interactions.	Focuses on procedures and functions.
Data and Behavior	Combines data (attributes) and behavior (methods).	Separates data and behavior into different entities.
Modularity	Emphasizes modularity through encapsulation and inheritance.	Less emphasis on modularity.
Code Reusability	Encourages code reuse through inheritance and polymorphism.	Code reuse is limited to functions and procedures.
Encapsulation	Wraps data and methods into a single unit (class).	No explicit support for encapsulation.
Inheritance	Supports inheritance, allowing classes to inherit attributes and methods from other classes.	Does not support inheritance.
Polymorphism	Supports polymorphism, allowing objects of different types to be treated as objects of a common superclass.	Polymorphism is achieved through function overloading.
Abstraction	Supports abstraction, hiding the complex implementation details and showing only essential features of an object.	Abstraction is limited to functions and procedures.
Message Passing	Objects communicate by passing messages between each other.	Functions communicate by passing parameters.
Data Hiding	Allows data hiding by restricting access to certain data members through access modifiers (e.g., private, protected).	No built-in support for data hiding.
Procedural Abstraction	Functions are used to achieve procedural abstraction, breaking down tasks into smaller, reusable procedures.	Focuses on breaking down tasks into smaller functions.
State and Behavior	Objects encapsulate both state (data) and behavior (methods) together.	Data and behavior are separate entities.
Extensibility	Supports extensibility through the addition of new classes and methods.	Extensibility is limited to adding new functions or procedures.
Complexity Management	Helps manage complexity through modular design and abstraction.	Complexity management relies on disciplined coding practices.
Error Handling	Provides built-in support for exception-handling mechanisms.	Error handling is implemented using error codes or return values.

TABLE 1.2
Comparison with other languages: Java vs Python vs C++

Feature/Aspect	Java	Python	C++
Nature of OOP Implementation	Strictly object-oriented; everything is an object.	Multi-paradigm, not strictly object-oriented.	Multi-paradigm, introduced OOP to C.
Class Definition and Inheritance	Single inheritance for classes, multiple for interfaces.	Supports multiple inheritances.	Supports multiple inheritances including private and protected inheritance.
Memory Management	Automatic with garbage collector.	Automatic with garbage collector.	Manual memory management.
Polymorphism and Method Overriding	Strict requires explicit @Override annotation.	Implicit due to dynamic typing.	Allows polymorphism, requires explicit management.
Ease of Learning and Use	Robust and consistent but can be verbose.	Simple syntax, beginner-friendly.	More challenging due to complexity.
Performance Considerations	Runs on JVM, portable but sometimes slower.	Generally slower, interpreted language.	High performance, compiles to native machine code.

1.6 INTRODUCTION TO JAVA

Java is a high-level programming language developed in 1995 by Sun Microsystems, later acquired by Oracle Corporation. Created by James Gosling and Patrick Naughton, Java's original name was "Oak" before being renamed as "Java" due to trademark issues. Unlike many programming languages, "Java" is not an acronym. Java is renowned for its platform independence, allowing programs written in Java to run on any hardware or software platform. Drawing from both C and C++, Java inherits its syntax from C and its object-oriented programming features from C++. The inaugural version of Java was labeled "Java 1.0," with subsequent editions incorporating numerous enhancements. The most recent iteration, Java SE 22, was introduced on March 19, 2024. Java platform comprises a Java Virtual Machine (VM) and an application programming interface (API). The Java Virtual Machine is a specialized program designed for specific hardware and software environments, enabling the execution of Java technology applications. The API serves as a set of software components facilitating the creation of various applications or software components.

1.6.1 Types of Java Applications

There are four types of Java applications:

1.6.1.1 Standalone Applications

Standalone applications, also known as desktop applications, are Java programs that run locally on a user's computer without the need for a web browser. These applications typically have graphical user interfaces (GUIs) and interact directly with the user. Java provides support for building standalone applications using various GUI frameworks such as Abstract Window Toolkit (AWT), Swing, and JavaFX. Standalone applications can range from simple utilities to complex software like IDEs and media players.

1.6.1.2 Enterprise Applications

Enterprise applications are large-scale software systems designed to meet the complex needs of organizations. These applications typically handle critical business processes, such as resource planning, customer relationship management, and supply chain management. Java is widely used for developing enterprise applications due to its platform independence, scalability, and robustness. Enterprise Java technologies such as Enterprise JavaBeans (EJB), Java Persistence API (JPA), and Java Message Service (JMS) are commonly used in building these applications.

1.6.1.3 Web Applications

Web applications are programs that run on web servers and are accessed by users through web browsers. They provide dynamic content and interactive features to users over the internet. Java offers several technologies for building web applications, including JavaServer Pages (JSP), Servlets, Spring Framework, and Hibernate. These technologies enable developers to create scalable, secure, and maintainable web applications for various purposes, such as e-commerce, social networking, and online banking.

1.6.1.4 Mobile Applications

Mobile applications are software programs designed to run on mobile devices such as smartphones and tablets. Java ME (Java Platform, Micro Edition) is a cross-platform framework that allows developers to create mobile applications that can run on a wide range of devices, regardless of the underlying hardware and operating system. Java ME provides libraries and APIs for developing mobile applications with features like graphics, networking, and user interface. These applications can be deployed on feature phones, smartphones, and embedded systems.

1.6.2 The Java Programming Language Platforms

There are four platforms of the Java programming language:

1.6.2.1 Java Platform, Standard Edition (Java SE)

Java SE defines the core components of the Java programming language, including basic types, objects, and control structures. It provides a runtime environment and a set of standard libraries that developers can use to build various types of applications, from command-line utilities to desktop GUI applications. Java SE includes essential packages for tasks such as networking, database access, XML parsing, and multithreading. It also offers tools for compiling, debugging, and running Java programs. Java SE serves as the foundation for higher-level Java platforms like Java EE and JavaFX.

1.6.2.2 Java Platform, Enterprise Edition (Java EE)

Java EE extends the capabilities of Java SE to support the development of large-scale enterprise applications. It provides a comprehensive API and runtime environment for building distributed, multi-tiered, and web-based applications. Java EE includes specifications and implementations for features such as web services, servlets, JavaServer Pages (JSP), Enterprise JavaBeans (EJB), Java Persistence API (JPA), and Java Message Service (JMS). It also offers tools and frameworks for building and deploying enterprise applications efficiently. Java EE applications are typically deployed on application servers that provide additional services such as security, transaction management, and scalability.

1.6.2.3 Java Platform, Micro Edition (Java ME)

Java ME is a platform for running Java applications on small, resource-constrained devices such as mobile phones, PDAs, and embedded systems. It provides a scaled-down version of the Java runtime environment optimized for devices with limited memory, processing power, and display capabilities. Java ME includes profiles and configurations tailored to specific types of devices, allowing developers to create applications that can run across a wide range of mobile and embedded platforms. Java ME applications can leverage libraries and APIs for tasks such as user interface development, networking, and data storage, enabling the development of mobile applications for various purposes.

1.6.2.4 JavaFX

JavaFX is a platform for building rich internet applications (RIAs) with a modern look and feel and high-performance graphics. It provides a set of APIs and tools for creating interactive, multimedia-rich user interfaces that can run on desktops, browsers, and mobile devices. JavaFX includes features such as a scene graph API, media playback, 2D and 3D graphics, animation, and effects. It also offers support for integrating with web services and accessing networked data sources. JavaFX applications can be deployed as standalone desktop applications or as applets embedded in web pages, offering developers flexibility in delivering compelling user experiences across different platforms.

1.6.3 Platform Independent

The Java compiler doesn't generate machine-specific executable code; instead, it produces bytecode, a platform-neutral format. This bytecode is executed by the Java Virtual Machine (JVM) based on predefined rules, making Java platform independent. Bytecode is universally interpretable by any JVM installed on diverse operating systems. As a result, Java source code is portable and can run seamlessly across various operating systems.

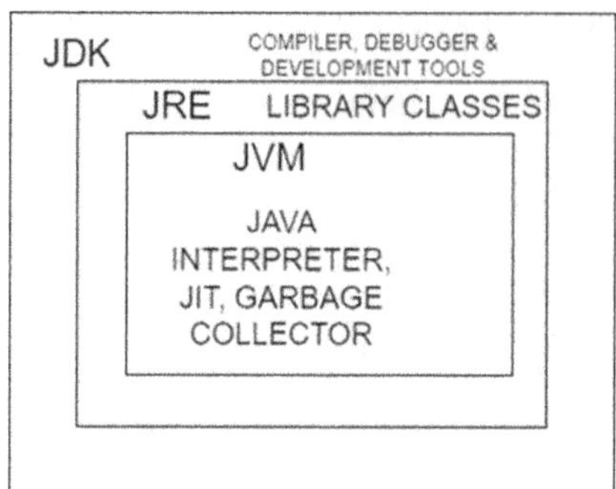

FIGURE 1.1 Components of Java.

1.7 JAVA ESSENTIAL COMPONENTS

Java programs are written in source code, which is human-readable but not understandable by the CPU. Figure 1.1 shows the relationship between JDK, JRE and JVM. To bridge this gap, Java employs three key components within its platform:

1.7.1 Java Development Kit (JDK)

The JDK, or Java Development Kit, is a comprehensive toolkit for Java developers available on various operating systems like Windows, macOS, Solaris, and Linux. It facilitates the execution of Java programs and allows the installation of multiple JDK versions on a single computer. Key functions of JDK include providing tools for Java programming, converting Java source code into bytecode using a compiler, and executing Java applications through a Java application launcher.

1.7.2 Java Virtual Machine (JVM)

The JVM, or Java Virtual Machine, acts as an engine that furnishes a runtime environment for Java applications. It plays a crucial role in translating Java bytecode into machine language. Unlike other programming languages where the compiler generates machine code specific to a system, in Java, the compiler produces bytecode intended for a Virtual Machine, namely the Java Virtual Machine. Notably, the JVM incorporates a Just-In-Time (JIT) compiler, which further optimizes performance by converting Java source code into low-level machine language dynamically.

1.7.3 Java Runtime Environment (JRE)

The JRE serves as software designed to execute other software. It encompasses essential components such as class libraries, loader class, and the JVM. By integrating both compiler and interpreter features, Java adopts a unique approach where the compiler compiles source code into bytecode, and the JVM interprets this bytecode into machine OS-dependent code, enabling platform independence.

1.8 JVM

The Java Virtual Machine (JVM) is an integral component of the Java Runtime Environment (JRE) responsible for providing a runtime environment for Java applications. It acts as an engine that interprets and executes Java bytecode, which is the intermediate representation of Java source code compiled by the Java compiler. The JVM abstracts the underlying hardware and operating system, enabling Java programs to run consistently across different platforms without the need for recompilation. Additionally, the JVM incorporates various features such as memory management, garbage collection, and dynamic class loading, contributing to the platform's portability, security, and performance. JVM can perform:

i. Reading Bytecode
ii. Verifying Bytecode
iii. Linking the Code With the Library

1.8.1 Reading Bytecode

The JVM is responsible for reading bytecode instructions generated by the Java compiler from .class files. Bytecode is a set of machine-readable instructions that represent the Java program's logic in a platform-independent manner. Upon receiving the bytecode, the JVM parses and interprets these instructions to execute the corresponding operations defined by the Java program.

1.8.2 Verifying Bytecode

Bytecode verification is a crucial process performed by the JVM to ensure the safety and integrity of Java programs. During bytecode verification, the JVM examines the bytecode instructions to detect potential security vulnerabilities, such as type mismatches, stack overflows, or illegal access to memory. By thoroughly analyzing the bytecode, the JVM can prevent harmful operations that could compromise the system's stability or security.

1.8.3 Linking the Code with the Library

The JVM is responsible for linking the bytecode instructions with the necessary libraries and runtime components required for program execution. This linking process involves resolving symbolic references in the bytecode to actual memory addresses or library functions. The JVM dynamically loads the required class files and libraries at runtime, ensuring that the Java program has access to the resources it needs to execute successfully. By linking the code with the library, the JVM facilitates seamless integration of Java applications with external resources, including system libraries, frameworks, and runtime environments.

1.8.4 How Java Virtual Machine Works?

The Java Virtual Machine (JVM) is a crucial component of the Java platform, responsible for executing Java bytecode and providing a runtime environment for Java applications. Here's an overview of how the JVM works:

1.8.4.1 Loading

When a Java program is executed, the JVM loads the compiled bytecode (.class files) into memory from the file system or network. The class loader subsystem of the JVM is responsible for loading classes into memory. It follows a hierarchical delegation model, where each class loader delegates the loading process to its parent class loader, and only loads classes that are not already loaded in memory.

1.8.4.2 Verification

Once the bytecode is loaded into memory, the JVM performs bytecode verification to ensure its integrity and security. During verification, the JVM examines the bytecode to detect any violations of Java's safety rules, such as type safety, memory access violations, or illegal operations. By verifying the bytecode, the JVM protects the runtime environment from potential security vulnerabilities and ensures the stability of Java applications.

1.8.4.3 Execution

After verification, the JVM begins executing the bytecode instructions. It uses an interpreter or a Just-In-Time (JIT) compiler to translate bytecode instructions into machine code that can be executed by the underlying hardware. In interpreted mode, the JVM interprets each bytecode instruction sequentially, executing the corresponding operations. In JIT compilation mode, the JVM dynamically compiles frequently executed bytecode sequences into native machine code for improved performance.

1.8.4.4 Memory Management

The JVM manages memory allocation and deallocation for Java objects using automatic memory management techniques, such as garbage collection. It divides the memory into different regions, such as the heap (for objects), the method area (for class metadata), and the runtime stack (for method invocations). The garbage collector periodically scans the heap to identify and reclaim memory occupied by unused objects, preventing memory leaks and optimizing memory usage.

1.8.4.5 Runtime Environment

The JVM provides a runtime environment for Java applications, including support for multi-threading, exception handling, and dynamic class loading. It implements the Java API (Application Programming Interface) for interacting with the underlying operating system and hardware, providing platform independence for Java programs. The JVM also manages the execution of Java threads, monitors synchronization, and handles exceptions thrown by Java code.

Bytecode, the compiled form of Java source code, is platform-independent and can be understood by any Java Virtual Machine (JVM) installed on any operating system. This characteristic of Java makes it highly portable across different environments.

1.8.5 Components of JVM

The JVM comprises two main components: the interpreter and the Just-In-Time (JIT) compiler. These components work together to execute Java bytecode efficiently.

1.8.5.1 Interpreter

The interpreter reads and executes bytecode instructions line by line. Due to its line-by-line execution approach, the interpreter may result in slower performance compared to native execution. When a method is called multiple times, the interpreter may need to re-interpret the bytecode each time, leading to overhead.

1.8.5.2 Just-In-Time (JIT) Compiler

The JIT compiler compiles the entire bytecode into native machine code at runtime. This native machine code is then used directly for repeated method calls, bypassing the need for interpretation. By compiling bytecode into native code, the JIT compiler significantly improves the performance of the system, especially for frequently executed code paths. The JIT compiler mitigates the overhead associated with repeated interpretation by generating optimized native code for hotspots in the program.

1.9 JAVA FEATURES

1.9.1 Object-Oriented Paradigm

Java adopts a robust object-oriented programming model, where everything is treated as an object. This paradigm facilitates easy extension and maintenance of codebases.

1.9.2 Platform Independence

Unlike traditional programming languages such as C and C++, Java compiles source code into platform-independent bytecode. This bytecode can run on any system equipped with a Java Virtual Machine (JVM), enabling cross-platform compatibility.

1.9.3 Simplicity

Java is designed to be user-friendly and easy to learn. Its object-oriented nature simplifies program development, making it accessible to novice programmers.

1.9.4 Security

Java's built-in security features enable the creation of robust, tamper-proof applications, thereby minimizing the risk of vulnerabilities and malware.

1.9.5 Architecture Neutrality

The Java compiler generates architecture-neutral bytecode, ensuring that compiled code can execute seamlessly across various hardware architectures.

1.9.6 Portability

Java's platform independence and absence of platform-specific dependencies make it highly portable. Its compiler, implemented in ANSI C, adheres to a clean portability boundary.

1.9.7 Robustness

Java prioritizes error prevention through rigorous compile-time and runtime checks, minimizing the occurrence of common programming errors.

1.9.8 Multithreading Support

Java's multithreading capabilities empower developers to create concurrent, responsive applications capable of executing multiple tasks concurrently.

1.9.9 Interpretation

Java bytecode is interpreted dynamically by the JVM at runtime, enabling rapid development and execution of code without the need for pre-compilation.

1.9.10 Performance Optimization

Leveraging Just-In-Time (JIT) compilers, Java achieves high performance by dynamically compiling bytecode into efficient native machine code.

1.9.11 Distributed Computing

Java is well-suited for distributed computing environments, making it ideal for developing networked applications for the internet.

1.9.12 Dynamism

Java exhibits dynamic behavior, allowing programs to adapt to evolving runtime conditions. Extensive runtime information enables runtime verification and resolution of object accesses.

1.10 JAVA 22 FEATURES

Java 22 introduces several significant improvements and features compared to previous versions, enhancing developer productivity, application performance, and language capabilities. Here's a summary of key improvements in Java 22 over earlier versions:

1.10.1 Project Amber: Language Enhancements

1.10.1.1 Statements Before `super(...)`

With JEP 447, developers can now place statements that do not reference the created instance before an explicit constructor invocation. This provides more flexibility in expressing constructor behavior and maintains the top-down execution order. Its explanation is given in Chapter 7 (Inheritance)

1.10.1.2 Unnamed Variables and Patterns

JEP 456 introduces unnamed variables and patterns, which improve code readability and maintainability by allowing variable declarations or nested patterns that are required but never used. Its explanation is given in Chapter 3 (Decision making) and Chapter 9 (Exception Handling).

1.10.1.3 String Templates

The second preview of JEP 459 simplifies string handling by allowing runtime-computed values within strings. This enhances security and readability when composing strings from user-provided values. Its explanation is given in Chapter 4 (Arrays).

1.10.1.4 Implicitly Declared Classes and Instance Main Methods

JEP 463, also in its second preview, makes it easier for beginners to write their first programs by simplifying single-class program declarations. This feature allows for a smooth transition from basic to more complex Java programs. Its explanation is given in Chapter 6 (Classes)

1.10.2 Concurrency Improvements: Project Loom

1.10.2.1 Structured Concurrency

JEP 462 introduces an API for structured concurrency, aiding developers in streamlining error handling, cancellation, and observability in concurrent programming. This helps eliminate risks like thread leaks and cancellation delays. Its explanation is given in Chapter 10 (Multithreading)

1.10.2.2 Scoped Values

The second preview of JEP 464 introduces scoped values, which allow the sharing of immutable data across threads. This feature enhances the ease of use, comprehensibility, performance, and robustness of concurrent code. Its explanation is given in Chapter 10 (Multithreading)

1.10.3 Native Interoperability: Project Panama

1.10.3.1 Foreign Function and Memory API

JEP 454 provides an API for Java programs to efficiently invoke foreign functions and access foreign memory without relying on JNI. This enhances the flexibility, safety, and performance of interfacing with native libraries and data.

1.10.3.2 Vector API

The seventh incubator of JEP 460 offers an API for expressing vector computations, which can be compiled into vector instructions on supported CPU architectures. This enables superior performance for numerical computations.

1.10.4 Core Libraries and Tools Enhancements

1.10.4.1 Class-File API

JEP 457, in preview, introduces a standard API for parsing, generating, and transforming Java class files, improving productivity for developers working with class files.

1.10.4.2 Launch Multi-File Source-Code Programs

JEP 458 enhances the Java application launcher, allowing programs supplied as multiple Java source files to be run directly, offering more flexibility in configuring build tools.

1.10.4.3 Stream Gatherers

The preview of JEP 461 enhances the Stream API with custom intermediate operations, making stream pipelines more flexible and expressive for efficient and maintainable code. Its explanation is given in Chapter 11 (File Handling).

1.10.5 Performance Improvements

1.10.5.1 Region Pinning for G1

JEP 423 introduces region pinning for the G1 garbage collector, reducing latency by allowing garbage collection during specific native library calls. This improvement helps maintain overall performance.

1.10.6 Cloud Support and Java Management Service

Java 22 is optimized for cloud deployment, particularly on Oracle Cloud Infrastructure (OCI), which supports Java 22 and offers free access to Oracle Java SE, Oracle GraalVM, and the Java SE Subscription Enterprise Performance Pack. Additionally, the Java Management Service (JMS) provides a unified console for managing Java runtimes and applications across on-premises and cloud environments.

These enhancements in Java 22 continue to evolve the language, making it more expressive, secure, and efficient for modern application development.

1.11 JAVA 21 VS JAVA22

Java 22 builds upon the foundation laid by Java 21, promoting several features from preview to standard status, introducing new preview and incubator features, and continuing to enhance performance, security, and the standard library. Table 1.3 tabulates the comparison of Java 21 and Java 22 features in a tabular form:

1.12 STRUCTURE OF JAVA PROGRAM

A Java program involves the following sections:

- Documentation Section
- Package Statement

TABLE 1.3
Comparison between Java 21 vs Java 22

Feature	Java 21	Java 22
Release Date	September 2023	March 2024
Sequenced Collections	Not Available	Available
Pattern Matching for Switch	Preview	Standard
Virtual Threads	Preview	Standard
Record Patterns	Preview	Standard
String Templates	Not Available	Preview
Foreign Function & Memory API	Second Incubator	Third Incubator
Scoped Values	Not Available	Incubator
Performance Improvements	Various minor improvements	Further enhancements and optimizations
Security Enhancements	Regular updates and patches	Additional updates and patches
Deprecations/Removals	Minor deprecations/removals	Additional deprecations/removals
Garbage Collectors	Various enhancements to existing GCs	Further enhancements to existing GCs
Platform APIs	Incremental updates and additions	Further updates and additions
Library Enhancements	Minor additions and improvements	Additional library enhancements
Preview Features	Pattern Matching for switch, Record Patterns, Virtual Threads	String Templates, Scoped Values
Standard Features	Various JEPs (JDK Enhancement Proposals)	Sequenced Collections, Pattern Matching for switch, Virtual Threads, Record Patterns

- Import Statements
- Interface Statement
- Class Definition
- Main Method Class
- Main Method Definition

1.12.1 Documentation Section

This section provides documentation about the program. It typically includes comments explaining the purpose of the program, its functionality, author information, and any other relevant details. Documentation is crucial for understanding the code and is often generated using tools like Javadoc.

```
/
* This program calculates the area of a circle.
* Author: Usharani Bhimavarapu
* Date: March 30, 2024
*/
```

1.12.2 Package Statement

The package statement is used to declare the package to which the Java file belongs. Packages are used for organizing classes into namespaces and preventing naming conflicts. It is the first statement in a Java file and is optional.

```
Eg: package com.example.myapp;
```

The statement `package com.example.myapp;` in Java is a declaration that specifies the package to which the current Java source file belongs.

1.12.3 Import Statements

Import statements are used to import classes or entire packages into the current Java file, allowing the programmer to use classes from those packages without fully qualifying their names. They come after the package statement (if present) and before the class definition.

```
Eg. import java.util.Scanner;
```

The statement import java.util.Scanner; in Java is used to import the Scanner class from the java.util package into the current Java source file.

1.12.4 Interface Statement

An interface statement defines a new interface in Java. Interfaces declare methods without providing implementations, serving as contracts that classes can implement. They are declared using the 'interface' keyword followed by the interface name and its method signatures.

```
public interface Drawable {
  void draw();
}
```

By defining interfaces, Java enables polymorphism, allowing objects of different classes to be treated uniformly based on their common behavior specified by the interface. This promotes code reusability, flexibility, and maintainability in Java programs.

1.12.5 Class Definition

A class definition defines a new class in Java, encapsulating data and behavior. It includes class modifiers, class name, superclass (if any), interfaces implemented (if any), class body, and constructors. Classes are the building blocks of Java programs and encapsulate data and methods.

```
public class Circle {
  private double radius;
    public Circle(double radius) {
this.radius = radius;
  }
    public double calculateArea() {
    return Math.PI * radius * radius;
  }
}
```

The class definition encapsulates the properties and behavior, providing a blueprint for creating and manipulating the objects within a Java program. Its high importance lies in its ability to model real-world entities and perform computations, demonstrating the fundamental principles of object-oriented programming and encapsulation.

1.12.6 Main Method Class

The main method class contains the main method, which serves as the entry point for Java applications. It typically has the 'public static void main(String[] args)' method signature, allowing the Java Virtual Machine (JVM) to execute the program.

```
   public class Main {
void main(String[] args) {
   // Program logic goes here
  }
}
```

1.12.6.1 Main Method Definition

The main method definition is where the execution of the Java program begins. It contains the main method, which must be declared as 'void main(String[] args)'. Inside the main method, the program logic is written, and other classes and methods are invoked as necessary.

```
void main(String[] args) {
  Circle circle = new Circle(5);
  double area = circle.calculateArea();
System.out.println("Area of the circle: " + area);
}
```

Example

```
package javapackage; // A package declaration
import java.util.*; // declaration of an import statement
   // This is a Comment Section
public class test{ // class name
int n = 4; // global variable
void main(String a[]) { // main method
test t = new test();//object  instantiation
t.display("Main");// method calling
    }
public void display(String s) { // method definition
System.out.println(s);
    }
}
```

This Java program encapsulates several essential elements of Java programming, providing a concise yet illustrative example. It begins with a package declaration, `javapackage`, indicating the organization of classes into a package. An import statement follows, importing the entire `java.util` package, which grants access to utilities and data structures. The program contains a class named `test`, denoted by the keyword `public`, indicating its visibility. Within this class, there is a global variable `n` initialized to `4`. The `main` method serves as the entry point of the program, where an instance of the `test` class is created, and its `display` method is invoked with the argument `"Main"`.The `display` method, defined within the `test` class, takes a string argument `s` and prints it to the console using `System.out.println()`. This method exemplifies encapsulation and modularity, as it performs a specific task separate from the main logic of the program.

1.13 CREATION AND EXECUTION OF JAVA PROGRAMS

Step 1:
Write a program on the notepad and save it with .java extension.

```
class test
{
void main(String a[])
{
System.out.println("this is to test");
}
}
```

Step 2:
Open Command Prompt.
Step 3:
Set the directory in which the .java file is saved. For example, the .java file is saved in C:\\java.
Step 4:
Use the javac command to compile the Java program. It generates a .class file in the same folder.

```
javac --enable-preview --source 22 filename.java
eg: javac --enable-preview --source 22 Test.java
```

Step 5:
Use the java command to run the Java program:

```
java --enable-preview --source 22 filename
eg: java --enable-preview --source 22 Test.java
```

1.14 FIRST SAMPLE PROGRAM

```
import java.io.*; // Importing classes from packages
public class test {// Main class
void main(String[] a)  // Main method
  {
     System.out.println("this is to test");// Print statement
  }
}
```

Output

```
this is to test
```

Explanation:

1. Comments: Comments are used for explaining code and are used in a similar manner, either in C or C++. Compilers ignore the comment entries and do not execute them. Comments can be of a single line(/) or multiple lines(/*….*/).

Single line Comments:

Syntax:

// Single line comment

Multi-line comments:

Syntax:

/* Multi line comments*/

2. import java.io.*: This statement imports all the classes from io package.
3. class: The class contains the data and methods to be used in the program.
4. static void Main(): static keyword tells us that this method is accessible without creating objects to the class. The void keyword tells that it is not going to return anything. The main() method is the starting point of the application.
6. System.in: This is the standard input stream that is used to read characters from the keyboard or any other standard input device.
7. System.out: This is the standard output stream that is used to produce the result of a program on an output device like a computer screen.
8. println(): This method displays text on the console.

Note: Everything in Java, is represented inside class.

1.15 SIMPLE JAVA PROGRAM USING JDK22

Step 1. Write the Java Program:
Write the Java program into a text editor and save it with the filename test.java.

```
class test
{
    void main(String[] args)
      {
      System.out.println("This is to test jdk22 main method ");
      }
}
```

Step 2. Open Command Prompt:
Open your command prompt or terminal.

Step 3. Navigate to the Directory:
Use the cd command to navigate to the directory where test.java is saved. For example:
bash
cd path\to\your\directory
Replace path\to\your\directory with the actual path where test.java is saved.

Step 4. Compile the Java Program:
To compile the Java program, use the javac command followed by the filename:

```
javac --release 22 --enable-preview test.java
```

This command compiles test.java and generates test.class file.

Step 5. Run the Java Program:

After successful compilation, use the java command to run the program:

```
java --source 22 --enable-preview test.java
```

```
Command Prompt
Microsoft Windows [Version 10.0.19045.4529]
(c) Microsoft Corporation. All rights reserved.

C:\Users\irp>cd \

C:\>cd jj

C:\jj>javac --release 22 --enable-preview test.java

C:\jj>java --source 22 --enable-preview test.java
This is to test jdk22 main method

C:\jj>java --version
java 22 2024-03-19
Java(TM) SE Runtime Environment (build 22+36-2370)
Java HotSpot(TM) 64-Bit Server VM (build 22+36-2370, mixed mode, sharing)
```

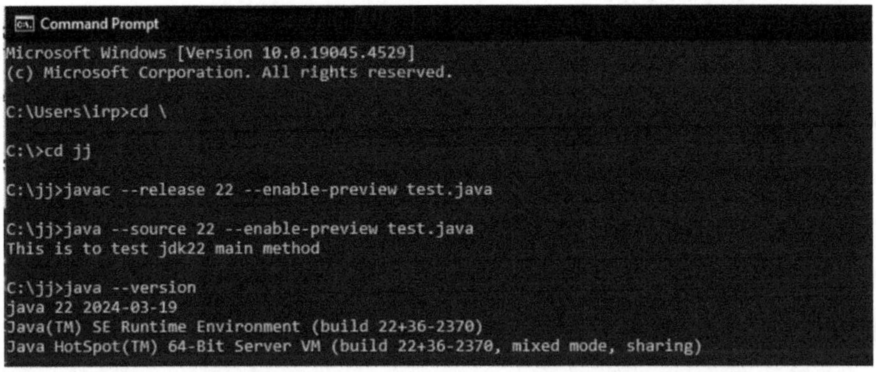

This command executes the test class and prints the message: This is to test jdk 22 main method.

2 Data Types and Operators in Java

2.1 INTRODUCTION

Data types are crucial in programming as they define the kind of data that a variable can hold, ensuring clarity, efficiency, and reliability in coding. The reasons for data types are:

- Clarity and Readability: Data types make code more understandable by indicating the type of data being manipulated. For instance, a variable declared as an integer (int) explicitly states that it holds whole numbers, enhancing code readability for other developers.
- Memory Allocation: Data types determine the amount of memory allocated to variables, optimizing memory usage and overall program performance. This ensures that only the necessary memory is reserved for each variable, reducing memory wastage.
- Type Safety: By enforcing strict data type rules, programming languages prevent errors caused by incompatible data assignments. This enhances the reliability and stability of programs, as type mismatches are caught during compilation rather than causing runtime errors.
- Compile-Time Checking: Data types enable compile-time checking, where the compiler verifies that operations performed on variables are valid according to their types. This helps identify errors early in the development process, minimizing debugging efforts and improving code quality.
- Optimization: Some data types are optimized for specific operations or hardware architectures, leading to improved performance in certain scenarios. For example, using primitive data types like int or double can be more efficient than using their object counterparts in terms of memory and processing overhead.

Despite their numerous advantages, data types also come with some limitations:

- Rigidness: Strict data typing can sometimes limit flexibility, especially in dynamically typed languages where variables can change types during runtime. Developers may find it cumbersome to work within the constraints of rigid-type systems, particularly in scenarios requiring more fluid data manipulation.
- Overhead: Using complex data types or objects can incur overhead in terms of memory and processing resources. This overhead becomes more pronounced in resource-constrained environments or when dealing with large-scale data structures.

DOI: 10.1201/9781003544319-2

- Learning Curve: Understanding and managing data types effectively require knowledge of their characteristics and behaviors, which can pose a learning curve for novice programmers. Misunderstandings or misuse of data types may lead to errors and inefficiencies in code.
- Compatibility Issues: In some cases, data types may not be compatible across different programming languages or platforms, requiring extra effort to ensure interoperability and data integrity when integrating components developed in disparate environments.

Despite these drawbacks, the benefits of using data types generally outweigh the challenges, contributing to the robustness, efficiency, and maintainability of software systems.

2.1.1 Predefined Keywords

Java has a set of predefined keywords that are reserved for specific purposes within the language. These keywords cannot be used as identifiers (such as variable names, method names, or class names) in Java programs. Here is a list of Java predefined keywords:

1. abstract: Used to declare a class as abstract or to declare a method without implementation.
2. assert: Used to assert the truth of a condition in debugging and testing.
3. boolean: Represents a data type that can hold one of two values: `true` or `false`.
4. break: Exits from the current loop or switch statement.
5. byte: Represents an 8-bit signed integer data type.
6. case: Defines a branch in a switch statement.
7. catch: Catches exceptions generated by try statements.
8. char: Represents a 16-bit Unicode character data type.
9. class: Defines a class.
10. const (not used): Reserved for future use.
11. continue: Skips the current iteration of loop and proceeds to the next iteration.
12. default: Specifies the default branch in a switch statement.
13. do: Starts a do-while loop.
14. double: Represents a double-precision 64-bit floating-point data type.
15. else: Specifies an alternative branch in an if statement.
16. enum: Declares an enumerated (enum) type.
17. extends: Indicates that a class is inheriting from another class or an interface is extending another interface.
18. final: Prevents inheritance (when applied to a class), modification (when applied to a method), or reassignment (when applied to a variable).
19. finally: Defines a block of code that will be executed after a try-catch block.
20. float: Represents a single-precision 32-bit floating-point data type.
21. for: Starts a for loop.
22. goto (not used): Reserved for future use.
23. if: Specifies a conditional statement.
24. implements: Indicates that a class is implementing an interface.
25. import: Imports other Java packages or classes.
26. instanceof: Tests whether an object is an instance of a specific class or interface.
27. int: Represents a 32-bit signed integer data type.
28. interface: Declares an interface.
29. long: Represents a 64-bit signed integer data type.
30. native: Specifies that a method is implemented in native code using JNI (Java Native Interface).
31. new: Creates new objects.
32. null: Represents a null reference, not referring to any object.

33. package: Declares a package.
34. private: Specifies that a member (method or variable) is accessible only within its own class.
35. protected: Specifies that a member is accessible within its own package and by subclasses.
36. public: Specifies that a member is accessible from any other class.
37. return: Exits from a method, optionally returning a value.
38. short: Represents a 16-bit signed integer data type.
39. static: Specifies that a member belongs to the class rather than any instance of the class.
40. strictfp: Restricts floating-point calculations to ensure portability.
41. super: Refers to the superclass.
42. switch: Specifies a multi-way branch statement.
43. synchronized: Specifies that a method can only be accessed by one thread at a time.
44. this: Refers to the current instance of a class.
45. throw: Throws an exception.
46. throws: Specifies that a method can throw exceptions.
47. transient: Specifies that a member variable is not part of the persistent state of an object.
48. try: Starts a block of code that will be tested for exceptions.
49. void: Specifies that a method does not return a value.
50. volatile: Specifies that a variable may be changed unexpectedly.
51. while: Starts a while loop.

These keywords are fundamental to Java syntax and serve specific roles in defining classes, controlling program flow, handling exceptions, and managing data types and access levels.

2.2 DATA TYPES IN JAVA

Data types in Java specify the nature of data that can be stored in variables. They define the size and format of the data, ensuring proper memory allocation and manipulation. Java supports two main categories of data types: primitive and non-primitive.

2.2.1 Primitive Data Types

Primitive data types represent basic values and are built into the Java language. They are used to store single values and have predefined sizes.
There are eight primitive data types in Java:

1. byte: Used for storing small integral values. Occupies 8 bits of memory. Represents integer values ranging from -128 to 127.Byte data type defaults to 0.
2. short: Used for storing small integral values, larger than `byte`. Occupies 16 bits of memory. Represents integer values ranging from -32,768 to 32,767.Short data type also defaults to 0.
3. int: Used for storing integral values. Typically used for storing whole numbers. Occupies 32 bits of memory. Represents integer values ranging from -2^{31} to 2^{31}-1.The int data type defaults to 0.
4. long: Used for storing large integral values. Used when `int` is not sufficient. Occupies 64 bits of memory. Represents integer values ranging from -2^{63} to 2^{63}-1. Long data type defaults to 0L.
5. float: Used for storing floating-point numbers. Occupies 32 bits of memory. Represents single-precision floating-point numbers. Float data type defaults to 0.0f.
6. double: Used for storing double-precision floating-point numbers. Occupies 64 bits of memory. Represents double-precision floating-point numbers. Double data type defaults to 0.0d.

7. char: Used for storing a single character or Unicode characters. Occupies 16 bits of memory. Represents single characters stored as Unicode values. Char data type has a default value of '\u0000'.
8. boolean: Used for storing `true` or `false` values. Occupies 1 bit of memory, but its size is not precisely defined. Represents true or false values. Boolean data type defaults to 'false'.

These primitive data types are fundamental to Java programming and are used extensively in variable declarations, method parameters, and return types. Each data type has its range and precision, catering to different needs in programming scenarios.

2.2.2 Non-Primitive Data Types

Non-primitive data types are also called reference types because they refer to objects in memory. They include:

a. Classes: Blueprint for creating objects. They define the properties and behaviors of objects.
b. Interfaces: Defines a contract for implementing classes. They specify a set of methods that a class must implement.
c. Arrays: Collection of similar data types arranged in contiguous memory locations. They provide a convenient way to store and manipulate multiple values of the same type.

2.3 PRIMITIVE DATATYPES

Primitive data types in Java are fundamental building blocks that represent basic data values directly in memory. They provide essential characteristics and capabilities crucial for efficient programming:
Advantages

- Efficiency: Primitive types are simple and occupy fixed amounts of memory, which allows for fast access and manipulation.
- Speed: Operations on primitive types are generally faster than operations on their corresponding wrapper classes (e.g., `int` vs `Integer`) because they do not involve the overhead of object creation and garbage collection.
- Memory Management: They are directly managed by the Java Virtual Machine (JVM), making memory allocation and deallocation straightforward.
- Predictable Behavior: Primitive types have well-defined ranges and behaviors, ensuring consistent results across different platforms and JVM implementations.
- Direct Access: They enable direct manipulation at the lowest level, which is essential for tasks like system programming, low-level data processing, and performance-critical applications.

Limitations

- Lack of Methods: Primitive types do not have methods or properties like objects. This limits their functionality in certain scenarios, such as performing operations on collections or leveraging object-oriented programming features directly.
- No Null Values: Primitive types cannot hold `null` values, which can be inconvenient when dealing with situations requiring the absence of a value. This necessitates the use of wrapper classes (`Integer`, `Double`, etc.) for nullable types.
- Limited Range: Each primitive type has a specific range of values it can hold. For instance, `byte` ranges from -128 to 127, which may not be sufficient for certain computations requiring larger numeric values.

- Not Extensible: Primitive types cannot be extended or customized. Their behavior and capabilities are fixed by the Java language specification, making them less flexible compared to objects and classes.

Despite these limitations, primitive data types remain crucial in Java programming due to their efficiency, speed, and suitability for a wide range of tasks from basic arithmetic operations to low-level system programming.

2.3.1 Byte Data Type

The `byte` data type in Java is used to store integer values within the range of -128 to 127. It is a primitive data type that occupies 8 bits or one byte of memory. This makes `byte` suitable for conserving memory when working with large arrays or when the range of values needed is within its limits. Commonly used in scenarios where memory efficiency is critical, such as in embedded systems or file processing where data size needs to be minimized. Despite its small range, `byte` is versatile for tasks like reading binary data, implementing low-level protocols, or handling streams efficiently. Its compact size also ensures faster data access and manipulation compared to larger data types, contributing to better performance in Java applications.

Program

```
class ByteExample {
void main(String[] a) {
byte b;
b = 121;
System.out.println(b);
  }
}
Output:121
```

The above Java program defines a class named ` ByteExample ` with a `main` method, which serves as the entry point for the program's execution. Within the `main` method, a variable `b` of type `byte` is declared and initialized with the value `121`. This variable `b` represents a small integer data type that can store values ranging from -128 to 127. After assigning the value to `b`, the program uses the `System.out.println()` method to print the value of `b` to the console. Consequently, when the program is executed, it will display `121` as the output, indicating the successful storage and retrieval of the assigned value to the byte variable `b`.

2.3.2 Short Data Type

It occupies 16 bits or 2 bytes of memory, making it larger than byte but smaller than int. The main benefit of using the short data type lies in its ability to conserve memory while still accommodating a broader range of integer values compared to byte. It allows developers to work with numbers ranging from -32,768 to 32,767, inclusive, which is suitable for many applications that require handling relatively small integers efficiently. By using short, developers can optimize memory usage in situations where the full range of int (which spans from -2,147,483,648 to 2,147,483,647) is unnecessary and excessive. This data type is particularly useful in environments where memory constraints are a concern or when dealing with arrays of integers that do not require the larger size of int.

Program

```
class ShortExample {
void main(String[] a) {
short temperature;
temperature = -200;
System.out.println(temperature);  // prints -200
  }
}
Output:
-200
```

The above Java program defines a class named ` ShortExample ` with a `main` method, which serves as the entry point for the program's execution. Inside the `main` method, a variable named `temperature` is declared of type `short`, which represents a data type capable of storing integer values within a larger range compared to `byte`, typically from -32,768 to 32,767. In this program, the variable `temperature` is assigned the value `-200`. Subsequently, the program utilizes the `System.out.println()` method to print the value of `temperature` to the console. Upon execution, the program will output `-200`, confirming that the assigned value has been successfully stored in the `short` variable `temperature`.

2.3.3 Java Int Data Type

The `int` data type in Java is essential for storing whole numbers within a specified range. It occupies 32 bits of memory and can represent values ranging from -2,147,483,648 to 2,147,483,647. This makes it suitable for calculations involving integers without the need for decimals, providing efficiency in terms of memory usage and computational speed. Its widespread use across Java programs ensures compatibility and interoperability, allowing for consistent numeric operations and data storage across different platforms and systems.

Program: Java int data type

```
class IntExample {
void main(String[] a) {
int n = 145;
System.out.println(n);  }
}
Output:145
```

The above Java program defines a class named ` IntExample ` with a `main` method, acting as the program's entry point. Within the `main` method, an integer variable `n` is declared and initialized with the value `145`. Following the initialization of `n`, the program utilizes the `System.out.println()` method to print the value of `n` to the console. Upon execution, the program will output `145`, confirming that the assigned value has been successfully stored in the `int` variable `n`, and subsequently printed to the console.

2.3.4 Java Long Data Type

The `long` data type in Java is crucial for handling large integers that exceed the range of the `int` type. It occupies 64 bits of memory, which allows it to store values from -9,223,372,036,854,775,808 to 9,223,372,036,854,775,807. This extended range makes `long` suitable for scenarios requiring precision and accuracy in calculations involving very large whole numbers, such as timestamps, large sums, or when dealing with astronomical or financial data. Its use ensures Java applications can manage and manipulate these large numerical values efficiently while maintaining platform compatibility and data integrity.

Program: Java long data type

```
class LongExample {
void main(String[] a) {
long n = -423322L;
System.out.println(n);
  }
}
Output:
-423322L
```

The above Java program defines a class named ` LongExample ` with a `main` method, which serves as the entry point for the program's execution. Within the `main` method, a variable named `n` is declared and initialized with the value `-423322L`. Here, `n` is of type `long`, a data type used to store large integer values within a broader range than `int`. The `long` data type can accommodate values ranging from -9,223,372,036,854,775,808-9,223,372,036,854,775,807, and the `L` suffix indicates that `-423322` is explicitly a `long` literal. Following the initialization, the program employs the `System.out.println()` method to print the value of `n` to the console. Upon execution, the program will output `-423322`, confirming that the assigned value has been successfully stored in the `long` variable `n`, and subsequently printed to the console.

2.3.5 Java Double Data Type

The `double` data type in Java is essential for representing floating-point numbers with double precision. It is a 64-bit type that allows for a wider range of values and greater precision compared to the `float` type. This makes `double` suitable for applications requiring accurate representation of decimal values, such as scientific calculations, financial computations, and graphics rendering. The `double` type adheres to the IEEE 754 standard, ensuring consistent behavior across different platforms. Its flexibility in handling both small and large fractional numbers with high precision makes it indispensable in Java programming for tasks demanding numerical accuracy and extensive mathematical operations.

Program: Java double data type

```
class Doublexample {
void main(String[] ar) {
  double n = -12.3;
System.out.println(n);
  }
}
Output:
-12.3
```

The above Java program defines a class named ` Doublexample ` with a `main` method, serving as the program's entry point. Within the `main` method, a variable named `n` is declared and initialized with the value `-12.3`. The data type of `n` is `double`, which represents floating-point numbers with double precision. Unlike the `float` data type, which has single precision, `double` provides

higher precision and can store larger decimal values with greater accuracy. After the initialization, the program utilizes the `System.out.println()` method to print the value of `n` to the console. Upon execution, the program will output
`-12.3`, confirming that the assigned value has been successfully stored in the `double` variable `n` and subsequently printed to the console.

2.3.6 Java Float Data Type

The `float` data type in Java is crucial for representing single-precision floating-point numbers. It occupies 32 bits of memory and is suitable for applications where memory efficiency and performance are critical. The `float` type is commonly used in scenarios such as scientific computations, real-time graphics, and embedded systems where precision requirements are moderate. It offers a wider range of values compared to integers and is capable of handling fractional numbers with reasonable precision. Although it provides less precision than the `double` type, it strikes a balance between accuracy and memory usage, making it suitable for various computational tasks in Java programming.

Program: Java float data type

```
class FloatExample {
void main(String[] a) {
  float n = -12.3f;
System.out.println(n);  }
}
Output:
-12.3
```

The above Java program defines a class named ` FloatExample` with a `main` method, which acts as the entry point for the program's execution. Within the `main` method, a variable named `n` is declared and initialized with the value `-12.3f`. The data type of `n` is `float`, which represents floating-point numbers with single precision. It's worth noting that in Java, floating-point literals are considered `double` by default, so appending the `f` suffix to `-12.3` explicitly indicates that it is a `float` literal. After initialization, the program employs the `System.out.println()` method to print the value of `n` to the console. Upon execution, the program will output `-12.3`, confirming that the assigned value has been successfully stored in the `float` variable `n` and subsequently printed to the console.

2.3.7 Java Char Data Type

The `char` data type in Java is essential for representing single 16-bit Unicode characters. It's used to store individual characters, such as letters, digits, and symbols, in Java programs. The `char` type allows for the manipulation and processing of textual data, enabling operations like comparisons, conversions, and transformations within strings and other text-based data structures. It supports a wide range of international characters due to its Unicode representation, making it suitable for multilingual applications and text processing tasks. In Java, `char` values are enclosed in single quotes (‘ ‘), distinguishing them from other data types. This data type is fundamental in user interfaces, file handling, and string manipulations where individual character-level operations are required.

Program: Java char data type

```
class CharExample {
void main(String[] a) {
char c = 'A';
```

```
System.out.println(c);
  }
}
```

Output:

```
A
```

The above Java program defines a class named ` CharExample ` with a `main` method, which serves as the starting point for the program's execution. Inside the `main` method, a variable named `c` is declared and assigned the character value `'A'`. The data type of `c` is `char`, representing a single 16-bit Unicode character. After the assignment, the program uses the `System.out.println()` method to print the value of `c` to the console. Upon execution, the program will output `'A'`, confirming that the assigned character has been successfully stored in the `char` variable `c`, and it's then printed to the console.

2.3.8 Boolean Data Type

The `boolean` data type in Java serves a crucial role in representing truth values, allowing for logical operations and decision-making within programs. It is used to store two possible states: `true` and `false`, which are the only values assignable to a `boolean` variable. This simplicity makes it efficient for conditions, loops, and branching statements, enabling developers to control program flow based on boolean expressions. In Java, boolean variables consume a single bit of memory, optimizing memory usage and enhancing performance, especially in large-scale applications. Its straightforward nature also facilitates clarity in code readability and debugging, ensuring that logical conditions are expressed in a concise and understandable manner throughout Java programs.

Program

```
class BooleanExample {
void main(String[] a) {
boolean flag = true;
System.out.println(flag);
}
}
```

Output:

```
true
```

In this program, we define a class named `BooleanExample`. Inside the class, we create a `main` method, which acts as the entry point for execution. We declare a boolean variable `flag` and assign it the value `true`. The program then outputs the value of `flag` using the `System.out.println` statement. As a result, the program prints `true` to the console. The use of the boolean data type allows us to work with true/false values efficiently.

2.3.9 Min and Max Values of All Java Datatypes

In Java, each primitive data type has specific ranges of values it can hold. These values are specified by the Java language and are crucial for understanding the limitations and capabilities of each data type when performing calculations, storing data, or designing algorithms.

Program: Program for min and max values of predefined java datatypes

```
public class Test
{
    void main(String[] args) {
```

```
System.out.println("int min:"+Integer.MIN_VALUE);
System.out.println("int max:"+Integer.MAX_VALUE);
System.out.println("byte min:"+Byte.MIN_VALUE);
System.out.println("byte max:"+Byte.MAX_VALUE);
System.out.println("short min:"+Short.MIN_VALUE);
System.out.println("short max:"+Short.MAX_VALUE);
System.out.println("long min:"+Long.MIN_VALUE);
System.out.println("long max:"+Long.MAX_VALUE);
System.out.println("float min:"+Float.MIN_VALUE);
System.out.println("float max:"+Float.MAX_VALUE);
System.out.println("double min:"+Double.MIN_VALUE);
System.out.println("double max:"+Double.MAX_VALUE);
      }
}
```

Output:

```
int min:-2147483648
int max:2147483647
byte min:-128
byte max:127
short min:-32768
short max:32767
long min:-9223372036854775808
long max:9223372036854775807
float min:1.4E-45
float max:3.4028235E38
double min:4.9E-324
double max:1.7976931348623157E308
```

The values of `MIN_VALUE` and `MAX_VALUE` represent the minimum and maximum possible values that can be stored within a particular primitive data type in Java. For the `int` data type, `Integer.MIN_VALUE` represents the smallest integer value that can be stored, which is -2^{31} or -2,147,483,648. On the other hand, `Integer.MAX_VALUE` denotes the largest integer value that can be stored, which is $2^{31} - 1$ or 2,147,483,647. The `byte` data type is an 8-bit signed integer, and `Byte.MIN_VALUE` indicates the smallest value that can be stored, which is -128. Conversely, `Byte.MAX_VALUE` signifies the largest value that can be stored, which is 127. For the `short` data type, `Short.MIN_VALUE` represents the smallest value, which is -2^{15} or -32,768. Conversely, `Short.MAX_VALUE` represents the largest value, which is $2^{15} - 1$ or 32,767. The `long` data type is a 64-bit signed integer, and `Long.MIN_VALUE` denotes the smallest value, which is -2^{63} or -9,223,372,036,854,775,808. Conversely, `Long.MAX_VALUE` denotes the largest value, which is $2^{63} - 1$ or 9,223,372,036,854,775,807. For the `float` data type, `Float.MIN_VALUE` represents the smallest positive nonzero value that can be stored, approximately 1.4×10^{-45}. On the other hand, `Float.MAX_VALUE` represents the largest finite positive value that can be stored, approximately 3.4028235×10^{38}. The `double` data type is a double-precision 64-bit floating-point number, and `Double.MIN_VALUE` represents the smallest positive nonzero value, approximately 4.9×10^{-324}. Conversely, `Double.MAX_VALUE` represents the largest finite positive value, approximately $1.7976931348623157 \times 10^{308}$.

2.4 TYPE CASTING

Type casting or type coercion converts data from one data type to another data type. By using casting, data cannot be changed but only the data type is changed.

Note: Type casting is not possible for a boolean data type.

There are two types of type casting

- Implicit casting
- Explicit casting

2.4.1 Implicit Casting

Implicit casting or widening casting converts data from a narrower range data type to a wider range data type. It also means converting a lower data type like an int to a higher data type like a double.

Implicit casting follows the order of conversion as shown in Figure 2.1.

Program

```
public class ImplictExample {
void main(String[] ar) {
int a = 20;
long b = a;    //implicit casting from int to long data type
double c = b;    // implicit casting from long to double data type
System.out.println(a);
System.out.println(b);
System.out.println(c);
  }
}
Output:
20
20
20.0
```

The above Java program, named " ImplictExample," demonstrates implicit type casting, also known as widening or automatic type conversion, within the context of primitive data types. It begins with the declaration of the main method, which serves as the entry point for program execution. Inside this method, an integer variable \`a\` is initialized with the value \`20\`. The program then showcases implicit casting by assigning the value of \`a\` to a \`long\` variable \`b\` and subsequently assigning the value of \`b\` to a \`double\` variable \`c\`. This process involves converting smaller data types to larger data types to accommodate the wider range or precision of the target data type. Following the implicit casting operations, the program prints the values of variables \`a\`, \`b\`, and \`c\` to the console using the \`System.out.println()\` method. Upon execution, the program demonstrates that the values of \`a\`, \`b\`, and \`c\` are automatically converted during assignment, showcasing the automatic conversion of an \`int\` to a \`long\` and then to a \`double\` data type.

2.4.2 Explicit Type Casting

Explicit type casting or narrowing type casting involves assigning a data type of high range to a lower range. For this casting, java supports the "()" operator. If the casting fails, a compile-time error will be returned by the compiler.

Explicit casting follows the order of conversion as shown in Figure 2.2.

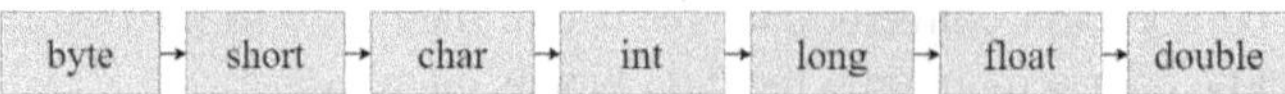

FIGURE 2.1 Implicit type casting.

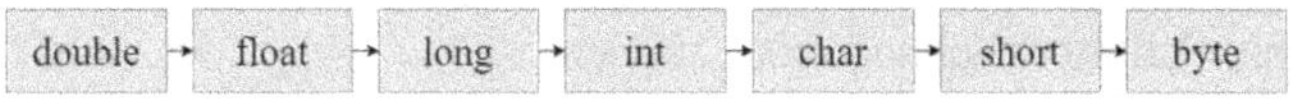

double → float → long → int → char → short → byte

FIGURE 2.2 Explicit type casting.

Program

```
public class ExplicitExample {
void main(String a[]) {
double d = 57.17;
int i = (int)d; // Explicit casting from long to int data type
System.out.println(d);
System.out.println(i); //fractional part lost
  }
}
Output:
57.17
57
```

In this program, we define a class named `ExplicitExample` with a `main` method. Inside the method, a `double` variable `d` is assigned the value `57.17`. We then explicitly cast the `double` value to an `int`, storing the result in the variable `i`. Since `int` only holds whole numbers, the fractional part of `d` is lost during the casting. The program first prints the original `double` value `57.17`, followed by the `int` value `57`, demonstrating the effect of explicit casting.

2.5 OPERATORS IN JAVA

Operators in Java are essential components that facilitate various computations and operations within programs.

Need for Operators in Java

- Expression Evaluation: Operators allow programmers to perform calculations and evaluate expressions efficiently. They enable basic arithmetic (e.g., `+`, `-`, `*`, `/`) and complex operations (e.g., bitwise operations, relational operations).
- Manipulating Data: Operators provide mechanisms to manipulate data stored in variables. For instance, assignment operators (`=`, `+=`, `-=`) modify the value of variables based on certain conditions or expressions.
- Control Flow: Logical operators (`&&`, `||`, `!`) are crucial for implementing conditional statements (`if`, `else`, `switch`) and loops (`for`, `while`, `do-while`). They control the flow of execution based on boolean expressions.
- Enhanced Functionality: Specialized operators like ternary (`?:`), increment (`++`), and decrement (`--`) operators provide concise ways to express conditional assignments and increment/decrement operations.
- Bit-Level Manipulation: Bitwise operators (`&`, `|`, `^`, `<<`, `>>`, `>>>`) allow manipulation of individual bits within integer types. They are essential for tasks like encoding, decoding, and performance optimization in low-level programming.

Advantages of Operators in Java

- Simplicity and Conciseness: Operators enable concise and readable code by condensing complex operations into compact expressions.

- Efficiency: Most operators in Java are highly optimized for performance, making computations and data manipulations faster and more efficient.
- Expressiveness: Operators enhance the expressiveness of the language, allowing programmers to convey their intentions clearly and effectively.
- Standardization: Operators provide a standardized way to perform common tasks across different programs and applications, promoting code reusability and familiarity.
- Versatility: Java's operators cater to a wide range of programming needs, from basic arithmetic to advanced bitwise operations, making the language versatile for various domains.

Limitations of Operators in Java

- Overload and Complexity: Overuse or misuse of operators can lead to complex and hard-to-understand code, diminishing code maintainability and readability.
- Potential for Errors: Incorrect usage of operators can introduce bugs and logical errors in the program, especially with bitwise and assignment operators.
- Limited Functionality: While Java provides a comprehensive set of operators, some specialized tasks may require additional libraries or custom implementations beyond standard operators.
- Learning Curve: Beginners may find certain operators, especially bitwise and ternary operators, challenging to grasp initially due to their specialized functionalities and syntax.
- Performance Considerations: Certain operators, especially those involving bit-level manipulations or complex expressions, may have varying performance impacts depending on the hardware and compiler optimizations.

Java provides a rich set of operators to perform operations on variables and values. These operators can be categorized into several types:

2.5.1 Arithmetic Operators

Used to perform basic arithmetic operations:

- Addition (`+`): Adds two operands.
- Subtraction (`-`): Subtracts the second operand from the first.
- Multiplication (`*`): Multiplies two operands.
- Division (`/`): Divides the numerator by the denominator.
- Modulus (`%`): Returns the remainder of division.

Program

```
public class ArithmeticOperators {
  void main(String[] args) {
    int ushaAge = 30;
    int raniAge = 25;
    int sum = ushaAge + raniAge; // Addition
    int difference = ushaAge - raniAge; // Subtraction
    int product = ushaAge * raniAge; // Multiplication
    int quotient = ushaAge / raniAge; // Division
    int remainder = ushaAge % raniAge; // Modulus
System.out.println("Sum: " + sum);
System.out.println("Difference: " + difference);
System.out.println("Product: " + product);
System.out.println("Quotient: " + quotient);
```

```
System.out.println("Remainder: " + remainder);
  }
}
Output:
Sum: 55
Difference: 5
Product: 750
Quotient: 1
Remainder: 5
```

In this program, we define a class called `ArithmeticOperators` where two integer variables, `ushaAge` and `raniAge`, are assigned the values 30 and 25, respectively. The program performs arithmetic operations on these values, calculating the sum, difference, product, quotient, and remainder. The sum of 30 and 25 is 55, the difference is 5, the product is 750, the quotient from dividing 30 by 25 is 1, and the remainder is 5. These results are printed to the console.

2.5.2 Unary Operators

Operate on a single operand:

- Unary plus (`+`): Indicates a positive value (usually redundant).
- Unary minus (`-`): Negates an expression.
- Increment (`++`): Increases the value of an operand by 1.
- Decrement (`--`): Decreases the value of an operand by 1.
- Logical complement (`!`): Inverts the value of a boolean.

Program

```
public class UnaryOperators {
  void main(String[] args) {
    int ushaAge = 30;
    int age = ushaAge; // Assignment
    age++; // Increment
System.out.println("Increment: " + age);
    age--; // Decrement
System.out.println("Decrement: " + age);
    age = -ushaAge; // Unary minus
System.out.println("Unary minus: " + age);
boolean isAdult = ushaAge> 18; // True
isAdult= !isAdult; // Logical complement
System.out.println("Logical complement: " + isAdult);
  }
}
Output:
Increment: 31
Decrement: 30
Unary minus: -30
Logical complement: false
```

In this program, we define a class named `UnaryOperators` with a `main` method that demonstrates the use of unary operators in Java. We begin by assigning the value `30` to the variable `ushaAge` and then assign it to `age`. We increment the value of `age` using `age++`, which results in `31`, and print it. Next, we decrement the value of `age` back to `30` using `age--`, and print it again.

The unary minus operator is applied to `ushaAge`, changing `age` to `-30`. Finally, we check if `ushaAge` is greater than 18 and store the result (`true`) in the `isAdult` variable. The logical complement operator `!` is used to reverse the value of `isAdult`, resulting in `false`, and we print that as well.

2.5.3 Relational Operators

Used to compare two values:

- Equal to (`==`): Checks if two values are equal.
- Not equal to (`!=`): Checks if two values are not equal.
- Greater than (`>`): Checks if the left operand is greater than the right.
- Less than (`<`): Checks if the left operand is less than the right.
- Greater than or equal to (`>=`): Checks if the left operand is greater than or equal to the right.
- Less than or equal to (`<=`): Checks if the left operand is less than or equal to the right

Program

```
public class RelationalOperators {
  void main(String[] args) {
    int ushaAge = 30;
    int raniAge = 25;
boolean isEqual = ushaAge == raniAge;
boolean isNotEqual = ushaAge != raniAge;
boolean isUshaOlder = ushaAge>raniAge;
boolean isRaniOlder = ushaAge<raniAge;
boolean isUshaAtLeastAsOld = ushaAge>= raniAge;
boolean isRaniAtMostAsOld = ushaAge<= raniAge;
System.out.println("Equal: " + isEqual);
System.out.println("Not equal: " + isNotEqual);
System.out.println("Usha is older: " + isUshaOlder);
System.out.println("Rani is older: " + isRaniOlder);
System.out.println("Usha is at least as old: " + isUshaAtLeastAsOld);
System.out.println("Rani is at most as old: " + isRaniAtMostAsOld);
  }
}
Output:
Equal: false
Not equal: true
Usha is older: true
Rani is older: false
Usha is at least as old: true
Rani is at most as old: false
```

This Java program, "RelationalOperators," meticulously assesses the age comparison between two individuals, Usha and Rani, through the lens of relational operators. Initializing Usha's age as 30 and Rani's age as 25, the program meticulously evaluates multiple relational expressions to determine the dynamic between their ages. It deduces whether Usha's age is equal to Rani's age, not equal, if Usha is older than Rani, if Rani is older than Usha, if Usha is at least as old as Rani, and if Rani is at most as old as Usha. Subsequently, the program presents the outcome of these comparisons; each conveyed through individual print statements. Upon execution, the program meticulously outputs the results, indicating that Usha's and Rani's ages are not equal, with Usha being older, and Rani being at least as old as Usha.

2.5.4 Logical Operators

Used to combine multiple boolean expressions:

- Logical AND (`&&`): Returns true if both operands are true.
- Logical OR (`||`): Returns true if at least one of the operands is true.
- Logical NOT (`!`): Inverts the value of a boolean.

Program

```
public class LogicalOperators {
  void main(String[] args) {
    int ushaAge = 30;
    int raniAge = 25;
boolean isUshaAdult = ushaAge>18;
boolean isRaniAdult = raniAge>18;
boolean bothAdults = isUshaAdult&&isRaniAdult;
boolean atLeastOneAdult = isUshaAdult || isRaniAdult;
boolean notUshaAdult= !isUshaAdult;
System.out.println("Both are adults: " + bothAdults);
System.out.println("At least one is adult: " + atLeastOneAdult);
System.out.println("Usha is not an adult: " + notUshaAdult);
  }
}
Output:
Both are adults: true
At least one is adult: true
Usha is not an adult: false
```

The above Java program, "LogicalOperators," explores the application of logical operators to assess the adulthood status of two individuals, Usha and Rani. By initializing Usha's age as 30 and Rani's age as 25, the program calculates whether each individual meets the adult age criteria (over 18 years old). It evaluates if Usha and Rani are both adults (`bothAdults`) using the logical AND operator (`&&`) to determine if both conditions are true. Additionally, it evaluates if at least one of them is an adult (`atLeastOneAdult`) using the logical OR operator (`||`), ensuring that either Usha or Rani (or both) fulfill the adult age criteria. Finally, it evaluates if Usha is not an adult (`notUshaAdult`) using the logical NOT operator (`!`), negating the result obtained for Usha's adulthood status. The program then prints the outcomes of these logical evaluations to the console, providing clear insights into the adulthood status of Usha and Rani based on the logical conditions applied.

2.5.5 Bitwise Operators

Operate on bits and perform bit-by-bit operations:

- Bitwise AND (`&`): Performs a bitwise AND.
- Bitwise OR (`|`): Performs a bitwise OR.
- Bitwise XOR (`^`): Performs a bitwise exclusive OR.
- Bitwise complement (`~`): Inverts each bit.
- Left shift (`<<`): Shifts bits to the left.
- Right shift (`>>`): Shifts bits to the right.
- Unsigned right shift (`>>>`): Shifts bits to the right without sign extension.

Program

```
public class BitwiseOperators {
  void main(String[] args) {
    int ushaAge = 30;
    int raniAge = 25;
    int bitwiseAnd = ushaAge&raniAge;
    int bitwiseOr = ushaAge | raniAge;
    int bitwiseXor = ushaAge ^ raniAge;
    int bitwiseComplement = ~ushaAge;
    int leftShift = ushaAge<<1;
    int rightShift = ushaAge>>1;
    int unsignedRightShift = ushaAge>>>1;
System.out.println("Bitwise AND: " + bitwiseAnd);
System.out.println("Bitwise OR: " + bitwiseOr);
System.out.println("Bitwise XOR: " + bitwiseXor);
System.out.println("Bitwise complement: " + bitwiseComplement);
System.out.println("Left shift: " + leftShift);
System.out.println("Right shift: " + rightShift);
System.out.println("Unsigned right shift: " + unsignedRightShift);
  }
}
Output:
Bitwise AND: 24
Bitwise OR: 31
Bitwise XOR: 7
Bitwise complement: -31
Left shift: 60
Right shift: 15
Unsigned right shift: 15
```

This Java program, named "BitwiseOperators," provides a comprehensive exploration of bitwise operators applied to the ages of two individuals, Usha and Rani. Initialized with Usha's age as 30 and Rani's age as 25, the program meticulously computes various bitwise operations on these age values. It calculates the bitwise AND (`bitwiseAnd`), bitwise OR (`bitwiseOr`), and bitwise XOR (`bitwiseXor`) between Usha's and Rani's ages, revealing the binary outcomes of these operations. Additionally, it computes the bitwise complement (`bitwiseComplement`) of Usha's age, effectively flipping all bits to their opposite values. Furthermore, the program demonstrates the left shift (`leftShift`), right shift (`rightShift`), and unsigned right shift (`unsignedRightShift`) operations applied to Usha's age, illustrating how these operations manipulate the binary representation of the age value. Finally, the program presents the results of these bitwise operations through print statements, providing a comprehensive overview of the bitwise manipulation performed on the age values of Usha and Rani.

2.5.6 Assignment Operators

Used to assign values to variables:

- Simple assignment (`=`): Assigns the right-hand operand to the left-hand variable.
- Add and assign (`+=`): Adds the right-hand operand to the left-hand variable and assigns the result to the left-hand variable.
- Subtract and assign (`-=`): Subtracts the right-hand operand from the left-hand variable and assigns the result to the left-hand variable.

- Multiply and assign (`*=`): Multiplies the right-hand operand by the left-hand variable and assigns the result to the left-hand variable.
- Divide and assign(`/=`): Divides the left-hand variable by the right-hand operand and assigns the result to the left-hand variable.
- Modulus and assign (`%=`): Takes the modulus using two operands and assigns the result to the left-hand variable.

Program

```
public class AssignmentOperators {
  void main(String[] args) {
    int ushaAge = 30;
    int raniAge = 25;
    int age = ushaAge;
    age += raniAge;
System.out.println("Add and assign: " + age);
    age -= raniAge;
System.out.println("Subtract and assign: " + age);
    age *= raniAge;
System.out.println("Multiply and assign: " + age);
    age /= raniAge;
System.out.println("Divide and assign: " + age);
    age %= raniAge;
System.out.println("Modulus and assign: " + age);
  }
}
Output:
Add and assign: 55
Subtract and assign: 30
Multiply and assign: 750
Divide and assign: 30
Modulus and assign: 5
```

In this program, we define a class named `AssignmentOperators` where various assignment operators are demonstrated. First, we assign the value `30` to `ushaAge` and `25` to `raniAge`. We then assign `ushaAge` to a new variable `age`. Then uses compound assignment operators to modify the value of `age` in various ways. The `+=` operator adds `raniAge` to `age`, resulting in `55`, which is printed. The `-=` operator subtracts `raniAge`, bringing `age` back to `30`. The `*=` operator multiplies `age` by `raniAge`, producing `750`. The `/=` operator divides `age` by `raniAge`, yielding `30`. Finally, the `%=` operator calculates the remainder of `age` divided by `raniAge`, giving `5`. These results are printed, showing the effects of each compound assignment operation.

2.5.7 Conditional Operator (Ternary)

A shorthand for `if-then-else` statements:

```
Ternary operator (`? :`): `condition ? if-true : if-false`
```

Program

```
public class ConditionalOperator {
  void main(String[] args) {
    int ushaAge = 30;
```

```
    int raniAge = 25;
      String olderPerson = (ushaAge>raniAge) ? "Usha" : "Rani";
System.out.println("Older person: " + olderPerson);
  }
}
```

Output:

```
Older person: Usha
```

In this program, we define a class named `ConditionalOperator` to demonstrate the use of the conditional (ternary) operator in Java. Two integer variables, `ushaAge` and `raniAge`, are assigned values 30 and 25, respectively. Then compares these two values using the conditional operator `(ushaAge > raniAge)`, which checks if `ushaAge` is greater than `raniAge`. If the condition is true, the result is "Usha"; otherwise, it is "Rani". The result is stored in the `olderPerson` variable and printed to the console, indicating who is older.

2.6 WRAPPER CLASSES

Wrapper classes in Java are part of the `java.lang` package and provide a way to use primitive data types (like `int`, `char`, `boolean`, etc.) as objects. Each of the eight primitive data types has a corresponding wrapper class:

- `byte` -> `Byte`
- `short` -> `Short`
- `int` -> `Integer`
- `long` -> `Long`
- `float` -> `Float`
- `double` -> `Double`
- `char` -> `Character`
- `boolean` -> `Boolean`

Benefits of Wrapper Classes

- Object-Oriented Features: Wrapper classes allow primitive data types to be used as objects, enabling the use of object-oriented features like generics and collection frameworks.
- Utility Methods: They provide a range of utility methods for converting between different data types, parsing strings, and performing other useful operations.
- Collections Framework: Many Java frameworks and APIs, such as the Collections Framework, require the use of objects. Wrapper classes enable primitives to be used in these contexts.
- Synchronization: Objects can be synchronized in multi-threaded programming, while primitive types cannot.
- Null Values: Wrapper classes can represent null values, which is useful in cases where a value might be undefined or missing. This is particularly helpful in database applications and collections.
- Type Conversion: They offer methods for type conversion (e.g., `Integer.parseInt`, `Double.parseDouble`).

Limitations of Wrapper Classes

- Performance Overhead: Wrapping primitives in objects introduces additional overhead in terms of memory and processing time.
- Memory Consumption: Objects require more memory than primitive types, leading to higher memory consumption.

- Unboxing and Boxing: Automatic conversion between primitives and wrapper objects (autoboxing and unboxing) can lead to unexpected `NullPointerException` and performance issues if not managed carefully.
- Complexity: Using wrapper classes can introduce complexity in code, especially in performance-critical applications.

Need for Wrapper Classes in Java Programming

- Generic Collections: Java's collection framework (like `ArrayList`, `HashMap`, etc.) works with objects. To store primitive types in these collections, we need their corresponding wrapper classes.
- Reflection: Java's reflection API works with objects. Wrapper classes allow primitive types to be manipulated using reflection.
- Data Structures: When working with data structures that require the use of objects, such as those found in many Java libraries and frameworks, wrapper classes are necessary.
- Interfacing with Libraries: Many libraries and APIs expect objects rather than primitives. Wrapper classes allow primitives to be passed and manipulated in such contexts.
- Utility Methods: Wrapper classes provide a variety of utility methods, such as `Integer.parseInt` and `Double.valueOf`, which are useful for converting between strings and primitive types.

2.7 SPECIAL CHARACTERS

In Java, special characters have various meanings and uses, often related to escaping sequences, character literals, and formatting. These special characters are used to represent characters that are not easily typed on a keyboard, such as newline characters, tabs, and Unicode characters. Understanding and utilizing these special characters allows for precise control over text representation and formatting in Java programs.

2.7.1 Escape Sequences

Escape sequences are used to represent certain special characters within string literals or character literals. Here are some common escape sequences in Java:

- `\'` - Single quote
- `\"` - Double quote
- `\\` - Backslash
- `\n` - Newline
- `\r` - Carriage return
- `\t` - Tab
- `\b` - Backspace
- `\f` - Form feed
- `\uXXXX` - Unicode character (where `XXXX` is the Unicode value in hexadecimal)

Usage of Special Characters

- String Literals: Special characters are often used within string literals to represent characters that cannot be typed directly.

```
String nameDetails ="Name: Usha\nQualification: B.Sc.";
      String filePath = "C:\\Users\\Usha\\Documents";
```

- Character Literals: Special characters can be used as character literals to represent single characters.

```
char newline = '\n';  // Newline character
   char tab = '\t';  // Tab character
```

- Unicode Characters: Unicode escape sequences allow for the representation of characters from different languages and symbols.

```
char omega = '\u03A9';  // Greek capital letter Omega (Ω)
             String smiley = "\u263A";  // Smiley face (☺)
```

- Formatting and Control Characters: Special characters are used in formatting text and controlling output.

```
System.out.println("First Line\nSecond Line");  // Output spans two lines
System.out.println("Column1\tColumn2");
```

Program

```
public class SpecialCharactersExample {
  void main(String[] args) {
    // String Literals
    String nameDetails = "Name: Usha\nQualification:Ph.D.";
    String filePath = "C:\\Users\\Usha\\Documents";
    // Displaying string literals
    System.out.println(nameDetails);
    System.out.println("File Path: " + filePath);
    // Character Literals
    char newline = '\n';  // Newline character
    char tab = '\t';  // Tab character
    // Displaying character literals
    System.out.println("Character Literals:");
    System.out.println("Newline character:" + newline + "After newline");
    System.out.println("Tab character:" + tab + "After tab");
    // Unicode Characters
    char omega = '\u03A9';  // Greek capital letter Omega (Ω)
    String smiley = "\u263A";  // Smiley face (☺)
    // Displaying Unicode characters
    System.out.println("Unicode Characters:");
    System.out.println("Omega: " + omega);
    System.out.println("Smiley face: " + smiley);
    // Formatting and Control Characters
    System.out.println("Formatted Output:");
    System.out.println("First Line\nSecond Line");
    System.out.println("Column1\tColumn2");
  }
}
```

Output:

```
Name: Usha
```

```
Qualification: Ph.D.
File Path: C:\Users\Usha\Documents
Character Literals:
Newline character:
After newline
Tab character:  After tab
Unicode Characters:
Omega: Ω
Smiley face: ☺
Formatted Output:
First Line
Second Line
Column1 Column2
```

In this program, we define a class named `SpecialCharactersExample` to demonstrate the use of special characters, escape sequences, and Unicode characters in Java. First, two string literals are defined: `nameDetails`, which includes a newline character (`\n`) to separate lines, and `filePath`, which uses escape sequences for the backslashes (`\\`) in a file path. These strings are printed to the console, showing how escape sequences format text. Next, we introduce character literals such as the newline (`\n`) and tab (`\t`) characters, displaying their effects when printed. Unicode characters are then demonstrated by printing the Greek letter Omega (`\u03A9`) and a smiley face (`\u263A`). Finally, the program uses formatted output with control characters to print text on separate lines and create columns using tabs.

2.8 JAVA VARIABLE SCOPE

In Java, the scope of a variable determines where the variable can be accessed within the code. Understanding variable scope is crucial for writing maintainable and bug-free programs. Java has different types of variable scopes:

- Local Scope
- Instance Scope
- Class Scope

2.8.1 Local Scope

Variables declared inside a method, constructor, or block are called local variables. They are only accessible within that method, constructor, or block.

Program

```
public class LocalScopeExample {
  public void display() {
    int localVar = 10; // local variable
    System.out.println("Local Variable: " + localVar);
  }
  void main(String[] args) {
    LocalScopeExample example = new LocalScopeExample();
    example.display();
    // localVar is not accessible here
    // System.out.println(localVar); // This will cause a compilation error
  }
}
```

```
Output:
Local Variable: 10
```

In this program, we define a class called `LocalScopeExample` that demonstrates the concept of local scope in Java. Inside the class, the `display` method is defined, where an integer variable `localVar` is declared and initialized with the value `10`. This variable is local to the `display` method, meaning it can only be accessed within that method. When `display` is called, it prints the value of `localVar` to the console. In the `main` method, an instance of `LocalScopeExample` is created, and the `display` method is invoked. The output shows the message indicating the value of the local variable. However, if you attempt to access `localVar` directly in the `main` method, it would result in a compilation error, as `localVar` is out of scope outside the `display` method.

2.8.2 Instance Scope

Instance variables (or fields) are declared within a class but outside any method, constructor, or block. They are accessible within all methods, constructors, and blocks of the class, and their values are unique to each instance of the class.

Program

```
public class InstanceScopeExample {
  private int instanceVar; // instance variable
public InstanceScopeExample() {
  }
  public InstanceScopeExample(int instanceVar) {
    this.instanceVar = instanceVar;
  }
  public void display() {
    System.out.println("Instance Variable: " + instanceVar);
  }
  void main(String[] args) {
    InstanceScopeExample example1 = new InstanceScopeExample(5);
    InstanceScopeExample example2 = new InstanceScopeExample(10);
    example1.display(); // Output: Instance Variable: 5
    example2.display(); // Output: Instance Variable: 10
  }
}
Output:
Instance Variable: 5
Instance Variable: 10
```

In this program, we define a class named `InstanceScopeExample` that illustrates the use of instance variables in Java. The class contains a private instance variable `instanceVar`, which is initialized through the constructor. When an object of `InstanceScopeExample` is created, the constructor assigns the passed value to the instance variable. The `display` method is defined to print the value of `instanceVar`. In the `main` method, two instances of the class are created: `example1` with an instance variable value of `5`, and `example2` with a value of `10`. When the `display` method is called on each instance, it prints the corresponding value of the instance variable.

2.8.3 Class Scope

Class variables (or static variables) are declared with the `static` keyword inside a class but outside any method, constructor, or block. They are accessible to all instances of the class and share the same value among all instances.

Program

```
public class ClassScopeExample {
  private static int classVar = 0; // class variable
  public ClassScopeExample() {
    classVar++;
  }
  public void display() {
    System.out.println("Class Variable: " + classVar);
  }
  void main(String[] args) {
    ClassScopeExample example1 = new ClassScopeExample();
    ClassScopeExample example2 = new ClassScopeExample();
    example1.display(); // Output: Class Variable: 2
    example2.display(); // Output: Class Variable: 2
  }
}
Output:
Class Variable: 3
Class Variable: 3
```

In this program, we define a class named `ClassScopeExample` that demonstrates the use of class (static) variables in Java. A private static variable `classVar` is declared and initialized to `0`. The constructor of the class increments this variable each time a new instance is created. The `display` method prints the value of the static variable. In the `main` method, two instances of `ClassScopeExample` are created: `example1` and `example2`. Each time a new instance is instantiated, the `classVar` is incremented. Therefore, by the time both instances are created, `classVar` becomes `3`. When the `display` method is called for both instances, it prints the same value for the class variable.

2.9 ACCESS AND NON-ACCESS MODIFIERS

In Java, a modifier is a keyword used to alter the properties of classes, methods, and variables, providing additional information to the compiler about how these entities should be treated. Modifiers can control the visibility, behavior, and characteristics of these entities.

Modifiers in Java are categorized into two main types: Access Modifiers and Non-Access Modifiers.

2.9.1 Access Modifiers in Java

Access modifiers in Java determine the visibility and accessibility of classes, methods, and variables. Java provides four access modifiers:

- `public`: The member is accessible from any other class.
- `protected`: The member is accessible within its own package and by subclasses.
- `default` (no modifier): The member is accessible only within its own package.
- `private`: The member is accessible only within its own class.

2.9.2 Non-Access Modifiers in Java

Non-access modifiers in Java provide additional functionality and characteristics to classes, methods, and variables. These include:

- `static`: Belongs to the class rather than an instance of the class.
- `final`: Prevents modification (e.g., a final class cannot be subclassed, a final method cannot be overridden, a final variable cannot be reassigned).
- `abstract`: Used to declare a class that cannot be instantiated or a method that must be implemented by subclasses.
- `synchronized`* Used to control access to a method or block, allowing only one thread to execute it at a time.
- `volatile`: Indicates that a variable's value may be changed unexpectedly by different threads.
- `transient`: Prevents serialization of the variable.
- `native`: Specifies that a method is implemented in native code using JNI (Java Native Interface).
- `strictfp`: Ensures floating-point calculations adhere to IEEE 754 standards.

2.9.2.1 Programs for Each Access Specifiers

1. `public` Access Specifier:
   The member is accessible from any other class.

Program

```
public class PublicAccess {
  public int publicVar = 10;  // Public variable
  public void publicMethod() { // Public method
    System.out.println("This is a public method.");
  }
void main(String[] args) {
    PublicAccess obj = new PublicAccess();
    System.out.println("Public Variable: " + obj.publicVar); // Accessible
    obj.publicMethod(); // Accessible
  }
}
```

Output

```
Public Variable: 10
This is a public method.
```

In this `PublicAccess` class, we demonstrate the use of the `public` access modifier in Java. The variable `publicVar` and the method `publicMethod()` are both declared as `public`, meaning they are accessible from anywhere, including other classes, packages, and even subclasses. This makes them universally accessible, regardless of where the accessing class is located. In the `main` method, we create an instance of the `PublicAccess` class. Since both `publicVar` and `publicMethod()` are public, we can easily access and print the value of `publicVar` and call the `publicMethod()`.

2. `protected` Access Specifier:
   The member is accessible within its own package and by subclasses.

Program

```
class ProtectedAccess {
  protected int protectedVar = 20;  // Protected variable
  protected void protectedMethod() { // Protected method
```

```
    System.out.println("This is a protected method.");
  }
  void main(String[] args) {
    ProtectedAccess obj = new ProtectedAccess();
    System.out.println("Protected  Variable:  "  +  obj.protectedVar);  //
       Accessible
    obj.protectedMethod(); // Accessible
  }
}
```

Output

```
Protected Variable: 20
This is a protected method.
```

In the above `ProtectedAccess` class, we demonstrate the use of the `protected` access modifier in Java. The variable `protectedVar` and the method `protectedMethod()` are both marked as `protected`, meaning they are accessible within the same package and can also be accessed by subclasses, even if they are in different packages. In the `main` method, we create an instance of `ProtectedAccess` and access both the `protectedVar` and `protectedMethod()` within the same class. This access is allowed because members with `protected` access are fully available within their own class and package. Additionally, any subclass of `ProtectedAccess`, even if located in a different package, would be able to access these protected members, making `protected` useful for providing controlled access in inheritance scenarios while still maintaining some level of encapsulation.

3. `default` (no modifier) Access Specifier:

   The member is accessible only within its own package.

Program

```
class DefaultAccess {
  int defaultVar = 30;  // Default (package-private) variable
  void defaultMethod() { // Default (package-private) method
    System.out.println("This is a default method.");
  }
  void main(String[] args) {
    DefaultAccess obj = new DefaultAccess();
    System.out.println("Default Variable: " + obj.defaultVar); // Accessible
    obj.defaultMethod(); // Accessible
  }
}
```

Output

```
Default Variable: 30
This is a default method.
```

In the above `DefaultAccess` class, we demonstrate the concept of the default (or package-private) access modifier in Java. The variable `defaultVar` and the method `defaultMethod()` are not explicitly marked with any access modifier, which means they have default access. This allows them to be accessed by any class within the same package but restricts access from classes in other packages. In the `main` method, we create an instance of `DefaultAccess` and access both the `defaultVar` and `defaultMethod()` from within the same class, which is always allowed. This example would work similarly for any other class within the same package, allowing those classes to access the `defaultVar` and `defaultMethod()`.

4. `private` Access Specifier:

   The member is accessible only within its own class.

Program

```
public class PrivateAccess {
  private int privateVar = 40;  // Private variable
  private void privateMethod() { // Private method
    System.out.println("This is a private method.");
  }
void main(String[] args) {
    PrivateAccess obj = new PrivateAccess();
    System.out.println("Private Variable: " + obj.privateVar);
    // Accessible within the class
    obj.privateMethod(); // Accessible within the class
  }
}
```

Output

```
Private Variable: 40
This is a private method.
```

In this `PrivateAccess` program, we demonstrate how the `private` access modifier works in Java. The `privateVar` variable and `privateMethod()` are both declared as `private`, meaning they are accessible only within the class where they are defined. No other class, including subclasses or classes in the same package, can directly access these members. In the `main` method, we create an instance of the `PrivateAccess` class. Since we are within the same class, we can access and print the value of the `privateVar` and call the `privateMethod()`. This shows that private members are fully accessible within the class but are completely hidden from the outside.

2.9.3 Programs for Each Non Access Specifiers

2.9.3.1 `static`

A static member belongs to the class rather than an instance of the class.

Program

```
public class StaticExample {
  static int staticVar = 100; // Static variable
  static void staticMethod() { // Static method
    System.out.println("This is a static method.");
  }
void main(String[] args) {
    System.out.println("Static Variable: " + staticVar);
    // Accessible without object creation
    staticMethod(); // Accessible without object creation
  }
}
```

Output

```
Static Variable: 100
This is a static method.
```

In this `StaticExample` program, we illustrate the use of the `static` keyword in Java, which indicates that a variable or method belongs to the class itself rather than to instances of the class. We declare a static variable `staticVar` initialized to 100, which is shared among all instances of the class. Additionally, we define a static method `staticMethod()`, which can be called without needing to create an instance of the class. This method simply prints a message to the console. In the `main` method, we access the static variable `staticVar` and print its value, demonstrating that it can be accessed directly from the class without object instantiation. We also call `staticMethod()`, further emphasizing that static methods can be invoked without creating an instance.

2.9.3.2 `final`

A final member cannot be changed once assigned, and a final class or method cannot be modified.

Program

```
public class FinalExample {
  final int finalVar = 50; // Final variable
  final void finalMethod() { // Final method
    System.out.println("This is a final method.");
  }
void main(String[] args) {
    FinalExample obj = new FinalExample();
    System.out.println("Final Variable: " + obj.finalVar);
    // Value can't be changed
    obj.finalMethod(); // Method can't be overridden
  }
}
```

Output

```
Final Variable: 50
This is a final method.
```

In this `FinalExample` program, we demonstrate the use of the `final` keyword in Java, which serves several purposes. The class defines a `final` variable `finalVar`, which is initialized to 50. Once assigned, this variable cannot be changed or reassigned, ensuring its value remains constant throughout the program. Additionally, we declare a `final` method named `finalMethod()`. Marking a method as `final` prevents it from being overridden by any subclasses, ensuring that its behavior remains unchanged and consistent. In the `main` method, we create an instance of `FinalExample` and print the value of `finalVar`, which demonstrates that it cannot be modified. We also call `finalMethod()`, showcasing that the method can be accessed normally, but cannot be altered in any subclass.

2.9.3.3 `abstract`

An abstract class cannot be instantiated, and an abstract method must be implemented by its subclasses.

Program

```
abstract class AbstractExample {
  abstract void abstractMethod(); // Abstract method
  void concreteMethod() {
    System.out.println("This is a concrete method in an abstract class.");
  }
}
class SubClass extends AbstractExample {
  void abstractMethod() {
    System.out.println("Abstract method implemented in subclass.");
  }
  void main(String[] args) {
```

```
    SubClass obj = new SubClass();
    obj.abstractMethod(); // Must be implemented
    obj.concreteMethod();
  }
}
```

Output

```
Abstract method implemented in subclass.
This is a concrete method in an abstract class.
```

This example demonstrates how abstract classes provide a base for subclasses to build upon, while abstract methods enforce that certain methods must be implemented by the subclasses. The class `AbstractExample` is declared as `abstract`, meaning it cannot be instantiated directly and may contain abstract methods—methods without an implementation that must be implemented by any subclass. Inside `AbstractExample`, we define an abstract method `abstractMethod()` without a body. Additionally, we have a concrete method `concreteMethod()`, which has an implementation and can be used directly by subclasses. The `SubClass` class extends `AbstractExample` and provides an implementation for the `abstractMethod()`. This is mandatory because any concrete subclass of an abstract class must implement all its abstract methods. In the `main` method of `SubClass`, we create an object of `SubClass` and call both the `abstractMethod()` (which is now implemented) and the inherited `concreteMethod()`. This example demonstrates how abstract classes provide a base for subclasses to build upon, while abstract methods enforce that certain methods must be implemented by the subclasses.

2.9.3.4 `synchronized`

The synchronized keyword ensures only one thread can access a block or method at a time.

Program

```
public class SynchronizedExample {
  synchronized void synchronizedMethod() {
    System.out.println("This is a synchronized method.");
  }
  void main(String[] args) {
    SynchronizedExample obj = new SynchronizedExample();
    obj.synchronizedMethod();
    // Only one thread can access this method at a time
  }
}
```

Output

```
This is a synchronized method.
```

In this `SynchronizedExample` program, we demonstrate the use of the `synchronized` keyword in Java, which is essential for ensuring thread safety in a multithreaded environment. The `synchronizedMethod()` is marked as `synchronized`, meaning that only one thread can access this method at a time for any given instance of the class. If multiple threads attempt to call this method simultaneously, they will be queued, and only one thread will execute the method at a time. This prevents race conditions and ensures that the shared resource or operation remains consistent and thread-safe. In the `main` method, we create an instance of `SynchronizedExample` and call the `synchronizedMethod()`. Since this program is single-threaded, the synchronization aspect isn't fully observable here, but in a multithreaded environment, this ensures that access to the method is controlled so that no two threads can access it concurrently on the same object, maintaining data integrity.

2.9.3.5 `volatile`

A volatile variable can be modified by multiple threads unpredictably.

Program

```
public class VolatileExample {
  volatile boolean flag = false; // Volatile variable
  public void setFlag() {
    flag = true;
  }
  void main(String[] args) {
    VolatileExample obj = new VolatileExample();
    obj.setFlag(); // Changing the volatile variable
    System.out.println("Volatile Flag: " + obj.flag);
  }
}
```

Output

```
Volatile Flag: true
```

In this `VolatileExample` program, we demonstrate the use of the `volatile` keyword in Java, which is primarily used in multithreaded environments to ensure the visibility of variable changes across threads. The `flag` variable is declared as `volatile`, which means that any modification to its value will be immediately visible to all threads. This ensures that the variable's value is always read directly from memory, rather than being cached by individual threads. In the `setFlag` method, we change the value of `flag` to `true`. The `main` method creates an instance of the `VolatileExample` class, calls the `setFlag` method to update the volatile variable, and then prints the current value of `flag`. Although this program is single-threaded, the `volatile` keyword ensures that if the program were to run in a multithreaded environment, all threads would see the updated value of `flag` as soon as it's modified, preventing potential inconsistencies or stale values.

2.9.3.6 `transient`

A transient variable is not serialized during object serialization.

Program

```
import java.io.Serializable;
public class TransientExample implements Serializable {
  transient int transientVar = 100; // Transient variable
  int normalVar = 200;
  void main(String[] args) {
    TransientExample obj = new TransientExample();
    System.out.println("Transient Variable: " + obj.transientVar);
    System.out.println("Normal Variable: " + obj.normalVar);
  }
}
```

Output

```
Transient Variable: 100
Normal Variable: 200
```

In this `TransientExample` program, we illustrate the use of the `transient` keyword, which impacts how certain variables are handled during the serialization process in Java. The class implements the `Serializable` interface, indicating that objects of this class can be serialized—converted into a byte stream for storage or transfer. We define two instance variables: `transientVar` (marked with the `transient` keyword) and `normalVar` (a regular variable). The key difference is that `transientVar` will not be serialized, meaning its value will be ignored during serialization, and when the object is deserialized, `transientVar` will reset to its default value (in this case, 0 for an `int`). Conversely, `normalVar` will be serialized and deserialized as expected, preserving its value. In the `main` method, we create an instance of `TransientExample` and print both variables to show their current values, demonstrating the behavior before any serialization process occurs.

2.9.3.7 `native`

A native method is implemented using native code (like C/C++) via JNI.
Note: JNI setup and external native library implementation are needed for this to work.

Program

```
public class NativeExample {
  native void nativeMethod(); // Declaration of native method
  static {
    System.loadLibrary("NativeLib"); // Load native library
  }
  void main(String[] args) {
    NativeExample obj = new NativeExample();
    obj.nativeMethod(); // This will call the native method
  }
}
```

In this `NativeExample` program, we declare a native method and demonstrate how to use Java Native Interface (JNI) to integrate native code (typically written in languages like C or C++) with Java. The native method `nativeMethod()` is declared in the class but not implemented in Java. The implementation of this method is expected to be provided in an external native code library, which is typically written in a language like C or C++ and compiled separately. In the static block, we call `System.loadLibrary("NativeLib")`, which loads the native library named "NativeLib" that contains the implementation of the `nativeMethod()`. The static block ensures that this library is loaded when the class is first loaded by the JVM. In the `main` method, we create an instance of the `NativeExample` class and call the `nativeMethod()` on the created object. This method will execute the corresponding native code in the external library. To fully run this program, you would need to set up the native code, compile it into a shared library (like `.dll` for Windows or `.so` for Linux), and ensure that the library is correctly loaded using the `System.loadLibrary()` call.

2.9.3.8 `strictfp`

Ensures that floating-point calculations follow IEEE 754 standards.

Program

```
public strictfp class StrictfpExample {
  void main(String[] args) {
    double num1 = 10e+10;
    double num2 = 6e+08;
    double result = num1 / num2;
    System.out.println("Strictfp Result: " + result); // Ensures IEEE 754
floating-point calculation standards
  }
}
```

Output

```
Strictfp Result: 166.66666666666666
```

In this `StrictfpExample` program, we declare the class using the `strictfp` keyword, which ensures that all floating-point arithmetic performed within the class strictly adheres to the IEEE 754 floating-point standard. This is particularly useful for maintaining consistency in floating-point calculations across different platforms, ensuring that the results will always be the same regardless of the hardware or environment. Inside the `main` method, we initialize two double-precision floating-point variables, `num1` and `num2`, with the values `10e+10` and `6e+08` respectively, which represent scientific notation for large numbers. We then divide `num1` by `num2` and store the result in the variable `result`. Finally, the program outputs the result of this division operation to the console. The use of `strictfp` guarantees that the floating-point calculations are performed consistently, following IEEE 754 standards for precision and rounding.

2.10 JAVA ENUMS

Enums in Java are a special type of class that represents a group of constants (unchangeable variables). They are used to define a collection of named values that can be treated as constants. Enums are commonly used when you have a fixed set of related constants, such as days of the week, months of the year, directions, etc.

2.10.1 Benefits of Using Enums

- **Type Safety**: Enums provide a type-safe way to define and use constant values, reducing the likelihood of errors compared to using int or string constants.
- **Readability**: Enums improve code readability by providing meaningful names for sets of values.
- **Built-in Methods**: Enums come with built-in methods such as values(), ordinal(), and valueOf(String name), which are useful for various operations.
- **Behavior Encapsulation**: Enums can have methods and fields, allowing you to encapsulate related behavior directly within the enum.

2.10.2 Limitations of Enums

- **Limited Extensibility**: Enums cannot be extended (inherited) because they implicitly extend java.lang.Enum.
- **Memory Overhead**: Each enum value is an instance of the enum class, which can have some memory overhead compared to using simple constants.

2.10.3 Defining an Enum

An enum is defined using the enum keyword.
Eg.

```
enum ComputerCourse {
  JAVA("Java Programming", "Beginner to Advanced"),
  PYTHON("Python Programming", "Beginner to Advanced"),
  WEB_DEVELOPMENT("Web Development", "HTML, CSS, JavaScript"),
  DATA_STRUCTURES("Data Structures", "In-depth Data Structures");
  private final String courseName;
```

```
  private final String description;
  ComputerCourse(String courseName, String description) {
    this.courseName = courseName;
    this.description = description;
  }
  public String getCourseName() {
    return courseName;
  }
  public String getDescription() {
    return description;
  }
}
```

Program

```
public class ComputerCourseExample {
  void main(String[] args) {
    // Print all courses
    for (ComputerCourse course : ComputerCourse.values()) {
      System.out.println(course.getCourseName() + ": " + course.
      getDescription());
    }
    // Select a specific course
    ComputerCourse selectedCourse = ComputerCourse.JAVA;
    System.out.println("\nSelected Course:");
    System.out.println("Course Name: " + selectedCourse.getCourseName());
    System.out.println("Description: " + selectedCourse.getDescription());
  }
}
```

Complete program

```
enum ComputerCourse {
  JAVA("Java Programming", "Beginner to Advanced"),
  PYTHON("Python Programming", "Beginner to Advanced"),
  WEB_DEVELOPMENT("Web Development", "HTML, CSS, JavaScript"),
  DATA_STRUCTURES("Data Structures", "In-depth Data Structures");
  private final String courseName;
  private final String description;
  ComputerCourse(String courseName, String description) {
    this.courseName = courseName;
    this.description = description;
  }
  public String getCourseName() {
    return courseName;
  }
  public String getDescription() {
    return description;
  }
}
public class ComputerCourseExample {
public ComputerCourseExample(){}
  void main(String[] args) {
    // Print all courses
    for (ComputerCourse course : ComputerCourse.values()) {
```

```
      System.out.println(course.getCourseName() + ": " + course.
      getDescription());
    }
    // Select a specific course
    ComputerCourse selectedCourse = ComputerCourse.JAVA;
    System.out.println("\nSelected Course:");
    System.out.println("Course Name: " + selectedCourse.getCourseName());
    System.out.println("Description: " + selectedCourse.getDescription());
  }
}
```

Output:

```
Java Programming: Beginner to Advanced
Python Programming: Beginner to Advanced
Web Development: HTML, CSS, JavaScript
Data Structures: In-depth Data Structures
Selected Course:
Course Name: Java Programming
Description: Beginner to Advanced
```

In this program, we define an enumeration called `ComputerCourse`, which encapsulates different computer courses and their corresponding descriptions. Each enum constant, such as `JAVA`, `PYTHON`, `WEB_DEVELOPMENT`, and `DATA_STRUCTURES`, is initialized with a course name and a description through a constructor. The private fields `courseName` and `description` store these values. To provide access to these properties, two public methods, `getCourseName` and `getDescription`, are implemented. The `ComputerCourseExample` class contains the `main` method, where we utilize the `values()` method of the enum to retrieve all defined courses. A for-each loop iterates over the enum constants, printing the name and description of each course to the console. Additionally, we selects the `JAVA` course explicitly, showcasing how to access individual enum instances and their properties. By doing so, it highlights the versatility of enums in Java, allowing for a structured approach to managing related data with built-in methods for easy retrieval and display.

2.11 MEDICAL APPLICATIONS

2.11.1 Case Study 1

Glucose detection involves measuring the concentration of glucose in the blood, which is crucial for diagnosing and managing conditions like diabetes. The parameters considered for glucose detection typically include the following:

- Measurement Units: Glucose levels are commonly measured in milligrams per deciliter (mg/dL) or millimoles per liter (mmol/L), with the former being more prevalent in the United States. The choice of units affects the interpretation of glucose levels.
- Normal Range: The normal range of blood glucose varies depending on factors such as fasting status (before meals or after fasting overnight) and the time since the last meal. For non-diabetic individuals, normal fasting blood sugar levels are generally between 70 and 99 mg/dL (3.9 to 5.5 mmol/L).
- Hypoglycemia Threshold: Hypoglycemia occurs when blood glucose levels fall below normal levels, typically below 70 mg/dL (3.9 mmol/L). Symptoms of hypoglycemia can range from mild shakiness and sweating to severe confusion and loss of consciousness.
- Hyperglycemia Threshold: Hyperglycemia refers to high blood glucose levels, usually above 180 mg/dL (10 mmol/L) in non-pregnant adults. Prolonged or frequent hyperglycemia can lead to complications such as diabetic ketoacidosis (DKA) in individuals with diabetes.

- Diagnosis and Monitoring: Glucose detection is essential for diagnosing diabetes mellitus, a chronic condition characterized by persistent elevated blood sugar levels. Monitoring glucose levels helps individuals with diabetes manage their condition through medication, diet, and lifestyle adjustments.

```
import java.util.Scanner;
public class GlucoseDetection {
  void main(String[] args) {
    Scanner scanner = new Scanner(System.in);
System.out.print("Enter the blood glucose level (mg/dL): ");
    int glucoseLevel = scanner.nextInt();
    // Check glucose level
    if (glucoseLevel< 70) {
System.out.println("Hypoglycemia detected!");
    } else if (glucoseLevel> 180) {
System.out.println("Hyperglycemia detected!");
    } else {
System.out.println("Normal glucose level.");
    }
  }
}
```

The Java program `GlucoseDetection` is designed to assess and classify blood glucose levels based on user input. Utilizing the `Scanner` class for input handling, the program prompts users to enter their blood glucose level in milligrams per deciliter (mg/dL). Upon receiving this input, the program evaluates the integer value against predefined thresholds to determine the user's health condition. The conditional checks in the program are straightforward: if the glucose level is below 70 mg/dL, it identifies hypoglycemia, a condition indicating low blood sugar. Conversely, if the glucose level exceeds 180 mg/dL, the program identifies hyperglycemia, which signifies high blood sugar. For values between 70 and 180 mg/dL, the program prints a message indicating a normal glucose level.

2.11.2 Case Study 2

Obesity detection typically involves assessing the Body Mass Index (BMI), a widely used indicator of body fatness and health risk associated with weight. The parameters considered for obesity detection are:

- Weight: The weight of an individual is measured in kilograms (kg). It serves as a primary input for calculating BMI, where higher weights contribute to a higher BMI.
- Height: Height is measured in centimeters (cm) and is used alongside weight to calculate BMI. Taller individuals tend to have higher BMIs for the same weight compared to shorter individuals.
- Body Mass Index (BMI): BMI is calculated using the formula:

$$BMI = \frac{weight\ (kg)}{(height\ (m) * height\ (m))}$$

- The calculation shifts the weight by 6 bits (equivalent to multiplying by 64) for precision before dividing by the square of the height in meters. A BMI greater than 30 indicates obesity.
- Obesity Threshold: A BMI of 30 or higher is generally recognized as indicative of obesity. Obesity increases the risk of various health problems, including cardiovascular diseases, diabetes, and certain cancers.
- Health Risks: Beyond BMI, other factors such as waist circumference, body fat distribution, and overall health conditions are also considered in clinical settings to assess obesity-related health risks comprehensively.

The program exemplifies a basic obesity detection system using BMI calculation based on user-provided weight and height inputs.

```
import java.util.Scanner;
public class ObesityDetection {
  void main(String[] args) {
    Scanner scanner = new Scanner(System.in);
System.out.print("Enter your weight (kg): ");
    int weight = scanner.nextInt();
System.out.print("Enter your height (cm): ");
    int height = scanner.nextInt();
    int bmi = (weight << 6) / (height * height);
    if (bmi> 30) {
System.out.println("Obesity detected!");
    } else {
System.out.println("No obesity detected.");
    }
  }
}
```

The Java program `ObesityDetection` is designed to assess obesity by calculating the Body Mass Index (BMI) based on user-inputted weight and height. Initially, the program utilizes a `Scanner` object to capture the user's weight in kilograms and height in centimeters. These values are then used to compute the BMI using the formula `(weight << 6) / (height * height)`, where `weight << 6` shifts the weight value left by 6 bits, effectively multiplying it by 64. This method leverages bit manipulation for efficient calculation. The calculated BMI is then evaluated through a conditional statement: if the BMI exceeds 30, the program outputs "Obesity detected!" indicating a high BMI associated with obesity. Otherwise, it prints "No obesity detected.", suggesting a BMI within a normal or underweight range.

3 Control Statements

3.1 INTRODUCTION

Decision-making statements and loop control statements are essential constructs in Java programming for controlling the flow of execution and iterating over code blocks.

3.1.1 Decision Making

Decision making in Java involves evaluating conditions and executing different code blocks based on the result of these evaluations. It allows the program to make choices and follow different paths of execution depending on various conditions at runtime. There are four main types:

- if statement: It executes a block of code if a specified condition is true. If the condition evaluates to false, the code block is skipped.
- if-else statement: This statement extends the if statement by providing an alternative block of code to execute if the condition is false.
- else if ladder statement: It is used when there are multiple conditions to be checked sequentially. Each condition is evaluated one by one, and the corresponding block of code is executed if the condition is true. If none of the conditions are true, a default block of code can be executed.
- switch statement: It allows the program to evaluate the value of a variable and execute different blocks of code based on different possible values of the variable.

Decision-making constructs in Java, such as if, else if, else, switch, and ternary operators, allow programs to execute specific blocks of code based on certain conditions. This capability is essential for creating dynamic and responsive applications that can adapt to varying inputs and states. Decision-making enables complex logic, error handling, and control over program flow, making it possible to implement features like user authentication, data validation, and game mechanics.

Advantages

- Flexibility: Allows the program to perform different actions based on different conditions.
- Control: Provides precise control over the flow of execution.
- Complexity Handling: Enables the implementation of complex logic and decision trees.
- Code Readability: Enhances code readability by clearly delineating different logical paths.
- Error Handling: Facilitates robust error checking and handling.

DOI: 10.1201/9781003544319-3

Limitations

- Complexity: Excessive use can lead to complex and hard-to-read code, often referred to as "spaghetti code."
- Performance: Nested decision structures can affect performance, especially if the conditions are computationally expensive.
- Maintenance: Complex decision-making structures can be difficult to maintain and debug.
- Scalability: Large-scale decision logic might require refactoring to more scalable solutions like state machines or strategy patterns.

3.1.2 Loops

Loops in Java are used to execute a block of code repeatedly as long as a specified condition is met. They are essential for tasks that require iteration, such as processing elements of an array or performing repeated calculations. There are three types of loops:

- for loop: It is an entry-controlled loop that repeats a block of code a specified number of times. It consists of initialization, condition, and increment/decrement expressions.
- while loop: It is also an entry-controlled loop that repeats a block of code as long as a specified condition is true. It checks the condition before each iteration.
- do-while loop: This loop is an exit-controlled loop that repeats a block of code at least once and then continues to repeat it as long as a specified condition is true. It checks the condition after each iteration.

Loops in Java, such as for, while, and do-while, allow code to be executed repeatedly based on a condition. This is essential for tasks that require repetition, such as iterating over data structures (arrays, lists), processing user inputs, or performing repetitive calculations. Loops reduce code duplication and make it possible to handle large datasets efficiently.

Advantages

- Efficiency: Enables the execution of repetitive tasks without duplicating code.
- Automation: Facilitates the automation of tasks that need to be repeated multiple times.
- Code Reduction: Significantly reduces the amount of code by handling repetitive operations through iteration.
- Flexibility: Provides mechanisms to iterate through collections, arrays, and ranges with ease.
- Dynamic Control: Allows dynamic adjustment of the number of iterations based on runtime conditions.

Limitations

- Infinite Loops: Poorly constructed loops can result in infinite loops, causing the program to hang.
- Complexity: Nested loops can lead to complex code that's difficult to read and maintain.
- Performance: Improper use of loops, especially nested loops, can lead to performance bottlenecks.
- Debugging: Errors within loops can be hard to debug, particularly if the loop conditions or iterations are complex.
- Memory Consumption: Excessive iterations may lead to high memory consumption and potential memory leaks if resources are not properly managed.

These statements are fundamental for implementing conditional logic and repetitive tasks in Java programs, enabling developers to create more dynamic and flexible applications.

3.2 CONDITIONAL STATEMENTS

Conditional statements in Java facilitate decision-making based on specific conditions. When a condition evaluates to true, a designated block of code is executed.

3.2.1 If Statement

The if statement is the cornerstone of conditional logic in Java and provides a powerful mechanism for controlling program flow based on dynamic conditions. This fundamental conditional statement in Java determines whether a specific block of code will be executed based on a condition. If the condition evaluates to true, the associated block of statements is executed; otherwise, it is skipped.

Syntax

```
if (condition) {
  // Code to execute if condition is true
}
Example:
int x = 10;
if (x > 5) {
System.out.println("x is greater than 5");
}
```

The above program demonstrates the usage of the `if` statement in Java for making decisions based on a specific condition. Within the `main` method, an integer variable `x` is initialized with the value 10. The `if` statement checks whether the value of `x` is greater than 5. If this condition evaluates to true, meaning `x` is indeed greater than 5, the statement within the block of the `if` statement is executed. In this case, the program prints the message "x is greater than 5" to the console. If the condition evaluates to false, indicating that `x` is not greater than 5, the statement within the block is skipped, and no output is produced. Thus, the `if` statement allows for conditional execution of code based on the outcome of a specified condition, providing flexibility and control over program behavior.

3.2.2 Nested If Statement

An `if` statement is nested within another. When the outer `if` condition evaluates to true, indicating its fulfillment, the program proceeds to evaluate the inner `if` condition. Subsequently, if the inner condition also evaluates to true, signifying that it meets the specified criteria, the corresponding block of code enclosed within the inner `if` statement is executed. This hierarchical arrangement of conditional statements allows for the sequential evaluation of multiple conditions and the execution of associated code blocks based on their outcomes.

Syntax

```
if (condition1) {
  // Code to execute if condition1 is true
  if (condition2) {
    // Code to execute if condition1 and condition2 are true
  }
}
```

Program

```
public class NestedIfExample {
  void main(String[] args) {
    int x = 10;
    int y = 20;
    if (x > 5) { // Outer if statement
      System.out.println("x is greater than 5");
      if (y > 15) { // Nested if statement
        System.out.println("y is greater than 15");
      } else {
        System.out.println("y is 15 or less");
      }
    }
  }
}
Output:
x is greater than 5
y is greater than 15
```

In this program, we define a ` NestedIfExample ` class with a `main` method that initializes two integer variables, `x` and `y`, with values 10 and 20, respectively. An outer `if` statement checks whether `x` is greater than 5; if true, it prints a message indicating that `x` is greater than 5. Within this outer block, a nested `if` statement evaluates whether `y` is greater than 15, printing a corresponding message based on the result. If `y` is not greater than 15, it prints that `y` is 15 or less.

3.2.3 If-Else Statement

If the condition holds, the code enclosed within the `if` statement will be executed; otherwise, the code within the `else` block will be executed.

Syntax

```
if (condition) {
  // Code to execute if condition is true
} else {
  // Code to execute if condition is false
}
```

Program

```
public class IfElseExample {
  void main(String[] args) {
    int n = 100; // Initialize variable
    if (n > 100) {
      System.out.println("Value is greater than 100");
    } else {
      System.out.println("Value is less than 100");
    }
  }
}
Output:
Value is less than 100
```

The program is written in Java and defines a class named " IfElseExample ". Within this class, there is a main method, which serves as the entry point of the program. Inside the main method, an integer variable "n" is declared and initialized with the value 100. Then, there's an `if` statement that checks if the value of "n" is greater than 100. If this condition is true, it prints the message "Value is greater than 100" to the console. Otherwise, if the condition is false, it prints the message "Value is less than 100" to the console.

3.2.4 Else If Ladder

The else if ladder in Java is a decision-making construct that allows for multiple conditions to be evaluated in sequence. It is useful when there are several potential paths of execution, each dependent on a different condition. The else if ladder starts with an if statement that evaluates the first condition; if it is true, the corresponding block of code is executed, and the ladder terminates. If the condition is false, control moves to the next else-if statement, where another condition is evaluated. This process continues until a true condition is found or until an optional else statement is encountered, which executes if none of the previous conditions are true. The else if ladder enhances code readability and maintainability by clearly outlining multiple conditional paths, making it easier to understand the flow of logic. It is particularly beneficial in scenarios requiring complex decision-making with several possible outcomes.

Syntax

```
if (condition1) {
  // Code to execute if condition1 is true
} else if (condition2) {
  // Code to execute if condition2 is true
} else if (condition3) {
  // Code to execute if condition3 is true
} else {
  // Code to execute if none of the above conditions are true
}
```

The above code snippet illustrates the syntax of a conditional statement structure. It begins with an `if` statement followed by optional `else if` statements, and concludes with an optional `else` statement. The `if` statement checks `condition1`. If `condition1` evaluates to `true`, the corresponding block of statements is executed. If `condition_1` is not met, the program moves to the next `else if` statement, which checks `condition2`. If `condition2` evaluates to `true`, the corresponding block of statements is executed. This sequence continues for each subsequent `else if` statement, checking conditions until a condition evaluates to `true`. If none of the conditions in the `if` or `else if` statements are met, the block of statements within the `else` clause is executed. Each block of statements represents the code that executes if the corresponding condition is true. This structure allows for the execution of different blocks of code based on the evaluation of multiple conditions. This structure allows for branching execution based on the outcomes of different conditions, providing flexibility in programming logic.

Program

```
import java.util.Scanner;
public class GradeMarks {
  void main(String[] args) {
    Scanner scanner = new Scanner(System.in);
```

```
    System.out.print("Enter the student's marks: ");
    int marks = scanner.nextInt();
    char grade;
    if (marks >= 90) {
      grade = 'A';
    } else if (marks >= 80&&marks <90) {
      grade = 'B';
    } else if (marks >= 70&&marks <80) {
      grade = 'C';
    } else if (marks >= 60&&marks <70) {
      grade = 'D';
    } else if (marks >= 50&&marks <60) {
      grade = 'E';
    } else {
      grade = 'F';
    }
    System.out.println("Grade =  " + grade);
    scanner.close();
  }
}
```

Output:

```
Enter the student's marks: 95
Grade = A
```

In this program, we define a `GradeMarks` class with a `main` method that prompts the user to enter a student's marks using a `Scanner` for input. Based on the marks entered, the program uses a series of conditional statements to determine the corresponding grade, assigning it to the `grade` variable: 'A' for 90 and above, 'B' for 80 to 89, 'C' for 70 to 79, 'D' for 60 to 69, 'E' for 50 to 59, and 'F' for any marks below 50. Finally, the program prints the determined grade to the console and closes the scanner to prevent resource leaks.

3.2.5 Switch Case

When confronted with various choices, Java offers the switch statement as a means of executing specific branches of code determined by the value of an expression. The switch construct operates effectively with primitive data types such as byte, short, char, and int. Additionally, it accommodates enumerated types, instances of the String class, and Wrapper classes. By assessing the expression, the switch statement directs program flow to the appropriate code block, thus facilitating decision-making processes within the program's logic.

Syntax

```
switch (expression) {
  case value1:
    // Code to execute if expression equals value1
    break;
  case value2:
    // Code to execute if expression equals value2
    break;
  // More cases...
  default:
    // Code to execute if expression does not match any case
}
```

Program

Switch Case without break statement:

```
public class test {
  void main(String[] args) {
    int n = 200; // Initialize variable
    switch (n) {
      case 100:
        System.out.println("Value of Case 1 is 100");
        // No break statement here
      case 200:
        System.out.println("Value of Case 2 is 200");
        // No break statement here
      default:
        System.out.println("Value of default is 200");
    }
  }
}
Output:
Value of Case 2 is 200
Value of default is 200
```

The above Java program defines a class named "test" with a main method serving as its entry point. Inside the main method, an integer variable "n" is declared and initialized with a value of 200. In the switch statement, there are three cases: case 100, case 200, and a default case. However, there is no `break` statement after each case block, which leads to a fall-through behavior. This means that when the value of "n" matches case 200, it will execute the code block for case 200 as well as the subsequent code blocks for the default case. As a result, when "n" is 200, the program will print the messages associated with case 200 ("Value of Case 2 is 200") and the default case ("Value of default is 200").

Program

Switch Case with break statement

```
public class test {
  void main(String[] args) {
    int n = 200; // Initialize variable
    switch (n) {
      case 100:
        System.out.println("Value of Case 1 is 100");
        break; // Prevent fall-through
      case 200:
        System.out.println("Value of Case 2 is 200");
        break; // Prevent fall-through
      default:
        System.out.println("Value of default is 200");
        break; // Prevent fall-through
    }
  }
}
Output:
Value of Case 2 is 200
```

The above Java program defines a class named "test" with a main method serving as its entry point. Inside the main method, an integer variable "n" is declared and initialized with a value of 200. In the switch statement, there are three cases: case 100, case 200, and a default case. Each case block contains a set of statements to execute when the value of "n" matches the corresponding case. Additionally, each case block is terminated by a `break` statement, ensuring that once a matching case is found and executed, the switch statement exits, preventing fall-through behavior. When the program runs, since the value of "n" is 200, the switch statement matches the case 200 and executes the code block associated with it. Consequently, the program prints the message "Value of Case 2 is 200" to the console.

3.3 LOOPS

A loop is a fundamental programming construct consisting of a series of statements that iteratively execute either for a predetermined number of repetitions or until certain conditions are satisfied. Loops provide a mechanism to automate repetitive tasks and streamline code execution. Depending on the specific loop construct used in a programming language, such as `for`, `while`, or `do-while`, the loop will continue executing until a specified condition becomes false or until a certain number of iterations have been completed. This iterative process allows programmers to efficiently handle tasks that involve repeated operations, enhancing code efficiency and readability.

The Need for Looping in Programming

Looping is a fundamental concept in programming that allows a set of instructions to be executed repeatedly based on a condition. It is essential for various reasons:

- Repetitive Tasks: Many programming tasks involve repetitive actions. Loops allow you to automate these tasks without writing redundant code.
- Efficiency: Looping enables you to perform tasks more efficiently by reducing code duplication.
- Dynamic Data Handling: When working with data structures like arrays or lists, loops allow you to process each element dynamically.
- Automation: Loops are essential for automating tasks that need to be performed multiple times, such as processing user inputs, generating reports, or handling file operations.

Benefits of Looping

- Code Reusability and Reduction: Loops allow you to write a block of code once and reuse it multiple times, reducing the amount of code you need to write and maintain.
- Simplifies Complex Tasks: Complex repetitive tasks can be simplified using loops, making the code more readable and easier to understand.
- Flexibility: Loops can handle varying numbers of iterations, making them flexible for different tasks such as iterating over data structures of unknown length.
- Automation: Loops enable the automation of repetitive tasks, which is crucial for tasks such as data processing, simulations, and batch processing.
- Dynamic and Real-time Processing: Loops allow programs to react to real-time data changes and process data dynamically as it becomes available.

Limitations of Looping

- Infinite Loops: If the loop's termination condition is not correctly defined, it can lead to infinite loops, causing the program to hang or crash.

- Performance Overhead: Loops, especially nested loops, can lead to performance overhead if not optimized properly. They can consume significant processing time and resources.
- Complexity: Overuse of loops or poorly designed loops can make the code complex and difficult to understand or maintain.
- Memory Consumption: Loops that create new objects or hold large data structures in memory can lead to increased memory consumption and potential memory leaks.
- Logical Errors: Incorrect loop conditions or improper use of loop control statements (like `break` and `continue`) can introduce logical errors that are hard to debug.

3.3.1 Examples of Looping in Java

1. For Loop

```
for (int i = 0; i < 10; i++) {
  System.out.println("Iteration: " + i);
}
This `for` loop will print "Iteration: 0" to "Iteration: 9".
```

2. While Loop

```
int i = 0;
while (i < 10) {
  System.out.println("Iteration: " + i);
  i++;
}
This `while` loop achieves the same result as the `for` loop above.
```

3. Do-While Loop

```
int i = 0;
do {
  System.out.println("Iteration: " + i);
  i++;
} while (i < 10);
This `do-while` loop ensures that the code block is executed at least once
before the condition is tested.
```

3.3.2 For Loop

The for loop is one of the most commonly used control flow statements in Java, allowing code to be executed repeatedly based on a condition. It is particularly useful when you know in advance how many times you want to execute a statement or a block of statements.

Syntax

```
for (initialization; condition; update) {
  // code to be executed
}
```

- **Initialization**: This part is executed once at the beginning of the loop. It is typically used to initialize a loop control variable.

- **Condition**: This part is evaluated before each iteration. If it evaluates to true, the loop's body is executed. If it evaluates to false, the loop terminates.
- **Update**: This part is executed after each iteration of the loop's body. It is generally used to update the loop control variable.

Program: for loop

```
public class test {
  void main(String[] args) {
    // For loop to iterate from 1 to 10
    for (int x = 1; x <= 10; x++) {
      System.out.println(x); // Print current value of x
    }
  }
}
```

Output:

```
1
2
3
4
5
6
7
8
9
10
```

The above Java program defines a class named "test" with a main method serving as its entry point. Inside the main method, a traditional for loop is used to iterate over a range of integer values from 1 to 10. The loop begins with the initialization of an integer variable "x" with a value of 1. It then executes the loop body, which prints the current value of "x" to the console using the `System.out.println()` method. After each iteration, the loop updates the value of "x" by incrementing it by 1. This process continues until the condition `x <= 10` is no longer satisfied, at which point the loop terminates. Consequently, when the program runs, it sequentially prints the numbers 1 through 10 to the console, each on its own line.

3.3.2.1 For-Each Loop

The Java for-each loop, also known as the enhanced for loop, is a convenient construct used to iterate over elements in an array or a collection type. It simplifies the process of traversing through the elements of these data structures by acting as an iterator. When using a for-each loop, you do not need to explicitly provide an increment or decrement statement. Instead, the loop automatically traverses through each element of the array or collection, returning them one by one for processing within the loop body. This streamlined syntax reduces the likelihood of errors and enhances code readability, making it easier for developers to work with arrays and collections in Java programs.

Syntax

```
for (dataType element : collectionOrArray) {
  // Code to execute for each element
}
```

The Java for-each loop, also known as the enhanced for loop, provides a concise and intuitive way to iterate over elements within an array or a collection. Its syntax consists of the keyword `for`, followed by parentheses containing the declaration of the loop variable, which represents each element in the array or collection, preceded by its data type, and then the array or collection itself. Within the loop body, encapsulated by curly braces, developers can define the actions to be performed on each element during iteration. Notably, unlike traditional for loops, there is no need to explicitly specify incrementation or decrementation of an index variable. Instead, the for-each loop handles iteration automatically, sequentially accessing each element until the end of the array or collection is reached. This streamlined syntax not only reduces the likelihood of errors but also enhances code readability, making it particularly useful when iterating through arrays or collections in Java programs.

Program: for-each loop

```
public class test {
  void main(String[] args) {
    int[] a = {1, 2, 3, 4, 5, 6, 7, 8, 9}; // Array of integers
    // For-each loop to iterate over the array
    for (int x : a) {
      System.out.println(x); // Print each value of x
    }
  }
}
```

Output:

```
1
2
3
4
5
6
7
8
9
```

The above Java program defines a class named "test" with a main method serving as its entry point. Inside the main method, an integer array "a" is declared and initialized with values 1 through 9. We utilized a for-each loop to iterate over each element in the array "a". During each iteration, the value of the current element is assigned to the loop variable "x". Within the loop body, we prints the value of "x" to the console using the `System.out.println()` method. Consequently, when the program runs, it iterates through the elements of the array "a" and prints each element's value to the console, producing the output of numbers 1 through 9 in consecutive lines.

3.3.2.2 When to Use

- Use a **for loop** when you:
  - Need precise control over the iteration process.
  - Need to manipulate the loop counter or iterate in a custom manner.
  - Require the index of each element.
- Use an **enhanced for loop** when you:
  - Need to iterate over all elements in a collection or array without modifying the structure.
  - Prefer cleaner and more readable code for simple iterations.
  - Don't need the index of elements during iteration.

3.3.2.3 Labeled For Loop in Java

The labeled `for` loop in Java is a construct that allows you to provide a label (an identifier followed by a colon) to a loop statement, enabling you to break or continue the execution of an outer loop from within an inner loop. This is particularly useful in situations where you have nested loops and need to control the flow of execution at an outer level rather than at the inner-most loop level.

Syntax

```
labelName:
for (initialization; condition; update) {
  // Loop body
}
```

In Java, a labeled `for` loop is a construct that enables developers to provide a unique label followed by a colon (`:`) to a standard `for` loop. This labeling allows for precise control over loop termination and continuation, particularly in scenarios involving nested loops. The syntax begins with the label name followed by a colon, followed by the traditional `for` loop structure enclosed within curly braces. Within the loop, initialization, condition, and increment/decrement statements dictate the loop's behavior. The labeled `for` loop is especially useful when developers need to break or continue the outer loop from within the inner loop, a task not achievable with regular loops. By utilizing labels, developers can specify the exact loop they wish to manipulate, enhancing code clarity and maintainability. This construct offers greater flexibility in managing complex control flow situations, making it an essential tool in Java programming, particularly in scenarios where nested loops are prevalent.

By labeling the outer loop, you can specify the target loop for `break` and `continue` statements, ensuring that the desired loop is affected.
For example:

```
public class LabeledForExample {
  void main(String[] args) {
    outerLoop: // Label for the outer loop
    for (int i = 1; i <= 3; i++) {
      for (int j = 1; j <= 3; j++) {
        if (i * j > 4) {
          System.out.println("Breaking out of outer loop");
          break outerLoop; // Exits the outer loop
        }
        System.out.println("i = " + i + ", j = " + j);
      }
    }
  }
}
```

Output:

```
i = 1, j = 1
i = 1, j = 2
i = 1, j = 3
i = 2, j = 1
i = 2, j = 2
Breaking out of outer loop
```

In this program, we define a ` LabeledForExample ` class with a `main` method that demonstrates the use of labeled loops in Java. The outer loop is labeled `outerLoop` and iterates three times with the variable `i`, while the inner loop iterates three times with the variable `j`. Inside the inner loop, a conditional statement checks if the product of `i` and `j` exceeds 4. If this condition is met, it prints a message indicating that it is breaking out of the outer loop and uses the `break outerLoop` statement to exit both loops immediately. If the condition is not met, it prints the current values of `i` and `j`.

Program: labeled for loop

```
public class InnerLabelLoopExample {
  void main(String[] args) {
    // Outer loop with label "lab1"
    lab1: for (int x = 1; x <= 5; x++) {

        // inner loop with label "lab2"
        lab2:for (int y = 1; y <= 4; y++) {
          if (x == 4 && y == 2) {
            System.out.println("Breaking out of inner loop");
            break lab2; // Breaks out of the outer loop
          }
          System.out.println("x = " + x + ", y = " + y);
        }
    }
  }
}
```

```
Output:
x = 1, y = 1
x = 1, y = 2
x = 1, y = 3
x = 1, y = 4
x = 2, y = 1
x = 2, y = 2
x = 2, y = 3
x = 2, y = 4
x = 3, y = 1
x = 3, y = 2
x = 3, y = 3
x = 3, y = 4
x = 4, y = 1
Breaking out of inner loop
x = 5, y = 1
x = 5, y = 2
x = 5, y = 3
x = 5, y = 4
```

In this program, we define the `InnerLabelLoopExample` class, which contains a `main` method demonstrating the use of labeled inner and outer loops. The outer loop, labeled `lab1`, iterates with the variable `x` from 1 to 5, while the inner loop, labeled `lab2`, iterates with the variable `y` from 1 to 4. Inside the inner loop, a conditional statement checks if `x` is 4 and `y` is 2. If this condition is met, it prints a message indicating that it is breaking out of the inner loop and executes `break lab2`, which exits only the inner loop. If the condition is not satisfied, the program prints the current values of `x` and `y`.

3.3.2.4 Nested For Loop in Java

Indeed, the Java nested `for` loop construct is exceptionally handy when dealing with situations where one or more `for` loops need to be placed inside each other. The nested structure allows for the execution of the inner loop(s) within the body of the outer loop. Each iteration of the outer loop triggers the complete execution of the inner loop(s), adhering to the condition(s) specified for each loop.

This nested arrangement is particularly useful for scenarios where a task needs to be performed for every combination of elements across multiple ranges or arrays. For instance, if you have a two-dimensional array representing a grid, nested loops can efficiently traverse through each cell of the grid, allowing you to process data or perform actions on each individual element.

The behavior of nested loops ensures that the inner loop(s) execute fully for every iteration of the outer loop, providing a systematic and organized approach to handling complex data structures or tasks. This construct offers flexibility and precision in controlling program flow, making it an indispensable tool in Java programming for tasks that require iteration across multiple dimensions or sets of data.

Program

```
public class test {
  void main(String[] args) {
    // Outer loop for each row
    for (int x = 1; x <= 7; x++) {
      // Inner loop for printing asterisks
      for (int y = 1; y <= x; y++) {
        System.out.print("* "); // Print asterisk followed by a space
      }
      System.out.println(); // Move to the next line after each row
    }
  }
}
Output:
*
* *
* * *
* * * *
* * * * *
* * * * * *
* * * * * * *
```

The above Java program defines a class named "test" with a main method serving as its entry point. Inside the main method, two nested `for` loops are utilized to generate a pattern of asterisks in the shape of a right triangle. The outer loop, controlled by the variable "x", iterates from 1 to 7, indicating the number of rows in the triangle. For each iteration of the outer loop, an inner loop, controlled by the variable "y", iterates from 1 to the current value of "x". This inner loop governs the number of asterisks printed in each row, ensuring that the number of asterisks increases with each subsequent row. Within the inner loop, an asterisk followed by a space is printed using `System.out.print()`, generating the pattern of asterisks for each row. After completing the inner loop for each row, the next line is moved to using `System.out.println()`, which causes subsequent rows to be printed on new lines. Consequently, when the program runs, a right triangle pattern of asterisks is generated, with each row containing an increasing number of asterisks, ranging from 1 to 7, forming the shape of a right triangle.

3.3.2.5 Infinite For Loop in Java

The Java infinite `for` loop serves as a valuable tool in scenarios where there's a requirement to continuously execute a specific block of code without a predetermined exit condition. This construct facilitates tasks such as creating background processes, implementing event listeners, or running server-side programs that need to remain active indefinitely.
The syntax of an infinite `for` loop is straightforward:

```
for (;;) {
  // Loop body
}
```

This loop lacks a condition in its parentheses, meaning it will continue iterating endlessly until it's explicitly interrupted by a `break` statement or by terminating the program's execution. Without a defined exit condition, the loop will execute its body repetitively, effectively creating an infinite loop.

While the infinite `for` loop is powerful, it should be used judiciously, with care taken to ensure that there's a way to terminate it when necessary. If not managed properly, an infinite loop can lead to resource exhaustion, system instability, or program crashes. Therefore, it's essential to implement appropriate mechanisms for breaking out of the loop when required, ensuring the program's reliability and stability.

Program

```
public class Main {
  void main(String[] args) {
    for (;;) {
      System.out.println("infinite");
      // To prevent overwhelming output, you might add a sleep statement
      or break condition in real scenarios
    }
  }
}
```

The above Java program defines a class named "test" with a main method serving as its entry point. Within the main method, an infinite `for` loop is employed, indicated by the absence of any initialization, condition, or iteration expression within the loop's parentheses. This lack of parameters signifies that the loop will execute indefinitely, continuously printing the string "infinite" to the console within its loop body. When the program is executed, the infinite loop begins, and the statement inside the loop body is repeatedly executed without interruption. As a result, the string "infinite" is continuously outputted to the console, reflecting the perpetual execution of the loop. Since there's no defined termination condition, the loop will continue to run indefinitely until the program is manually terminated or interrupted externally.

3.3.3 The While Loop

The while loop in Java serves as an entry-controlled loop, meaning it evaluates the test expression or condition before executing the loop body. The syntax of a while loop is straightforward: it begins with the keyword `while`, followed by the test expression enclosed within parentheses, and the loop body enclosed within curly braces. The loop body may consist of a single statement, multiple statements enclosed within curly braces (a compound statement), or it may be empty.

During each iteration of the while loop, the test expression is evaluated. If the expression evaluates to true, indicating that the condition is still satisfied, the loop body is executed. Subsequently, the loop variable, if present, must be initialized before the loop begins, and it should be updated within the loop body to ensure proper control flow.

The loop continues to execute as long as the test expression remains true. Once the test expression evaluates to false, signifying that the condition is no longer met, program control passes to the line immediately following the end of the loop body.

This control flow characteristic of the while loop makes it ideal for situations where the number of iterations is not known beforehand and depends on some condition being satisfied. By properly initializing, updating, and evaluating loop variables within the loop body, developers can effectively utilize the while loop construct to create flexible and dynamic looping behavior in Java programs.

Syntax

```
while (condition) {
  // Loop body
}
```

In a while loop, the loop body may contain a single, compound or an empty statement. The loop repeats while the test expression or condition evaluates to true. When the expression becomes false, the program control passes to the line just after the end of the loop body code. In a while loop, a loop variable must be initialized before the loop begins. And the loop variable should be updated inside the while loop's body.

Program

```
public class Main {
  void main(String[] args) {
    long i, fact = 1; // Variables for factorial calculation
    long n = 5; // Number to calculate factorial of
    // Loop to calculate factorial
    while (n != 0) {
      fact *= n; // Update factorial
      n--; // Decrement n
    }
    // Output the result
    System.out.println("Factorial of 5 is " + fact);
  }
}
Output:
The factorial of 5 is: 120
```

In this program, we calculate the factorial of the number 5 using a while loop. We initialize the variables `fact` to 1 and `n` to 5, then enter a loop that continues until `n` becomes zero. Inside the loop, we multiply `fact` by `n` to update the factorial value and decrement `n` by 1. Finally, we print the result, which shows that the factorial of 5 is 120.

A while loop also has several variations.

3.3.3.1 Empty While Loop

An empty while loop does not contain any statement in its body. It just contains a null statement, which is denoted by a semicolon after the while statement:

```
public class Main {
  void main(String[] args) {
    long w = 0; // Variable for time delay
    // Time delay loop
    while (w < 10000) {
      w++; // Increment w
      // No operation in loop body (empty loop)
    }
    // Output message indicating completion of delay
    System.out.println("Delay completed.");
  }
}
Output:
Delay completed.
```

The above code is a time delay loop. The time delay loop is useful for pausing the program for some time. It demonstrates the usage of an empty while loop for creating a time delay. In this example, a long integer variable "w" is initialized to 0. The while loop is constructed with a condition that increments "w" by 1 until its value becomes less than 10000. However, the loop body consists only of a null statement, indicated by the semicolon immediately following the while statement. The purpose of this empty while loop is to introduce a time delay in the program execution. By continually incrementing "w" until it reaches the specified value (10000 in this case) without executing any meaningful code within the loop body, the program effectively pauses or delays its execution for a certain period. Time delay loops like this one can be useful in scenarios where you need to introduce a controlled pause in program execution, such as in timing-sensitive applications, simulations, or scenarios requiring synchronization with external events. However, it's important to note that the effectiveness and accuracy of such time delay loops may vary depending on factors such as hardware, system load, and compiler optimizations. Additionally, busy-waiting loops like this can consume CPU resources, so they should be used judiciously and in appropriate contexts.

3.3.3.2 Infinite While Loop

A while loop can be an infinite loop if there are no update statement inside its body.

Program

```
public class InfiniteWhileExample {
  void main(String[] args) {
    int j = 0; // Initialize the variable j
    // Infinite while loop
    while (j <= 10) {
      System.out.println("Square of " + j + " is " + (j * j));
      // Missing increment statement (j++)
    }
    // This statement will never be reached
    j++;
  }
}
```

A class named " InfiniteWhileExample " is defined, with a main method serving as its entry point. Inside the main method, an integer variable "j" is initialized to 0. Subsequently, a while loop is utilized with the condition "j <= 10", indicating that the loop will execute as long as the value of "j" is less than or equal to 10. Within the while loop's body, the square of the current value of "j" is printed to the console using the `System.out.println()` method. However, there's an issue in the loop structure: the loop variable "j" is not being incremented within the loop body. As a result, the loop continues to execute indefinitely with "j" always equal to 0, resulting in an infinite loop. Additionally, there is a statement `j++;` placed outside the while loop. However, this statement will never be reached due to the infinite loop preceding it. Consequently, this statement will have no effect on the program execution.

3.3.4 The Do-While Loop

The do-while loop is an exit-controlled loop. It evaluates the test expression at the bottom of the loop after executing the statements in the loop body.
Note: do-while loop always executes at least once.

In the for and while loops, the condition is evaluated before executing the loop -body. The loop body never executes if the test expression evaluates to false for the first time itself.

Syntax

```
do {
  // Statements to be executed
} while (condition);
```

The braces { } are not necessary when the loop body contains a single statement.

Program

```
public class Test {
  void main(String[] args) {
    char c = 'A'; // Initialize the character variable
    // Do-while loop to print characters from 'A' to 'Z'
    do {
      System.out.print(c + " "); // Print the current character followed
                                    by a space
      c++; // Increment the character
    } while (c <= 'Z'); // Continue loop while c is less than or equal to 'Z'
  }
}
Output:
A B C D E F G H I J K L M N O P Q R S T U V W X Y Z
```

The above Java program defines a class named "test" with a main method serving as its entry point. Inside the main method, a character variable "c" is initialized to the character 'A'. A do-while loop is utilized to print characters from 'A' to 'Z', inclusively. The current value of "c" is printed to the console, followed by a space, using the `System.out.println()` method within the body of the do-while loop. Then, the value of "c" is incremented by one. This process continues as long as the value of "c" is less than or equal to the character 'Z', as specified by the condition "c <= 'Z' " in the do-while loop. Since characters in Java are represented as numeric Unicode values, the loop effectively iterates through the character codes from 'A' to 'Z', incrementing "c" by one in each iteration until it reaches the character 'Z'. Once "c" exceeds 'Z', the loop terminates, and the program execution ends. Therefore, when the program is executed, it prints the uppercase letters of the English alphabet from 'A' to 'Z', each separated by a space, to the console.

3.4 LOOP CONTROL STATEMENTS

Control statements in Java are fundamental constructs that allow programmers to alter the normal sequential flow of execution within a program. Java supports several control statements, two of which are the break statement and the continue statement.

- Break Statement: The break statement is used to prematurely terminate the execution of a loop or switch statement. When encountered within a loop or switch, the break statement causes the program control to exit the loop or switch immediately, transferring execution to the statement that follows the loop or switch block. This allows programmers to effectively control the flow of their program by exiting loops or switch statements based on certain conditions.
- Continue Statement: The continue statement is utilized within loops to skip the remaining code within the loop's body and immediately retest the loop's condition before proceeding to the next iteration. Unlike the break statement, which exits the loop entirely, the continue statement allows the loop to continue iterating but skips the remaining code in the current iteration. This can be useful for skipping certain iterations based on specific conditions without terminating the loop altogether.

Both the break and continue statements provide programmers with powerful tools for controlling the flow of execution within loops and switch statements in Java, allowing for greater flexibility and efficiency in program design and implementation.

3.4.1 Break

In Java, the break statement is used to terminate the execution of a loop or switch statement prematurely. When the break statement is encountered within a loop (such as a for, while, or do-while loop), it causes the loop to exit immediately, and control is transferred to the statement following the loop. Similarly, within a switch statement, the break statement ends the execution of the current case and exits the switch block, preventing the execution from falling through to subsequent cases. The break statement enhances control over the flow of a program, allowing for more precise management of loops and switch cases, thus improving readability and reducing the risk of errors.

Syntax

```
break;
```

Program

```
public class Test {
  void main(String[] args) {
    // For loop to iterate from 1 to 5
    for (int i = 1; i <= 5; i++) {
      if (i == 4) {
        break; // Terminate the loop if i equals 4
      }
      System.out.println(i); // Print the value of i
    }
  }
}
```

Output:

```
1
2
3
```

The above Java program defines a class named "test" with a main method serving as its entry point. Inside the main method, a for loop is utilized to iterate over a range of integer values from 1 to 5. The loop variable "i" is initialized to 1, and the loop continues as long as "i" is less than or equal to 5During each iteration of the for loop, it is checked if the current value of "i" is equal to 4 using an if statement. If the condition is met, a break statement is encountered, causing the loop to terminate prematurely, and control moves to the statement immediately following the loop, skipping any remaining iterations. However, if the condition in the if statement is not satisfied, the code inside the if statement's block is executed, which prints the value of "i" to the console using the `System.out.println()` method, resulting in the values of "i" being printed for each iteration of the loop, except when "i" equals 4. Consequently, when the program is executed, the numbers 1, 2, and 3 are printed to the console, each on its own line, before the loop is terminated prematurely when "i" becomes equal to 4. In the above program, the for loop is used to print the value of "i" in each iteration. The statement,

```
if (i == 4) {
  break; // Terminate the loop if i equals 4
}
```

This means when the value of i is equal to 4, the loop terminates. Hence we get the output with values less than 5 only.

3.4.1.1 Labeled Break Statement

In Java, a labeled break statement is used to break out of a specific outer loop or block of code, rather than just the innermost loop. This is particularly useful when dealing with nested loops or complex code blocks where you need to exit from multiple levels of loops.

Here's how it works:

- **Label**: You can label a block of code (usually a loop) by placing an identifier followed by a colon before the block.
- **Break Statement**: When you use the break statement with the label, it terminates the execution of the labeled block, not just the innermost loop.

Syntax

```
labelName: // Label for the loop
while (condition) {
  // Code inside the outer loop
  while (condition) {
    // Code inside the inner loop
    // To break out of the outer loop from within the inner loop
    break labelName;
  }
}
```

Program: labeled break statement

```
public class Test {
  void main(String[] args) {
    // Label for the outer loop
    first:
    for (int i = 1; i < 5; i++) {
      // Label for the inner loop
      second:
      for (int j = 1; j < 3; j++) {
```

```
        // Print the current values of i and j
        System.out.println("i: " + i + ", j: " + j);
        // Check if i is equal to 2
        if (i == 2) {
          // Break out of the outer loop labeled "first"
          break first;
        }
      }
    }
    // Code here will execute after breaking out of the outer loop
    System.out.println("Exited both loops");
  }
}
```

Output

```
i: 1, j: 1
i: 1, j: 2
i: 2, j: 1
Exited both loops
```

In this program, we define a `Test` class with a `main` method serving as its entry point. Within the main method, we labeled nested for loops. The outer loop, labeled as "first", initializes an integer variable "i" to 1 and continues as long as "i" is less than 5. During each iteration of the outer loop, the inner loop, labeled as "second", initializes an integer variable "j" to 1 and continues as long as "j" is less than 3. Within the inner loop's body, the current values of "i" and "j" are printed to the console using the `System.out.println()` method, displaying each combination of "i" and "j". Additionally, there's an if statement that checks if the value of "i" is equal to 2. If this condition is met, a break statement is encountered with the label "first", causing the outer loop labeled "first" to terminate immediately. However, as soon as the value of "i" becomes equal to 2, the outer loop labeled "first" breaks, causing the program control to exit both loops entirely.

3.4.2 Continue

In Java, the continue statement is used within loops to skip the current iteration and proceed directly to the next iteration of the loop. This is particularly useful when you need to bypass certain parts of the loop's body under specific conditions without exiting the loop entirely.

How it Works:

- When the continue statement is encountered, the remaining statements in the current iteration are ignored, and control is transferred to the next iteration of the loop.
- For "for" loops, the control moves to the update statement (usually the increment or decrement statement).
- For while and do-while loops, the control moves to the loop's condition evaluation.

Syntax

```
continue;
```

Program: Java continue statement

```
public class Main {
  void main(String[] args) {
    // Iterate over a range of integer values from 1 to 5
```

```
        for (int i = 1; i <= 5; i++) {
          // Check if the current value of i is equal to 4
          if (i == 4) {
            // Skip the rest of the loop body for this iteration
            continue;
          }
          // Print the value of i to the console
          System.out.println(i);
        }
    }
}
```

Output:

```
1
2
3
5
```

In this program, we define a ` Main ` class and within this main method, a for loop is employed to iterate over a range of integer values from 1 to 5, inclusive. During each iteration of the loop, it is checked if the current value of the loop variable "i" is equal to 4 using an if statement. If the condition evaluates to true, indicating that "i" is equal to 4, a continue statement is encountered. This statement causes the remaining code within the loop's body for the current iteration to be skipped, and control proceeds directly to the next iteration of the loop. As a result, when the loop variable "i" is equal to 4, the print statement within the loop body is skipped, and execution continues with the next iteration. However, for all other values of "i" (1, 2, 3, and 5), the print statement is executed, printing the value of "i" to the console using the `System.out.println()` method. Consequently, when the program is executed, the numbers 1, 2, 3, and 5 are printed to the console, each on its own line. The number 4 is excluded from the output due to the continue statement, which skips the print statement for that iteration.

In the above program, the for loop prints the value of i in each iteration. The statement,

```
if (i == 4) {
  // Skip the rest of the loop body for this iteration
  continue;
}
```

Here, the continue statement is executed when the value of i becomes 4. It then skips the print statement for those values. Hence, the output skips the values 4.

3.4.2.1 Labeled Continue Statement

A labeled continue statement in Java provides a way to control the flow of nested loops more precisely. It allows you to skip the current iteration of an outer loop from within an inner loop. By using a label with the continue statement, you can specify which loop to continue.

How It Works:

- A label is defined by an identifier followed by a colon (:) before a loop statement.
- Using Labeled continue: When the continue statement is used with a label, it skips the current iteration of the labeled loop, not just the innermost loop.

Syntax

```
continue label;
```

Program: labeled continue statement

```
public class Main {
  void main(String[] args) {
ttt: // Label for the outer loop
    for (int i = 1; i <= 5; i++) {
      for (int j = 1; j <= 5; j++) {
        if (i == 3&& j == 4) {
          // Continue to the next iteration of the outer loop
          continue ttt;
        }
        System.out.println("i = " + i + ", j = " + j);
      }
    }
  }
}
Output:
i = 1, j = 1
i = 1, j = 2
i = 1, j = 3
i = 1, j = 4
i = 1, j = 5
i = 2, j = 1
i = 2, j = 2
i = 2, j = 3
i = 2, j = 4
i = 2, j = 5
i = 3, j = 1
i = 3, j = 2
i = 3, j = 3
i = 4, j = 1
i = 4, j = 2
i = 4, j = 3
i = 4, j = 4
i = 4, j = 5
i = 5, j = 1
i = 5, j = 2
i = 5, j = 3
i = 5, j = 4
i = 5, j = 5
```

In this program, an outer loop labeled "ttt" iterates over the variable `i` from 1 to 5, while an inner loop iterates over the variable `j` from 1 to 5. Within the inner loop, there is a condition that checks if `i` equals 3 and `j` equals 4. If this condition is met, the program encounters a `continue` statement that applies to the outer loop, causing the program to skip the remaining code in the inner loop and jump directly to the next iteration of the outer loop. Consequently, when `i` is 3 and `j` is 4, the print statement is bypassed, and no output is generated for that specific iteration. For all other combinations of `i` and `j`, the program prints the current values of `i` and `j` to the console. As a result, when executed, the program will print the values of `i` and `j` for all pairs except for (3, 4). The number 4 is excluded from the output due to the continue statement, which skips the print statement for that iteration.

In the above example, the labeled continue statement is used to skip the current iteration of the loop labeled as ttt. The statement if (i == 3 || j == 4) continuettt;

Here, the outermost for loop is labeled as ttt,

```
ttt: // Label for the outer loop
    for (int i = 1; i <= 5; i++) {  ...}
```

The iteration of the outer for loop is skipped if the value of i is 3 or the value of j is 4. In the above example, the labeled continue statement is utilized to control the iteration flow within a nested loop structure. The outermost for loop is labeled as "ttt", allowing precise targeting of loop control statements. The iteration of this outer loop is governed by the loop variable "i", which ranges from 1 to 4. Within the nested loop structure, there's an if statement containing a labeled continue statement: `if (i == 3 || j == 4) continue ttt;`. This statement checks two conditions: if the value of "i" is equal to 3 or if the value of "j" is equal to 4. If either condition evaluates to true during an iteration of the nested loop, the labeled continue statement causes the program to skip the remainder of the inner loop's body and immediately proceed to the next iteration of the outer loop labeled as "ttt".Consequently, the labeled continue statement allows the program to selectively bypass certain iterations of the outer loop based on specified conditions. By labeling the outer loop, precise control over the flow of execution within nested loops is achieved, providing flexibility and granularity in loop control mechanisms.

3.5 UNNAMED VARIABLES

In Java 22, the concept of unnamed variables and patterns refers to a feature introduced to enhance the language's flexibility and readability when dealing with variables and patterns that are required syntactically but not necessarily used directly in the code logic. This feature allows developers to use underscore (_) as a placeholder for variables that are needed for syntactic purposes, such as in declarations, pattern matching, or destructuring assignments, but where the actual value is not of interest or is unused in the subsequent code. The introduction of unnamed variables and patterns in Java 22 addresses several key needs in software development, particularly in terms of improving code readability, reducing verbosity, and enhancing maintainability.

Needs for Unnamed Variables in Java 22

- Enhanced Readability: Unnamed variables and patterns allow developers to ignore or discard values that are not needed in certain contexts, such as variable declarations, lambda expressions, or pattern matching. This improves code clarity by eliminating the need to invent or use arbitrary variable names for values that are irrelevant to the current logic.
- Reduced Code: Before Java 22, developers often had to declare variables or patterns with names that were not meaningful or used only to satisfy syntax requirements. Unnamed variables and patterns eliminate this code, making the intent of the code more evident and reducing visual clutter.
- Simplified Pattern Matching: The ability to use unnamed variables in pattern matching allows for more concise and expressive code when handling complex data structures. It enables developers to focus on the relevant parts of the pattern without being distracted by unnecessary variable declarations.
- Improved Maintainability: By reducing the amount of unused or irrelevant variable declarations, unnamed variables and patterns contribute to cleaner codebases that are easier to maintain and modify. This enhancement aligns with modern programming practices that emphasize simplicity and code that is easier to reason about.
- Compatibility with Functional Programming: Functional programming paradigms often involve operations where certain values or results are discarded. Unnamed variables and

patterns support these paradigms by allowing developers to express operations more naturally without unnecessary variable naming overhead.

3.5.1 Using Unnamed Variables in For Loops

Java allows the developers to use an underscore (_) as an unnamed variable within a for loop. This signifies the developers are not interested in the specific value being iterated over, but only in the loop's execution.

Program

```
public class Demo {
  void main(String[] args) {
    int[] numbers = {1, 2, 3, 4, 5};
    int total = 0;
    for (int _ : numbers) {
      total++;
    }
    System.out.println("Total numbers: " + total);
  }
}
Output:
Total numbers: 5
```

This Java program calculates the total number of elements in the `numbers` array and prints the result. It initializes an array `numbers` with integers, iterates through each element using an unnamed variable in the enhanced for-loop, increments a counter `total` for each iteration, and finally prints the total count of numbers in the array.

3.6 MEDICAL APPLICATIONS

3.6.1 Case Study 1

SymptomChecker can quickly identify symptoms that might indicate a more serious condition (e.g., persistent fever or a combination of symptoms), prompting users to seek timely medical help, which is crucial in preventing complications like flu. The SymptomChecker program considers the following parameters for symptom detection:

- **Fever**: Fever is a common symptom indicating various infections or illnesses.
- **Cough**: Cough is another prevalent symptom associated with respiratory tract infections.

The program checks the combination of fever and cough to suggest the possibility of a cold or flu. If only fever or cough is present, it advises consulting a doctor. If no definitive diagnosis is made after up to three rounds of questioning, the program advises that the symptoms might be minor and suggests considering home remedies or consulting a doctor if symptoms persist.

```
import java.util.Scanner;
public class SymptomChecker {
  void main(String[] args) {
  Scanner scanner = new Scanner(System.in);
System.out.println("Do you have a fever (Y/N)?");
  String hasFever = scanner.nextLine();
```

```
System.out.println("Do you have a cough (Y/N)?");
  String hasCough = scanner.nextLine();
boolean diagnosed = false;
  for (int i = 0; i< 3 && !diagnosed; i++) {
    if (hasFever.equalsIgnoreCase("Y") && hasCough.equalsIgnoreCase("Y")) {
        System.out.println("You might have a cold or flu. Please consult a
        doctor.");
            diagnosed = true;
    } else if (hasFever.equalsIgnoreCase("Y")) {
      System.out.println("You might have a fever. Please consult a doctor.");
            diagnosed = true;
    } else if (hasCough.equalsIgnoreCase("Y")) {
      System.out.println("You might have a cough. Please consult a doctor
      for diagnosis.");
            diagnosed = true;
    }
    if (i< 2 && !diagnosed) {
        System.out.println("Do you have any other symptoms (Y/N)?");
            String hasOtherSymptoms = scanner.nextLine();
            if (hasOtherSymptoms.equalsIgnoreCase("Y")) {
        System.out.println("Please consult a doctor for a complete diagnosis.");
              diagnosed = true;
    }
    }
  }
  if (!diagnosed) {
      System.out.println("Your symptoms might be minor. Consider home rem-
      edies or consult a doctor if they persist.");
  }
  }
}
```

The program `SymptomChecker` allows users to assess their health condition based on input regarding fever and cough symptoms. It begins by prompting the user to input whether they have a fever and cough, then proceeds to evaluate these inputs to determine potential health implications. If the user reports both fever and cough, it suggests they might have a cold or flu, prompting them to consult a doctor. If only one symptom is reported, it advises consultation for that specific symptom. Additionally, the program allows for up to two rounds of querying for other symptoms, emphasizing the importance of seeking medical advice if necessary. If no significant symptoms are identified, it recommends home remedies or further consultation if symptoms persist, aiming to provide preliminary health guidance effectively.

3.6.2 Case Study 2

Proper medication adherence is directly linked to better health outcomes. By supporting patients in adhering to their prescribed treatment plans, medication reminders contribute to improved disease management, reduced complications, and overall better health. The reminder system provides a convenient way for users to manage their medication schedules without relying solely on memory. It allows users to input their medication details and receive timely reminders, integrating seamlessly into their daily routines.

- Medication Name: Users input the name of the medication they need to take.
- Dosage: Users specify the dosage details, such as "1 tablet" or "2 capsules."

- Dosage Frequency: The program prompts users to enter how many times per day they need to take the medication. This ensures that users can set reminders for each required dosage throughout the day.
- Dose Times: For each dosage frequency entered, the program asks users to specify the exact time of day (in 24-hour format) when each dose should be taken. This helps in setting precise reminders aligned with the user's daily routine.
- Reminder Messages: After collecting all the necessary information, the program generates reminder messages for each dose time entered. These messages include details such as the medication name, dosage, and scheduled time to ensure users remember to take their medication at the correct times.
- Data Validation: Throughout the interaction, the program ensures that user inputs are validated to prevent errors, such as negative dosage frequencies or invalid time formats.

```
import java.util.Scanner;
public class MedicationReminder {
  void main(String[] args) {
  Scanner scanner = new Scanner(System.in);
System.out.println("Enter medication name:");
  String medicationName = scanner.nextLine();
System.out.println("Enter dosage (e.g., 1 tablet):");
  String dosage = scanner.nextLine();
  int dosageTimes = 0;
  do {
System.out.println("How many times per day do you need to take " +
medicationName + "? (Enter 0 to finish)");
dosageTimes = scanner.nextInt();
  } while (dosageTimes< 0); // Ensure non-negative value
  for (int i = 0; i<dosageTimes; i++) {
System.out.println("Enter time for dose " + (i + 1) + " in 24-hour format
(HH:MM):");
    String time = scanner.nextLine();
System.out.println("Reminder: Take " + dosage + " of " + medicationName +
" at " + time);
  }
System.out.println("Medication details saved.");
  }
}
```

The `MedicationReminder` program is designed to assist users in managing their medication schedule effectively. It begins by prompting the user to input the medication name and dosage information. Then, it enters a loop where it asks the user how many times per day they need to take the medication, ensuring that a non-negative value is entered. After obtaining this information, the program iterates through a loop for each dose time entered by the user, prompting them to specify the time in 24-hour format (HH:MM). For each dose time specified, it generates a reminder message detailing the medication name, dosage, and the scheduled time for the dose.

3.6.3 Case Study 3

"Allergy Checker" aims to help users identify potential allergies, understand their triggers, and encourage them to seek professional medical advice for accurate diagnosis and treatment. It leverages user input and a predefined list of common allergies to provide informative feedback tailored to the user's situation.

```
import java.util.Scanner;
public class AllergyChecker {
  void main(String[] args) {
  Scanner scanner = new Scanner(System.in);
String[] allergies = {"pollen", "dust", "nuts", "pets"};
System.out.println("Do you have any allergies? (Y/N)");
  String hasAllergies = scanner.nextLine();
  if (hasAllergies.equalsIgnoreCase("Y")) {
System.out.println("Enter your allergies separated by commas (e.g., pollen,
dust):");
    String userAllergies = scanner.nextLine();
booleanallergyFound = false;
    for (String allergy : allergies) {
    if (userAllergies.toLowerCase().contains(allergy)) {
allergyFound = true;
System.out.println("You might be allergic to " + allergy + ".");
String[] triggers = null;
      switch (allergy) {
      case "pollen":
        triggers = new String[]{"spring", "flowers", "grass"};
break;
      case "dust":
        triggers = new String[]{"dust mites", "pet dander", "mold"};
break;
      }
      if (triggers != null) {
System.out.println("Potential triggers for " + allergy + " allergy:");
      for (String trigger : triggers) {
System.out.println("- " + trigger);
      }
      }
      break; // Exit loop after finding an allergy
    }
    }
    if (!allergyFound) {
System.out.println("Your entered allergies don't match our list.");
    }
  } else {
System.out.println("You might be less prone to allergic reactions.");
  }
  }
}
```

The "AllergyChecker" program helps users assess potential allergies based on their input. It begins by asking if the user has any allergies, expecting a yes (Y) or no (N) response. If the user confirms having allergies (Y), they are prompted to input their specific allergies separated by commas. The program then checks against a predefined list of common allergies such as pollen, dust, nuts, and pets.Using a loop, the program compares the user-inputted allergies with the predefined list. If a match is found, it informs the user of the potential allergy and lists associated triggers, such as spring, flowers, and grass for pollen allergies, using a switch-case statement. After displaying the allergy information, the program concludes this part of the process by recommending consulting a doctor for further advice.If none of the user-inputted allergies match those in the predefined list, the program informs the user that their entered allergies do not match and advises consulting a doctor. If the user indicates they do not have any allergies (N), the program suggests they might be less prone to allergic reactions.

3.6.4 Case Study 4

The "BMI Calculator" is essential for promoting awareness of weight-related health risks and encouraging individuals to take proactive steps towards maintaining a healthy lifestyle. The BMI (Body Mass Index) is a widely used indicator of body fatness and helps in categorizing individuals into different weight categories: underweight, normal weight, overweight, and obese. This assessment provides valuable information about potential health risks associated with weight. It empowers users with information to make informed decisions about their health and well-being. The parameters considered are:

- BMI Calculation: Using the formula `weight / (height * height)`, the program computes the BMI value
- Specific weight categories:
  - Underweight: BMI < 18.5
  - Normal Weight: 18.5 <= BMI < 25
  - Overweight: 25 <= BMI < 30
  - Obese: BMI >= 30

After displaying the BMI and its corresponding category, the program advises the user to consult a doctor.

```
import java.util.Scanner;
public class BMICalculator {
  void main(String[] args) {
  Scanner scanner = new Scanner(System.in);
  // User input
System.out.println("Enter your height in meters (e.g., 1.75):");
  double height = scanner.nextDouble();
System.out.println("Enter your weight in kilograms (e.g., 70):");
  double weight = scanner.nextDouble();
  // Calculate BMI
  double bmi = weight / (height * height);
  // BMI category using else-if ladder
System.out.println("Your BMI is: " + String.format("%.2f", bmi));
  if (bmi< 18.5) {
System.out.println("You are in the underweight category.");
  } else if (bmi>= 18.5 &&bmi< 25) {
System.out.println("You are in the normal weight category.");
  } else if (bmi>= 25 &&bmi< 30) {
System.out.println("You are in the overweight category.");
  } else {
System.out.println("You are in the obese category.");
  }
System.out.println("Consult a doctor");
  }
}
```

The “BMICalculator” program computes a person’s Body Mass Index (BMI) based on their input of height and weight. It starts by prompting the user to enter their height in meters and weight in kilograms using the Scanner class. After receiving these inputs, it calculates the BMI using the formula weight / (height * height). The BMI value is then displayed with two decimal places for accuracy.Next, the program categorizes the BMI into four categories—underweight, normal weight, overweight, and obese—using an else if ladder. Each category corresponds to a specific range of BMI values, providing the user with an understanding of their weight status relative to health guidelines.

4 Arrays

4.1 INTRODUCTION

An array in programming is indeed a data structure that allows you to store multiple elements of the same data type in contiguous memory locations. This means that all elements are stored one after another, making it easy to access them sequentially using indexing. Each element in the array is identified by its index, starting from zero. This data structure is particularly useful when you need to work with a collection of elements of the same type, such as a list of numbers or strings. Figure 4.1 shows the array storage representation.

The syntax for declaring an array is:

```
datatype arrayname = new datatype[size];
```

Benefits

- **Storage of Multiple Values:** Arrays enable users to store and access multiple values of the same data type efficiently.
- **Sequential Access:** Elements in an array are stored sequentially in memory, which allows for fast access using index positions.
- **Optimized Memory Usage:** Arrays are a contiguous block of memory, making them efficient in terms of memory usage compared to other data structures for storing similar types of data.
- **Ease of Iteration:** Arrays provide a straightforward way to iterate through elements using loops like for-each or traditional for loops.
- **Passing Multiple Values:** Arrays allow you to pass multiple values as parameters to methods or return multiple values from methods.

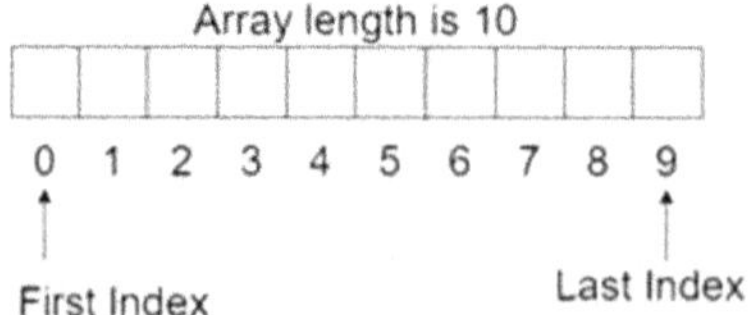

FIGURE 4.1 Array representation.

DOI: 10.1201/9781003544319-4

Limitations

- **Fixed Size:** Arrays have a fixed size defined at the time of declaration, which cannot be changed dynamically at runtime.
- **Homogeneous Elements:** Arrays can only store elements of the same data type, limiting their flexibility compared to other data structures.
- **Memory Management:** Inefficient memory usage when the array size is much larger than required or when resizing is needed (requires creating a new array and copying elements).

4.1.1 Categories of Arrays in Java

In Java, arrays can be categorized based on several criteria, each serving different purposes and offering specific functionalities. Here are the main categories of arrays in Java:

- Zero-Length Arrays: Arrays with zero elements.
- Single-Dimensional Arrays: Arrays that store elements of the same data type in a single row or column.
- Multi-Dimensional Arrays: Arrays that store elements in multiple rows and columns, creating a grid-like structure.
- Dynamic Arrays (ArrayList): A resizable array-like structure provided by the `ArrayList` class in Java's `java.util` package.
- Jagged Arrays: Arrays where each row can have a different number of elements.
- Arrays of Objects: Arrays where each element is an object reference rather than a primitive data type.

Each category of arrays in Java serves specific needs and offers distinct advantages depending on the type of data being stored, the required operations, and memory efficiency considerations. Understanding these categories helps in choosing the right type of array for different programming tasks and optimizing performance in Java applications.

4.2 ZERO-LENGTH ARRAYS

A zero-length array in Java is an array that contains zero elements.

Program

```
public class ZeroLengthArrayExample {
  void main(String[] args) {
  int[] emptyArray = new int[0];
  System.out.println("Length of the emptyArray: " + emptyArray.length);
  for (int i = 0; i < emptyArray.length; i++) {
    System.out.println("Element at index " + i + ": " + emptyArray[i]);
  }
  }
}
Output:
Length of the emptyArray: 0
```

The Java program ZeroLengthArrayExample illustrates the concept and behavior of zero-length arrays in Java. In Java, a zero-length array is an array that has been instantiated with a size of zero, denoted by int[] emptyArray = new int[0];. This means the array does not contain any elements, and its length property returns 0. In the program, after initializing emptyArray, it prints the length of the array using emptyArray.length, which outputs 0. The subsequent for loop attempts to iterate over the array indices (0 to emptyArray.length - 1), but since there are no elements in the array, the loop body does not execute. As a result, the program does not produce any output when iterating over the array indices.

4.3 ONE-DIMENSIONAL ARRAYS

In Java, an array with one dimension is indeed referred to as a 1D array. In a 1D array, all elements are of the same data type. This allows for the efficient storage and retrieval of a collection of values of the same kind.

For example, you can declare a 1D array of integers like this:

int[] numbers = new int[5]; // Declares an integer array of size 5

In this example, `numbers` is a 1D array of integers, and all elements within the array are integers. Each element in the array can be accessed using its index, starting from 0 to `length - 1`, where `length` is the size of the array.

Syntax

In Java, one can declare an array using any of the three syntaxes:

1. `dataType[] arrayName;`
2. `dataType []arrayName;`
3. `dataType arrayName[];`

All three syntaxes achieve the same result, which is declaring an array of the specified data type. Here's an explanation of each syntax:

1. dataType[] arrayName;: This syntax is the most commonly used and preferred convention in Java. It explicitly specifies the data type of the array (`dataType`) followed by square brackets `[]`, which denote that `arrayName` is an array. This syntax is concise and easy to read.
2. dataType []arrayName;: This syntax places the square brackets `[]` adjacent to the data type `dataType`, which also indicates that `arrayName` is an array of elements of type `dataType`. While less common than the first syntax, it is still valid in Java.
3. dataType arrayName[];: This syntax is less common and less preferred in Java. It declares the array name `arrayName` followed by square brackets `[]` and then the data type `dataType`. While it is syntactically correct, it is not as readable or commonly used as the other two syntaxes.

All three syntaxes achieve the same result of declaring an array in Java, but the first syntax (`dataType[] arrayName;`) is the most commonly used and recommended convention.

4.3.1 Instantiation of an Array

Instantiation of an array refers to the process of creating an instance of an array data structure in memory, specifying its size and type. This allows for the allocation of space to store multiple elements of the same data type, enabling organized data management.

1. array a=**new** datatype[size];

In the above syntax, ‘a’ is the instance for the array with size ‘size’

Program

```
import java.util.Scanner;
public class Main {
```

```
  void main(String[] args) {
  // Declare and initialize an array of size 5
  int[] a = new int[5];
  Scanner sc = new Scanner(System.in);
  // Prompt the user to input 5 numbers
  System.out.println("Please enter 5 numbers:");
  // Loop to store the user input in the array
  for (int i = 0; i < a.length; i++) {
    a[i] = sc.nextInt();  // Store user input in array
  }
  // Print elements at even positions (indices 0, 2, 4)
  System.out.println("Elements at even positions (0, 2, 4):");
  for (int i = 0; i < a.length; i++) {
    if (i % 2 == 0) {  // Check if the index is even
      System.out.print(a[i] + " ");
    }
  }
  }
}
```

Output:

```
Please enter 5 numbers:
1 2 3 4 5
Elements at even positions (0, 2, 4):
1 3 5
```

The above program prints the even position array elementsi.e 0,2, and 4 location elements. Program begins by importing the `Scanner` class from the `java.util` package to facilitate user input. Within the `main` method, an integer array `a` of size 5 is declared and initialized. A `Scanner` object `sc` is instantiated to capture user input. The program then prompts the user to input 5 numbers using the `println` method. Following this, a `for` loop iterates through the array, assigning each element a value inputted by the user via the `nextInt()` method of the `Scanner` class. Once all numbers are inputted, another `for` loop is employed to iterate through the array again. Within this loop, each element undergoes a check for evenness using the modulus operator `%`. If the remainder when dividing the element by 2 is 0, indicating it's even, the number is printed using the `print` method.

Program

Array initialization and declaration

```
public class Main {
  void main(String[] args) {
  // Initialize an array of integers with a length of 5
  int[] a = new int[5];
  // Assign values 1 through 5 to the elements of the array
  for (int i = 0; i < a.length; i++) {
    a[i] = i + 1;  // Assigning values 1 to 5
  }
  // Use a for-each loop to print each element of the array
  for (int i : a) {
    System.out.print(i + " ");  // Print each element followed by a space
  }
  }
}
```

Output

```
1 2 3 4 5
```

In this program, an integer array of size 5 is initialized to hold values. A loop populates the array with integers from 1 to 5, assigning each value to the corresponding index. After filling the array, a for-each loop is utilized to iterate through the array and print each element, followed by a space.

Program

Program: array initialization at the time of declaration

```
public class Main {
  void main(String[] args) {
  // Initialize the array with values 1 through 5 directly
  int[] a = {1, 2, 3, 4, 5};
  // Use a for-each loop to iterate over and print each element
  for (int i : a) {
    System.out.print(i + " ");  // Print each element followed by a space
  }
  }
}
```

Output

```
1 2 3 4 5
```

The above Java program initializes an array `a` of integers with the values 1 through 5 directly in the array declaration. A for-each loop is then used to iterate over each element `i` in the array `a`. During each iteration, the value of the current element `i` is printed to the console, followed by a space using the `System.out.print()` method. As a result, when the program is executed, it prints the numbers 1 through 5, separated by spaces, on a single line.

4.4 TWO-DIMENSIONAL ARRAYS

In Java, a 2D array is structured as rows and columns, much like a matrix. It's represented using the syntax `data_type array_name[rows][columns];`. This syntax specifies the data type of the elements in the array, followed by the array name and the dimensions in terms of rows and columns enclosed in square brackets. For example, to declare a 2D array of integers with three rows and four columns, the syntax would be `int[][] myArray = new int[3][4];`. This creates a 2D array with 3 rows and 4 columns, where each element is initialized to the default value for the data type, which is `0` for integers.

Syntax

data_typearray_name[rows][columns];

Program

```
public class Main {
  void main(String[] args) {
  // Initialize a 2D array with different row lengths
  int[][] a = {
    {1, 2, 3},      // First row with 3 elements
    {4, 5, 6, 7},  // Second row with 4 elements
    {8, 9}        // Third row with 2 elements
  };
  // Print the length of each row
  for (int i = 0; i < a.length; i++) {
    System.out.println("Length of row " + i + ": " + a[i].length);
  }
  }
}
```

Output:
```
Length of row 0: 3
Length of row 1: 4
Length of row 2: 2
```

In the `main` method, a 2D array `a` is initialized with three rows, each containing a different number of elements. The first row has three elements, the second row has four elements, and the third row has two elements. The lengths of each row are retrieved using the `length` property of the array. Each row's length is printed individually with `System.out.println()`, providing clear feedback on the dimensions of the array structure. Upon execution, the program outputs the length of each row, indicating the number of elements in each row.

4.5 3D ARRAYS

In Java programming, 3D arrays offer a powerful means to organize and manipulate data in a three-dimensional space, akin to sculpting intricate forms in a digital landscape.

Syntax

dataType[][][] arrayName = newdataType[row][column][height];

The syntax declares a 3D array named `arrayName` of type `dataType`, with dimensions specified by `row`, `column`, and `height`.

Program

Program for Reading to 3D array and print 3D array elements in java

```
import java.util.Scanner;
public class Main {
  void main(String[] args) {
  // Initialize a 3D array with varying sizes for each row
  int[][][] a = new int[2][][];
  // First 2D array has 3 rows with varying sizes
  a[0] = new int[3][];
  a[0][0] = new int[2];  // First row has 2 elements
  a[0][1] = new int[3];  // Second row has 3 elements
  a[0][2] = new int[1];  // Third row has 1 element
  // Second 2D array has 2 rows with varying sizes
  a[1] = new int[2][];
  a[1][0] = new int[4];  // First row has 4 elements
  a[1][1] = new int[2];  // Second row has 2 elements
  Scanner sc = new Scanner(System.in);
  // Prompt the user to enter values for each element
  System.out.println("Enter values for the 3D array:");
  for (int i = 0; i < a.length; i++) {
    for (int j = 0; j < a[i].length; j++) {
      for (int k = 0; k < a[i][j].length; k++) {
        System.out.printf("a[%d][%d][%d]: ", i, j, k);
        a[i][j][k] = sc.nextInt();
      }
    }
  }
  // Print the entered values and separate each sub-array
  System.out.println("Entered values of the 3D array:");
  for (int[][] array2D : a) {
    for (int[] array1D : array2D) {
```

```
      for (int element : array1D) {
        System.out.print(element + " ");
      }
      System.out.println();
    }
    System.out.println("----------"); // Line of dashes to separate sub-arrays
  }
  }
}
```

Output:

```
Enter values for the 3D array:
a[0][0][0]: 1
a[0][0][1]: 2
a[0][1][0]: 3
a[0][1][1]: 4
a[0][1][2]: 5
a[0][2][0]: 6
a[1][0][0]: 7
a[1][0][1]: 8
a[1][0][2]: 9
a[1][0][3]: 10
a[1][1][0]: 11
a[1][1][1]: 12
Entered values of the 3D array:
1 2
3 4 5
6
----------
7 8 9 10
11 12
----------
```

The above Java program initializes a three-dimensional array `a` to store integer values. The array has dimensions [2][3][], [2][2][], and [2][]. Used nested for loops to iterate over each element of the array and prompt the user to enter values for each element. The array is dynamically allocated with varying sizes for each dimension. Once the user enters the values, the program prints the entered elements using nested for-each loops to iterate over each dimension of the array. After printing the elements of each sub-array, a line of dashes is printed to separate each sub-array for better readability.

4.6 JAGGED ARRAYS

Jagged arrays in Java are arrays of arrays where each row of the array can have a different length. Unlike regular multi-dimensional arrays (like 2D arrays), jagged arrays allow for more flexibility in representing data structures where the number of elements can vary between rows.

Syntax

```
dataType[][] arrayName = new dataType[rowSize][];
arrayName[0] = new dataType[numberOfColumnsInFirstRow];
arrayName[1] = new dataType[numberOfColumnsInSecondRow];
```

Example

```
int[][] jaggedArray = new int[3][];
jaggedArray[0] = new int[]{1, 2, 3};
jaggedArray[1] = new int[]{4, 5};
jaggedArray[2] = new int[]{6, 7, 8, 9};
```

Benefits

- Memory Efficiency: Jagged arrays consume memory only as needed, which can be more efficient compared to regular multi-dimensional arrays.
- Flexibility: Each row can have a different number of elements, allowing for irregular data structures to be represented accurately.

Limitations

- Access Complexity: Accessing elements can be less straightforward due to varying row lengths, requiring additional bounds checking.
- Initialization Overhead: Initializing and managing jagged arrays can be more complex, especially when dimensions change dynamically.

Program

```
public class JaggedArrayExample {
  void main(String[] args) {
      int[][] jaggedArray = new int[3][];
  jaggedArray[0] = new int[]{1, 2, 3};
  jaggedArray[1] = new int[]{4, 5};
  jaggedArray[2] = new int[]{6, 7, 8, 9};
  for (int i = 0; i < jaggedArray.length; i++) {
    for (int j = 0; j < jaggedArray[i].length; j++) {
      System.out.print(jaggedArray[i][j] + " ");
    }
    System.out.println();    }
  }
}
Output:
1 2 3
4 5
6 7 8 9
```

In this program "JaggedArrayExample", a jagged array named `jaggedArray` is declared and initialized with three rows, where each row can have a different number of elements. The first row is initialized with three elements (1, 2, 3), the second row with two elements (4, 5), and the third row with four elements (6, 7, 8, 9). Nested for loops are then used to iterate through the jagged array, printing each element followed by a space. After completing the inner loop for each row, a new line is printed to separate the rows visually in the output.

4.7 ARRAY OF OBJECTS

In Java, an "array of objects" refers to an array where each element is an object of a class or a subclass. Unlike arrays of primitive data types, which store values directly, arrays of objects store references (or pointers) to objects on the heap.

Benefits

- **Flexible Data Structure:** Arrays of objects allow you to store multiple instances of different classes or subclasses in a single data structure. This flexibility is useful when you need to manage collections of related objects.
- **Dynamic Size:** Arrays in Java have a fixed size once created. However, by using dynamic data structures like ArrayList (which internally uses an array), developers can achieve resizable arrays of objects, accommodating varying numbers of elements as needed.
- **Efficient Access:** Accessing elements in an array (both primitive and objects) is efficient because it involves direct indexing. This makes arrays of objects suitable for scenarios where quick access to elements by index is necessary.

Limitations

- **Fixed Size:** Arrays have a fixed size once created. If you need to add or remove elements dynamically, you would need to create a new array or use resizable data structures like ArrayList, which internally manages array resizing.
- **Homogeneous Elements:** Arrays in Java are homogeneous, meaning they can only store elements of the same type (either the specified class or its subclasses). This limits the direct storage of objects of different classes or types within the same array without using superclass references or generics.
- **Type Safety:** Arrays of objects can lead to type safety issues if not used carefully. Since arrays store references to objects, casting or improper type handling can result in ClassCastException at runtime.

Program

```
public class Example {
  void main(String[] args) {
  Object[] jaggedArray = {
    new int[]{1, 2, 3},
    new String[]{"Usha", "Rani"},
    new double[]{3.14, 2.71}
  };
        for (Object obj : jaggedArray) {
    if (obj instanceof int[]) {
      int[] intArr = (int[]) obj;
      System.out.print("int array: ");
      for (int num : intArr) {
        System.out.print(num + " ");
      }
      System.out.println();
    } else if (obj instanceof String[]) {
      String[] strArr = (String[]) obj;
      System.out.print("String array: ");
      for (String str : strArr) {
        System.out.print(str + " ");
      }
      System.out.println();
    } else if (obj instanceof double[]) {
      double[] doubleArr = (double[]) obj;
      System.out.print("double array: ");
```

```
      for (double num : doubleArr) {
        System.out.print(num + " ");
      }
      System.out.println();
    }
  }
  }
}
```

Output:

```
int array: 1 2 3
String array: Usha Rani
double array: 3.14 2.71
```

This Java program demonstrates the use of a jagged array (`jaggedArray`) which stores arrays of different types (`int[]`, `String[]`, `double[]`). It iterates through each element of `jaggedArray`, checks its type using `instanceof`, and prints the elements of each nested array accordingly, categorizing them as `int array`, `String array`, or `double array`.

4.8 COMMAND-LINE ARGUMENTS

Java command-line arguments are parameters passed to a Java program when it is executed from the command line. These arguments are specified after the name of the Java class file to be executed. In Java, command-line arguments are received by the `main` method of the class specified as the entry point of the program. The `main` method must accept an array of strings as its parameter, which represents the command-line arguments passed to the program.
For example, consider the following command to run a Java program:

```
java MyProgram arg1 arg2 arg3
```

In this command:

- `MyProgram` is the name of the Java class file to be executed.
- `arg1`, `arg2`, and `arg3` are the command-line arguments being passed to the program.

Within the Java program, these arguments are accessed through the `args` parameter of the `main` method:

Program

```
public class MyProgram {
  void main(String[] args) {
  // Access and process command-line arguments
  for (String arg : args) {
    System.out.println("Argument: " + arg);
  }
  }
}
```

Output

```
C:\jj>java --enable-preview --source 22 MyProgram.java testing
Argument: testing
```

In this example, the `args` parameter is an array of strings containing the command-line arguments passed to the program. The program can then iterate over this array to access and process each argument as needed. When executing a Java program from the command-line, developers have the option to pass additional information known as command-line arguments. These arguments are provided as strings separated by spaces and are accessible within the Java program via the `args[]` parameter of the `main` method. The `args[]` array contains all the command-line arguments passed to the program, with each argument stored as a separate element in the array. To access the command-line arguments, developers can use the `args[]` array within the `main` method. The length of the `args[]` array can be determined using the `length` property, allowing developers to ascertain the number of command-line arguments provided. Each individual argument is accessed by indexing the `args[]` array, with `args[0]` representing the first argument, `args[1]` representing the second argument, and so on.

Program

```
public class Test {
  void main(String[] a) {
    // Check if any command-line arguments are provided
    if (a.length > 0) {
      // Print the first command-line argument
      System.out.println(a[0]);
    } else {
      // Print an error message if no arguments are provided
      System.out.println("No command-line arguments provided.");
    }
  }
}
```

Output

```
C:\jj>java --enable-preview --source 22 Test.java usharani
usharani
```

The above Java program defines a class named `Test` with a single method `main`. This method takes a single parameter `a`, which is an array of strings representing command-line arguments. Within the `main` method, the program prints the first element of the `a` array using `System.out.println(a[0])`. When the program is run, the first command-line argument provided by the user will be printed to the console. If no arguments are provided, the program will throw an `ArrayIndexOutOfBoundsException` because accessing `a[0]` would be out of bounds for an empty array.

Program

Sum of two numbers using command-line arguments

```
public class Test {
  void main(String[] args) {
  // Check if there are at least two arguments provided
  if (args.length >= 2) {
    try {
      // Parse the first command-line argument as an integer
      int a = Integer.parseInt(args[0]);
      // Parse the second command-line argument as an integer
      int q = Integer.parseInt(args[1]);
      // Calculate the sum of the two numbers
      int sum = a + q;
      // Print the result
      System.out.println("The sum is: " + sum);
    } catch (NumberFormatException e) {
```

```
      // Handle the case where the input is not a valid integer
      System.out.println("Please provide valid integers as command-line
arguments.");
    }
  } else {
    // Handle the case where less than two arguments are provided
    System.out.println("Please provide two command-line arguments.");
  }
  }
}
```

Output

```
C:\jj>java --enable-preview --source 22 Test.java 10 20
The sum is: 30
```

The above Java program attempts to perform addition using command-line arguments passed to the program. Firstly, the `main` method takes an array of strings `a` as its parameter to represent command-line arguments. Within the method, the program tries to parse the first command-line argument `a[0]` as an integer and assign it to a variable `a`. Similarly, it tries to parse the second command-line argument `a[1]` as an integer and assign it to a variable `q`.

Program

Fibonacci Series program using command-line arguments

```
public class FibonacciGenerator {
  void main(String[] args) {
  // Check if the command-line argument is provided
  if (args.length > 0) {
    try {
      // Parse the command-line argument as an integer
      int n = Integer.parseInt(args[0]);
      // Initialize the first two Fibonacci numbers
      int f1 = 0;
      int f2 = 1;
      // Print the Fibonacci sequence
      System.out.println("Fibonacci sequence up to " + n + " terms:");
      // Handle the case where n is 1
      if (n >= 1) {
        System.out.print(f1 + " ");
      }
      // Print the remaining terms if n is greater than 1
      for (int i = 1; i < n; i++) {
        System.out.print(f2 + " ");
        int s = f1 + f2; // Calculate the next Fibonacci number
        f1 = f2;      // Update f1 to the current f2
        f2 = s;      // Update f2 to the next Fibonacci number
      }
      // Print a newline for better formatting
      System.out.println();
    } catch (NumberFormatException e) {
      // Handle the case where the input is not a valid integer
      System.out.println("Please provide a valid integer as a command-line
argument.");
    }
  } else {
```

```
    // Handle the case where no arguments are provided
    System.out.println("Please provide the number of terms as a command-
line argument.");
    }
  }
}
```

Output

```
C:\jj>java --enable-preview --source 22 FibonacciGenerator.java 10
Fibonacci sequence up to 10 terms:
0 1 1 2 3 5 8 13 21 34
```

This Java program aims to generate the Fibonacci sequence up to a specified number of terms, with the number of terms provided as a command-line argument. The program first parses the command-line argument `a[0]` as an integer, representing the number of terms in the Fibonacci sequence. It initializes two variables `f1` and `f2` to 0 and 1, respectively, which are the first two numbers of the Fibonacci sequence. Using a `for` loop, the program iterates from the second term (`i = 1`) up to the specified number of terms (`n`). Within each iteration, it prints the current Fibonacci number `f1`, calculates the next Fibonacci number `s` by adding `f1` and `f2`, updates the values of `f1` and `f2` to progress to the next numbers in the sequence. The loop continues until the desired number of terms is reached. At each iteration, the program prints the Fibonacci number `f1`, generating the Fibonacci sequence in the console output. The Fibonacci sequence starts with 0 and 1, and each subsequent term is the sum of the two preceding terms.

4.9 STRING

Strings serve as a fundamental data type in Java, allowing the storage of text or sequences of characters. While Java also provides the primitive data type `char` for single-character storage, it becomes insufficient for handling names or longer character sequences. There are two primary methods for storing sequences of characters in Java: using a `char[]` array and utilizing the `String` class. The first method involves creating a `char[]` array, where each element of the array represents an individual character. For instance:

Program

```
public class Main {
  void main(String[] args) {
  // Declare and initialize a character array
  char[] c = {'t', 'e', 's', 't', 'i', 'n', 'g'};
  // Print the character array
  System.out.println(c);  // This will print "testing"
  // Alternatively, declare and print a string literal
  String s = "testing";
  System.out.println(s);  // This will also print "testing"
  }
}
```

Output:

```
testing
testing
```

Within the `main` method, a character array (`char[] c`) is declared and initialized with the individual characters 't', 'e', 's', 't', 'i', 'n', and 'g'. Subsequently, a `System.out.println()` statement is employed to output the contents of the character array to the console. When attempting to print a character array using `System.out.println()`, Java automatically converts the array to its string representation, resulting in the concatenation of the individual characters. Therefore, the output of this program will be the string "testing. Alternatively, the second method utilizes the `String` class, which allows for the direct declaration of a sequence of characters enclosed within double quotes:

Program

```
public class Main {
  void main(String[] args) {
  // Declare and initialize a string variable
  String sname = "usharani";
  // Print the content of the string variable
  System.out.println(sname);  // This will print "usharani"
  }
}
Output:
Usharani
```

Inside the `main` method, a string variable named `sname` is declared and assigned the value "usharani." Subsequently, a `System.out.println()` statement is utilized to output the content of the string variable to the console. The result of executing this program will be the display of the string "usharani" in the console.

A `String` variable is essentially an object capable of storing character values. Strings in Java, being 16 bits using UTF-16 encoding, act similarly to an array of characters. The creation of strings can be achieved through two ways: using string literals or employing the `new` keyword.

u	s	h	a	r	a	n	i	\0

- String Literal: This method optimizes memory by referencing existing objects in the String constant pool if they match the content.

```
String s = "testing";
```

- Using new Keyword: In this approach, a new string object is created in the normal heap memory, and the literal is placed in the String constant pool.

```
String demoString = new String("testing");
```

Program

```
public class Main {
  void main(String[] args) {
  // Declare and initialize string variables
  String s1 = "Dr.";
  String s2 = "Usharani";
  String s3 = "Bhimavarapu";
  // Print the strings concatenated on the same line
  System.out.print(s1);  // Prints "Dr."
  System.out.print(s2);  // Prints "Usharani" immediately after "Dr."
```

```
  System.out.print(s3); //   Prints   "Bhimavarapu"   immediately   after
"Usharani"
  }
}
```

Output:

```
Dr. Usharani Bhimavarapu
```

The program begins by declaring and initializing three string variables: `s1` with the value "Dr.", `s2` with "Usharani," and `s3` with "Bhimavarapu." Following this, a sequence of `System.out.print()` statements is employed to display these strings consecutively on the same line. The use of `System.out.print()` instead of `System.out.println()` ensures that each string is printed without moving to a new line. Consequently, the output of the program will be the concatenation of the three strings, appearing as a single line: "Dr.UsharaniBhimavarapu."

Interfaces and Classes in Strings in Java

- CharBuffer: The `CharBuffer` class implements the `CharSequence` interface and is designed to enable the use of character buffers in place of `CharSequences`. This is particularly useful in scenarios like regular expression handling in the `java.util.regex` package.
- String: The `String` class in Java represents an immutable sequence of characters. Objects of the `String` class are constant and cannot be modified once created. Operations like converting to uppercase or lowercase return a new object rather than modifying the original. Strings in Java are automatically thread-safe.

```
String str = "testing";
// or
String str = new String("testing");
```

- CharSequence Interface: The `CharSequence` interface is employed for representing character sequences in Java. Classes implemented using this interface, such as `String`, `StringBuffer`, and `StringBuilder`, provide various functionalities like substring extraction, finding occurrences, concatenation, converting to uppercase, and converting to lowercase.
- StringBuffer: The `StringBuffer` class is a peer class of `String` and offers functionalities similar to strings. However, `StringBuffer` represents growable and writable character sequences, making it mutable. It is thread-safe, suitable for multi-threaded environments where shared objects need protection. It is created using the following syntax:

```
StringBuffer demoString = new StringBuffer("testing");
```

- StringBuilder: The `StringBuilder` class represents a mutable sequence of characters, providing an alternative to the immutable `String` class. Unlike `StringBuffer`, it is not thread-safe, making it more suitable for single-threaded programs. It is created using the following syntax:

```
StringBuilder demoString = new StringBuilder();
demoString.append("testing");
```

- StringTokenizer: The `StringTokenizer` class is used to break a string into tokens. It internally maintains a current position within the string for tokenization. Tokens are substrings of the original string.
- StringJoiner: The `StringJoiner` class in the `java.util` package constructs a sequence of characters separated by a delimiter, optionally starting with a provided prefix and ending with a supplied suffix. It simplifies the process of joining strings with a delimiter.

```
StringJoiner joiner = new StringJoiner(",");
```

- String Literal and String Constant Pool: In Java, strings can be created using string literals. The JVM checks the String constant pool for the existence of the string. If the string is not present, a new instance is created and placed in the pool. If the string exists, the reference to the existing instance is returned.

4.9.1 Memory Allocation of Strings

When a String object is created using a literal, it is allocated in the String constant pool. This enables the JVM to optimize the initialization of String literals for better memory management.

For instance:

```
String s = "testing";
```

In contrast, if a String is created using the `new` operator, indicating dynamic allocation, it is assigned a new memory location in the heap. Strings created in this manner are not automatically added to the String constant pool.
For example:

```
String s = new String("testing");
```

If there is a desire to store a dynamically allocated string in the constant pool, the `intern()` method can be used:

```
String s1 = s.intern();// This will add the string to the String con-
stant pool.
```

It is generally recommended to use String literals, as it allows the JVM to optimize memory allocation and enhances overall performance. This approach ensures that commonly used strings are efficiently managed in the constant pool, contributing to better memory utilization.

4.9.2 Immutable Strings

A String serves as an essential data type in any application, frequently utilized for storing critical attributes such as usernames and passwords. In the Java programming language, String objects exhibit the property of immutability, meaning that once a String object is created, its content or state cannot be altered. Instead, any attempt to modify a String results in the creation of a new String object, leaving the original unaffected. This characteristic of immutability enhances the reliability and security of stored data, ensuring that String values remain constant once assigned, thereby preventing unintended modifications or tampering.

Program

```
public class Main {
  void main(String[] args) {
  // Declare and initialize a string variable
  String s = "Usharani";
  // Attempt to concatenate another string
  s.concat(" Bhimavarapu");
  // Print the original string
  System.out.println(s);  // This will print "Usharani"
  }
}
Output:
Usharani
```

Inside the `main` method, a String variable `s` is declared and initialized with the value "Usharani." Subsequently, the `concat()` method is invoked on the string `s`, attempting to append the string " Bhimavarapu" to it. However, it's important to note that the `concat()` method does not modify the original string; instead, it returns a new string that represents the concatenation. In this program, the result of the `concat()` method is not assigned to any variable, and the original string `s` remains unchanged. As a consequence, when the program prints the value of `s` using `System.out.println()`, it will display "Usharani" because strings in Java are immutable, meaning their values cannot be altered once assigned. If the intention is to capture the result of the concatenation, the statement `s = s.concat(" Bhimavarapu");` should be used to update the variable `s` with the new concatenated value.

Program

```
public class Main {
  void main(String[] args) {
  // Declare and initialize a string variable
  String s = "Usharani";
  // Concatenate and update the string variable
  s = s.concat(" Bhimavarapu");
  // Print the updated string
  System.out.println(s);  // This will print "Usharani Bhimavarapu"
  }
}
Output:
Usharani Bhimavarapu
```

Within the `main` method, a String variable `s` is declared and initialized with the value "Usharani." The `concat()` method is then invoked on the string `s`, aiming to append the string " Bhimavarapu" to it. Unlike certain string methods, the `concat()` method does not modify the original string in-place; instead, it returns a new String representing the concatenation. In this program, the result of the `concat()` operation is correctly assigned back to the variable `s`, effectively updating its value to "Usharani Bhimavarapu." Finally, the program prints the modified value of `s` using `System.out.println()`, resulting in the output "Usharani Bhimavarapu."

Java employs the concept of String literals, wherein multiple reference variables can point to the same String object. If one reference variable modifies the object's value, this change will be reflected across all other reference variables pointing to the same object. This characteristic of shared mutability underscores the immutability of String objects in Java.

Several features contribute to the immutability of String objects:

- ClassLoader Usage: String objects are often used as arguments for ClassLoader in Java. If these String objects were modifiable, the loaded class might be different due to changes in their values. To prevent potential misinterpretations and inconsistencies, String objects are designed to be immutable.
- Thread Safety: String immutability ensures thread safety. Since String objects cannot be modified once created, developers don't need to worry about synchronization issues when sharing these objects across multiple threads.
- Security Considerations: Immutable String objects enhance security in applications. For instance, in scenarios like banking software, where usernames and passwords are sensitive information, the immutability of String objects prevents unauthorized modifications, making the application more secure.
- Heap Space Efficiency:String immutability contributes to efficient heap space utilization. When creating a new String object, the Java Virtual Machine (JVM) checks if the value already exists in the String pool. If it does, the existing value is assigned to the new object, reducing memory consumption and promoting efficient use of heap space.

4.9.3 Methods in String

In Java, the `String` class provides a rich set of methods for manipulating and processing strings. One of the most commonly used methods is `length()`, which returns the number of characters in a string. The `charAt(int index)` method allows access to a specific character at the given index, while `substring(int beginIndex, int endIndex)` extracts a portion of the string between specified indices. For searching, methods like `indexOf(String str)` and `lastIndexOf(String str)` are available to find the first or last occurrence of a substring. String comparison is facilitated by `equals(Object obj)` for content equality and `compareTo(String anotherString)` for lexicographical comparison.

To modify strings, `toUpperCase()` and `toLowerCase()` convert the string to upper or lower case, respectively, while `trim()` removes any leading or trailing whitespace. The `replace(char oldChar, char newChar)` method allows for the replacement of specific characters within the string. Additionally, `split(String regex)` breaks the string into an array based on a given delimiter. The immutability of strings in Java means that operations return new string instances rather than modifying the original string, which is a key aspect of string handling in Java. These methods enable robust string manipulation, making it easier to handle textual data in applications.

Program

```
public class Main {
  void main(String[] args) {
  // Declare and initialize a string variable
  String s = "testing";
  // Retrieve the character at index 3
  char c = s.charAt(3);
  // Print the retrieved character
  System.out.println(c);  // This will print 't'
  }
}
Output:
t
```

Inside the `main` method, a String variable `s` is declared and initialized with the value "testing." The `charAt()` method on the String `s` retrieves and stores the character at the specified index, in this case, the character at index 3. The retrieved character is assigned to a char variable `c`. Subsequently, the `System.out.println()` prints the value of the char variable `c` to the console. In this instance, the output of the program will be the character at index 3 of the string "testing," which is 't'.

Program

```
public class Main {
  void main(String[] args) {
  // Declare and initialize string variables
  String s1 = "usha";
  String s2 = "usha";
  String s3 = "rani";
  // Compare strings using compareTo()
  int result1 = s1.compareTo(s2);  // Comparing s1 with s2
  int result2 = s1.compareTo(s3);  // Comparing s1 with s3
  int result3 = s2.compareTo(s3);  // Comparing s2 with s3
  int result4 = s2.compareTo(s1);  // Comparing s2 with s1
  // Print comparison results
  System.out.println("s1.compareTo(s2): " + result1);
  // 0 (s1 and s2 are equal)
  System.out.println("s1.compareTo(s3): " + result2);
  // Positive value (s1 < s3)
  System.out.println("s2.compareTo(s3): " + result3);
  // Positive value (s2 < s3)
  System.out.println("s2.compareTo(s1): " + result4);
  // 0 (s2 and s1 are equal)
  }
}
```

Output:

```
s1.compareTo(s2): 0
s1.compareTo(s3): 3
s2.compareTo(s3): 3
s2.compareTo(s1): 0
```

The above Java program defines a class named `Main` with a `main` method that compares three strings, `s1`, `s2`, and `s3`, using the `compareTo()` method. The method evaluates the lexicographical order of the strings, providing integer results based on the ASCII values of corresponding characters. In the comparisons, `s1` and `s2` being identical ("usha") result in a 0, indicating equality. Comparisons with `s3` yield positive values as "usha" precedes "rani" in lexicographical order. The program prints these comparison results to the console, demonstrating how the `compareTo()` method facilitates string comparisons in Java. s1.compareTo(s2): Since both s1 and s2 have the same content ("usha"), the result is 0. s1.compareTo(s3): The lexicographical order places "usha" before "rani," so the result is a positive value.s2.compareTo(s3): Similar to the previous comparison, "usha" is lexicographically before "rani," resulting in a positive value.s2.compareTo(s1): As both strings are equal, the result is 0.

Program

```
public class Main {
  void main(String[] args) {
  // Declare and initialize a string variable
  String s = "testing";
  // Check if substrings are contained within the string s
  boolean result1 = s.contains("test");
  boolean result2 = s.contains("in");
```

```
  boolean result3 = s.contains("tin");
  // Print the results of contains method
  System.out.println(result1);  // This will print true
  System.out.println(result2);  // This will print false
  System.out.println(result3);  // This will print true
  }
}
```

Output:

```
true
true
true
```

Within the `main` method, a String variable `s` is declared and initialized with the value “testing.” The `contains()` method on the String `s` checks for the presence of specific substrings within it. The `contains()` method returns a boolean value, indicating whether the specified substring is present in the original string. In this program, three `System.out.println()` statements are used to print the results of different `contains()` method invocations. The first statement checks if the substring “test” is present in the original string “testing,” and since it is, the result is `true`. The second statement checks for the substring “in,” which is not present, resulting in `false`. Finally, the third statement checks for the substring “tin,” and since it is part of “testing,” the result is `true`.

Program

```
public class Main {
  void main(String[] args) {
  // Declare and initialize a string variable
  String s = "testing";
  // Check if the string ends with specific suffixes
  boolean result1 = s.endsWith("ing");
  boolean result2 = s.endsWith("ting");
  // Print the results of endsWith method
  System.out.println(result1);
  System.out.println(result2);
  }
}
```

Output:

```
true
true
```

Inside the `main` method, a String variable `s` is declared and initialized with the value “testing.” The `endsWith()` method on the String `s` determines if it ends with specific suffixes. The `endsWith()` method returns a boolean value, indicating whether the original string ends with the specified suffix. In this program, two `System.out.println()` statements are employed to print the results of different `endsWith()` method invocations. The first statement checks if the string “testing” ends with the suffix “ing,” and since it does, the result is `true`. The second statement checks for the suffix “ting,” and although “testing” contains this substring, the `endsWith()` method specifically evaluates the suffix and, in this case, the result is `false`.

Program

```
public class Main {
  void main(String[] args) {
  // Declare and initialize string variables
```

```
  String s1 = "usharani";
  String s2 = "usharani";
  String s3 = "USHARANI";
  String s4 = "usha";
  // Compare strings using equals() method and print results
  System.out.println(s1.equals(s2)); // true, as both are "usharani"
  System.out.println(s1.equals(s3)); // false, due to case sensitivity
  System.out.println(s1.equals(s4)); // false, as "usharani" is not equal
                                        to "usha"
  }
}
```

Output:

```
true
false
false
```

Inside the `main` method, four String variables, namely `s1`, `s2`, `s3`, and `s4`, are declared and initialized with different values. The `equals()` method compares pairs of these strings and prints the results to the console. The `equals()` method in Java is used to check whether two strings have the same content. If the content is identical, the method returns `true`; otherwise, it returns `false`. In this program, the following comparisons are made and the results are printed:

1. `s1.equals(s2)`: Since both `s1` and `s2` contain the same content ("usharani"), the result is `true`.
2. `s1.equals(s3)`: Although the content is the same, the `equals()` method is case-sensitive, so "usharani" is not considered equal to "USHARANI," resulting in `false`.
3. `s1.equals(s4)`: The content of `s1` ("usharani") is not the same as `s4` ("usha"), so the result is `false`.

The output of the program will be a series of `true` and `false` values, indicating the equality or inequality of the compared strings.

Program

```
public class Main {
  void main(String[] args) {
  // Initialize string and numeric variables
  String s = "usharani";
  double num1 = 1.1142;
  double num2 = 123456.5763636;
  // Format the strings
  String s1 = String.format("name is %s", s);
  String s2 = String.format("value is %.6f", num1);
  String s3 = String.format("value is %35.31f", num2);
  // Print the formatted strings
  System.out.println(s1); // Output: name is usharani
  System.out.println(s2); // Output: value is 1.114200
  System.out.println(s3); // Output: value is 123456.5763636000000000000
                              00000000000
  }
}
```

Output:

```
name is usharani
```

```
value is 1.114200
value is 123456.5763636000000000000000000000
```

Inside the `main` method, a String variable `s` is declared and initialized with the value "usharani." The `String.format()` method creates formatted strings, incorporating the value of `s` and other numeric values. In the program, three `String.format()` statements are used to create formatted strings `s1`, `s2`, and `s3`. The first statement formats a string with the placeholder "%s," and the value of `s` is substituted into this placeholder, resulting in the formatted string "name is usharani." The second statement formats a string with the placeholder "%f," and the numeric value 1.1142 is substituted, yielding the formatted string "value is 1.114200." Lastly, the third statement formats a string with the placeholder "%35.31f," and the numeric value 123456.5763636 is substituted. The resulting string is printed to the console. The output of the program will be the three formatted strings, demonstrating the flexibility of the `String.format()` method in creating strings with specified formats, including placeholders for variable substitution.

Program

```
public class Main {
  void main(String[] args) {
  // Initialize the string
  String s = "Usharani";
  // Convert the string to a byte array
  byte[] byteArray = s.getBytes();
  // Print the byte values
  System.out.println("Byte values:");
  for (byte b : byteArray) {
    System.out.println(b);
  }
  // Declare a character array with length 10
  char[] c = new char[10];
  // Extract characters from index 1 to 6 of the string
  s.getChars(1, 7, c, 0);
  // Print the extracted characters
  System.out.println("Extracted characters:");
  System.out.println(c);
  }
}
Output:
Byte values:
85
115
104
97
114
97
110
105
Extracted characters:
sharan
```

Inside the `main` method, a String variable `s` is declared and initialized with the value "Usharani." The `getBytes()` method on the String `s` obtains the corresponding byte array representation of the string. A `for` loop is employed to iterate through the elements of the byte array, and each byte value is printed to the console. This showcases the conversion of characters in the string to their corresponding byte values. Additionally, a character array `c` is declared with a length of 10. The `getChars()` method is utilized on the string `s` to extract a portion of characters (from index 1 to 6) and copy them into the character array `c` starting at index 0. The extracted characters are then printed to the console using `System.out.println(c)`. The output of the program will be a sequence of byte values representing the ASCII values of characters in the string "Usharani," followed by the extracted characters "sharan" from the original string, demonstrating how these methods facilitate character and byte manipulation in Java. The `getChars()` method allows for a selective extraction of characters from a string into an array.

Program

```
public class Main {
  void main(String[] args) {
  // Declare and initialize string variables
  String s1 = "Usharani";
  String s2 = "Bhimavarapu";
  // Get the lengths of the strings
  int length1 = s1.length();
  int length2 = s2.length();
  // Print the lengths of the strings
  System.out.println("string length is: " + length1);
  System.out.println("string length is: " + length2);
  }
}
Output:
string length is: 8
string length is: 11
```

Inside the `main` method, two String variables, `s1` and `s2`, are declared and initialized with the values "Usharani" and "Bhimavarapu," respectively. The `length()` method on each String variable determines and print the lengths of the respective strings. The `length()` method in Java is used to find the number of characters in a String, effectively providing the length of the string. In this program, two `System.out.println()` statements are employed to print the lengths of `s1` and `s2` to the console. The output of the program will be lines indicating the lengths of the strings, such as "string length is: 8" for "Usharani" and "string length is: 11" for "Bhimavarapu".

Program

```
public class Main {
  void main(String[] args) {
  // Declare and initialize string variable
  String s = "testing";
  // Extract and print substrings
  // Extract substring from index 2 (inclusive) to 4 (exclusive)
  System.out.println(s.substring(2, 4)); // Output: st
  // Extract substring from index 2 to the end of the string
  System.out.println(s.substring(2)); // Output: sting
  }
}
Output:
st
sting
```

Within the `main` method, a String variable `s` is declared and initialized with the value "testing." The `substring()` method on the String `s` extracts and prints substrings based on specified indices. The first `System.out.println()` statement demonstrates the use of the two-argument version of the `substring()` method, where the starting index is inclusive (2) and the ending index is exclusive (4). This operation extracts the substring "st" from the original string "testing" and prints it to the console. The second `System.out.println()` statement uses the one-argument version of the `substring()` method, where only the starting index (2) is provided. In this case, the method extracts the substring starting from index 2 until the end of the string, resulting in "sting" being printed to the console.

Program

```
public class Main {
  void main(String[] args) {
  // String initialization
  String s = "testing";
  // Convert the string to a character array
  char[] c = s.toCharArray();
  // Print each character in the array
  for (char ch : c) {
    System.out.print(ch); // Output: testing
  }
  System.out.println(); // New line for separation
  // Convert string to lowercase and print
  String s1 = "USHARANI";
  System.out.println(s1.toLowerCase()); // Output: usharani
  // Convert string to uppercase and print
  String s2 = "bhimavarapu";
  System.out.println(s2.toUpperCase()); // Output: BHIMAVARAPU
  }
}
```

Output:

```
testing
usharani
BHIMAVARAPU
```

Within the `main` method, several string-related operations are performed on different string variables. Firstly, declared a string variable `s` and utilized the `toCharArray()` method to convert it into a character array `c`. Then used a `for` loop to iterate through the elements of the character array and printed each character to the console. This demonstrates the conversion of a string to a character array and subsequent character-wise processing. Next, declared a string `s1` containing uppercase letters and used the `toLowerCase()` method to convert all the characters to lowercase. The result, "usharani," is printed to the console. This highlights the transformation of uppercase characters to lowercase. Similarly, another string `s2` containing lowercase letters is declared, and the `toUpperCase()` method is applied to convert all characters to uppercase. The result, "BHIMAVARAPU," is printed to the console.

Program

```
public class Main {
  void main(String[] args) {
  // Initialize the string
  String s = "Dr. Usha rani Bhimavarapu";
```

```
    // Split the string based on whitespace
    String[] w = s.split("\\s");
    // Print each word from the array
    for (String word : w) {
      System.out.println(word);
    }
    }
}
```

Output:

```
Dr.
Usha
rani
Bhimavarapu
```

Inside the `main` method, a String variable `s` is declared and initialized with the value "Dr. Usha rani Bhimavarapu." The `split()` method on the String `s` splits it into an array of words based on whitespace characters. The `split()` method takes a regular expression as its argument, and in this case, the regular expression "\\s" is used to match any whitespace character, including spaces and tabs. The resulting array of words is stored in the String array `w`. A `for` loop is then employed to iterate through the elements of the array, and each word is printed to the console using `System.out.println()`. The output of the program will be each word from the original string printed on a new line. The words "Dr.," "Usha," "rani," and "Bhimavarapu" are printed separately.

Program

```
import java.util.List;
import java.util.stream.Collectors;
public class Main {
  void main(String[] args) {
  // Initialize strings
  String s = "Dr. USha rani Bhimavarapu";
  String s1 = "TESTING";
  String s2 = "  Andhra Pradesh State  ";
  String s3 = "Vijayawada City\n";
  String s4 = "usha";
  // Check if the string is blank
  System.out.println(s.isBlank()); // false
  s = "";
  System.out.println(s.isBlank()); // true
  // Convert s1 into a stream of lines and collect into a list
  List<String> lines = s1.lines().collect(Collectors.toList());
  System.out.println(lines); // [TESTING]
  // Strip whitespace and print with '#' characters
  System.out.println("#" + s2.strip() + "#"); // #Andhra Pradesh State#
  System.out.println("#" + s2.stripLeading() + "#"); //  #Andhra  Pradesh
                                                        State  #
  System.out.println("#" + s2.stripTrailing() + "#"); //        # Andhra
                                                         Pradesh State#
  // Repeat strings and print
  System.out.println(s3.repeat(3)); // Vijayawada City\nVijayawada City\
                                    nVijayawada City\n
  System.out.println(s4.repeat(2)); // ushausha
  }
}
```

Output:
```
false
true
[TESTING]
#Andhra Pradesh State#
#Andhra Pradesh State  #
#  Andhra Pradesh State#
Vijayawada City
Vijayawada City
Vijayawada City
ushausha
```

The program begins by initializing a string `s` with the value "Dr. USha rani Bhimavarapu." The `isBlank()` method is then applied to check if the string is empty or consists only of whitespace characters. The result is printed to the console, and the sets `s` to an empty string and performs the `isBlank()` check again, illustrating the behavior of this method. Next, a string `s1` containing the uppercase word "TESTING" is printed to the console. The `lines()` method is then utilized to convert `s1` into a stream of lines, and the `collect()` method from the `Collectors` class is applied to gather these lines into a `List`. The resulting list is printed to demonstrate the usage of the `lines()` method in breaking a string into lines. Another string `s2` with leading and trailing whitespace is initialized, and various methods related to whitespace handling are showcased. The original string, modified with `strip()`, `stripLeading()`, and `stripTrailing()` methods, is printed with surrounding '#' characters to visualize the whitespace manipulation. Subsequently, a string `s3` containing the text "Vijayawada City" followed by a newline character is used with the `repeat()` method. The `repeat(3)` call generates a string by repeating the original string three times, demonstrating the repetition capability of the `repeat()` method. Additionally, another string `s3` with the value "usha" is repeated twice using `repeat(2)`.

4.10 STRING BUFFER

Java's StringBuffer class is employed for the creation of mutable (modifiable) String objects, allowing for dynamic changes to the content. Unlike the String class, which is immutable, StringBuffer provides the flexibility to modify its content as needed. It is noteworthy that the StringBuffer class is thread-safe, meaning that multiple threads cannot access it simultaneously, ensuring orderly and synchronized operations.

Mutable strings are those that can be altered or modified, and for this purpose, Java provides the StringBuffer and StringBuilder classes. These classes offer various methods to manipulate and update the content of a string:

- `append()` Method: The `append()` method concatenates the specified argument with the current string represented by the StringBuffer.
- `insert()` Method: The `insert()` method inserts the given string at the specified position within the current StringBuffer.
- `replace()` Method: The `replace()` method replaces a portion of the string, specified by the beginIndex and endIndex, with the provided string.
- `delete()` Method: The `delete()` method removes characters from the StringBuffer, starting from the beginIndex to the endIndex.
- `reverse()` Method: The `reverse()` method reverses the characters of the current StringBuffer.
- `capacity()` Method: The `capacity()` method returns the current capacity of the StringBuffer. If the number of characters exceeds the current capacity, it automatically increases the capacity by a specific formula (oldcapacity*2)+2.

- ensureCapacity()` Method: The `ensureCapacity()` method ensures that the given capacity becomes the minimum capacity for the current StringBuffer. If the specified capacity is greater than the current capacity, it increases the capacity using the same formula as mentioned in the `capacity()` method.

In essence, the StringBuffer class provides a mutable alternative to the immutable String class in Java, allowing for dynamic modifications and ensuring thread-safe operations when accessed by multiple threads.

Program
manipulation of strings in a mutable manner.

```
public class Main {
  void main(String[] args) {
  // Initialize a StringBuffer object with the initial value "testing"
  StringBuffer sb = new StringBuffer("testing");
  // Use the append() method to concatenate "stringbuffer" to the existing
  content
  sb.append(" stringbuffer");
  // Print the modified string
  System.out.println(sb.toString());
  }
}
Output:
testing stringbuffer
```

Within the `main` method, a `StringBuffer` object named `sb` is instantiated and initialized with the initial value "testing." The `append()` method is then employed on the `StringBuffer` object `sb` to concatenate the string "stringbuffer" to its existing content. Importantly, the `StringBuffer` class allows for mutable strings, meaning that the original string can be altered. In this case, the `append()` method modifies the content of the `sb` object by appending the specified string. Concluded with the use of `System.out.println()` to print the modified string, resulting in the output: "testing stringbuffer.".

Program

```
public class Main {
  void main(String[] args) {
  // Initialize a StringBuffer object with the initial value "test"
  StringBuffer sb = new StringBuffer("test");
  // Use the insert() method to insert "Java" at index 3
  sb.insert(3, "Java");
  // Print the modified string
  System.out.println(sb.toString());
  }
}
Output:
tesJavat
```

Within the `main` method, a `StringBuffer` object named `sb` is instantiated and initialized with the initial value "test." The `insert()` method is then utilized on the `StringBuffer` object `sb` to insert the string "Java" at the specified position, which in this case is the index 3. Unlike immutable strings, the `StringBuffer` class allows for dynamic modifications, and the `insert()` method provides a means to insert new content at a specified position within the string. In this program, the original string "test" is altered, and the specified string "Java" is inserted at index 3, resulting in the modified string "testJava." The modified string is printed using `System.out.println()`, resulting in the output " tesJavat."

Program

```
public class Main {
  void main(String[] args) {
  // Initialize a StringBuffer object with the initial value "usharani"
  StringBuffer sb = new StringBuffer("usharani");
  // Use the replace() method to replace characters from index 2 to 4
  with "test"
  sb.replace(2, 4, "test");
  // Print the modified string
  System.out.println(sb.toString());
  }
}
```

Output

```
ustestrani
```

Within the `main` method, a `StringBuffer` object named `sb` is instantiated and initialized with the initial value "usharani." The `replace()` method is then applied to the `StringBuffer` object `sb` to substitute a portion of the string. In this case, the characters at positions 2 to 4 (exclusive) are replaced with the string "test." Unlike immutable strings, the `StringBuffer` class supports such dynamic modifications, enabling the alteration of specific segments within the string. After the `replace()` operation, the original string "usharani" is modified, and the specified replacement "test" is inserted in the designated position, resulting in the modified string "utestrani." The modified string is printed using `System.out.println()`, producing the output " ustestrani."

Program

```
public class Main {
  void main(String[] args) {
  // Initialize a StringBuffer object with the initial value "testing"
  StringBuffer sb = new StringBuffer("testing");
  // Use the delete() method to remove characters from index 2 to 4
  (exclusive)
  sb.delete(2, 5); // Deletes characters from index 2 to 4
  // Print the modified string
  System.out.println(sb.toString());
  }
}
```

Output:

```
teng
```

Within the `main` method, a `StringBuffer` object named `sb` is instantiated and initialized with the initial value "testing." The program utilizes the `delete()` method on the `StringBuffer` object `sb` to remove a specified portion of the string. In this instance, the characters at positions 2 to 4 (exclusive) are deleted, altering the original string "testing." After the execution of the `delete()` operation, the modified string is now "teng." The `System.out.println()` statement is then employed to print the updated string to the console.

Program

```
public class Main {
  void main(String[] args) {
  // Initialize a StringBuffer object with the initial value "testing"
  StringBuffer sb = new StringBuffer("testing");
  // Use the reverse() method to reverse the characters in the StringBuffer
  sb.reverse();
  // Print the reversed string
  System.out.println(sb.toString());
  }
}
Output:
gnitset
```

Inside the `main` method, a `StringBuffer` object named `sb` is instantiated and initialized with the initial value "testing." The `reverse()` method on the `StringBuffer` object `sb` reverses the characters within the string. Unlike immutable strings, `StringBuffer` allows for dynamic modifications, and the `reverse()` method provides a straightforward way to invert the order of characters in the string. Upon executing the `reverse()` operation, the original string "testing" is modified, resulting in the reversed string "gnitset." The modified string is printed to the console using `System.out.println()`, resulting in the output "gnitset."

Program

```
public class Main {
  void main(String[] args) {
  // Initialize a StringBuffer object without initial content
  StringBuffer sb = new StringBuffer();
  // Print the initial capacity of the StringBuffer
  System.out.println(sb.capacity());
  // Append the string "Usharani" to the StringBuffer
  sb.append("Usharani");
  // Print the capacity after appending the first string
  System.out.println(sb.capacity());
  // Append the string "Bhimavarapu" to the StringBuffer
  sb.append("Bhimavarapu");
  // Print the final capacity after appending the second string
  System.out.println(sb.capacity());
  }
}
Output:
16
16
34
```

Within the `main` method, a `StringBuffer` object named `sb` is instantiated without any initial content. The `capacity()` method determines and print the initial capacity of the `StringBuffer` object, which by default is 16 characters. Following this, the the `append()` method adds the string "Usharani" to the `StringBuffer` object. Subsequently, the updated capacity of the `StringBuffer` object is printed, which may have changed if the length of the appended string exceeded the initial capacity. Finally, another string, "Bhimavarapu," is appended to the existing content of the

`StringBuffer`, and then prints the final capacity of the `StringBuffer`. The output of the program will display the initial capacity, the capacity after appending the first string, and the final capacity after adding the second string. i.e. (Initial capacity*2)+2.

4.11 STRING BUILDER

The StringBuilder in Java is employed for managing a modifiable sequence of characters. In contrast to the String class, which generates an unchangeable sequence of characters, the StringBuilder class serves as a mutable alternative, allowing dynamic modifications to the character sequence. The functionality of the StringBuilder closely parallels that of the StringBuffer class, as both offer alternatives to the immutable nature of the String class by facilitating the creation of mutable character sequences. Nevertheless, the StringBuilder class diverges from the StringBuffer class in terms of synchronization. Unlike the StringBuffer class, the StringBuilder class does not ensure synchronization. Consequently, it is intended for seamless substitution in scenarios where the StringBuffer was originally utilized in a single-threaded context, as is typically the case. In situations where synchronization is unnecessary, it is advisable to prefer the StringBuilder class over StringBuffer, as it tends to exhibit superior performance across most implementations. Instances of StringBuilder lack thread safety and are not designed for concurrent use by multiple threads. In cases where synchronization is imperative, the StringBuffer class is recommended. StringBuilder is acknowledged for its non-thread-safe nature and notable performance advantages when compared to the StringBuffer class.

Program

```
public class Main {
  void main(String[] args) {
  // Create and initialize a StringBuilder with the string "Usha"
  StringBuilder sb = new StringBuilder("Usha");
  // Append the string "rani" to the StringBuilder
  sb.append("rani");
  System.out.println(sb); // Output: Usharani
  // Insert the string "Dr." at the beginning of the StringBuilder
  sb.insert(0, "Dr.");
  System.out.println(sb); // Output: Dr.Usharani
  // Replace the substring from index 7 to 11 (exclusive) with "Rani"
  sb.replace(7, 11, "Rani");
  System.out.println(sb); // Output: Dr.UshaRani
  // Print the current capacity of the StringBuilder
  System.out.println(sb.capacity()); // Output: 20 (Capacity may vary)
  // Delete the substring from index 7 to 11 (exclusive)
  sb.delete(7, 11);
  System.out.println(sb); // Output: Dr.Usha
  // Reverse the content of the StringBuilder
  sb.reverse();
  System.out.println(sb); // Output: ahsU.rD
  }
}
```

Output:

```
Usharani
Dr.Usharani
Dr.UshaRani
20
Dr.Usha
ahsU.rD
```

Inside the `main` method, a StringBuilder object named `sb` is created and initialized with the string "Usha". Firstly, the `append` method concatenates the string "rani" to the existing StringBuilder, resulting in the string "Usharani". The StringBuilder is then printed, displaying the updated content. Next, the `insert` method is employed to insert the prefix "Dr." at the beginning of the StringBuilder, transforming it into "Dr.Usharani". The StringBuilder is printed again to showcase the modification. The `replace` method is utilized to replace the substring from index 7 to 11 (exclusive) with the string "Rani". This operation changes the StringBuilder content to "Dr.UshaRani", and the modified StringBuilder is printed. Later is printed the current capacity of the StringBuilder using the `capacity` method.. Subsequently, the `delete` method is applied to remove the substring from index 7 to 11 (exclusive), resulting in the StringBuilder content "Dr.Usha". The modified StringBuilder is printed after this operation. Finally, the `reverse` method is used to reverse the characters within the StringBuilder, resulting in the string "ahsU. rD". The program prints the final content of the StringBuilder after this reversal.

4.12 STRING TOKENIZER

The StringTokenizer class in Java serves the purpose of dividing a string into distinct tokens. Internally, a StringTokenizer object maintains a current position within the string being tokenized, and certain operations cause this position to advance beyond the processed characters. This class plays a crucial role in the initial stage of the parsing process, often referred to as the lexer or scanner.

Java's String Tokenization involves the utilization of the StringTokenizer class, allowing applications to dissect strings into tokens effectively. The class implements the enumeration interface, facilitating the enumeration of tokens. It is primarily employed for parsing data, requiring the specification of both an input string and a string containing delimiters. Delimiters, in this context, are characters that act as separators between tokens. Each character within the delimiter string is recognized as a valid delimiter. By default, common whitespace characters such as spaces, new lines, and tabs serve as delimiters. In essence, the StringTokenizer class provides a mechanism for breaking down strings into manageable tokens based on specified delimiters, offering a fundamental step in the parsing process within Java applications.

Program

```
import java.util.StringTokenizer;
public class Main {
  void main(String[] args) {
  // Initialize a StringTokenizer with the string "This is to test."
  StringTokenizer tokenizer = new StringTokenizer("This is to test.");
  // Initialize a counter for token index
  int tokenIndex = 1;
  // Iterate over the tokens
  while (tokenizer.hasMoreTokens()) {
    // Retrieve the next token
    String token = tokenizer.nextToken();
    // Print the token with its index
    System.out.println("Token " + tokenIndex + ": " + token);
    // Increment the token index
    tokenIndex++;
  }
  }
}
```

Output:

```
Token 1: This
Token 2: is
Token 3: to
```

```
Token 4: test.
```

Inside the `main` method, an instance of the `StringTokenizer` class is created, initialized with the string "This is to test." The `StringTokenizer` class is part of the `java.util` package and is commonly used to break a string into tokens. A `for` loop is employed to iterate over the tokens obtained from the `StringTokenizer` instance. The loop condition checks if there are more tokens to process using the `hasMoreTokens()` method. If a token is available, the `nextToken()` method is called to retrieve and print the token along with its corresponding index. The output of the program will display each token in the given string along with its index.

4.13 STRING TEMPLATES

The introduction of String Templates in Java 22 addresses several practical needs in modern software development, particularly in enhancing code readability, improving security, and simplifying the process of string interpolation.

Needs for String Templates in Java 22

- Improved Readability and Expressiveness: String Templates provide a more natural and readable way to embed expressions within string literals. This feature allows developers to directly include variables and expressions in strings without using complex concatenation or formatting methods, thereby making the code more concise and easier to understand.
- Enhanced Security: When constructing strings from user-provided or dynamically computed values, developers often need to ensure that the resulting strings are correctly formatted and secure against injection attacks (such as SQL injection or script injection). String Templates promote secure coding practices by automatically handling escaping and formatting, reducing the risk of security vulnerabilities.
- Simplified String Concatenation: Before Java 22, concatenating strings with variables or expressions required explicit handling of concatenation operators (`+`) and conversion of non-string values to strings. String Templates streamline this process by allowing developers to directly embed expressions within `${}` placeholders, eliminating the need for manual conversion and concatenation.
- Facilitates Internationalization (i18n): String Templates support the process of internationalization by allowing developers to embed localized variables and expressions directly within string literals. This makes it easier to manage and maintain localized versions of applications without modifying the structure of the original strings.
- Compatibility with Modern Programming Patterns: String Templates align with modern programming patterns and frameworks that emphasize readability, simplicity, and developer productivity. They facilitate the adoption of declarative programming styles by providing a straightforward way to include variables and expressions within strings.

Program

```
class Demo {
  void main(String[]a) {
  String name="Usharani";
  String greeting = STR."Hello, \{name}!";
  System.out.println(greeting);
  }
}
Output:
Hello, Usharani!
```

The above program creates a greeting message using a string template and prints it to the console. It uses the name "Usharani" to generate the greeting message "Hello, Usharani!".

Program

```
class Demo {
  void main(String[] args) {
  int a=10,b=20;
  String result = STR."The sum of \{a} and \{b} is \{a + b}.";
  System.out.println(result);
  }
}
Output:
The sum of 10 and 20 is 30.
```

This program calculates the sum of two integers and prints the result using a string template. It uses variables a and b to generate the message "The sum of 10 and 20 is 30".

Program

```
class Demo {
  void main(String[] args) {
double price=24.56;
  String formattedPrice = STR."The price is \{String.format("%.2f", price)}
  dollars.";
  System.out.println(formattedPrice);
  }
}
Output
The price is 24.56 dollars.
```

This program uses a string template to include a formatted price within a message. Specifically, it formats the price to two decimal places using String.format.

4.14 JAVA REGULAR EXPRESSION

In Java, regular expressions (regex) provide a powerful way to search, manipulate, and validate strings based on patterns. Regular expressions are powerful tools for string manipulation and validation in Java, offering a versatile way to handle text processing tasks effectively.

4.14.1 Benefits of Regular Expressions in Java

- Flexibility: Allows complex pattern matching and manipulation of strings.
- Efficiency: Provides optimized matching algorithms.
- Consistency: Helps maintain uniform data validation across applications.
- Expressiveness: Concisely defines patterns for searching and replacing text.

4.14.2 Basics of Regular Expressions in Java

4.14.2.1 Creating a Pattern

In Java, regular expressions are represented by the `Pattern` class from the `java.util.regex` package. You can create a pattern using the `Pattern.compile()` method, which compiles the regex into a `Pattern` object.

Program

```
import java.util.regex.*;
public class RegexExample {
  void main(String[] args) {
  String regex = "ab+c";
  Pattern pattern = Pattern.compile(regex);
  System.out.println(pattern);
  }
}
Output
ab+c
```

In this program, a regular expression pattern "ab+c" is defined and compiled using the `Pattern.compile()` method. The program then prints the compiled pattern, which confirms the creation of the regex object. The output reflects the regular expression itself.

4.14.2.2 Matching and Searching

Once you have a `Pattern` object, you can use it to create a `Matcher` object that can perform various operations like matching, searching, and replacing strings based on the pattern.

Program

```
import java.util.regex.*;
public class RegexExample {
  void main(String[] args) {
  String regex = "ab+c";
  Pattern pattern = Pattern.compile(regex);
  String input = "abbbc";
  Matcher matcher = pattern.matcher(input);
  boolean matches = matcher.matches(); // true if whole input matches
                                          the regex
  boolean found = matcher.find(); // true if regex pattern is found in
                                    the input
System.out.println(matches);
System.out.println(found);
  }
}
Output
true
false
```

In "RegexExample" example, a regular expression `ab+c` is compiled into a pattern. The input string `"abbbc"` is then tested against this pattern using a matcher. The `matches()` method checks if the entire input string matches the regex, while the `find()` method looks for any occurrence of the pattern within the input. The results are printed, indicating whether the full match or any match was found.

4.14.2.3 Regex Methods

- `matches()`: Checks if the entire input string matches the regex pattern.
- `find()`: Searches for occurrences of the regex pattern within the input string.

- `group()`: Returns the string that matched the regex pattern.
- `start()` and `end()`: Return the start and end index of the matched substring.

4.14.2.4 Common Regex Patterns

- `.`: Matches any single character.
- `[abc]`: Matches any character within the brackets.
- `[^abc]`: Matches any character not within the brackets.
- `\d`: Matches any digit (equivalent to `[0-9]`).
- `\w`: Matches any word character (equivalent to `[a-zA-Z0-9_]`).
- -`\s`: Matches any whitespace character.
- `*`, `+`, `?`: Quantifiers that specify how many times a character or group can occur (`*` zero or more, `+` one or more, `?` zero or one).

4.14.2.5 Example: Validating an Email

Program

```
import java.util.regex.*;
public class EmailValidator {
  void main(String[] args) {
  String email = "usharanibhimavarapu@gmail.com";
  String regex = "^[a-zA-Z0-9_]+@[a-zA-Z0-9]+\\.[a-zA-Z]{2,}$";
  Pattern pattern = Pattern.compile(regex);
  Matcher matcher = pattern.matcher(email);
  if (matcher.matches()) {
    System.out.println("Valid email format.");
  } else {
    System.out.println("Invalid email format.");
  }
  }
}
```

Output:

```
Valid email format.
```

In this program, an email validation logic is implemented using regular expressions. The regex pattern `^[a-zA-Z0-9_]+@[a-zA-Z0-9]+\\.[a-zA-Z]{2,}$` is designed to match a valid email format, which includes alphanumeric characters and underscores before the "@" symbol, a domain name, and a top-level domain with at least two characters. The input email address `"usharanibhimavarapu@gmail.com"` is tested against this pattern using a matcher. If the email format matches the regex, the program prints "Valid email format."; otherwise, it prints "Invalid email format." The program prints "Valid email format." since the email address `"usharanibhimavarapu@gmail.com"` matches the specified regex pattern for valid email formats.

4.15 MEDICAL APPLICATIONS

4.15.1 Case Study 1

Buerger's disease, also known as thromboangiitis obliterans, is a rare disease of the arteries and veins in the arms and legs. Symptoms may include pain in the hands and feet, which may be severe, and claudication.

- Symptoms of Buerger's disease: An array of predefined symptoms associated with Buerger's disease (buergersSymptoms).

The program prompts the user to enter symptoms experienced by the patient, compares these symptoms with the predefined symptoms of Buerger's disease, and outputs whether Buerger's disease is detected or not based on matching symptoms.

```
import java.util.Scanner;
public class BuergersDiseaseDetection {
  void main(String[] args) {
  Scanner scanner = new Scanner(System.in);
  // Symptoms of Buerger's disease
  String[] buergersSymptoms = {"Pain in hands and feet", "Claudication",
     "Pale, red or blue toes or fingers"};
  // Patient symptoms array
  String[] patientSymptoms = new String[3];
  // Input patient symptoms
  System.out.println("Enter symptoms experienced by the patient:");
  for (int i = 0; i < patientSymptoms.length; i++) {
    System.out.print("Symptom " + (i + 1) + ": ");
    patientSymptoms[i] = scanner.nextLine();
  }
  // Check for Buerger's disease
  boolean hasBuergers = checkBuergers(buergersSymptoms, patientSymptoms);
  // Output the result
  System.out.println("Buergers Disease Detection Result:");
  System.out.println(hasBuergers ? "Buergers Disease Detected" : "Buergers
  Disease Not Detected");
  }
// Method to check for Buerger's disease based on symptoms
private static boolean checkBuergers(String[] buergersSymptoms, String[]
patientSymptoms) {
  for (String buergersSymptom : buergersSymptoms) {
    for (String patientSymptom : patientSymptoms) {
      if (patientSymptom.equalsIgnoreCase(buergersSymptom)) {
        return true;
      }
    }
  }
  return false;
  }
}
```

The Java program "BuergersDiseaseDetection" is designed to assist in detecting Buerger's disease based on user-input symptoms. It begins by initializing an array named buergersSymptoms with typical symptoms associated with Buerger's disease, such as pain in hands and feet, claudication, and discoloration of toes or fingers. The user is then prompted to enter their symptoms, which are stored in the patientSymptoms array using a for loop that iterates through each index of the array.

Following this, the program employs a method named checkBuergers to compare the symptoms entered by the user (patientSymptoms) with the predefined symptoms of Buerger's disease (buergersSymptoms). This method utilizes nested loops to iterate through both arrays and checks for any matching symptoms, disregarding case sensitivity. If a match is found during this comparison process, the program sets a boolean variable hasBuergers to true, indicating the possible presence of Buerger's disease based on the symptoms entered.

Once the comparison is completed, the program outputs the result of the disease detection. If hasBuergers is true, it prints "Buergers Disease Detected", suggesting that the symptoms entered by the user match those commonly associated with Buerger's disease. Conversely, if no matches are found, it prints "Buergers Disease Not Detected", implying that the entered symptoms do not align with the typical symptoms of the disease.

4.15.2 Case Study 2

Crohn's disease is a chronic inflammatory condition that primarily affects the gastrointestinal tract, causing inflammation and damage to the lining of the digestive system. It is a type of inflammatory bowel disease (IBD) and can affect any part of the gastrointestinal tract, from the mouth to the anus. The parameters considered are:

- CRP (C-Reactive Protein) Level: CRP is a marker of inflammation in the body. Elevated levels of CRP can indicate inflammation, which is common in Crohn's disease due to the chronic inflammation of the gastrointestinal tract.
- ESR (Erythrocyte Sedimentation Rate): ESR measures how quickly red blood cells settle at the bottom of a test tube. Higher ESR levels suggest the presence of inflammation in the body, which can be indicative of Crohn's disease.
- WBC (White Blood Cell) Count: WBCs are a part of the immune system and an elevated WBC count can indicate inflammation or infection, which is often seen in Crohn's disease flare-ups.
- Hemoglobin Level: Hemoglobin is a protein in red blood cells that carries oxygen. Low levels of hemoglobin (anemia) can occur in Crohn's disease due to blood loss from inflamed intestines or malnutrition.
- Albumin Level: Albumin is a protein made by the liver. Low albumin levels can indicate malnutrition or severe inflammation, which can occur in Crohn's disease if there is poor nutrient absorption or chronic inflammation affecting the liver.

The thresholds are based on typical clinical findings and may vary depending on the healthcare provider's assessment.

- CRP Threshold: Elevated CRP levels (>10.0 mg/L) indicate inflammation.
- ESR Threshold: Elevated ESR levels (>20.0 mm/hr) indicate inflammation.
- WBC Threshold: Elevated WBC counts (>11.0 x10^9/L) suggest an immune response.
- Hemoglobin Threshold: Low hemoglobin levels (<12.0 g/dL) indicate anemia.
- Albumin Threshold: Low albumin levels (<3.5 g/dL) indicate malnutrition or inflammation.

If a patient's test results exceed these thresholds in a manner consistent with Crohn's disease patterns then the "Crohn's Disease Detected". Otherwise, "Crohn's Disease Not Detected".

```
import java.util.Scanner;
public class CrohnsDiseaseDetection {
  void main(String[] args) {
```

```
  Scanner scanner = new Scanner(System.in);
  // Input blood test parameters
  System.out.println("Enter CRP level (mg/L): ");
  double crp = scanner.nextDouble();
  System.out.println("Enter ESR level (mm/hr): ");
  double esr = scanner.nextDouble();
  System.out.println("Enter WBC count (x10^9/L): ");
  double wbc = scanner.nextDouble();
  System.out.println("Enter Hemoglobin level (g/dL): ");
  double hemoglobin = scanner.nextDouble();
  System.out.println("Enter Albumin level (g/dL): ");
  double albumin = scanner.nextDouble();
  // Determine if the patient has Crohn's disease based on thresholds
  boolean hasCrohns = detectCrohnsDisease(crp, esr, wbc, hemoglobin,
  albumin);
  // Output the result
  System.out.println("Crohn's Disease Detection Result:");
  System.out.println(hasCrohns ? "Crohn's Disease Detected" : "Crohn's
  Disease Not Detected");
  scanner.close();
  }
  private static boolean detectCrohnsDisease(double crp, double esr, double
  wbc, double hemoglobin, double albumin) {
  // Define thresholds for detecting Crohn's disease
  double crpThreshold = 10.0;      // CRP level (mg/L)
  double esrThreshold = 20.0;      // ESR level (mm/hr)
  double wbcThreshold = 11.0;      // WBC count (x10^9/L)
  double hemoglobinThreshold = 12.0;  // Hemoglobin level (g/dL)
  double albuminThreshold = 3.5;    // Albumin level (g/dL)
  // Check if the patient's parameters exceed the thresholds
  if (crp > crpThreshold && esr > esrThreshold && wbc > wbcThreshold &&
    hemoglobin < hemoglobinThreshold && albumin < albuminThreshold) {
    return true;
  }
  return false;
  }
}
```

The program "CrohnsDiseaseDetection" facilitates the detection of Crohn's disease based on inputted test parameters. It begins by initializing a `Scanner` object to receive user input for biomarkers associated with Crohn's disease. The user is prompted to enter levels of CRP (C-reactive protein), ESR (erythrocyte sedimentation rate), WBC (white blood cell count), hemoglobin, and albumin. Each parameter is stored as a double variable for subsequent evaluation.

Following input collection, the program invokes the `detectCrohnsDisease` method, which compares the entered values against predefined thresholds known to indicate Crohn's disease. These thresholds include CRP levels above 10.0 mg/L, ESR levels above 20.0 mm/hr, WBC counts above 11.0 x10^9/L, and low levels of hemoglobin (below 12.0 g/dL) and albumin (below 3.5 g/dL). If all conditions are met based on the entered values, the method returns `true`, indicating a potential presence of Crohn's disease.

The program then outputs the detection result based on the method's return value. If `hasCrohns` is `true`, it prints "Crohn's Disease Detected", suggesting that the test parameters entered align with the diagnostic thresholds for Crohn's disease. Conversely, if no conditions are met, it prints "Crohn's Disease Not Detected".

5 Java Methods

5.1 INTRODUCTION

In Java, a method is a block of code that performs a specific task or operation. It encapsulates a set of instructions within a defined scope and can be invoked or called from other parts of the program to execute its functionality. Methods enable code reuse, modularization, and abstraction, making programs more organized, efficient, and maintainable.

Advantages of Methods

- Code Reusability: Methods facilitate the reuse of code, reducing duplication and promoting consistency across the program.
- Modularity:Methods enhance code organization by breaking down complex tasks into smaller, more manageable units, improving readability and maintainability.
- Abstraction: Methods abstract away implementation details, providing a clear interface for interacting with functionality without needing to understand its internal workings.
- Parameterization: Methods can accept parameters, allowing them to operate on different data inputs, thus increasing flexibility and adaptability.
- Encapsulation: Methods encapsulate functionality, promoting data hiding and ensuring that only relevant information is exposed to other parts of the program.

Limitations of Methods

- Performance Overhead: Invoking methods incurs a slight performance overhead due to method call overhead and parameter passing, although modern JVMs optimize this to a large extent.
- Complexity: Excessive use of methods can lead to code fragmentation and increased complexity, making the program harder to understand and maintain.
- Overhead: Defining and managing a large number of methods can introduce overhead in terms of memory consumption and program size.
- Debugging: Debugging methods can sometimes be challenging, especially if they are overly complex or if errors occur deep within nested method calls.

Despite these limitations, the benefits of methods generally outweigh their drawbacks, making them an indispensable tool for writing clean, efficient, and maintainable Java code.

DOI: 10.1201/9781003544319-5

Syntax

```
accessModifier returnType methodName(parameterType parameter1, parameterType
parameter2, ...) {
  // Method body
  // Statements
  return value; // Optional return statement
}
```

- Access Modifier: Specifies the accessibility of the method (e.g., `public`, `private`, `protected`, or default access).
- Return Type: Specifies the data type of the value returned by the method. Use `void` if the method does not return a value.
- Method Name: The name of the method, which must be a valid Java identifier.
- Parameters: Input data passed to the method. Parameters are optional, and a method may have zero or more parameters.
- Method Body: Contains the statements that define the behavior of the method.
- Return Statement: Optional statement used to return a value from the method. It is not required for methods with `void` return type.

Program

```
public class Calculator {
    // Method to add two integers
  public int add(int num1, int num2) {
    return num1 + num2;
  }
  // Method to subtract two integers
  public int subtract(int num1, int num2) {
    return num1 - num2;
  }
  // Method to multiply two integers
  public int multiply(int num1, int num2) {
    return num1 * num2;
  }
  // Method to divide two integers
  public double divide(int num1, int num2) {
    if (num2 != 0) {
      return (double) num1 / num2;
    } else {
      throw new IllegalArgumentException("Cannot divide by zero");
    }
  }
  // Main method to test the Calculator class
  void main(String[] args) {
    Calculator calculator = new Calculator();
    System.out.println("Addition: " + calculator.add(10, 5));
    System.out.println("Subtraction: " + calculator.subtract(10, 5));
    System.out.println("Multiplication: " + calculator.multiply(10, 5));
    System.out.println("Division: " + calculator.divide(10, 5));
  }
}
```

```
Output:
Addition: 15
Subtraction: 5
Multiplication: 50
Division: 2.0
```

In this program, a `Calculator` class is created to perform basic arithmetic operations. The class includes four methods: `add`, `subtract`, `multiply`, and `divide`, each designed to take two integer parameters and return the result of the respective operation. The `divide` method includes error handling to prevent division by zero by throwing an `IllegalArgumentException`. The `main` method creates an instance of the `Calculator` class and tests the arithmetic methods using the values 10 and 5. It prints the results of each operation—addition, subtraction, multiplication, and division—to the console. The results are as follows: the addition of 10 and 5 gives 15, the subtraction results in 5, the multiplication yields 50, and the division results in 2.0. This demonstrates the functionality of the `Calculator` class effectively.

Methods can be called from within the same class or from other classes by creating an object of the class containing the method. A method can have zero or more parameters. The order, number, and data types of the parameters must match when calling the method. Methods can be overloaded, meaning a class can have multiple methods with the same name but different parameter lists. A method can optionally have a return statement to return a value to the caller. If the return type is `void`, no value is returned. A method's accessibility can be controlled using access modifiers (`public`, `private`, `protected`, or default access).

5.2 TYPES OF METHODS

In Java, methods can be categorized as user-defined or predefined based on how they are created and their purpose.

5.2.1 User-Defined Methods

User-defined methods are created by the programmer to perform specific tasks within a Java program. These methods are defined within classes and can be invoked by the programmer as needed.

Program

```
Program of User-Defined Method:
public class MyClass {
  // User-defined method
  public void greet() {
    System.out.println("This is to test");
  }
  void main(String[] args) {
    MyClass obj = new MyClass();
    obj.greet(); // Calling user-defined method
  }
}
Output:
This is to test
```

In this program, a class named `MyClass` is defined, which contains a user-defined method called `greet()`. This method, when called, prints the message "This is to test" to the console.

In the `main` method, an instance of `MyClass` is created, and the `greet()` method is invoked using this instance. This execution results in the output of the greeting message. The program demonstrates how to define and call methods within a class in Java. When run, the output will be:This is to test.

5.2.2 Predefined Methods (Built-in Methods)

Predefined methods, also known as built-in methods, are provided by Java's standard libraries or external libraries. These methods are available for use without the programmer needing to define them explicitly.

Program

```
public class PredefinedMethodExample {
  void main(String[] args) {
    String str = "Usharani!";
    int length = str.length();
    System.out.println("Length of the string: " + length);
  }
}
Output:
Length of the string: 9
```

In this program, a class named `PredefinedMethodExample` is defined, which contains a `main` method that demonstrates the use of a predefined method in Java. A string variable `str` is initialized with the value "Usharani!". Then called the `length()` method on this string to determine the number of characters it contains. The length is stored in the variable `length`, which is subsequently printed to the console. The output of the program will be: Length of the string: 9. This indicates that the string "Usharani!" has 9 characters, including the exclamation mark.

In Java, there are several types of methods, each serving a different purpose. Here are the most common types of methods:

5.2.2.1 Instance Methods

Instance methods are associated with objects of a class and can access instance variables and other instance methods of the class. They are invoked using object references.

```
public class MyClass {
  private int value;
  // Instance method
  public void setValue(int newValue) {
    value = newValue;
  }
  // Another instance method
  public int getValue() {
    return value;
  }
}
```

In this program, a class named `MyClass` is defined, featuring a private instance variable called `value`. The class includes two instance methods: `setValue(int newValue)` and `getValue()`. The `setValue` method is responsible for assigning a new integer value to the private variable `value`, allowing external code to modify it in a controlled manner. Conversely, the `getValue` method retrieves the current value of the `value` variable, enabling access without direct manipulation. This approach exemplifies encapsulation in object-oriented programming, ensuring that the internal state of the class is managed through dedicated methods, promoting data integrity and controlled access.

5.2.2.2 Static Methods

Static methods belong to the class rather than to any specific instance. They can be invoked using the class name without creating an object.

```
public class MathUtils {
  // Static method
  public static int add(int a, int b) {
    return a + b;
  }
  // Another static method
  public static int subtract(int a, int b) {
    return a - b;
  }
}
```

In this program, a class named `MathUtils` is defined, containing two static methods: `add(int a, int b)` and `subtract(int a, int b)`. The `add` method takes two integer parameters and returns their sum, while the `subtract` method takes two integer parameters and returns the result of subtracting the second parameter from the first. By being declared as static, these methods can be called without needing to create an instance of the `MathUtils` class, making them easily accessible for performing basic arithmetic operations directly. This design promotes code reusability and simplicity, as users can invoke these methods directly using the class name.

5.2.2.3 Constructor Methods

Constructor methods are special methods invoked when an object of a class is created using the `new` keyword. They initialize the object's state.

```
public class test {
  private String name;
  // Constructor method
  public test(String initialName) {
    name = initialName;
  }
}
```

In this program, a class named `test` is defined with a private instance variable `name`. The class includes a constructor method that takes a single parameter, `initialName`, which is used to initialize the `name` variable when an object of the class is created. This constructor ensures that the `name` field is set to a specific value at the time of instantiation, encapsulating the data and providing a controlled way to initialize objects of the `test` class. By using a constructor, the program establishes a clear and structured method for initializing the state of an object, promoting good object-oriented design principles.

5.2.2.4 Getter and Setter Methods

Getter methods retrieve the values of private instance variables, and setter methods set the values of private instance variables. They are often used to encapsulate access to instance variables.

```
public class Employee {
  private String name;
  // Getter method
  public String getName() {
    return name;
  }
  // Setter method
  public void setName(String newName) {
    name = newName;
```

```
  }
}
```

In this program, a class named `Employee` is defined with a private instance variable `name`. The class provides a getter method, `getName()`, which allows access to the value of the `name` variable, and a setter method, `setName(String newName)`, which enables modification of the `name` variable. This design follows the principles of encapsulation in object-oriented programming, allowing controlled access and modification of the private data. The getter and setter methods ensure that the `name` variable can be safely accessed and updated while maintaining the integrity of the `Employee` object's state.

5.2.2.5 Instance Initialization Blocks

Instance initialization blocks are used to initialize instance variables. They are executed each time an object of the class is created.

```
public class MyClass {
  private int value;
  // Instance initialization block
  {
    value = 10;
  }
}
```

In this program, the class `MyClass` contains a private instance variable named `value`. An instance initialization block is defined within the class, which sets the `value` variable to 10 whenever an object of `MyClass` is created. This instance initialization block runs before the constructor of the class, ensuring that the `value` is initialized to 10 for every instance of `MyClass` without needing explicit initialization in the constructor. This approach provides a convenient way to set default values for instance variables when an object is instantiated.

5.2.2.6 Static Initialization Blocks

Static initialization blocks are used to initialize static variables. They are executed when the class is loaded into memory.

```
public class MyStaticClass {
  private static int count;
  // Static initialization block
  static {
    count = 0;
  }
}
```

In this program, the class `MyStaticClass` includes a private static variable named `count`. A static initialization block is defined to initialize `count` to 0. This block executes when the class is first loaded into memory, ensuring that the `count` variable is set to 0 before any instances of the class are created or any static methods are called. Using a static initialization block allows for complex initialization logic for static variables if needed, while providing a clear and organized way to set default values for static members.

5.2.2.7 Abstract Methods

Abstract methods are declared without an implementation in abstract classes or interfaces. Subclasses must provide a concrete implementation for abstract methods.

```
public abstract class Shape {
  // Abstract method
  public abstract double area();
}
```

In this program, the class `Shape` is defined as an abstract class, which means it cannot be instantiated directly. It includes an abstract method named `area()`, which does not have a body and must be implemented by any subclass that extends `Shape`. This design enforces a contract for subclasses, requiring them to provide their own implementation of the `area()` method, allowing for polymorphism. By using an abstract class, the program establishes a framework for different shapes to define their area calculation, promoting code reusability and flexibility in handling various shape types.

5.2.2.8 Final Methods

Final methods cannot be overridden in subclasses. They can be declared in any class, including abstract classes.

```
public class Parent {
  // Final method
  public final void display() {
    System.out.println("Parent class");
  }
}
```

In this program, the class `Parent` defines a method named `display()` as a final method. This means that the method cannot be overridden by any subclasses that inherit from the `Parent` class. The `display()` method prints "Parent class" to the console when called. By declaring the method as final, the program ensures that its behavior remains consistent across all instances of the `Parent` class and its subclasses, preventing any modifications that could change the intended output. This design is useful for maintaining the integrity of the method's functionality in an inheritance hierarchy.

These are the main types of methods in Java, each serving a different purpose and providing different levels of flexibility and control in programs.

5.3 PARAMETERS AND RETURN TYPE

In Java, parameters and return types of methods can be categorized based on their data types and whether they are primitive types, reference types, or void. Here are the main categories:

5.3.1 Primitive Type Parameters and Return Types

Primitive types are basic data types in Java, such as `int`, `double`, `boolean`, etc. Methods can accept parameters and return values of primitive types.

```
public class MathUtils {
  // Method with primitive type parameters and return type
  public static int add(int a, int b) {
    return a + b;
```

```
    }
}
```

In this program, the class `MathUtils` contains a static method named `add`, which takes two parameters of the primitive type `int`. The method calculates the sum of these two integers and returns the result as an integer. By defining the method as static, it can be called without creating an instance of the `MathUtils` class. This approach is common for utility classes that provide mathematical operations, allowing for easy access to the addition functionality from other parts of the program.

5.3.2 Reference Type Parameters and Return Types

Reference types include classes, interfaces, arrays, and enums. Methods can accept parameters and return values of reference types.

```
public class StringUtils {
  // Method with reference type parameters and return type
  public static String concat(String str1, String str2) {
    return str1 + str2;
  }
}
```

In this program, the class `StringUtils` features a static method called `concat`, which takes two parameters of the reference type `String`. The method concatenates these two strings and returns the combined result as a new `String`. By defining `concat` as a static method, it can be invoked without needing to instantiate the `StringUtils` class, making it convenient for string manipulation tasks. This approach is commonly used in utility classes to provide reusable methods for string operations, allowing for efficient and clear code when combining string values in various applications.

5.3.3 Void Return Type

A method with a `void` return type does not return any value. It is used when a method performs an action but does not need to return a result.

```
public class Printer {
  // Method with void return type
  public static void printMessage(String message) {
    System.out.println(message);
  }
}
```

In this program, the `Printer` class defines a static method called `printMessage`, which has a `void` return type. This method takes a single parameter of type `String` named `message`. When invoked, it prints the provided message to the console using `System.out.println()`. The use of a void return type indicates that this method does not return any value; its purpose is solely to perform an action—specifically, to display the message. This design is common in utility classes that handle output operations, allowing for clear and straightforward message printing without the need for additional return handling.

5.3.4 Multiple Parameters

Methods can accept multiple parameters of the same or different data types.

```
public class Calculator {
  // Method with multiple parameters
  public static int add(int a, int b, int c) {
    return a + b + c;
  }
}
```

In this code, a `Calculator` class is created with a method called `add`. The `add` method accepts three integer parameters: `a`, `b`, and `c`. It performs the addition of these three integers and returns the result.

5.3.5 Varargs Parameters

Varargs (variable-length arguments) allow methods to accept a variable number of arguments of the same type.

```
public class VarargsExample {
  // Method with varargs parameter
  public static int sum(int... numbers) {
    int total = 0;
    for (int num : numbers) {
      total += num;
    }
    return total;
  }
}
```

In this code, a `VarargsExample` class is defined with a method called `sum` that uses a varargs parameter (`int... numbers`). The varargs parameter allows the method to accept a variable number of arguments. Inside the method, a `for-each` loop iterates over the passed `numbers`, and the total sum is calculated by adding each number to a `total` variable. Finally, the method returns the calculated total. This approach simplifies passing multiple arguments without having to explicitly define the number of parameters in the method signature.

Program

```
public class Test
{
  static void display(int ...v)
  {
System.out.print("Number of arguments = " + v.length + ", Contents = ");
  if(v.length==0)
System.out.println("none");
for(int x : v)
    {
System.out.print(x + "  ");
    }
System.out.println();
  }
    void main(String[] args) {
      int n1[] = { 10 };
    int n2[] = { 1, 2, 3 };
    int n3[] = { };
    display(n1);
```

```
    display(n2);
    display(n3);
      }
}
Output:
Number of arguments = 1, Contents = 10
Number of arguments = 3, Contents = 1  2  3
Number of arguments = 0, Contents = none
```

This program demonstrates the usage of varargs in Java to handle a variable number of arguments efficiently. The `display`, method takes a variable number of integer arguments using the varargs syntax (`int ...v`). Within the `display` method, the number of arguments is printed along with their contents. If there are no arguments, it prints "none." Then, it iterates over the provided arguments and prints each integer value followed by a space. After printing all the arguments, it adds a newline character to move to the next line. In the `main` method, three arrays of integers (`n1`, `n2`, and `n3`) are declared and initialized with different sets of integer values. These arrays are then passed as arguments to the `display` method in three separate function calls. The first call passes `n1`, which contains a single integer (10), the second call passes `n2`, which contains three integers (1, 2, and 3), and the third call passes `n3`, an empty array. Upon execution, the program will output the number of arguments along with their contents for each function call. For `n1`, it will print "Number of arguments = 1, Contents = 10." For `n2`, it will print "Number of arguments = 3, Contents = 1 2 3." For `n3`, since it has no arguments, it will print "Number of arguments = 0, Contents = none."

5.3.6 Array Parameters

Methods can accept arrays as parameters, allowing them to process multiple values of the same type.

```
public class ArrayExample {
  // Method with array parameter
  public static int findMax(int[] numbers) {
    int max = numbers[0];
    for (int i = 1; i < numbers.length; i++) {
      if (numbers[i] > max) {
        max = numbers[i];
      }
    }
    return max;
  }
}
```

In this code, the `ArrayExample` class defines a method named `findMax` that takes an array of integers (`int[] numbers`) as a parameter. The method finds the maximum value within the considered array by initializing the `max` variable with the first element of the array and then iterating through the rest of the elements. For each element, it checks if the current value is greater than `max`; if so, it updates the `max` value. After completing the loop, the method returns the maximum value found in the array.

5.3.7 Object Parameters

Methods can accept objects of a class as parameters, allowing them to operate on objects' state or behavior.

```
public class Person {
  private String name;
  // Method with object parameter
  public void setName(Person p) {

  }
}
```

In this code, the `Person` class has a private field `name` and a method `setName` that takes a `Person` object as its parameter. The method is intended to receive an object of the `Person` class.

5.4 CALL BY VALUE

In call by value, a copy of the actual value of the argument is passed to the method. Any changes made to the parameter within the method do not affect the original value of the argument outside the method.

Program

```
public class CallByValueExample {
  void main(String[] args) {
    int num = 10;
    System.out.println("Before calling method: " + num);
    increment(num);
    System.out.println("After calling method: " + num);
  }
  public static void increment(int x) {
    x++;
    System.out.println("Inside method: " + x);
  }
}
Output:
Before calling method: 10
Inside method: 11
After calling method: 10
```

In the above code, the concept of "call by value" is illustrated. An integer variable named `num` is initialized with a value of 10. The program first prints the value of `num` before invoking the method `increment`. When the `increment` method is called, the value of `num` is passed as an argument to the method. Inside the `increment` method, the parameter `x` (which holds the value of `num`) is incremented by 1, and the updated value is printed. However, since Java uses call by value, the modification made to `x` inside the method does not affect the original `num` variable outside the method. After the method execution, the value of `num` remains unchanged, and the program prints this unchanged value, demonstrating that the original variable is not altered by changes made inside the method when primitive types are used.

5.4.1 Call by Reference

In call by reference, a reference to the memory address of the argument is passed to the method. This means any changes made to the parameter within the method affect the original value of the argument outside the method.

Program

```
public class CallByReferenceExample {
  void main(String[] args) {
    StringBuilder str = new StringBuilder("Usha");
    System.out.println("Before calling method: " + str);
    appendtext(str);
    System.out.println("After calling method: " + str);
  }
  public static void appendtext(StringBuilder sb) {
    sb.append(" Rani");
    System.out.println("Inside method: " + sb);
  }
}
```

Output:

```
Before calling method: Usha
Inside method: Usha Rani
After calling method: Usha Rani
```

In the above program, a `StringBuilder` object named `str` is created and initialized with the value "Usha." First is printed the initial value of `str` before any modifications are made. The `appendtext` method is then called, passing the `StringBuilder` object as an argument. Inside the `appendtext` method, the string " Rani" is appended to the original string. The modified value of `str` is printed inside the method, showing the change. Finally is printed the value of `str` again after the method call, demonstrating that the original object was modified, resulting in the final output being "Usha Rani."

5.5 METHOD OVERLOADING

Method overloading allows a class to define multiple methods with the same name, but different headers.

Three ways to overload a method:

In order to overload a method, the argument lists of the methods must differ in either of these:

1. Number of Parameters.
   sum(int, int)
   sum(int, int, int)
2. Data Type of Parameters.
   sum(int, int)
   sum(int, float)
3. Sequence of Data Type of Parameters.
   sum(int, float)
   sum(float, int)

Program

Program for overload static methods

```
public class test {
  static void display(int n)
  {
System.out.println("one int argu");
  }
```

```
  static void display(int n,int m)
  {
System.out.println("two int argu");
  }
  static void display(float n)
  {
System.out.println("one float argu");
  }
  void main(String[] args) {
display(10);
display(10,10);
    display((float)10.5);
  }
}
```

Output:

```
one int argu
two int argu
one float argu
```

The above Java program demonstrates method overloading, where multiple methods named `display` have different parameter lists. The `display` method is overloaded to accept either a single integer, two integers, or a single float. In the `main` method, the `display` method is called three times with different arguments: once with a single integer (which prints "one int argu"), once with two integers (which prints "two int argu"), and once with a float (which prints "one float argu").

Program

Program for final class method overloading in java

```
final class test
{
  void display()
  {
System.out.println("0 parameter display()");
  }
  void display(int i)
  {
System.out.println("1 int parameter display()"+i);
  }
  void display(String s)
  {
System.out.println("1 string parameter display()"+s);
  }
  void display(int i,int j)
  {
System.out.println("2 int parameter display()"+i+" "+j);
  }
}
class sample
{
  void main(String a[])
  {
    test t=new test();
t.display();
t.display(10);
t.display("testing");
```

```
t.display(100,200);
  }
}
```

Output:

```
0 parameter display()
1 int parameter display()10
1 string parameter display()testing
2 int parameter display()100 200
```

The above Java program demonstrates method overloading within a `final` class named `test`. The `test` class contains four overloaded `display` methods: one without parameters, one with a single integer parameter, one with a single string parameter, and one with two integer parameters. Each method prints a specific message indicating which version of `display` was called along with any provided arguments. In the `main` method of the `sample` class, an instance of the `test` class is created, and each overloaded `display` method is called in turn, showcasing the different outputs based on the method's parameters.

Program

Program for Static method overloading and calling those methods from different class in java

```
class test
{
static  void display()
  {
System.out.println("0 parameter display()");
  }
  static void display(int i)
  {
System.out.println("1 int parameter display()"+i);
  }
  static void display(String s)
  {
System.out.println("1 string parameter display()"+s);
  }
    static void display(int i,int j)
  {
System.out.println("2 int parameter display()"+i+" "+j);
  }
}
class sample {
  void main(String a[])
  {
test.display();
test.display(10);
test.display("testing");
test.display(100,200);
  }
}
```

Output

```
0 parameter display()
1 int parameter display()10
1 string parameter display()testing
2 int parameter display() 100 200
```

The above Java program demonstrates method overloading with static methods in the `test` class. The `test` class contains four overloaded static `display` methods: one without parameters, one with a single integer parameter, one with a single string parameter, and one with two integer parameters. Each method prints a message indicating which version of `display` was called, along with arguments. In the `main` method of the `sample` class, each overloaded `display` method is called on the `test` class without creating an instance, showcasing different outputs based on the parameters.

Program

Program for writing more than one main method in java

```
public class sample{
  void main(String[] args) {
System.out.println("main(String[] args)");
  }
  void main(String arg1) {
System.out.println("main(String arg1)");
  }
  void main(String arg1, String arg2) {
System.out.println("main(String arg1, String arg2)");
  }
}
Output:
main(String[] args)
```

The above Java program demonstrates overloading of the `main` method in the `sample` class. There are three `main` methods, each with different parameter lists: one with a `String[]` parameter, one with a single `String` parameter, and one with two `String` parameters. When the program is run, the `main` method with the `String[]` parameter is executed by default, printing "main(String[] args)". The other `main` methods can be called from within the program, but they will not be executed automatically by the Java runtime.

Program

Program for over loading the main method in java with string[],string parameters

```
public class sample {
  void main(String[] args) {
System.out.println("main(String[] args)");
    main("test");
  }
  void main(String arg1) {
System.out.println("main(String arg1)");
    main("test","ing");
  }
  void main(String arg1, String arg2) {
System.out.println("main(String arg1, String arg2)");
  }
}
Output:
main(String[] args)
main(String arg1)
main(String arg1, String arg2)
```

The above Java program demonstrates overloading and chaining of the `main` method in the `sample` class. The `main(String[] args)` method is the entry point and prints "main(String[] args)". It then calls `main("test")`, which prints "main(String arg1)" and calls `main("test", "ing")`. The final `main(String arg1, String arg2)` method prints "main(String arg1, String arg2)".

Program

Program for over loading the main method in java class with string and int paramters

```
public class JavaApplication {
  void main(int a){
System.out.println(a);
  }
  void main(String args[]){
System.out.println("main() method invoked");
main(100);
  }
}
Output:
main() method invoked
100
```

The above Java program demonstrates overloading of the `main` method in the `JavaApplication` class. The standard `main(String[] args)` method is the entry point and prints "main() method invoked". It then calls the overloaded `main(int a)` method, passing the integer `100` as an argument. The `main(int a)` method prints the integer `100`.

Program

Program for over loading the main method with vargs in java

```
public class JavaApplication {
    static public void main(String [] args)
    {
main( 50, 60, 70 );
          JavaApplication t = new JavaApplication( );
        String [] message  = { "java", "Programming","language" };
t.main(50);
t.main( 10, message );
    }
    static void main(int ... args)
    {
System.out.println( "In the static main called by JVM's main" );
for( int i : args )
        {
System.out.println( i );
        }
    }
    public void main(int x)
    {
System.out.println( "In the overloaded  non-static main with int with value
  " + x );
    }
    public void main(int x,String [] args)
```

```
    {
System.out.println( "In the overloaded  non-static main with int with value
   " + x );
        for (String s:args)
        {
System.out.println(s);
        }
    }
}
```

Output:

```
In the static main called by JVM's main
50
60
70
In the overloaded  non-static main with int with value 50
In the overloaded  non-static main with int with value 10
java
Programming
Language
```

The above Java program demonstrates the overloading of the `main` method in both static and non-static forms within the `JavaApplication` class. The static `main(String[] args)` method serves as the entry point and calls various overloaded versions of the `main` method. It calls the static `main(int... args)` with three integers, the non-static `main(int x)` with a single integer, and the non-static `main(int x, String[] args)` with an integer and a string array. Each `main` method prints specific messages and iterates through the given arguments, showcasing different ways to overload and utilize the main method in Java.

Program:

Program for over loading the main method in java with out main(string []args)

```
public class JavaApplication {
  void main(String... args)
  {
System.out.println("in main");
    main("test");
main(10);
  }
  void main(int i)
  {
System.out.println("int value"+i);
  }
  void main(String s)
  {
System.out.println("String "+s);
  }
}
```

Output:

```
in main
String test
int value10
```

The above Java program demonstrates overloading of the `main` method in the `JavaApplication` class. The main entry point is the `main(String... args)` method, which prints "in main". It then calls the overloaded `main(String s)` method with the argument `"test"`, printing "String test". Next, it calls the overloaded `main(int i)` method with the argument `10`, printing "int value10".

5.6 PASSING ARRAYS TO METHODS

In Java, passing arrays to methods allows for the efficient handling and manipulation of array data within a program.

```
public class RectangleArea {
  void main(String[] args) {
    double[] dimensions = {5.0, 10.0};
    double area = calculateRectangleArea(dimensions);
    System.out.println("Area of the rectangle: " + area);
  }
  public static double calculateRectangleArea(double[] dimensions) {
    if (dimensions.length != 2) {
      throw new IllegalArgumentException("Invalid dimensions array. Expected
      length and width.");
    }
    double length = dimensions[0];
    double width = dimensions[1];
    return length * width;
  }
}
Output:
Area of the rectangle: 50.0
```

We passed the array as an argument to the `calculateRectangleArea` method, which calculates the area of the rectangle based on the considered dimensions. The `calculateRectangleArea` method accepts an array of type `double[]`, ensuring that it contains exactly two elements representing the length and width of the rectangle. If the dimensions array does not meet this requirement, an `IllegalArgumentException` is thrown. Within the method, the length and width are extracted from the dimensions array, and the area of the rectangle is calculated using the formula: `area = length * width`.Finally, the calculated area is returned to the `main` method, where it is displayed to the user.

5.7 RETURNING ARRAYS FROM METHODS

In Java, methods can also return arrays, providing flexibility in data handling and manipulation.

```
public class RectangleArea {
  void main(String[] args) {
      double[] dimensions = {5.0, 10.0};
    double[] result = calculateRectangleArea(dimensions);
    System.out.println("Area of the rectangle: " + result[0]);
    System.out.println("Length of the rectangle: " + result[1]);
    System.out.println("Width of the rectangle: " + result[2]);
  }
  public static double[] calculateRectangleArea(double[] dimensions) {
    if (dimensions.length != 2) {
      throw new IllegalArgumentException("Invalid dimensions array. Expected
      length and width.");
    }
```

```
        double length = dimensions[0];
        double width = dimensions[1];
        double area = length * width;
          double[] result = {area, length, width};
        return result;
    }
}
```

Output:

```
Area of the rectangle: 50.0
Length of the rectangle: 5.0
Width of the rectangle: 10.0
```

We passed an array as an argument to the `calculateRectangleArea` method, which calculates the area of the rectangle based on the considered dimensions and returns an array containing the area, length, and width. The `calculateRectangleArea` method accepts an array of type `double[]` as a parameter, ensuring that it contains exactly two elements representing the length and width of the rectangle. If the dimensions array does not meet this requirement, an `IllegalArgumentException` is thrown. Within the method, the length and width are extracted from the dimensions array, and the area of the rectangle is calculated using the formula: `area = length * width`.A new array `result` is created to store the calculated area, length, and width, and it is returned to the `main` method.In the `main` method, the returned array `result` is accessed to display the calculated area, length, and width of the rectangle.

5.8 RECURSION

Recursion is a programming technique where a function or method calls itself directly or indirectly to solve a problem by breaking it down into smaller instances of the same problem. This process continues until a base case is reached, which is a condition that stops the recursion from continuing indefinitely.

Benefits of Recursion for Arrays

- Simplicity: Allows you to handle arrays and collections in a straightforward and elegant manner.
- Flexibility: Can be used to solve problems that involve nested structures or variable sizes (like trees and graphs).
- Reduction of Complexity: Breaks down complex problems into simpler sub-problems, enhancing readability and maintainability.

Limitations

- Stack Overflow: If not carefully managed (e.g., with proper base cases), recursion can lead to stack overflow errors due to excessive function calls.
- Performance: Recursive solutions may sometimes be less efficient in terms of time and space complexity compared to iterative solutions.

Example

```
public class RecursionExample {
  void main(String[] args) {
    int[] arr = {1, 2, 3, 4, 5};
    printArray(arr, 0);
  }
```

```
  public static void printArray(int[] arr, int index) {
    // Base case: Stop recursion when index is out of bounds
    if (index >= arr.length) {
      return;
    }
    // Print current element
    System.out.println("Element at index " + index + ": " + arr[index]);
    // Recursive call to print the next element
    printArray(arr, index + 1);
  }
}
```

Output:

```
Element at index 0: 1
Element at index 1: 2
Element at index 2: 3
Element at index 3: 4
Element at index 4: 5
```

In the above program, a recursive method is implemented to print the elements of an integer array. The `main` method initializes an array called `arr` with the values {1, 2, 3, 4, 5} and calls the `printArray` method, starting with an index of 0. The `printArray` method checks if the current index is within the bounds of the array. If the index is greater than or equal to the length of the array, the recursion stops (base case). If the index is valid, the method prints the current element at that index and then calls itself with the next index (index + 1). This continues until all elements of the array are printed, resulting in the output showing each element along with its corresponding index.

5.9 MEDICAL APPLICATIONS

5.9.1 Case Study 1

Liver functioning refers to the liver's ability to perform its vital functions, which are crucial for maintaining overall health and well-being. The parameters considered for liver functioning are:

- Liver Enzymes:
  - Alanine Aminotransferase (ALT): Elevated ALT levels indicate liver inflammation or damage. Normal range: 7–56 U/L.
  - Aspartate Aminotransferase (AST): Elevated AST levels suggest liver damage but are less specific than ALT. Normal range: 10–40 U/L.
  - Alkaline Phosphatase (ALP): Elevated ALP levels may indicate liver disease or bile duct obstruction. Normal range varies by age and sex.

- Bilirubin Levels:
  - Total Bilirubin: Elevated levels can indicate liver disease or problems with bile ducts. Normal range: 0.1–1.2 mg/dL.
  - Direct Bilirubin: Elevated direct bilirubin levels suggest issues with bile ducts or liver function. Normal range: 0–0.3 mg/dL.

```
public class LiverFunctionTest {
  //Method to check liver function based on ALT (Alanine Aminotransferase) levels
  public static void checkLiverFunction(double alt) {
    if (alt < 7 || alt > 56) {
```

```
      System.out.println("ALT levels are abnormal. Liver function may be
      impaired.");
    } else {
      System.out.println("ALT levels are normal.");
    }
  }
  public static void checkLiverFunction(double ast, double alt) {
    if (ast < 10 || ast > 40) {
      System.out.println("AST levels are abnormal. Liver function may be
      impaired.");
    } else {
      System.out.println("AST levels are normal.");
    }
    checkLiverFunction(alt);
  }
  public static void checkLiverFunction(double totalBilirubin, double
directBilirubin, double ast, double alt) {
    if (totalBilirubin < 0.1 || totalBilirubin > 1.2) {
      System.out.println("Total Bilirubin levels are abnormal. Liver
      function may be impaired.");
    } else {
      System.out.println("Total Bilirubin levels are normal.");
    }
    if (directBilirubin < 0 || directBilirubin > 0.3) {
      System.out.println("Direct Bilirubin levels are abnormal. Liver
      function may be impaired.");
    } else {
      System.out.println("Direct Bilirubin levels are normal.");
    }
    checkLiverFunction(ast, alt);
  }
  void main(String[] args) {
    checkLiverFunction(45); // Check using ALT levels
    checkLiverFunction(30, 50);
    checkLiverFunction(1.1, 0.2, 35, 45);
  }
}
```

The LiverFunctionTest class provides methods to assess liver function. The first method, checkLiverFunction(double alt), evaluates the ALT (Alanine Aminotransferase) level. If the ALT value falls outside the normal range of 7 to 56, it indicates potential impairment of liver function. The second method, checkLiverFunction(double ast, double alt), additionally checks the AST (Aspartate Aminotransferase) level. An abnormal AST level (below 10 or above 40) suggests liver function impairment. This method then calls the ALT check to further assess liver health. The third method, checkLiverFunction(double totalBilirubin, double directBilirubin, double ast, double alt), includes checks for total and direct bilirubin levels. Abnormal values for total bilirubin (less than 0.1 or more than 1.2) or direct bilirubin (less than 0 or more than 0.3) indicate potential liver dysfunction. It subsequently calls the AST and ALT checks for a comprehensive liver function evaluation. Each method outputs diagnostic messages indicating whether the tested parameters are within normal ranges or if there are indications of impaired liver function.

5.9.2 Case Study 2

Migraine is a neurological disorder characterized by recurrent, moderate to severe headaches often accompanied by other symptoms such as nausea, vomiting, sensitivity to light, and sensitivity to sound. These headaches typically affect one side of the head, pulsate or throb, and can last from a few hours to several days if untreated. Migraines are often debilitating, causing significant disruption to daily life and activities.

Here are some of the parameters commonly considered:

1. C-Reactive Protein (CRP):
   CRP is a marker of inflammation. Elevated levels may indicate inflammation in the body, which could be associated with migraine attacks.
2. Serotonin Levels:
   Serotonin is a neurotransmitter that plays a role in regulating mood and pain sensation. Fluctuations in serotonin levels have been linked to migraine pathophysiology.
3. Estrogen Levels:
   Hormonal changes, particularly fluctuations in estrogen levels, are known triggers for migraine attacks, especially in women.
4. Glucose Levels:
   Abnormal glucose metabolism or fluctuations in blood glucose levels have been observed in migraine patients.
5. White Blood Cell (WBC) Count:
   Changes in WBC count can indicate systemic inflammation or immune system responses, which may be associated with migraine attacks.
6. Other Markers:
   Additional parameters such as cytokines (e.g., interleukins), neuropeptides (e.g., calcitonin gene-related peptide – CGRP), and other biomarkers related to oxidative stress or mitochondrial dysfunction are also under investigation.

```
import java.util.Scanner;
public class MigraineDetection {
  void main(String[] args) {
    Scanner scanner = new Scanner(System.in);
    System.out.println("Migraine Detection System");
    System.out.println("-------------------------");
    System.out.print("Enter CRP level (mg/L): ");
    double crp = scanner.nextDouble();
    System.out.print("Enter Serotonin level (ng/mL): ");
    double serotonin = scanner.nextDouble();
    System.out.print("Enter Estrogen level (pg/mL): ");
    double estrogen = scanner.nextDouble();
    System.out.print("Enter Glucose level (mg/dL): ");
    double glucose = scanner.nextDouble();
    System.out.print("Enter WBC count (x10^9/L): ");
    double wbc = scanner.nextDouble();
    boolean hasMigraine = detectMigraine(crp, serotonin, estrogen, glu-
    cose, wbc);
    if (hasMigraine) {
      System.out.println("Based on the blood test results, Migraine
      detected.");
    } else {
```

```
      System.out.println("Based on the blood test results, No Migraine
      detected.");
    }
    scanner.close();
  }
  private static boolean detectMigraine(double crp, double serotonin,
  double estrogen, double glucose, double wbc) {
    double crpThreshold = 5.0;
    double serotoninThreshold = 100.0;
    double estrogenThreshold = 50.0;
    double glucoseThreshold = 100.0;
    double wbcThreshold = 8.0;
    if (crp > crpThreshold || serotonin < serotoninThreshold || estrogen <
    estrogenThreshold ||
      glucose < glucoseThreshold || wbc < wbcThreshold) {
      return true;
    } else {
      return false;
    }
  }
}
```

The `MigraineDetection` begins by prompting the user to enter levels of CRP, Serotonin, Estrogen, Glucose, and WBC count. These values are then evaluated against predefined thresholds within the `detectMigraine` method to determine if migraine is detected. If any parameter exceeds its respective threshold, the program concludes that migraine is present. The results are displayed accordingly, indicating whether migraine is detected based on the input.

6 Java Classes

6.1 INTRODUCTION

Java adopts the paradigm of object-oriented programming (OOP), which emphasizes the decomposition of intricate issues into manageable entities called objects. The foundation of Java programming revolves around the concepts of classes and objects, each encapsulating attributes and behaviors.

6.1.1 ENCAPSULATION

Encapsulation in object-oriented programming refers to the bundling of data (attributes or properties) and methods (functions or procedures) that operate on the data into a single unit, known as a class. It is one of the fundamental principles of object-oriented design, alongside inheritance and polymorphism.

Key Aspects of Encapsulation

- Data Hiding: Encapsulation allows data to be hidden within a class and accessed only through its public methods. This restricts direct access to the data from outside the class, which helps prevent accidental modification and ensures consistency in the object's state.
- Access Control: Through encapsulation, access modifiers (like `private`, `protected`, `public`) can be used to specify the visibility of class members. This controls how data is accessed and modified by other parts of the program, promoting security and maintainability.

Need for Encapsulation

- Modularity: Encapsulation promotes modularity by grouping related data and methods together, making the code more organized and easier to understand.
- Security: By hiding internal state and requiring access through controlled methods, encapsulation prevents external code from directly manipulating sensitive data, reducing the risk of unintended side effects.
- Flexibility and Maintenance: Encapsulation allows implementation details to be changed without affecting other parts of the program, as long as the public interface remains unchanged. This supports easier maintenance and updates.

DOI: 10.1201/9781003544319-6

Benefits of Encapsulation

- Controlled Access: Ensures that the internal state of objects is accessed and modified only through defined methods, maintaining data integrity and reducing bugs.
- Code Reusability: Encapsulation supports code reuse by providing a clear and standardized interface for interacting with objects, facilitating easier integration into larger systems.
- Enhanced Testing: Encapsulation makes it easier to test individual components of a program independently, leading to more robust and reliable software.

Limitations of Encapsulation

- Overhead: Implementing encapsulation may introduce additional overhead, as more effort is required to design and maintain class interfaces and ensure proper data access.
- Complexity: It can sometimes be challenging to determine the appropriate level of encapsulation, leading to overly complex designs or unnecessary restrictions on data access.
- Performance: Directly accessing data through getter and setter methods (rather than directly) can incur a slight performance overhead, although modern Java compilers and runtime optimizations mitigate this impact.

6.2 CLASSES

A class in Java encapsulates data and behavior within a single unit, providing a blueprint for creating objects with consistent attributes and operations. By organizing fields, methods, constructors, and other components within a class, Java promotes code reusability, modularity, and maintainability in object-oriented programming. In the realm of object-oriented programming, a class acts as a cohesive unit that consolidates both data members and methods. These elements collectively form a shared blueprint for all instances associated with the class.

- Fields: Fields, also known as attributes or variables, represent the data associated with an object of the class. They define the state of the object by storing values that characterize its properties. Fields can have different access modifiers (e.g., public, private, protected) to control their visibility and accessibility from other classes.
- Methods: Methods are functions defined within a class that define the behavior of objects of that class. They encapsulate the operations that can be performed on the class's data (fields) or modify its state. Methods can perform various tasks, including data manipulation, computation, or interaction with other objects.
- Constructors: Constructors are special methods used for initializing objects of a class. They have the same name as the class and are called automatically when an object is created. Constructors initialize the state of newly created objects by assigning initial values to the class's fields. They can be parameterized to accept arguments for initialization.
- Blocks: Java supports three types of blocks within a class: initialization blocks, static blocks, and instance blocks. Initialization blocks are used to initialize instance variables, static blocks are executed when the class is loaded into memory, and instance blocks are executed when an object of the class is created.

Need for Classes

- Abstraction: Classes provide a way to abstract complex systems by encapsulating related data and behavior into a single unit.
- Modularity: They help in organizing code into manageable units, making it easier to understand, maintain, and reuse.

- Code Reusability: Classes facilitate code reuse through inheritance and composition, allowing developers to extend or compose existing classes to build new functionality.
- Encapsulation: They support encapsulation by hiding implementation details and exposing a well-defined interface for interacting with objects.
- Polymorphism: Classes enable polymorphism, allowing objects of different classes to be treated uniformly through inheritance and method overriding.

Advantages of Classes

- Organization: Classes help in organizing code into logical units, making it easier to manage and understand.
- Encapsulation: They support encapsulation by bundling data and methods together, protecting data integrity and providing a clear interface for interacting with objects.
- Reusability: Classes promote code reuse through inheritance and composition, reducing duplication and enhancing maintainability.
- Abstraction: They allow for abstraction by hiding implementation details and exposing only essential features to users of the class.
- Inheritance: Classes facilitate inheritance, enabling the creation of hierarchical relationships between classes and promoting code reuse and extensibility.
- Polymorphism: They enable polymorphism, allowing objects of different classes to be treated uniformly through inheritance and method overriding.

Limitations of Classes

- Inflexibility: Once a class is defined, its structure and behavior are fixed, which may limit adaptability to changing requirements.
- Overhead: Classes introduce some overhead in terms of memory and performance due to the creation of objects and method invocations.
- Complexity: Large class hierarchies and complex class relationships can lead to increased complexity, making code harder to understand and maintain.
- Inheritance Issues: Improper use of inheritance can lead to issues such as tight coupling, code duplication, and violation of encapsulation.
- Encapsulation Violation: Public access to fields and methods of a class can lead to encapsulation violations and potential misuse of the class.

Despite these limitations, classes are fundamental building blocks in Java programming, providing a powerful mechanism for organizing, encapsulating, and reusing code. When used appropriately, classes contribute to the creation of modular, maintainable, and scalable software systems.

Syntax

```
access-specifier class<class_name>
{
field;
method;
}
```

The class declarations can include these components:

- Modifiers: A class can be public or has default access.
- Class keyword: class keyword is used to create a class.

- Class name: The name should begin with an initial letter (capitalized by convention).
- Body: The class body surrounded by braces, {}.
- Constructors play a pivotal role in initializing newly created objects in Java. Each Java class must possess at least one constructor. In cases where a Java class doesn't explicitly define any constructor, the Java compiler autonomously supplies a no-argument constructor, often referred to as the default constructor. This default constructor invokes the no-argument constructor of the class's superclass.

6.3 ACCESSING VARIABLES

In Java, instance variables (also known as non-static fields) are specific to each instance of a class, while class variables (also known as static fields) are shared among all instances of the class.

Example: Accessing instance variables

Instance variables are accessed using object references. Each object has its own copy of instance variables.

Program

```
public class Test {
  // Instance variables
  private String name;
  private int age;
public Test() {
  }
  // Constructor to initialize instance variables
  public Test(String name, int age) {
    this.name = name;
this.age = age;
  }
  // Method to display instance variables
  public void displayDetails() {
System.out.println("Name: " + name + ", Age: " + age);
  }
  void main(String[] args) {
    // Creating objects of Test class
Test obj = new Test();
    Test obj1 = new Test("Usharani", 30);
    Test obj2 = new Test("Bhimavarapu", 25);
    // Accessing instance variables via methods
    obj1.displayDetails();
    obj2.displayDetails();
  }
}
Output:
Name: Usharani, Age: 30
Name: Bhimavarapu, Age: 25
```

In this program, a class named `Test` is defined with two instance variables: `name` (of type String) and `age` (of type int). The class includes a default constructor that initializes no values and a parameterized constructor that sets the `name` and `age` based on provided arguments. A method named `displayDetails` is implemented to print the values of the instance variables to the console in a formatted string. Within the `main` method, two objects of the `Test` class are created using the parameterized constructor: `obj1` with the name "Usharani" and age 30, and `obj2` with the name

"Bhimavarapu" and age 25. The program then calls the `displayDetails` method for both objects, resulting in the output displaying the names and ages of each object.

Example: Accessing class variables

Class variables are accessed using the class name or object references.

Program

```
public class Test {
  // Class variable (static field)
  private static int instanceCount = 0;
  // Constructor to increment the instance count
  public Test() {
instanceCount++;  // Increment the static variable
  }
  // Static method to get the instance count
  public static int getInstanceCount() {
    return instanceCount;
  }
  void main(String[] args) {
    // Creating objects of Test class
    Test obj1 = new Test();
    Test obj2 = new Test();
    // Accessing class variable via class name
System.out.println("Numberofinstancescreated: "+Test.getInstanceCount());
  }
}
Output:
Number of instances created: 3
```

In the above program, a class named `Test` is designed with a static variable `instanceCount` that tracks how many instances (objects) of the class have been created. Every time the constructor of the `Test` class is called, it increments this static variable by 1, ensuring that the total number of created instances is stored in `instanceCount`. A static method `getInstanceCount` is provided to retrieve the value of `instanceCount`. `. Finally, the value of `instanceCount` is printed using the static method.

6.4 ACCESSING METHODS

In Java, instance methods are methods that belong to an instance of a class, and they can access instance variables and other instance methods. Class methods, also known as static methods, belong to the class itself and can access class variables and other static methods.

Example for accessing instance methods:

```
public class Test {
private String name;
private int age;
Test(){}
public Test(String name, int age) {
this.name = name;
this.age = age;
  }
public void displayDetails() {
System.out.println("Name: " + name + ", Age: " + age);
```

```
  }
void main(String[] args) {
Test obj1=new Test("Usharani", 30);
Test obj2=new Test("Bhimavarapu", 25);
    obj1.displayDetails();
    obj2.displayDetails();
  }
}
```

Output:

```
Name: Usharani, Age: 30
Name: Bhimavarapu, Age: 25
```

In the above program, we have created a class named `Test` that contains two private instance variables: `name` and `age`. A parameterized constructor is defined to initialize the `name` and `age` fields when an object is created. A method `displayDetails()` is used to print the values of `name` and `age` to the console. In the `main` method, two objects of the `Test` class are instantiated using the parameterized constructor with different values for `name` and `age`. Finally, the `displayDetails()` method is called on both objects to display their respective details.

Example for accessing class methods:

Program

```
public class Test {
private static int instanceCount=0;
public Test() {
instanceCount++;
  }
public static int getInstanceCount() {
return instanceCount;
  }
void main(String[] args) {
Test obj1=new Test();
Test obj2=new Test();
Test obj3=new Test();
System.out.println("Total instances: " + Test.getInstanceCount());
  }
}
```

In this program, a class named `Test` is defined with a static field `instanceCount`, which keeps track of how many objects of the class have been created. Each time a new `Test` object is instantiated, the `instanceCount` is incremented in the constructor. The `getInstanceCount()` method is a static method used to return the current value of `instanceCount`. The static field ensures that the count is shared across all instances of the `Test` class.

Output:

```
Total instances: 4
```

6.5 CREATING OBJECTS

An object is an instance of a class, representing a specific occurrence of the class's structure and behavior. In Java, objects are created from classes. To instantiate an object of a class, the class name is specified, followed by the object name, and the keyword `new` is used. This process allocates memory for the object and invokes the class's constructor to initialize its state.

Syntax

```
className object = new className();
```

An instance of a class is referred to as an object in Java. To create an object, the 'new' keyword is essential, followed by a call to the class constructor. The process involves thee steps: declaration, instantiation, and initialization.
In the object creation process in Java, there are three fundamental steps:

- Declaration: This step involves declaring a variable with a specific object type. It defines a reference variable that can hold the reference to an object of a particular class.
- Instantiation: In this step, the 'new' keyword is used to create a new instance of the class. It allocates memory for the object and initializes its state.
- Initialization: After instantiation, the constructor of the class is invoked using the 'new' keyword followed by any required arguments in parentheses. This initializes the newly created object with initial values or performs any necessary setup operations.

These steps are essential for creating objects in Java and are integral to the object-oriented programming paradigm. They provide a structured approach to creating and initializing objects, allowing for efficient memory management and flexible object creation. There exist various methods to instantiate objects in Java:

- Using the 'new' Keyword: This is the standard and most frequently used approach. It involves creating an object by invoking the class constructor.

  ```
  Test object = new Test();
  ```

- Using Class.forName(String className) Method: The Class.forName(String className) method in the java.lang package returns the class object associated with a given string class name. This method is used to dynamically load and instantiate classes.

  ```
  Test obj = (Test) Class.forName("com.example.Test").newInstance();
  ```

- Using the clone() Method: The clone() method is part of the Object class and creates a copy of the object. It is used to generate a new object that is an exact copy of the original object.

  ```
  Test obj1 = new Test();
  Test obj2 = (Test) obj1.clone();
  ```

- Deserialization: Deserialization involves reading an object from its saved state in a file. It recreates the object from its serialized form stored in a file.

  ```
  FileInputStream file = new FileInputStream(filename);
  ObjectInputStream in = new ObjectInputStream(file);
  Object obj = in.readObject();
  ```

- Anonymous Object: An anonymous object is one without a reference. It is created at the time of object instantiation and can be used for a single operation.

```
new Test(); // Anonymous object
Method Invocation through a Reference:
test t = new Test();
t.method(); // Method invocation through a reference
```

6.6 CONSTRUCTOR

In Java, a constructor is a special method that is automatically called when an object of a class is instantiated using the `new` keyword. It is used to initialize the object's state. A constructor in Java:

- Has the same name as the class.
- Does not have a return type, not even `void`.
- Can be overloaded (multiple constructors with different parameter lists).
- Can invoke another constructor using `this()` (constructor chaining).

6.6.1 Types of Constructors

Constructors in Java are special methods used to initialize objects. They have the same name as the class and do not have a return type. There are six main types of constructors in Java:

1. Default Constructor
   - Automatically provided by Java if no other constructors are defined.
   - Initializes the object with default values.
2. No-Argument Constructor
   - A constructor that does not take any parameters.
   - Can be explicitly defined by the programmer.
3. Parameterized Constructor
   - Takes one or more parameters to initialize the object with specific values.
4. Copy Constructor
   - Used to create a new object as a copy of an existing object.
   - Not a built-in feature in Java, but can be implemented by defining a constructor that takes an object of the same class as a parameter.
5. Private Constructor
   - Used to restrict instantiation of a class from outside.
   - Commonly used in Singleton design patterns or utility classes.
6. Static Constructor (Static Initialization Block)
   - Java does not support static constructors.
   - Static initialization blocks are used instead to initialize static variables.
7. Protected Constructor
   - Used to restrict instantiation of a class

These constructors allow for various ways to instantiate and initialize objects in Java, providing flexibility and control over the object creation process.

6.6.1.1 Default/ No-Argument Constructor

- A constructor with no parameters.
- Automatically provided by Java if no other constructors are defined.
- Initializes instance variables to their default values (e.g., `0` for numeric types, `null` for objects).

Program

```
public class Test {
     public Test() {
       // Default constructor
System.out.println("Default constructor called.");
     }
     void main(String[] args) {
       Test obj = new Test(); // Creating an object, default constructor called
     }
   }
Output:
Default constructor called.
Default constructor called.
```

In this program, a class named `Test` is defined with a default constructor. The default constructor is a parameterless constructor that prints a message, "Default constructor called," when it is invoked. Inside the `main` method, an object of the `Test` class is created by calling the default constructor. When the object (`obj`) is instantiated, the default constructor is automatically called, and the message is printed to indicate that the constructor has been executed.

6.6.1.2 Parameterized Constructor

- A constructor with parameters.
- Used to initialize instance variables with specified values at the time of object creation.

Program

```
  public class Test {
     private int id;
     private String name;
public Test() {
         }
     public Test(int id, String name) {
       // Parameterized constructor
       this.id = id;
       this.name = name;
     }
     void main(String[] args) {
Test obj1 = new Test();
       Test obj = new Test(1, "Usharani"); //  Creating an object with
                                           parameters
System.out.println("ID: " + obj.id + ", Name: " + obj.name);
     }
   }
Output:
ID: 1, Name: Usharani
```

In this program, we define a class `Test` that contains two instance variables: `id` and `name`. The class includes two constructors. The first one is a default constructor and the second is a parameterized constructor that accepts two arguments, `id` and `name`, and assigns them to the corresponding instance variables using the `this` keyword to differentiate between the constructor parameters and the class fields. Within the `main` method, we create two objects. The first object, `obj1`, is created using the default constructor and the second object, `obj`, is created using the parameterized constructor, assigning `id` the value `1` and `name` the value `"Usharani"`. The program then prints the values of the `id` and `name` fields of the `obj` object.

6.6.1.3 Copy Constructor

- Constructs a new object by copying the values of an existing object of the same class.
- Helps in creating a new object with the same state as an existing object.

Program

```
public class Test {
  private int id;
  private String name;
  public Test() {
      }
  public Test(int id, String name) {
    // Parameterized constructor
    this.id = id;
    this.name = name;
  }
  public Test(Test another) {
    // Copy constructor
    this.id = another.id;
    this.name = another.name;
  }
  void main(String[] args) {
    Test obj = new Test();
    Test obj1 = new Test(1, "Usharani"); // Creating an object
    Test obj2 = new Test(obj1);     // Using copy constructor to create obj2
System.out.println("ID: " + obj2.id + ", Name: " + obj2.name);
  }
}
Output:
ID: 1, Name: Usharani
```

In this program, we have created a class `Test` with two instance variables, `id` and `name`. The class has three constructors. The default constructor allows object creation without initializing the instance variables. The parameterized constructor takes two arguments, `id` and `name`, and assigns them to the instance variables. This allows us to initialize objects with specific values. Additionally, the class includes a copy constructor that accepts an object of the same class and duplicates its `id` and `name` values into a new object. In the `main` method, we first create an object `obj1` using the parameterized constructor, assigning it the values `1` for `id` and `"Usharani"` for `name`. Next, we create another object `obj2` using the copy constructor, copying the values from `obj1`. Finally, the program outputs the `id` and `name` of `obj2`, which are the same as those of `obj1`.

6.6.1.4 Static Constructor (Static Initialization Block)

- Block of code inside a class that is executed only once when the class is loaded into memory.
- Used for static initialization of static variables or other static tasks.

Program

```
public class Test {
  private static int count;
```

```
      static {
        // Static initialization block
        count = 0;
System.out.println("Static block initialized.");
      }
      public Test() {
        count++;
System.out.println("Constructor called, Count: " + count);
      }
      void main(String[] args) {
Test obj = new Test();
        Test obj1 = new Test();
        Test obj2 = new Test();
      }
    }
```

Output:

```
Static block initialized.
Constructor called, Count: 1
Constructor called, Count: 2
Constructor called, Count: 3
Constructor called, Count: 4
```

In this program, we have a class `Test` that includes a static variable `count` to track the number of objects created. The program uses a static initialization block to initialize the `count` variable to 0 and print a message when the class is first loaded into memory. The static block is executed only once, before any objects are created or constructors are called. The constructor of the `Test` class increments the `count` each time an object is created and prints the current value of `count`. With each object creation, the value of `count` increases, and the program prints the corresponding count value. The static block runs only once when the class is loaded, while the constructor runs every time a new object is instantiated.

These types of constructors provide flexibility in Java programming for initializing objects based on different requirements and scenarios. Each type serves a specific purpose in object creation and initialization.

6.6.1.5 Private Constructor

A private constructor in Java is a constructor declared with the private access modifier. This means the constructor can only be accessed from within the same class and cannot be invoked from outside the class, including from its subclasses.

```
class Main {
  private Main() {
System.out.println("private Constructor");
  }
  void main(String[] args) {
        Main obj = new Main();
  }
}
```

Output:

```
private Constructor
private Constructor
```

In this program, the `Main` class contains a private constructor, which restricts the instantiation of the class from outside the class itself. The constructor prints "private Constructor" when it is called. In the `main` method, an attempt is made to create an instance of the `Main` class using `new

Main()`. Since the constructor is private, this instantiation is allowed only within the class itself. This pattern of using a private constructor is often seen in the Singleton design pattern, where the goal is to restrict the creation of multiple instances of a class. In this case, the program will create an instance of the `Main` class inside the `main` method, which is valid because it is within the class scope, and the message "private Constructor" will be printed as the constructor is called.

6.6.1.6 Protected Constructor

A protected constructor in Java is a constructor that is accessible within its own package and also by subclasses (inheritors) of its class, regardless of whether they are in the same package or different packages.

Program

```
public class proc {
  protected proc() {
System.out.println("Protected Constructor");
  }
  void main(String[] args) {
          proc obj = new proc();
  }
}
Output:
Protected Constructor
```

In this program, the `proc` class features a protected constructor, which allows the constructor to be accessed within the same package and by subclasses, even if they are in different packages. The constructor prints "Protected Constructor" when invoked. Inside the `main` method, an instance of the `proc` class is created using `new proc()`. Since the `main` method is part of the same class, it has access to the protected constructor. Therefore, when the object is instantiated, the message "Protected Constructor" will be printed to the console.

6.6.2 Constructor Overloading

Constructor overloading in Java refers to the ability to define multiple constructors within a class, each with a different parameter list. This allows objects to be initialized in different ways depending on the arguments provided at the time of instantiation.

Benefits

- Multiple Initializations: Constructor overloading allows objects to be initialized in different ways based on the parameters passed. This flexibility enables developers to create objects with varying initial states without needing multiple factory methods or setter calls.
- Cleaner Code: By providing multiple constructors, you can encapsulate different initialization logic within the class itself, making the code cleaner and more readable.
- Convenient Initialization: It provides a convenient way to initialize objects with commonly used configurations, reducing the need for repetitive code.
- Enhanced Flexibility: Allows subclasses to leverage superclass constructors and extend their functionality by adding additional parameters or custom initialization logic.

Limitations

- Complexity: Having multiple constructors can potentially lead to code complexity and maintenance overhead, especially when dealing with large classes or when constructors have many parameters.
- Ambiguity: Overloading can sometimes make the code less clear if the purpose of each constructor is not well-documented or if the parameter lists are not carefully chosen.
- Compile-time Errors: Incorrect parameter lists or ambiguous overloaded constructors can lead to compile-time errors, especially if the compiler cannot determine the best match for a given set of arguments.

6.6.2.1 Private Constructor Overloading

Private constructor overloading refers to the practice of defining multiple private constructors within a class, each with a different parameter list. Unlike public or protected constructors, private constructors are not accessible from outside the class and are typically used for controlling object creation within the class itself or for Singleton design patterns.

Program

```
public class proc {
  private proc() {
System.out.println("private Constructor");
  }
private proc(int i) {
System.out.println("1 param private Constructor");
  }
  void main(String[] args) {
          proc obj = new proc();
proc obj1 = new proc(1);
  }
}
Output:
private Constructor
1 param private Constructor
```

In this program, the `proc` class contains two private constructors. The first constructor is a default constructor that prints "private Constructor" when called. The second constructor takes an integer parameter and prints "1 param private Constructor." Inside the `main` method, an instance of the `proc` class is created using the default constructor, which outputs "private Constructor." Then, an attempt is made to create another instance using the parameterized constructor.

6.6.2.2 Protected Constructor Overloading

Protected constructor overloading in Java provides flexibility and customization in object creation within the class hierarchy, ensuring that subclasses can use constructors with varying parameter sets to suit their specific needs while maintaining encapsulation and controlled access levels.

Program

```
Program for protected constructor overloading in java
class test {
  // Protected constructor with no parameters
  protected test() {
```

```
    System.out.println("protected constructor");
  }
  // Protected constructor with an integer parameter
  protected test(int num) {
    System.out.println("protected constructor with int " + num);
  }
  // Protected constructor with a string parameter
  protected test(String str) {
    System.out.println("protected constructor with string " + str);
  }
}
public class Main {
  void main(String[] args) {
    // Creating instances of the 'test' class using different constructors
    test t = new test();         // Calls the no-argument constructor
    test t1 = new test(100);      // Calls the constructor with an integer
                                  argument
    test t2 = new test("testing");  // Calls the constructor with a string
                                    argument
  }
}
```

Output:

```
protected constructor
protected constructor with int 100
protected constructor with string testing
```

This Java program consists of two classes: "test" and "Main".The "test" class defines three constructors, all of which are declared with the "protected" access modifier. The first constructor is parameterless and prints "protected constructor" when invoked. The second constructor takes an integer parameter and prints "protected constructor with int" followed by the value of the integer parameter. The third constructor takes a string parameter and prints "protected constructor with string" followed by the value of the string parameter. In the "Main" class's main method, three instances of the "test" class are created using different constructors. The first instance, "t", is created using the parameterless constructor, and it prints "protected constructor" to the console. The second instance, "t1", is created using the constructor that accepts an integer parameter with the value 100, and it prints "protected constructor with int 100" to the console. The third instance, "t2", is created using the constructor that accepts a string parameter with the value "testing", and it prints "protected constructor with string testing" to the console.

6.6.3 Constructor Chaining

Constructor chaining refers to the practice of calling one constructor from another constructor within the same class or from a constructor in a superclass. This technique is used to avoid code duplication and to ensure that a series of initializations occurs in a specific order. Constructor chaining can be achieved using the this() keyword for chaining within the same class or the super() keyword for chaining to the superclass constructor.

Benefits of Constructor Chaining

- Code Reusability: By chaining constructors, common initialization code can be written once and reused across multiple constructors. This reduces redundancy and makes the code easier to maintain.

- Consistency in Initialization: Constructor chaining ensures that all constructors in a class or across related classes consistently perform the necessary initializations, reducing the risk of errors due to incomplete initialization.
- Simplified Code Structure: Using chaining, the code structure becomes more organized and readable, as related initialization tasks are grouped together.
- Inheritance Hierarchies: In inheritance hierarchies, constructor chaining allows the base class to initialize its fields before the derived class adds its own initializations, ensuring a logical order of operations.

Limitations of Constructor Chaining

- Complexity: Overusing constructor chaining, especially in classes with many fields or complex initialization logic, can make the code difficult to understand and debug.
- Tightly Coupled Code: Constructor chaining can lead to tightly coupled code, where changes in one constructor may require changes in all chained constructors, making the code less flexible.
- Error Handling: Handling exceptions during constructor chaining can be challenging, as the constructors must handle any exceptions that occur within the chain.
- Limited Flexibility: Constructor chaining can limit the flexibility to initialize objects in different ways, as the constructors become dependent on the chained sequence.

Program

```
public class Test {
  int x;
  int y;
  int z;
  public Test() {
this(0, 0, 0);
System.out.println("Default constructor called");
  }
  public Test(int x) {
this(x, 0, 0);
System.out.println("Constructor with one parameter called");
  }
  public Test(int x, int y) {
this(x, y, 0);
System.out.println("Constructor with two parameters called");
  }
  public Test(int x, int y, int z) {
this.x = x;
this.y = y;
this.z = z;
System.out.println("Constructor with three parameters called");
  }
  public void display() {
System.out.println("x: " + x + ", y: " + y + ", z: " + z);
  }
  void main(String[] args) {
    Test obj1 = new Test();
    obj1.display();
    Test obj2 = new Test(10);
    obj2.display();
    Test obj3 = new Test(10, 20);
```

```
    obj3.display();
    Test obj4 = new Test(10, 20, 30);
    obj4.display();
  }
}
```

Output:

```
Constructor with three parameters called
Default constructor called
Constructor with three parameters called
Default constructor called
x: 0, y: 0, z: 0
Constructor with three parameters called
Constructor with one parameter called
x: 10, y: 0, z: 0
Constructor with three parameters called
Constructor with two parameters called
x: 10, y: 20, z: 0
Constructor with three parameters called
x: 10, y: 20, z: 30
```

In this program, the `Test` class showcases the concept of constructor chaining through multiple constructors designed to initialize three instance variables: `x`, `y`, and `z`. The default constructor (`Test()`) initializes all three variables to zero by calling the constructor that takes three parameters, and it prints "Default constructor called." The constructor with one parameter (`Test(int x)`) sets `x` to the provided value while initializing `y` and `z` to zero, displaying the message "Constructor with one parameter called." Similarly, the constructor with two parameters (`Test(int x, int y)`) sets `x` and `y` to the given values, with `z` defaulted to zero, and it prints "Constructor with two parameters called." The constructor that accepts three parameters (`Test(int x, int y, int z)`) directly initializes the instance variables and prints "Constructor with three parameters called." In the `main` method, four objects of the `Test` class are created, demonstrating the functionality of each constructor. After each object creation, the `display` method outputs the current values of `x`, `y`, and `z`.

6.6.3.1 Private Constructor Chaining

Private constructor chaining refers to the practice of invoking one private constructor from another within the same class. This is done using the this() keyword. Private constructor chaining helps to manage and streamline the initialization process within a single class, allowing for better code reuse and encapsulation.

Program

```
public class proc {
  private proc() {
this (10);
System.out.println("private Constructor");
  }
private proc(int i)
{System.out.println(" 1 parameter private Constructor");
}
  void main(String[] args) {
        proc obj = new proc();
  }
}
```

```
Output:
1 parameter private Constructor
private Constructor
1 parameter private Constructor
private Constructor
```

In this program, the `proc` class demonstrates the use of private constructors and constructor chaining. The class contains two constructors: a default constructor (`proc()`) and a parameterized constructor (`proc(int i)`). The default constructor calls the parameterized constructor using `this(10)`, which initializes the class with a default integer value of `10` before printing "private Constructor." The parameterized constructor prints "1 parameter private Constructor" when invoked. In the `main` method, an instance of the `proc` class is created using the default constructor. Since both constructors are private, this limits the instantiation of the class to within its own scope, effectively preventing access from outside the class.

6.6.3.2 Protected Constructor Chaining

Protected constructor chaining refers to the practice of invoking one constructor from another within the same class or between classes that are part of the same package or subclasses. This is done using the this() keyword for chaining within the same class

Program

```
Program for protected constructor chaining in java
class test {
  // Protected constructor with no parameters
  protected test() {
    this(10);  // Invokes the constructor with an integer parameter
    System.out.println("protected constructor");
  }
  // Protected constructor with an integer parameter
  protected test(int num) {
    this("testing");  // Invokes the constructor with a string parameter
    System.out.println("protected constructor with int " + num);
  }
  // Protected constructor with a string parameter
  protected test(String str) {
    System.out.println("protected constructor with string " + str);
  }
}
public class Main {
  void main(String[] args) {
    // Creating an instance of the 'test' class, triggering constructor
    chaining
    test t = new test();  // This will chain through all the constructors
  }
}
Output:
protected constructor with string testing
protected constructor with int 10
protected constructor
```

This Java program defines a class named "test" and another class named "Main". Within the "test" class, three constructors are defined, all marked with the "protected" access modifier. The first constructor, lacking parameters, initiates constructor chaining by invoking the constructor accepting an integer parameter using "this(10)". Inside this constructor, it prints "protected constructor with int 10" to the console. The second constructor, taking an integer parameter, further chains by invoking the constructor with a string parameter using "this("testing")". Inside this constructor, it prints "protected constructor with string testing" to the console. Lastly, the third constructor, accepting a string parameter, directly prints "protected constructor with string" followed by the value of the string parameter.

6.7 INITIALIZATION BLOCKS

Initialization blocks in Java are blocks of code that are used to initialize instance variables of a class. There are two types of initialization blocks: (a) Instance initialization block (b) static initialization block.

Instance initialization blocks are executed each time an instance of the class is created, whereas static initialization blocks are executed only once when the class is loaded into memory. Understanding these blocks helps in managing class initialization and ensuring proper variable initialization in Java programs.

6.7.1 Instance Initialization Block

- An instance initialization block is a block of code enclosed within curly braces `{...}` inside a class, but not inside any method, constructor, or static block.
- It runs each time an instance of the class is created.
- It is mainly used to initialize instance variables that require complex initialization logic or to share common initialization code across multiple constructors.
- Instance initialization blocks are executed in the order they appear in the class, immediately after the call to the superclass constructor (if applicable).

Instance initialization block example:

Program

```
public class TestInstanceBlock {
  // Instance variable
  private int number;
  // Instance initialization block
  {
    number = 10;
System.out.println("Instance initialization block: number = " + number);
  }
  // Constructor
  public TestInstanceBlock() {
System.out.println("Constructor called: number = " + number);
  }
  void main(String[] args) {
TestInstanceBlockobj = new TestInstanceBlock();
  }
}
Output:
Instance initialization block: number = 10
Constructor called: number = 10
Instance initialization block: number = 10
Constructor called: number = 10
```

In this example, the instance initialization block initializes the `number` variable to 10 each time an instance of `TestInstanceBlock` is created. The output demonstrates that the instance initialization block runs before the constructor.

6.7.2 Static Initialization Block

- A static initialization block is a block of code enclosed within `{...}` and preceded by the `static` keyword.
- It is executed only once when the class is loaded into the JVM (Java Virtual Machine).
- It is typically used to initialize static variables or to perform one-time initialization tasks for the entire class.
- Static initialization blocks are executed in the order they appear in the class, after static variable initialization and before the first use of the class.

Static initialization block example:

Program

```
public class TestStaticBlock {
  // Static variable
  private static int count;
  // Static initialization block
  static {
    count = 5;
System.out.println("Static initialization block: count = " + count);
  }
  void main(String[] args) {
System.out.println("Main method is called.");
  }
}
```

Output:

```
Static initialization block: count = 5
Main method is called.
```

In this example, the static initialization block initializes the static variable `count` to 5 when the class `TestStaticBlock` is loaded into memory. The static block runs before the `main` method, demonstrating its role in initializing static variables.

6.8 PASSING AND RETURNS OBJECTS

Passing objects as parameters in Java allows methods to manipulate and operate on existing objects, enabling efficient reuse and modification of object state without needing to duplicate data or create new instances. Returning objects from methods facilitates encapsulation and abstraction by hiding the details of object creation within the method, promoting cleaner code and separation of concerns in software design. These practices enhance code readability, maintainability, and performance by minimizing redundant object creation and promoting modular, reusable code components.

6.8.1 Passing Objects as Parameters

Passing objects as parameters and returning objects in Java involves using object references to manipulate and interact with objects passed into methods or returned from methods. Allows methods to operate on existing objects without needing to create new ones. Changes made to the object inside the method affect the original object.

Program

```
Passing Objects as Parameters
class Rectangle {
  private double width;
  private double height;
  // Constructor to initialize Rectangle object
  public Rectangle(double width, double height) {
this.width = width;
this.height = height;
  }
  // Method to calculate area of rectangle
  public double calculateArea() {
    return width * height;
  }
  // Getter method for width
  public double getWidth() {
    return width;
  }
  // Getter method for height
  public double getHeight() {
    return height;
  }
}
// Utility class with method to perform geometry calculations
class GeometryUtil {
  // Method to calculate and return area of a Rectangle object passed as
  parameter
  public static double doubleArea(Rectangle rect) {
    double area = rect.calculateArea();
    return area * 2;
  }
}
// Test class to demonstrate passing objects as parameters
public class TestPassingObjectsAsParameters {
  void main(String[] args) {
    // Creating a Rectangle object
    Rectangle rectangle = new Rectangle(5.0, 3.0);
    // Calling the doubleArea method of GeometryUtil class
    double doubledArea = GeometryUtil.doubleArea(rectangle);
    // Displaying the original and doubled area
System.out.println("Original Rectangle:");
System.out.println("Width: " + rectangle.getWidth() + ", Height: " +
rectangle.getHeight());
System.out.println("Area: " + rectangle.calculateArea());
System.out.println("\nDoubled Area:");
System.out.println("Area * 2: " + doubledArea);
  }
}
```

Output:

```
Original Rectangle:
Width: 5.0, Height: 3.0
Area: 15.0
Doubled Area:
Area * 2: 30.0
```

In this program, a `Rectangle` class is defined to represent a rectangle with properties for width and height, initialized through its constructor. The class includes a method to calculate the area of the rectangle and getter methods for the width and height. Additionally, a `GeometryUtil` utility class is created, containing a method `doubleArea` that takes a `Rectangle` object as a parameter, calculates its area, and returns double that area. The `TestPassingObjectsAsParameters` class demonstrates the functionality by creating an instance of `Rectangle` and invoking the `doubleArea` method. It then prints the rectangle's width, height, original area, and the doubled area to the console.

6.8.2 Returning Objects

Methods can create new objects based on existing ones and return them. This allows for encapsulation and abstraction, where details of object creation are hidden inside the method.

Program

```
class Rectangle {
  private double width;
  private double height;
  // Constructor to initialize Rectangle object
  public Rectangle(double width, double height) {
this.width = width;
this.height = height;
  }
  // Method to create and return a new Rectangle object that is double
  in size
  public Rectangle createDoubleSizeRectangle() {
    double newWidth = width * 2;
    double newHeight = height * 2;
    return new Rectangle(newWidth, newHeight);
  }
  // Getter method for width
  public double getWidth() {
    return width;
  }
  // Getter method for height
  public double getHeight() {
    return height;
  }
}
// Utility class with method to perform operations on Rectangle objects
class RectangleUtil {
  // Method to create and return a double size Rectangle based on a given
  Rectangle
  public static Rectangle createDoubleSizeRectangle(Rectangle rect) {
    return rect.createDoubleSizeRectangle();
  }
}
// Test class to demonstrate returning objects
public class TestReturningObjects {
void main(String[] args) {
    // Creating a Rectangle object
    Rectangle rectangle = new Rectangle(5.0, 3.0);
    // Calling the createDoubleSizeRectangle method of Rectangle class
    Rectangle doubleSizeRectangle = rectangle.createDoubleSizeRectangle();
    // Displaying the original and double size rectangles
```

```
System.out.println("Original Rectangle:");
System.out.println("Width: " + rectangle.getWidth() + ", Height: " + rect-
angle.getHeight());
System.out.println("\nDouble Size Rectangle:");
System.out.println("Width: " + doubleSizeRectangle.getWidth() + ", Height: "
   + doubleSizeRectangle.getHeight());
  }
}
```

Output:

```
Original Rectangle:
Width: 5.0, Height: 3.0
Double Size Rectangle:
Width: 10.0, Height: 6.0
```

In this program, a `Rectangle` class is defined to represent a rectangle with properties for width and height, which are initialized through its constructor. The class includes a method, `createDoubleSizeRectangle`, that creates and returns a new `Rectangle` object with dimensions double those of the original rectangle. The utility class, `RectangleUtil`, provides a static method to generate a double-sized rectangle based on a given rectangle instance, although it utilizes the `Rectangle` class's method directly. The `TestReturningObjects` class serves as the main testing class, where an instance of `Rectangle` is created with specific dimensions. It then calls the `createDoubleSizeRectangle` method to obtain a new rectangle that is double the size and prints both the original and the double-sized rectangle's dimensions to the console.

6.9 ARRAY OF OBJECTS

An array of objects in Java refers to an array where each element is an object of a class rather than a primitive data type. This allows for storing multiple instances of objects in a structured way, similar to how arrays store primitive data types. Each element of the array can hold a reference to an object of the specified class, enabling operations and manipulations on each object through array indexing.

Program

```
public class Test {
  private int id;
  private String name;
  public Test(int id, String name) {
    this.id = id;
    this.name = name;
  }
  public void displayDetails() {
System.out.println("ID: " + id + ", Name: " + name);
  }
  void main(String[] args) {
    // Creating an array of Test objects
Test[] testArray = new Test[3];
    // Initializing objects in the array
testArray[0] = new Test(1, "Dr.");
testArray[1] = new Test(2, "Usharani");
testArray[2] = new Test(3, "Bhimavarapu");
    // Accessing and using objects in the array
    for (Test test :testArray) {
test.displayDetails();
```

```
        }
    }
}
```

Output:

```
ID: 1, Name: Dr.
ID: 2, Name: Usharani
ID: 3, Name: Bhimavarapu
```

In this program, a `Test` class is defined with two instance variables: `id` and `name`, which are initialized through the constructor. The class includes a method, `displayDetails`, which prints the values of these variables. The `main` method serves as the entry point for the program, where an array of `Test` objects is created with a fixed size of three. Each element in the array is initialized with a new `Test` object, each having a unique `id` and `name`. After initializing the array, a for-each loop is used to iterate over the array, calling the `displayDetails` method for each `Test` object to print its information to the console.

6.10 THIS KEYWORD

In Java, this keyword is a reference to the current instance of a class. It can be used within instance methods or constructors to refer to the current object on which the method is being invoked or the constructor is being called.

Types of this Keyword

1. Referencing Current Object: Within an instance method or constructor, this refers to the current object instance. It can be used to access instance variables and invoke other methods of the same object.
2. Chaining Constructors: this() can be used to invoke one constructor from another constructor in the same class. This is known as constructor chaining.
3. Passing this to Other Methods: The this keyword can be passed as an argument to other methods or constructors, allowing methods of other objects to operate on the current object.

Benefits of this Keyword

- Disambiguation: It helps disambiguate between instance variables and parameters with the same name within constructors or methods.
- Constructor Chaining: Allows one constructor to call another constructor in the same class, reducing code duplication and ensuring initialization logic is centralized.
- Method Chaining: Enables fluent interfaces where method calls can be chained together on the same object.

Limitations of this Keyword

- Scope: This can only be used within non-static contexts (instance methods or constructors). It cannot be used in static methods.
- Clarity: Overuse or misuse of this can sometimes make code less readable or maintainable, especially in scenarios where method chaining or constructor overloading becomes complex.

6.10.1 Referring Variables

In Java, the `this` keyword refers to the current instance of the class. It is used primarily to distinguish between instance variables and local variables or method parameters that share the same name. By using `this`, you can explicitly indicate that you are referring to an instance variable of the current object, which helps avoid naming conflicts and ensures clarity in code readability and maintenance.

Program

```
public class Test {
  private int number;
public Test() {
    }
  public Test(int number) {
this.number = number; // 'this' refers to the current object instance
    }
  public void displayNumber() {
System.out.println("Number: " + this.number);
  }
  void main(String[] args) {
Test obj = new Test();
    Test obj1 = new Test(10);
obj1.displayNumber();
  }
}
```

Output:

```
Number: 10
```

In this program, the `Test` class is defined with a private instance variable `number`. It includes a default constructor that initializes the object without setting any value for `number`. Additionally, there is a parameterized constructor that takes an integer parameter to initialize the `number` variable, using `this` to refer to the current instance. The class also has a method called `displayNumber`, which prints the value of `number` to the console. In the `main` method, a `Test` object is created using the default constructor, followed by another object created with the parameterized constructor, passing the value `10`. Finally, the `displayNumber` method is called on the second object, which outputs the initialized number to the console.

6.10.2 Referring Methods

In Java, the `this` keyword is used to refer to methods of the current object within its own class. This is particularly useful when you want to call another constructor from within a constructor (constructor chaining), or to call an instance method from another instance method of the same class. By using `this.methodName()`, you explicitly invoke the method of the current object, which can simplify code and improve readability, especially in scenarios involving method overloading or complex object initialization logic.

Program

```
public class Test {
  private int number;
public Test() {
  }
  public Test(int number) {
this.number = number;
  }
  public void displayNumber() {
```

```
System.out.println("Number: " + this.getNumber());
  }
  private int getNumber() {
    return this.number;
  }
  void main(String[] args) {
Test obj = new Test();
    Test obj1 = new Test(10);
obj1.displayNumber(); // Output: Number: 10
  }
}
```

Output:

```
Number: 10
```

In this program, a class named `Test` is defined with a private instance variable `number`. The class has two constructors: a default constructor and a parameterized constructor that initializes `number` with a given value. The `displayNumber` method prints the value of `number` by calling a private method `getNumber`, which returns the value of `number`. In the `main` method, two objects of the `Test` class are created: one using the default constructor and another using the parameterized constructor with the value `10`. Finally, the `displayNumber` method is called on the second object, which outputs "Number: 10."

6.10.3 Invoking Another Constructor

In Java, you can invoke one constructor from another using the `this()` keyword. For instance, in a no-argument constructor, you can call a parameterized constructor like this: `this(10);`. This invocation must be the first statement in the constructor. After the call, any additional logic for that constructor can follow, making it an efficient way to reuse code within the class.

Program

```
public class Test {
private int number;
public Test() {
this(0); // Invoking parameterized constructor using 'this'  }
}
public Test(int number) {
this.number = number;
  }
public void displayNumber() {
System.out.println("Number: " + this.number);
  }
void main(String[] args) {
Test obj1=new Test();
    obj1.displayNumber(); // Output: Number: 0
Test obj2=new Test(10);
    obj2.displayNumber(); // Output: Number: 10
  }
}
```

Output:

```
Number: 0
Number: 10
```

In this program, the `Test` class demonstrates the use of constructors in Java, including a default constructor and a parameterized constructor. The default constructor initializes the `number` field to `0` by invoking the parameterized constructor with `this(0)`. This ensures that any instance of `Test` created without a specified number will default to `0`. The parameterized constructor allows for setting the `number` to a specified value. The `displayNumber` method prints the value of `number`. In the `main` method, two `Test` objects are created: `obj1` uses the default constructor, displaying "Number: 0," while `obj2` uses the parameterized constructor, displaying "Number: 10."

6.10.4 Object as Parameter

When using Java, the `this` keyword can be employed to refer to the current object instance within its own class, which is particularly useful when passing the current object instance as a parameter to another method or constructor. This approach allows for cleaner and more concise code, especially in scenarios where you need to pass the current object's state or behavior to another method for further processing or initialization. It helps in maintaining object-oriented principles by encapsulating related functionality within the object itself, promoting modular and reusable code design.

Program

```
public class Test {
  private int value;
public Test() {
  }
  public Test(int value) {
this.value = value;
  }
  public void display() {
System.out.println("Value: " + this.value);
  }
  public void processThisAsParameter() {
anotherMethod(this); // Passing current object as parameter
  }
  private void anotherMethod(Test obj) {
System.out.println("Passed value: " + obj.value);
  }
  void main(String[] args) {
Test obj1 = new Test();
    Test obj = new Test(42);
obj.display(); // Output: Value: 42
obj.processThisAsParameter(); // Calling method with this as parameter
  }
}
Output:
Value: 42
Passed value: 42
```

In this program, the `Test` class illustrates the use of constructors, method calls, and passing the current object as a parameter. The class has a private field `value`, which is initialized through a parameterized constructor. The default constructor allows the creation of an object without setting a value. The `display` method prints the value of the `value` field. The `processThisAsParameter` method demonstrates how the current object can be passed as a parameter to another method, specifically `anotherMethod`. This method takes a `Test` object as an argument and prints its `value`. In the `main` method, an object `obj` is created with a value of `42`, and both the `display` method and the `processThisAsParameter` method are called on it. The output shows the value of the object and the value passed to the `anotherMethod`, demonstrating the use of `this` to refer to the current instance.

6.10.5 Returning Current Object

In Java, you can return the current object from a method using the `this` keyword. This is useful in method chaining, where multiple method calls on the same object are strung together. For example, inside a method, you can write `return this;`, which returns the current instance of the class. This allows other methods to be called on the same object without needing to create a new instance.

Syntax

```
public class MyClass {
  public MyClass doSomething() {
    // perform some actions
    return this;  // returns the current object
  }
}
```

This allows you to chain methods like `obj.doSomething().doSomethingElse();`.

Program

```
public class Test {
private int number;
public Test() {
  }
public Test(int number) {
this.number = number;
  }
public Test increment() {
this.number++;
return this; // Returning current object instance
  }
public void displayNumber() {
System.out.println("Number: " + this.number);
  }
void main(String[] args) {
Test obj1=new Test(5);
Test obj=new Test(5);
obj.increment().increment().increment().displayNumber();                    //
Output: Number: 8
  }
}
Output:
Number: 8
```

In this program, the `Test` class demonstrates method chaining and object manipulation using constructors and instance methods. It has a private field `number`, which can be initialized via a parameterized constructor. The class includes an `increment` method that increments the `number` field by one and returns the current object instance (`this`). This allows for method chaining, enabling multiple calls to `increment` in a single statement. The `displayNumber` method outputs the current value of `number`. In the `main` method, an instance of `Test` is created with an initial value of `5`. The `increment` method is called three times in succession, resulting in the value of `number` being increased to `8`. Finally, the `displayNumber` method is invoked to print the updated value.

6.11 STATIC KEYWORD

In Java, the static keyword is used to define class-level entities that belong to the class itself rather than to instances (objects) of the class.

Benefits of Static

- **Memory Efficiency:** Static variables are stored in a fixed location in memory, reducing memory usage when multiple instances of the class are created.
- **Utility Methods:** Static methods can be used to create utility functions that don't require object instantiation, promoting code reusability.
- **Global Constants:** Constants declared as static final are effectively global constants, accessible throughout the class and by other classes.

Limitations of Static

- **Statelessness:** Static members do not maintain state across instances. They are shared among all instances of the class, which can lead to unexpected behavior if not managed carefully.
- **Testing and Mocking:** Static methods and variables can be challenging to mock in unit tests because their behavior is tied to the class itself rather than instances.
- **Inheritance:** Static methods are not polymorphic. They cannot be overridden in subclasses but can be shadowed with a method of the same signature.

6.11.1 Types of Static

6.11.1.1 Static Variables (Class Variables)

- Static variables are shared among all instances (objects) of a class.
- They are initialized only once, at the start of the execution, and are stored in the static memory.
- Accessed using the class name (ClassName.variableName) rather than an instance.

```
public class Example {
static int count=0; // Static variable
}
```

In this code, the `Example` class contains a static variable named `count`, initialized to `0`. Being a static variable, `count` is shared across all instances of the `Example` class, meaning it belongs to the class itself rather than any individual object. This allows it to maintain a single value that can be accessed and modified by any method within the class or by other classes. Static variables are often used for counters, configuration settings, or shared resources that should be consistent across all instances.

6.11.1.2 Static Methods

- Static methods belong to the class rather than any specific instance.
- They can be called using the class name (ClassName.methodName), without needing to instantiate the class.

- They cannot directly access instance variables or instance methods (without an object reference), but can access static variables and other static methods.

Program

```
public class MathUtils {
  public static int add(int a, int b) {
    return a + b; // Static method to add two integers
  }
  public static double squareRoot(double x) {
    return Math.sqrt(x); // Static method to calculate square root
  }
  void main(String[] args) {
    int sum = MathUtils.add(5, 3);
System.out.println("Sum: " + sum);
    double sqrt = MathUtils.squareRoot(16);
System.out.println("Square root: " + sqrt);
  }
}
Output:
Sum: 8
Square root: 4.0
```

In this program, the `MathUtils` class contains two static methods: `add` and `squareRoot`. The `add` method takes two integers as parameters and returns their sum, while the `squareRoot` method computes the square root of a given double value using the built-in `Math.sqrt` function. The `main` method demonstrates how to use these static methods by calling them directly through the class name without needing to create an instance of `MathUtils`. It calculates the sum of `5` and `3`, then prints the result, followed by calculating and printing the square root of `16`.

6.11.1.3 Static Blocks

Static blocks are used for static initialization of a class.
They are executed only once when the class is loaded into memory.
Useful for initializing static variables or performing any one-time setup tasks.

Program

```
public class InitializationExample {
  private static int randomNumber;
  static {
randomNumber = (int) (Math.random() * 100);
  }
  void main(String[] args) {
System.out.println("Random number: " + InitializationExample.randomNumber);
  }
}
Output:
Random number: 2
```

In this program, the `InitializationExample` class demonstrates the use of a static initialization block to initialize a static variable, `randomNumber`. This variable is assigned a random integer value between `0` and `99` by multiplying a random number generated by `Math.random()` (which returns a value between `0.0` and `1.0`) by `100`, and then casting it to an integer. The static block is executed when the class is loaded, ensuring that `randomNumber` is initialized before any instance of the class is created or any static methods are called. In the `main` method, the program prints the value of `randomNumber`, showcasing the result of the random initialization.

6.12 IMPLICITLY DECLARED CLASSES AND INSTANCE MAIN METHODS

The introduction of Implicitly Declared Classes and Instance Main Methods in Java 22 addresses several needs in software development, particularly in simplifying the learning curve for beginners, improving code readability, and enhancing the modularity of Java programs.

Needs for Implicitly Declared Classes and Instance Main Methods in Java 22

- Simplified Entry Point for Beginners: For novice programmers learning Java, the traditional requirement of explicitly declaring a class with a `main` method can be a barrier. Implicitly Declared Classes allow beginners to focus on writing executable code without the initial need to understand class declarations and static methods.
- Reduced Code: In many cases, Java programs start as single-class applications with a `main` method. Implicitly Declared Classes eliminate the need for explicit class declarations and static `main` methods, reducing code and making the entry point to the application more concise and readable.
- Enhanced Modularity and Readability: By allowing Java programs to start execution from an instance `main` method within a regular class, rather than a static context, code organization and modularity are improved. This feature supports a more object-oriented approach to application design, where the main functionality can be encapsulated within an instance of a class.
- Gradual Skill Progression: For learners progressing from simple single-class applications to more complex multi-class projects, Instance Main Methods provide a smoother transition. Beginners can start with a straightforward structure and gradually introduce more advanced Java features and design patterns as their skills develop.
- Support for Interactive and Exploratory Programming: Implicitly Declared Classes facilitate interactive and exploratory programming in Java environments. Developers can quickly write and execute code snippets without the overhead of class declarations, enabling rapid prototyping and experimentation.

Program

```
// Implicitly Declared class with an instance main method
public class Main {
  // Instance main method
  public void main(String[] args) {
System.out.println("This is to test Java 22 version!");
  }
  // Additional methods and fields can be defined here
  public void greet() {
System.out.println("Welcome to Java!");
  }
}
Output:
This is to test Java 22 version!
```

In this example, the `main` method is declared as an instance method within the `Main` class, rather than a static method. This approach allows the program to be executed directly from an instance of the `Main` class. This feature simplifies the initial setup of Java programs, enhances code modularity, and supports a more object-oriented style of programming from the application's entry point.

Program

```
void main() {
System.out.println("This is to test!");
}
```

Output

```
This is to test!
```

This program prints the message "This is to test!" to the console using the `println` method of the `System.out` object.

Program

```
void main() {
  int a = 5;
  int b = 10;
System.out.println("Sum: " + (a + b));
}
```

Output:

```
Sum: 15
```

This program initializes two integer variables, `a` and `b`, with values 5 and 10 respectively. It then calculates their sum and prints it along with the message "Sum: " using concatenation within the `println` statement.

Program

```
void main() {
  String name = "Usharani";
System.out.println("Hello, " + name + "!");
}
```

Output:

```
Hello Usharani
```

This program defines a variable `name` with the value "Usharani" and prints a greeting message "Hello, Usharani!" using concatenation within the `println` statement.

Program

```
void main() {
  int n = 5;
  int factorial = 1;
  for (int i = 1; i<= n; i++) {
    factorial *= i;
  }
System.out.println("Factorial: " + factorial);
}
```

Output:

```
Factorial: 120
```

This program calculates the factorial of the number 5 using a loop, initializing `factorial` to 1, iterating from 1 to 5, and multiplying each iteration's value to `factorial`, then printing the result "Factorial: 120"

Program

```
void main() {
  double celsius = 25.0;
  double fahrenheit = (celsius * 9/5) + 32;
System.out.println("Fahrenheit: " + fahrenheit);
}
Output:
Fahrenheit: 77.0
```

This program calculates and converts a temperature from Celsius to Fahrenheit using the formula $Fahrenheit = \left(Celsius \times \frac{9}{5}\right) + 32$. It initializes a Celsius value of 25.0, computes its Fahrenheit equivalent, and prints the result using standard output.

6.13 MEDICAL APPLICATIONS

6.13.1 Case Study 1

The primary parameters considered for gestationaldiabetes detection:

- **Fasting Blood Glucose:** This is the blood sugar level measured after a period of fasting (typically overnight). Elevated fasting blood glucose levels (usually above 126 mg/dL) are indicative of diabetes.
- **Postprandial Blood Glucose:** This refers to blood sugar levels measured after consuming a meal. Postprandial levels above 200 mg/dL, measured 2 hours after eating, are considered indicative of diabetes.
- **HbA1c (Glycated Hemoglobin):** HbA1c reflects average blood glucose levels over the past 2–3 months. Levels of 6.5% or higher indicate diabetes.

```
import java.util.Scanner;
class Patient {
  private String name;
  private int age;
  private String gender;
  public Patient(String name, int age, String gender) {
    this.name = name;
this.age = age;
this.gender = gender;
  }
  public String getName() {
    return name;
  }
  public int getAge() {
    return age;
  }
  public String getGender() {
    return gender;
  }
  @Override
```

```
  public String toString() {
    return "Patient{" +
        "name='" + name + '\'' +
        ", age=" + age +
        ", gender='" + gender + '\'' +
        '}';
  }
}
class GestationalDiabetesDetector {
    public booleanisDiabetesDetected(double fastingBloodSugar) {
    return fastingBloodSugar>= 92;
  }
  public   booleanisDiabetesDetected(double   fastingBloodSugar,   double
     postprandialBloodSugar) {
    return fastingBloodSugar>= 92 || postprandialBloodSugar>= 153;
  }
  public   booleanisDiabetesDetected(double   fastingBloodSugar,   double
     postprandialBloodSugar, double hbA1c) {
    return fastingBloodSugar>= 92 || postprandialBloodSugar>= 153 || hbA1c
>= 5.7;
  }
}public class GestationalDiabetesDetection {
  void main(String[] args) {
    Scanner scanner = new Scanner(System.in);
System.out.print("Enter patient name: ");
    String name = scanner.nextLine();
System.out.print("Enter patient age: ");
    int age = scanner.nextInt();
scanner.nextLine();
System.out.print("Enter patient gender: ");
    String gender = scanner.nextLine();
    Patient patient = new Patient(name, age, gender);
GestationalDiabetesDetectordiabetesDetector = new
   GestationalDiabetesDetector();
System.out.print("Enter fasting blood sugar level (mg/dL): ");
    double fastingBloodSugar = scanner.nextDouble();
System.out.print("Do you want to enter postprandial blood sugar level (yes/
  no)? ");
    String response = scanner.next();
boolean detected = false;
    if (response.equalsIgnoreCase("yes")) {
System.out.print("Enter postprandial blood sugar level (mg/dL): ");
      double postprandialBloodSugar = scanner.nextDouble();
System.out.print("Do you want to enter HbA1c level (yes/no)? ");
      response = scanner.next();
      if (response.equalsIgnoreCase("yes")) {
System.out.print("Enter HbA1c level (%): ");
        double hbA1c = scanner.nextDouble();
        detected  =  diabetesDetector.isDiabetesDetected(fastingBloodSugar,
           postprandialBloodSugar, hbA1c);
      } else {
        detected  =  diabetesDetector.isDiabetesDetected(fastingBloodSugar,
           postprandialBloodSugar);
      }
    } else {
```

```
      detected = diabetesDetector.isDiabetesDetected(fastingBloodSugar);
    }
System.out.println("Patient details: " + patient);
System.out.println("Gestational diabetes detection result: " + (detected ?
"Diabetes detected" : "No diabetes detected"));
  }
}
```

The above program begins by prompting the user to enter the patient's name, age, and gender, which are encapsulated into a `Patient` object upon instantiation. Three overloaded methods within `GestationalDiabetesDetector` assess different combinations of fasting blood sugar, postprandial blood sugar, and HbA1c levels to determine if diabetes is present. Using a `Scanner` for input, the program gathers fasting blood sugar levels and optionally postprandial blood sugar and HbA1c levels based on user responses. Depending on the provided data, it evaluates whether gestational diabetes is detected and outputs the patient's details alongside the diagnostic result.

6.13.2 Case Study 2

Forbes' disease, also known as Glycogen Storage Disease Type III (GSD III), is a rare genetic disorder characterized by the body's inability to break down glycogen properly in certain tissues, particularly the liver and muscles. This leads to the accumulation of abnormal amounts of glycogen in these tissues, causing symptoms such as muscle weakness, enlarged liver (hepatomegaly), and hypoglycemia (low blood sugar levels).

Parameters Considered for Forbes' Disease Detection

- **Muscle Weakness:** Patients with Forbes' disease often experience muscle weakness due to the abnormal glycogen accumulation in muscle tissues.
- **Liver Enlargement:** Hepatomegaly, or an enlarged liver, is a common sign of Forbes' disease. The liver accumulates excess glycogen, leading to its enlargement and potential complications.
- **Hypoglycemia:** Individuals with Forbes' disease may have episodes of hypoglycemia, especially during fasting or prolonged periods without food intake. This occurs because the liver cannot properly release glucose stored as glycogen.

```
import java.util.Scanner;
import java.util.function.Predicate;
public class ForbesDiseaseDetection {
  static class Patient {
    private String name;
    private int age;
    private String gender;
    private booleanhasMuscleWeakness;
    private booleanhasLiverEnlargement;
    private booleanhasHypoglycemia;
    public Patient(String name, int age, String gender,
       booleanhasMuscleWeakness, booleanhasLiverEnlargement,
       booleanhasHypoglycemia) {
      this.name = name;
this.age = age;
this.gender = gender;
this.hasMuscleWeakness = hasMuscleWeakness;
this.hasLiverEnlargement = hasLiverEnlargement;
this.hasHypoglycemia = hasHypoglycemia;
```

```
    }
    public String getName() {
      return name;
    }
    public int getAge() {
      return age;
    }
    public String getGender() {
      return gender;
    }
    public booleanhasMuscleWeakness() {
      return hasMuscleWeakness;
    }
    public booleanhasLiverEnlargement() {
      return hasLiverEnlargement;
    }
    public booleanhasHypoglycemia() {
      return hasHypoglycemia;
    }
    @Override
    public String toString() {
      return "Patient{" +
          "name='" + name + '\'' +
          ", age=" + age +
          ", gender='" + gender + '\'' +
          ", hasMuscleWeakness=" + hasMuscleWeakness +
          ", hasLiverEnlargement=" + hasLiverEnlargement +
          ", hasHypoglycemia=" + hasHypoglycemia +
          '}';
    }
  }
  void main(String[] args) {
    Scanner scanner = new Scanner(System.in);
System.out.print("Enter patient name: ");
    String name = scanner.nextLine();
System.out.print("Enter patient age: ");
    int age = scanner.nextInt();
scanner.nextLine();
System.out.print("Enter patient gender: ");
    String gender = scanner.nextLine();
System.out.print("Has muscle weakness (true/false): ");
booleanhasMuscleWeakness = scanner.nextBoolean();
System.out.print("Has liver enlargement (true/false): ");
booleanhasLiverEnlargement = scanner.nextBoolean();
System.out.print("Has hypoglycemia (true/false): ");
booleanhasHypoglycemia = scanner.nextBoolean();
    Patient patient = new Patient(name, age, gender, hasMuscleWeakness, 
hasLiverEnlargement, hasHypoglycemia);
    Predicate<Patient>muscleWeaknessPredicate = p ->p.hasMuscleWeakness();
    Predicate<Patient>liverEnlargementPredicate = p ->p.
hasLiverEnlargement();
    Predicate<Patient>hypoglycemiaPredicate = p ->p.hasHypoglycemia();
booleanhasForbesDisease = muscleWeaknessPredicate.test(patient) && 
liverEnlargementPredicate.test(patient) && 
hypoglycemiaPredicate.test(patient);
```

```
System.out.println("Patient details: " + patient);
System.out.println("Forbes' disease detection result: " + (hasForbesDisease
? "Forbes' disease detected" : "No Forbes' disease detected"));
  }
}
```

The program `ForbesDiseaseDetection` begins by prompting the user to enter details such as the patient's name, age, and gender, followed by boolean inputs indicating whether the patient has muscle weakness, liver enlargement, or hypoglycemia. Using this input, a `Patient` object is instantiated, encapsulating all provided data. The detection logic employs lambda expressions and predicates to evaluate if the patient exhibits symptoms indicative of Forbes' disease, namely muscle weakness, liver enlargement, and hypoglycemia.

7 Java Inheritance

7.1 INTRODUCTION

Data hiding is a fundamental concept in object-oriented programming (OOP) that refers to the practice of restricting direct access to certain components of an object's state (its data) from outside the object's definition. In Java, this is typically achieved by using access modifiers (`private`, `protected`, `public`) to control visibility and access to class members.

7.1.1 Key Aspects of Data Hiding

- Access Control: By marking certain fields (`private`) or methods (`private` or `protected`) within a class, access from outside the class is restricted. This prevents unintended modification or access to internal state.
- Encapsulation: Data hiding is closely related to encapsulation, where data and methods that operate on the data are bundled together within a class. Encapsulation ensures that the object's state is accessed and modified only through controlled methods.

7.1.2 Need for Data Hiding

- Security: Protects sensitive data from unauthorized access and manipulation, reducing the risk of accidental corruption or security breaches.
- Maintainability: Encourages a clear separation between the internal implementation details of a class and its public interface, making it easier to modify and refactor code without affecting other parts of the program.
- Flexibility: Allows classes to evolve independently, as changes to internal implementation details (private fields, methods) do not affect code that relies on the public interface.

7.1.3 Advantages of Data Hiding

- Enhanced Security: Prevents direct modification of sensitive data, ensuring that it is only accessed and modified through controlled methods. This reduces the risk of unintended side effects or security vulnerabilities.
- Improved Maintainability: Encourages better code organization and modular design by enforcing a clear separation between implementation details and public interface. This makes code easier to understand, debug, and maintain.
- Promotes Reusability: Encapsulation and data hiding facilitate code reuse, as objects can be integrated into different contexts without exposing their internal workings.

DOI: 10.1201/9781003544319-7

7.1.4 Limitations of Data Hiding

- Access Overhead: Requires additional effort to design and implement class interfaces (`getters` and `setters`) for accessing private data, which can increase code complexity and overhead.
- Potential Misuse: Over-restricting access to data can lead to overly complex designs or hinder legitimate use cases where direct access might be appropriate.
- Performance Considerations: Indirectly accessing data through getter and setter methods may incur a slight performance overhead compared to direct field access. However, modern JVM optimizations often mitigate this impact.

Example of data hiding in Java

```
public class Student {
  private String name;
  private int age;
  public Student(String name, int age) {
    this.name = name;
    this.age = age;
  }
  public String getName() { // Getter method
    return name;
  }
  public void setAge(int age) { // Setter method
    if (age > 0) {
      this.age = age;
    }
  }
}
```

In this example`name` and `age` are private fields, inaccessible directly from outside the `Student` class. `getName()` and `setAge(int age)` provide controlled access to `name` and `age`, respectively, ensuring that age is set only if it is positive.

7.1.5 Inheritance

Inheritance in Java is a fundamental concept that allows one class to inherit the properties and behaviors (fields and methods) of another class. This mechanism is one of the key features of object-oriented programming (OOP), enabling the creation of hierarchical classifications. It promotes code reuse and can make the system more modular and easier to manage.

Key Concepts of Java Inheritance

1. Superclass (Parent Class): The class whose properties and methods are inherited. It is also known as the base class or parent class.
2. Subclass (Child Class): The class that inherits the properties and methods of another class. It is also known as the derived class or child class.

In Java, inheritance is implemented using the `extends` keyword. When a class extends another class, it inherits all the non-private members (fields and methods) of the superclass.

7.1.5.1 Benefits of Inheritance

1. Code Reusability: Allows for the reuse of existing code, reducing redundancy and improving maintainability.

2. Method Overriding: Subclasses can provide specific implementations for methods defined in their superclasses.
3. Polymorphism: Enables a single interface to represent different underlying forms (objects). For instance, a method can accept a superclass type, allowing it to work with any subclass type as well.
4. Hierarchical Organization: Helps in organizing and structuring the code in a hierarchical manner, which is more intuitive and easier to understand.

7.1.5.2 Limitations of Inheritance

1. Tight Coupling: Inheritance creates a tight coupling between the superclass and subclass, making the system less flexible.
2. Fragile Base Class Problem: Changes in the superclass can affect all subclasses, sometimes in unintended ways.
3. Single Inheritance Limitation: Java supports only single inheritance, meaning a class can inherit from only one superclass. This can be restrictive in certain scenarios.
4. Increased Complexity: Deep inheritance hierarchies can become difficult to manage and understand.

Program

```
// Superclass named test
class test {
  // Method in the test class
  void display() {
    System.out.println("Parent class method");
  }
}
// Main class that extends test
public class Main extends test {
void main(String[] args) {
    // Create an instance of the test class
    test t = new test();
    // Call the display() method using the test object
    t.display();  // This will call the method from the test class
  }
}
```

Output:

```
Parent class method
```

The Java program consists of two classes: "test" and "Main." The "test" class contains a single method named "display()" that prints the message "Parent class method" to the console when called. The method does not return any value. The "Main" class extends the "test" class, indicating that it inherits the "display()" method from its superclass. Within the main method of the "Main" class, an instance of the "test" class is created using the statement "test t = new test();". This creates an object of the "test" class, which is then used to invoke the "display()" method. When the program is executed, the "display()" method of the "test" class is called using the object "t", resulting in the message "Parent class method" being printed to the console.

7.2 THE EXTENDS KEYWORD

In Java, inheritance is a fundamental principle of object-oriented programming, enabling classes to inherit and leverage data members and properties from parent or base classes. In this paradigm, subclasses, also referred to as child classes, are created by extending or inheriting from their parent class. This inheritance mechanism allows child classes to access and utilize the variables and methods defined in their parent class. The inclusion of the "extends" keyword in a child class declaration signals to the compiler that the child class inherits the attributes and behaviors of its parent class. By leveraging inheritance, Java developers can create hierarchies of classes, promoting code reusability, modularity, and extensibility in their applications.

Syntax

```
class super
{
------
-----
-----
}
class sub extends super
{
------
-----
-----
}
```

The "extends" keyword in Java indicates inheritance, where a subclass inherits the data members and methods of a superclass. When a class is declared using the syntax `class Sub extends Super`, it means that the class `Sub` is inheriting from the class `Super`. In this scenario:

- `Super` is referred to as the superclass or parent class.
- `Sub` is referred to as the subclass or child class.

The structure of the subclass declaration follows a specific format. The class keyword is followed by the name of the subclass, then the extends keyword, and finally the name of the parent class from which the subclass is inheriting. Inside the subclass, you define data members (variables) and methods that are unique to the subclass, in addition to those inherited from the parent class. This syntax allows the subclass to access and utilize the data members and methods of its parent class, enhancing code reuse and promoting a hierarchical structure in object-oriented programming.

Program

```
// Base class
class Base {
  // Method in the Base class
  void display() {
    System.out.println("Base Class Method");
  }
}
// Derived class that extends Base
class Derived extends Base {
  // Method in the Derived class
  void put() {
```

```
    System.out.println("Derived Class Method");
  }
}
// Test class with the main method
public class Test {
  void main(String[] args) {
    // Create an object of the Derived class
    Derived d = new Derived();
    // Call the display() method from the Base class
    d.display(); // Output: "Base Class Method"
    // Call the put() method from the Derived class
    d.put();    // Output: "Derived Class Method"
  }
}
```

Output:

```
Base Class Method
Derived Class Methods
```

The above Java program consists of three classes: "Base", "Derived", and "Test". The "Base" class contains a method named "display()", which prints the message "Base Class Method" to the console. The "Derived" class extends the "Base" class and defines a method named "put()", which prints the message "Derived Class Methods" to the console.The "Test" class contains the main method. Within the main method, an object of the "Derived" class named "d" is created using the statement "Derived d = new Derived();". Then, the "display()" method is called on the "d" object, resulting in the message "Base Class Method" being printed to the console. Next, the "put()" method is called on the same object, resulting in the message "Derived Class Method" being printed to the console. When the program is executed, it creates an object of the "Derived" class, demonstrating inheritance where the "Derived" class inherits the "display()" method from its superclass "Base".

7.3 PARENT CLASS CATEGORIES

In Java, any class can act as a parent class, serving as the foundation for inheritance hierarchies. Parent classes can further classify into two types based on their relationship with other classes: direct parent classes and indirect parent classes.

7.3.1 Direct Parent Class

A parent class is termed as a direct parent class if it is explicitly mentioned in the list of parent classes for a subclass. In other words, when a subclass directly extends or inherits from a parent class, the parent class is considered as the direct parent. For example:

```
class Test {
}
class Sample extends Test {
}
```

In this example, "Test" is the direct parent class of "Sample" since "Sample" explicitly extends "Test".

7.3.2 Indirect Parent Class

An indirect parent class, on the other hand, is a class that is not directly mentioned in the inheritance hierarchy but is inherited from another parent class. In this case, the subclass extends a class that itself extends another class. For example:

```
class Test {
}
class Sample extends Test {
}
class First extends Sample {
}
```

In the above example, “Test” is the direct parent class of “Sample” since “Sample” extends “Test”. However, for the class “First”, “Sample” is the direct parent class while “Test” becomes an indirect parent class. This is because “First” extends “Sample”, which in turn extends “Test”.

Program: Indirect parent class

```
// Parent class "test"
class Test {
  // Method in the "test" class
  void display() {
    System.out.println("Parent class method");
  }
}
// Child class "sample" that extends "test"
class Sample extends Test {
  // Method in the "sample" class
  void put() {
    System.out.println("Child class method");
  }
}
// Subchild class "test1" that extends "sample"
class Test1 extends Sample {
  // Method in the "test1" class
  void printing() {
    System.out.println("Subchild class method");
  }
}
// Subsubchild class "test2" that extends "test1"
class Test2 extends Test1 {
  // Method in the "test2" class
  void method() {
    System.out.println("Subsubchild class method");
  }
}
// Main class
public class Main {
  void main(String[] args) {
    // Create an object of "test2"
    Test2 t = new Test2();
    // Call methods from each class
    t.display();  // Output: "Parent class method"
    t.put();    // Output: "Child class method"
    t.printing();    // Output: "Subchild class method"
    t.method();    // Output: "Subsubchild class method"
  }
}
Output:
Parent class method
```

```
Child class method
Subchild class method
Subsubchild class method
```

The above Java program consists of several classes, including “test”, “sample”, “test1”, “test2”, and a public class named “Main”.The “test” class defines a method named “display()” that prints “Parent class method” to the console. The “sample” class extends the “test” class and defines a method named “put()” that prints “child class method” to the console. The “test1” class extends the “sample” class and defines a method named “printing()” that prints “subchild class method” to the console. The “test2” class extends the “test1” class and defines a method named “method()” that prints “subsubchild class method” to the console. Finally, the “Main” class extends the “sample” class. Within its main method, an instance of the “test2” class is created using the statement “test2 t = new test2();”. This object is used to call the “display()”, “put()”, “printing()”, and “method()” methods.When the program is executed, each of the methods from the “test”, “sample”, “test1”, and “test2” classes is invoked on the “t” object.

7.4 ACCESSING PARENT CLASS MEMBERS

In Java, the accessibility of a parent class is determined by the access modifiers applied to its members, including variables, methods, and constructors. These access modifiers specify how these members can be accessed from within the class itself and from other classes in the same or different packages. There are four main access modifiers:

1. Default:
   The default access modifier is automatically applied when no explicit access modifier is specified. It restricts access to the parent class only within the same package, preventing access from outside the package.
2. Public:
   The public access modifier allows unrestricted access to the parent class from any other class, regardless of the package. This modifier enables broad accessibility, making the parent class accessible to all classes in the application.
3. Protected:
   The protected access modifier limits access to the parent class to its subclasses, allowing access only within the same package or from subclasses in different packages. This modifier is useful for creating a level of accessibility that extends beyond the class itself but remains restricted to its subclasses.
4. Private:
   The private access modifier provides the strictest level of access control, restricting access to the parent class's members exclusively within the class itself. This modifier ensures that the members are accessible only from within the class and not from any external classes or subclasses.

By applying these access modifiers appropriately, Java programmers can manage the visibility and accessibility of parent class members, ensuring appropriate encapsulation and controlling the interactions between classes in the application.

7.4.1 Accessing Protected Members

Protected members of a parent class can be accessed directly by the child class, as they are visible to subclasses and classes in the same package.

Program

```
public class InheritanceExample {
  static class Base {
    protected String baseField;
    public Base() {
      baseField = "Base field";
    }
    protected void baseMethod() {
      System.out.println("Base method");
    }
    protected void displayBase() {
      System.out.println("Base Field: " + baseField);
    }
  }
  static class Child extends Base {
    protected String childField;
    public Child() {
      childField = "Child field";
    }
    protected void childMethod() {
      System.out.println("Child method");
    }
}
    void main(String[] args) {
      // Creating an instance of the Child class
      Child childInstance = new Child();
      // Accessing protected members from the base class
      System.out.println("Accessing Base Field from Child: " + childInstance.
         baseField);
      childInstance.baseMethod();
      // Accessing protected members from the child class
      System.out.println("Accessing Child Field from Child: " + childInstance.
         childField);
      childInstance.childMethod();
      // Displaying both base and child fields
      childInstance.displayBase();
  }
}
```

Output:

```
Accessing Base Field from Child: Base field
Base method
Accessing Child Field from Child: Child field
Child method
Base Field: Base field
```

The `InheritanceExample` class, which contains a base class `Base` and a derived class `Child`. The `Base` class defines a protected field `baseField` and two protected methods, `baseMethod()` and `displayBase()`. The constructor of the `Base` class initializes the `baseField` with the value "Base field." The `baseMethod()` prints a message "Base method," and `displayBase()` outputs the value of `baseField`.The `Child` class extends the `Base` class, inheriting its members, and adds its own protected field `childField` and method `childMethod()`. The constructor of the `Child` class initializes `childField` with "Child field," and `childMethod()` prints "Child method." In the `main` method, we create an instance of the `Child` class and access both the inherited and child-specific members. The instance allows us to access the `baseField` and `baseMethod()` from the `Base` class, as well as the `childField` and `childMethod()` from the `Child` class. Additionally, the `displayBase()` method is invoked to print the `baseField` value.

7.4.2 Accessing Private Members

Private members of a parent class cannot be accessed directly by the child class. To access private members, you need to use public or protected getter and setter methods in the parent class.

Program

```
class Parent {
  private int privateField;
  // Constructor to initialize privateField
  public Parent(int privateField) {
    this.privateField = privateField;
  }
  // Method to access privateField
  public int getPrivateField() {
    return privateField;
  }
}
class Child extends Parent {
  private int childPrivateField;
  public Child(int privateField, int childPrivateField) {
    super(privateField); // Calling parent class constructor
    this.childPrivateField = childPrivateField;
  }
  // Method to access parent's privateField indirectly
  public int getParentPrivateField() {
    return getPrivateField(); // Calling parent class method to access
                                privateField
  }
    // Method to access child's privateField directly
  public int getChildPrivateField() {
    return childPrivateField;
  }
}
public class Main {
  void main(String[] args) {
    Child child = new Child(10, 20);
    // Accessing parent's privateField indirectly
    System.out.println("Parent's privateField: " + child.
       getParentPrivateField());
    // Accessing child's privateField directly
    System.out.println("Child's privateField: " + child.
getChildPrivateField());
  }
}
Output:
Parent's privateField: 10
Child's privateField: 20
```

In the above program, we demonstrate inheritance and access to private fields through getter methods in Java. We define a `Parent` class with a private field `privateField`, which cannot be directly accessed from outside the class. To initialize this field, a constructor is provided, and a public method `getPrivateField()` is used to return its value. The `Child` class extends the `Parent` class, adding its own private field `childPrivateField`. In the `Child` constructor, the `super()` call is used to invoke the `Parent` class constructor, initializing the `privateField`. The `Child` class also provides two methods: `getParentPrivateField()` to access the parent's private field indirectly via the parent's `getPrivateField()` method, and `getChildPrivateField()` to access its own private field directly. In the `Main` class, we create an instance of the `Child` class, passing values 10 and 20 for the parent's and child's private fields, respectively. Using the instance, we access the parent's private field through the `getParentPrivateField()` method and the child's private field directly through the `getChildPrivateField()` method. The output confirms that the parent's private field holds the value 10, while the child's private field holds the value 20.

Program: Program for private constructor in inheritance in Java

```
// Base class
class Base {
  // Private constructor in Base class
  private Base() {
    System.out.println("private parent constructor");
  }
  // Parameterized constructor that calls the private constructor
  Base(int i) {
    this(); // Calls the private constructor
  }
}
// Child class that extends Base class
class Child extends Base {
  // Parameterized constructor in Child class
  Child(int i) {
    System.out.println("child constructor");
super(i); // Calls the parameterized constructor of the Base class
  }
}
// Sample class with main method
public class Sample {
    void main(String[] args) {
    // Create an instance of Child class
    Child c = new Child(10); // This calls the constructor chain
  }
}
Output:
child constructor
private parent constructor
```

This Java program consists of three classes: "base", "child", and "sample". The "base" class contains a private constructor, which prints "private parent constructor" when invoked, and a parameterized constructor that calls the private constructor using "this()".The "child" class extends the "base" class and defines its own parameterized constructor. This constructor invokes the superclass constructor prints "child constructor" to the console and using "super(i)".In the "sample" class's main method, an object of the "child" class is created using the statement "child c = new child(10);". This statement creates an instance of the "child" class with the parameter "10". As a result, the parameterized constructor of the "child" class is invoked. Inside this constructor, the superclass constructor is invoked first, which prints "private parent constructor", followed by the message "child constructor" being printed to the console.

7.5 TYPES OF INHERITANCE

Inheritance in Java allows one class to inherit the properties and methods of another class, promoting code reuse and a hierarchical class structure. Here are the various types of inheritance in Java:

- Single Inheritance:
  Single inheritance is when a class inherits from one and only one parent class. This is the simplest form of inheritance, where a derived class extends a single base class.

- Multilevel Inheritance:
  Multilevel inheritance involves a class being derived from another class, which is itself derived from another class, forming a chain of inheritance. This creates a multilevel hierarchy of classes.

- Hierarchical Inheritance:
  Hierarchical inheritance occurs when multiple classes inherit from a single-parent class. This allows for the creation of multiple derived classes from a single base class, forming a tree structure.

- Multiple Inheritance (Through Interfaces):
  Java does not support multiple inheritance with classes to avoid complexity and ambiguity (the diamond problem). However, multiple inheritance can be achieved through interfaces, where a class can implement multiple interfaces. It will be discussed in Chapter 8.

- Hybrid Inheritance (Using Interfaces):
  Hybrid inheritance is a combination of two or more types of inheritance. While Java does not support hybrid inheritance involving multiple classes, it can be achieved using a mix of classes and interfaces. This allows for a flexible combination of inheritance types, leveraging the strengths of both classes and interfaces.

7.5.1 Single Inheritance

Single inheritance is a fundamental concept in object-oriented programming, where a child class can inherit methods and data members from exactly one parent class. In this paradigm, the child class extends the functionality of the parent class by inheriting its attributes and behaviors.

In single inheritance, there exists a clear hierarchical relationship between the parent class and the child class. The child class can access and utilize the methods and data members defined in the parent class, enhancing code reuse and promoting modularity.

This inheritance relationship enables developers to create specialized classes that build upon the functionality provided by their parent classes. By inheriting from a single parent class, the child class can benefit from the encapsulation, abstraction, and polymorphism principles of object-oriented programming, leading to more modular and maintainable code.

Syntax

```
class super
{
// variables and methods
```

```
}
class sub extends super
{
// variables and methods
}
```

The syntax represents the structure of two Java classes: “superclass” and “subclass,” showcasing single inheritance. In this syntax, “superclass” is defined as the parent class, while “subclass” extends or inherits from the “superclass,” serving as the child class. The syntax follows the convention of class declaration in Java, where each class is declared using the “class” keyword followed by the class name.

Within the “superclass” and “subclass” definitions, developers can include variables and methods specific to each class. The “subclass” inherits all public and protected variables and methods from the “superclass,” enabling code reuse and extension. This inheritance relationship is established through the “extends” keyword, which indicates that the “subclass” inherits from the “superclass.”

By extending the “superclass,” the “subclass” gains access to its attributes and behaviors, allowing developers to build upon and enhance the functionality provided by the parent class. This promotes code modularity, encapsulation, and code reuse, essential principles of object-oriented programming. The syntax encapsulates the concept of single inheritance, where a child class inherits from exactly one parent class, forming a hierarchical relationship between the classes.

Note: The declaration of a single derived class is the same as that of the ordinary java class.

The subclass, a fundamental concept in object-oriented programming, comprises several components that define its structure and inheritance relationship with its superclass:

1. The Keyword Class: The subclass declaration begins with the keyword “class,” denoting the definition of a new class within the Java programming language.
2. The Name of the Subclass: Following the “class” keyword is the name of the subclass, which identifies the subclass within the program. This name typically reflects the nature or purpose of the subclass.
3. Extends Keyword: After specifying the name of the subclass, the “extends” keyword is used to indicate that the subclass extends or inherits from another class, known as its superclass. This establishes an inheritance relationship between the subclass and its superclass.
4. The Name of the Superclass: Following the “extends” keyword is the name of the superclass from which the subclass inherits. This superclass provides the blueprint or template for the subclass, allowing it to inherit attributes and behaviors.
5. The Remainder of the Subclass Definition: After specifying the superclass, the remainder of the subclass definition includes additional components such as member variables, methods, and constructors specific to the subclass. These components define the unique characteristics and functionalities of the subclass, which may complement or extend those inherited from the superclass.

Together, these components form the structure of the subclass, establishing its inheritance relationship with its superclass and defining its unique attributes and behaviors within the Java program.

Program

Single Inheritance with variables and methods

```
// Parent class "test"
class Test {
  // String variable in the "test" class
  String name = "parent";
  // Method in the "test" class
  void display() {
```

```
    System.out.println("Parent class method");
  }
}
// Child class "sample" that extends "test"
class Sample extends Test {
  // String variable in the "sample" class
  String name1 = "sub";
  // Method in the "sample" class
  void put() {
    System.out.println("Child class method");
    // Access the "name" variable from "test" class and "name1" variable
from "sample" class
    System.out.println("Name from parent class: " + name);
    System.out.println("Name from child class: " + name1);
  }
}
// Main class
public class Main {
void main(String[] args) {
    // Create an object of the "sample" class
    Sample s = new Sample();
    // Call the "display()" method from the "test" class
    s.display(); // Output: "Parent class method"
    // Call the "put()" method from the "sample" class
    s.put();    // Output: "Child class method", followed by the names
  }
}
```

Output:

```
Parent class method
Child class method
Name from parent class: parent
Name from child class: sub
```

The Java program consists of three classes: "test", "sample", and "Main". The "test" class defines a string variable "name" with the value "parent" and a method named "display()". The "display()" method prints "Parent class method" to the console when called. The "sample" class extends the "test" class, inheriting the "name" variable and the "display()" method. Additionally, it declares a new string variable "name1" with the value "sub" and defines a method named "put()". The "put()" method prints "child class method" to the console and accesses both the "name" and "name1" variables, printing their values along with respective messages. The "Main" class extends the "sample" class, inheriting all its variables and methods. Within the main method, an instance of the "sample" class is created using the statement "sample s = new sample();". This object is used to call the "display()" method inherited from the "test" class and the "put()" method defined in the "sample" class.When the program is executed, the "display()" method prints "Parent class method" to the console, followed by the "put()" method printing "child class method". Additionally, it accesses and prints the values of both "name" and "name1" variables, demonstrating the inheritance and access to variables across classes in Java inheritance hierarchy.

Program

```
// Base class with a private constructor
class Base {
  // Private constructor
```

```
  private Base() {
    System.out.println("Private Base constructor");
  }
  // Protected constructor for use by Child class
  protected Base(boolean flag) {
    System.out.println("Protected Base constructor");
  }
  // Static factory method to create an instance of Base
  public static Base createBase() {
    return new Base();
  }
}
// Child class extending Base
class Child extends Base {
  // Protected constructor in Child class
  protected Child() {
    System.out.println("Protected Child constructor");
super(true); // Call the protected constructor of Base
  }
}
// Test class with the main method
public class Test {
  void main(String[] args) {
    // Creating an instance of Base using the static factory method
    Base base = Base.createBase();
    // Creating an instance of Child
    Child child = new Child();  // This will call the protected constructor
of Child
  }
}
```

Output:

```
Private Base constructor
Protected Child constructor
Protected Base constructor
```

In the above program, the `Base` class has a private constructor and a protected constructor, with a static factory method to create an instance. The `Child` class extends `Base` and uses the protected constructor of `Base` within its own protected constructor. When creating an instance of `Child`, it first prints messages from the `Base` constructors and then from the `Child` constructor, showing the sequence of constructor calls. The output reflects this sequence, indicating that `Base`'s private constructor is invoked through the static factory method and `Child`'s protected constructor is called directly.

7.5.2 Multilevel Inheritance

In multilevel inheritance, a subclass inherits from another subclass, forming a chain of inheritance where each subclass becomes a parent class for subsequent subclasses. This creates a hierarchical relationship among the classes, allowing attributes and behaviors to be passed down the inheritance chain.

For example

```
class Grandparent {
  // Grandparent class members
```

```
}
class Parent extends Grandparent {
  // Parent class members
}
class Child extends Parent {
  // Child class members
}
```

In the above syntax, "Parent" class inherits from "Grandparent" class, and "Child" class inherits from "Parent" class. Consequently, "Child" class indirectly inherits from "Grandparent" class through the intermediate class "Parent". This forms a multilevel inheritance chain, where each class inherits attributes and behaviors from its parent class, ultimately leading to the inheritance of features from all classes up the hierarchy.

Multilevel inheritance facilitates code reuse, promotes modularity, and allows for the creation of complex class hierarchies in object-oriented programming. However, it's essential to use inheritance judiciously to maintain code clarity and prevent excessive coupling between classes.

Program

```
// Parent class "test"
class Test {
  // Method in the "test" class
  void display() {
    System.out.println("Parent class method");
  }
}
// Child class "sample" that extends "test"
class Sample extends Test {
  // Method in the "sample" class
  void put() {
    System.out.println("Child class method");
  }
}
// Main class
public class Main {
  void main(String[] args) {
    // Create an object of the "sample" class
    Sample s = new Sample();
    // Call the "display()" method from the "test" class
    s.display(); // Output: "Parent class method"
    // Call the "put()" method from the "sample" class
    s.put();    // Output: "Child class method"
  }
}
Output:
Parent class method
Child class method
```

The above Java program consists of three classes: "test", "sample", and "Main". The "test" class contains a method named "display()", which simply prints "Parent class method" to the console. The "sample" class extends the "test" class, inheriting the "display()" method, and defines a method named "put()", which prints "child class method" to the console. The "Main" class extends the "sample" class. Within its main method, an object of the "sample" class is created using the statement "sample s = new sample();". Then, the "display()" and "put()" methods are called using this object "s".Upon execution, the program prints "Parent class method" followed by "child class method" to the console, demonstrating the inheritance of methods from the superclass ("test") to the subclass ("sample").

7.5.3 Hierarchical Inheritance

Hierarchical inheritance in Java involves a class hierarchy where multiple subclasses inherit from a common superclass.

Program

```
// Superclass
class base {
  void f1() {
    System.out.println("base");
  }
}
// Subclass 1
class child extends base {
  void f2() {
    System.out.println("child");
  }
}
// Subclass 2
class subchild extends base {
  void f3() {
    System.out.println("subchild");
  }
}
public class Main {
  void main(String[] args) {
    // Creating objects of subclasses
child c=new child();
  subchild s=new subchild();
  c.f1();
c.f2();
s.f1();
s.f3();
  }
}
Output:
base
child
base
subchild
```

The above Java program illustrates hierarchical inheritance with a superclass named `base` and two subclasses named `child` and `subchild`. The `base` class contains a method `f1()` that prints "base", which is inherited by both subclasses. Each subclass also defines its own unique method: `f2()` in `child` and `f3()` in `subchild`, printing "child" and "subchild" respectively. In the `Main` class, objects of the `child` and `subchild` classes are instantiated. Through inheritance, both subclasses inherit the `f1()` method from the superclass `base`. Additionally, methods `f2()` and `f3()` are invoked on objects of `child` and `subchild` respectively, demonstrating how each subclass can have its own behavior in addition to what is inherited from the superclass.

7.6 CONSTRUCTOR CHAINING

Constructor chaining in inheritance refers to the process where a derived (child) class constructor calls the constructor of its base (parent) class. This ensures that the parent class is properly initialized before the child class adds its own properties and methods. In Java, this is typically achieved using the `super` keyword.

It is divided into two types:

(a) parameterless constructor chaining
(b) parameterized constructor chaining

7.6.1 Parameterless Constructor Chaining

It occurs when constructors without parameters are used to establish the chain of calls from the child class to the parent class. In Java, if a subclass constructor does not explicitly call a superclass constructor, the Java compiler automatically inserts a call to the parameterless constructor of the superclass using `super()`.

Program

```
class Parent {
  Parent() {
    System.out.println("Parent class parameterless constructor");
  }
}
class Child extends Parent {
  Child() {
    // Implicit call to super()
    System.out.println("Child class parameterless constructor");
  }
}
public class ConstructorChainingExample {
  void main(String[] args) {
    System.out.println("Creating Child instance:");
    Child child = new Child();
  }
}
Output:
Creating Child instance:
Parent class parameterless constructor
Child class parameterless constructor
```

In the above program, we demonstrate constructor chaining in Java, where a child class constructor implicitly calls the parent class constructor. The `Parent` class contains a parameterless constructor, which prints a message indicating that the parent class constructor has been invoked. The `Child` class extends the `Parent` class and also defines a parameterless constructor. Although there is no explicit call to `super()`, Java implicitly calls the parent class constructor when the child class constructor is invoked. This ensures that the parent class constructor is executed first, followed by the child class constructor. In the `Child` constructor, a message is printed to indicate that the child class constructor has been invoked. In the `ConstructorChainingExample` class, we create an instance of the `Child` class. This triggers the constructor chaining process: first, the parent class constructor is called, printing "Parent class parameterless constructor," and then the child class constructor is executed, printing "Child class parameterless constructor."

7.6.2 Parameterized Constructor

Parameterized constructor chaining in inheritance involves calling a specific constructor of the superclass from a subclass with the 'super()'.

Program

```
class Parent {
  Parent(String message) {
    System.out.println("Parent class constructor: " + message);
  }
}
class Child extends Parent {
  Child(String message) {
    System.out.println("Child class constructor: " + message);
super(message); // Explicit call to the parameterized constructor of Parent
  }
}
public class ConstructorChainingExample {
  void main(String[] args) {
    System.out.println("Creating Child instance:");
    Child child = new Child("Child");
  }
}
Output:
Creating Child instance:
Child class constructor: Child
Parent class constructor: Child
```

This program demonstrates constructor chaining in Java with inheritance, where the `Child` class extends the `Parent` class. The `Parent` class has a parameterized constructor that prints a message. The `Child` class also has a parameterized constructor that calls the `Parent` constructor using the `super` keyword and then prints its own message. The `ConstructorChainingExample` class contains the `main` method, which creates an instance of the `Child` class with a message. When executed, the program prints messages from both the `Parent` and `Child` constructors, showing the order of constructor calls.

7.6.2.1 Another Example with Multiple Constructors

Program

```
class Parent {
  Parent() {
    System.out.println("Parent class default constructor");
  }
  Parent(String message) {
    System.out.println("Parent class parameterized constructor: " +
       message);
  }
}
class Child extends Parent {
  Child() {
    System.out.println("Child class default constructor");
```

```
    super(); // Explicit call to the default constructor of Parent
  }
  Child(String message) {
      System.out.println("Child  class  parameterized  constructor:  " +
         message);
super(message); // Explicit call to the parameterized constructor of Parent
  }
}
public class ConstructorChainingExample {
  void main(String[] args) {
    System.out.println("Creating Child instance with default constructor:");
    Child child1 = new Child();
    System.out.println("\nCreating  Child  instance  with  parameterized
       constructor:");
    Child child2 = new Child("Usharani");
  }
}
```

Output:

```
Creating Child instance with default constructor:
Child class default constructor
Parent class default constructor
Creating Child instance with parameterized constructor:
Child class parameterized constructor: Usharani
Parent class parameterized constructor: Usharani
```

The above program demonstrates constructor chaining in Java using inheritance. The `Parent` class defines a default constructor and a parameterized constructor that prints respective messages. The `Child` class extends `Parent` and also defines both default and parameterized constructors, each explicitly calling the corresponding constructor of the `Parent` class using the `super` keyword. The `ConstructorChainingExample` class contains the `main` method, which creates instances of the `Child` class using both the default and parameterized constructors, illustrating how constructor calls are propagated up the inheritance hierarchy. When executed, it prints messages indicating the order of constructor calls for both the `Parent` and `Child` classes.

Program: Program for constructor chaining using super in multilevel inheritance

```
// Base class with two constructors
class Base {
  Base() {
    System.out.println("Base class no-argument constructor");
  }
  Base(String str) {
    System.out.println("Base class parameterized constructor: " + str);
  }
}
// Child class extending Base with two constructors
class Child extends Base {
  Child() {
    System.out.println("Child class no-argument constructor");
    super();  // Calls Base class no-argument constructor
  }
  Child(String str) {
       System.out.println("Child class parameterized constructor: " + str);
  super(str);  // Calls Base class parameterized constructor
```

```
  }
}
// Sub class extending Child with two constructors
class Sub extends Child {
  Sub() {
        System.out.println("Sub class no-argument constructor");
  super(); // Calls Child class no-argument constructor
  }
  Sub(String str) {
        System.out.println("Sub class parameterized constructor: " + str);
super(str); // Calls Child class parameterized constructor
  }
}
// Test class to demonstrate the constructors
public class Test {
  void main(String[] args) {
    // Create an object of Sub class without parameters
    Sub s1 = new Sub();
    // Create an object of Sub class with a "test" parameter
    Sub s2 = new Sub("test");
  }
}
```

Output:

```
Sub class no-argument constructor
Child class no-argument constructor
Base class no-argument constructor
Sub class parameterized constructor: test
Child class parameterized constructor: test
Base class parameterized constructor: test
```

The above Java program consists of three classes: `base`, `child`, and `sub`. The `base` class contains two constructors, one without parameters and one with a `String` parameter. Both constructors print messages indicating their invocation. The `child` class extends the `base` class and also contains two constructors, one without parameters and one with a `String` parameter. The constructors of the `child` class invoke the corresponding constructors of the `base` class using the `super` keyword and then print messages indicating their execution. The `sub` class extends the `child` class and contains similar constructors as the `child` class, invoking the superclass constructors and printing messages accordingly. In the `Test` class's `main` method, two `sub` objects are instantiated, one without parameters and one with a `"test"` parameter, demonstrating the invocation of constructors and their respective messages.

Program: Program for constructor chaining using super

```
// Base class with three constructors
class Base {
  Base() {
    System.out.println("Base class no-argument constructor");
  }
  Base(String str) {
    System.out.println("Base class parameterized constructor with String: "
        + str);
  }
  Base(int num) {
```

```
    System.out.println("Base class parameterized constructor with int: "
       + num);
  }
}
// Child class extending Base with two constructors
class Child extends Base {
  Child() {
    System.out.println("Child class no-argument constructor");
  super("test"); // Calls Base class constructor with String parameter
  }
  Child(String str) {
    System.out.println("Child class parameterized constructor with String: "
       + str);
super("test"); // Calls Base class constructor with String parameter
  }
}
// Test class to demonstrate constructor invocation
public class Test {
  void main(String[] args) {
    // Creating a Child object with no arguments
    Child c1 = new Child();
    // Creating a Child object with a String argument
    Child c2 = new Child("test");
  }
}
```

Output:

```
Child class no-argument constructor
Base class parameterized constructor with String: test
Child class parameterized constructor with String: test
Base class parameterized constructor with String: test
```

The above Java program includes two classes: `base` and `child`. The `base` class has three constructors, each with different parameters. The constructors print messages indicating their invocation. The `child` class extends the `base` class and contains two constructors, one without parameters and one with a `String` parameter. In both constructors, the `super` keyword is used to call the appropriate constructor from the superclass, passing `"test"` as an argument. After invoking the superclass constructor, messages indicating the constructor execution are printed. In the `Test` class's `main` method, two `child` objects are instantiated, one without parameters and one with a `"test"` parameter, demonstrating the constructor invocation and message printing.

7.7 STATEMENTS BEFORE 'SUPER(...)'

In Java 22, the feature allowing statements before `super(...)` in constructors addresses a long-standing limitation in the language's constructor invocation rules. Traditionally, constructors in Java required that any statement involving the instance being constructed (via `this`) must appear after the `super(...)` call or implicit `super()` call. This restriction often led to unnatural constructor code and made it challenging to adhere to best practices, such as initializing fields before invoking superclass constructors.

7.7.1 NEED FOR STATEMENTS BEFORE `SUPER(...)`

- Initialization Flexibility: Prior to this feature, constructors were constrained to initialize fields and perform other logic only after calling `super(...)`. This restriction could lead to complex workarounds and less readable code when initialization order mattered, especially in subclasses where superclass constructors needed specific setup.

- Field Initialization: With the ability to place statements before `super(...)`, developers can initialize fields or perform other tasks that do not depend on superclass state or construction. This improves clarity and allows for more natural ordering of initialization steps, aligning with typical coding practices and reducing the risk of errors due to incorrect initialization sequences.
- Enhanced Readability: By allowing statements before `super(...)`, constructors become more readable and intuitive. Developers can place preparatory logic at the beginning of constructors, making it clearer what setup is performed before the superclass's constructor is invoked.
- Subclass Constructor Benefits: Subclasses benefit significantly from this feature when they need to perform operations that are logically independent of superclass initialization. For instance, setting default values or validating parameters can now be done before invoking `super(...)`, ensuring that superclass constructors receive valid data.
- Consistency with Initialization Order: Modernizing the constructor invocation rules aligns Java with other programming languages, where constructor logic is more flexible and adheres to a natural flow of initialization. This change improves the language's usability without compromising compatibility with existing codebases.

Program

```
class Base {
  Base(String message) {
    System.out.println(message);
  }
}
class Child extends Base {
  Child() {
    System.out.println("Child constructor starts.");
    super("Base call from child");
  }
}
public class Test {
  void main(String[] args) {
    Child c= new Child();
  }
}
Output:
Child constructor starts.
Base call from child
```

This program works only in java22 for other versions it will throw an error because we used super() in the child class constructor after the println() statement. In this explanation, we demonstrate the use of constructors in a parent-child class relationship and how the `super()` call can be used in Java. We define a `Base` class that has a constructor accepting a `String` parameter. When this constructor is called, it prints the message passed to it. The `Child` class extends the `Base` class. In its constructor, the first line prints the message "Child constructor starts." However, the `super()` call that invokes the parent class constructor is placed after this print statement, which is valid in Java 22. In the `Test` class, when a `Child` instance is created, the `super("Base call from child")` statement in the child class constructor will invoke the parent class constructor, passing the string "Base call from child" to the `Base` constructor, which will print this message. Then, the child class constructor will continue, printing "Child constructor starts."

Program

```
class Logger {
  static void log(String message) {
    System.out.println(message);
  }
}
class Base {
  Base() {
    System.out.println("Base initialized");
  }
}
class Child extends Base {
  Child() {
    Logger.log("Logging before super()");
    super();
  }
}
public class Test {
  void main(String[] args) {
    Child c= new Child();
  }
}
```

Output:

```
Logging before super()
Base initialized
```

This program works in java22; for other versions it will throw an error because we used super() in the child class constructor after the println() statement. In this program, we demonstrate constructor chaining along with logging. The `Logger` class contains a static method `log()` used to print a message to the console. The `Base` class defines a constructor that prints "Base initialized" when an object of this class is created. The `Child` class extends `Base` and includes its own constructor. Initially, the program attempts to log a message using `Logger.log("Logging before super()")` before calling the parent class constructor with `super()`. However, this approach is valid in Java 22 and the compiler first prints logging the message and later initializes the base class by printing "Base initialized.

Program

```
class Base {
  Base(int number) {
    System.out.println("Number: " + number);
  }
}
class Child extends Base {
  Child() {
    int x = 10;
    System.out.println("Calculating x: " + x);
    super(x);
  }
}
public class Test {
void main(String[] args) {
    Child c= new Child();
  }
}
```

Output

```
Calculating x: 10
Number: 10
```

This program works in java22; for other versions it will throw an error because we used super() in the child class constructor after the println() statement. In this program, we demonstrate how a child class constructor can pass values to the parent class constructor using the `super()` keyword. The `Base` class has a constructor that accepts an integer parameter, and when invoked, it prints "Number: " followed by the value of the integer passed to it. In the `Child` class, the constructor first calculates a value `x`, sets it to 10, and prints "Calculating x: 10". After this, the `super(x)` call is made to pass the value of `x` (which is 10) to the `Base` class constructor. This triggers the parent class's constructor, which prints "Number: 10."When the `Test` class creates an instance of `Child`, the `Child` constructor runs first, printing "Calculating x: 10". Then, the `Base` class constructor is called via `super(x)`, which prints "Number: 10".

Program

```
class Base {
  Base(double value) {
    System.out.println("Value: " + value);
  }
}
class Child extends Base {
  Child() {
    double pi = Math.PI;
    System.out.println("Pi: " + pi);
    super(pi);
  }
}
public class Test {
  void main(String[] args) {
    Child c= new Child();
  }
}
```

Output

```
Pi: 3.141592653589793
Value: 3.141592653589793
```

This program works in java22 for other versions it will throw error because we used super() in the child class constructor after the println() statement. In this program, we demonstrate how a child class can pass computed values to the parent class constructor. The `Base` class has a constructor that accepts a `double` parameter, and it prints the value of this parameter prefixed with "Value:". In the `Child` class, the constructor first calculates the value of π (Pi) using `Math.PI` and prints "Pi: " followed by the computed value. After printing, the `super(pi)` call passes this value to the `Base` class constructor, which then prints "Value: " followed by the same value of Pi. When the `Test` class creates an instance of `Child`, the sequence of execution begins with the `Child` constructor, which prints "Pi: 3.141592653589793". Immediately after this, the `Base` class constructor is invoked via `super(pi)`, which prints "Value: 3.141592653589793".

Program

```
class Base {
  Base(String name, int age) {
    System.out.println("Name: " + name + ", Age: " + age);
```

```
    }
}
class Child extends Base {
    Child() {
        String name = "Usharani";
        int age = 25;
        System.out.println("Assigning values");
        super(name, age);
    }
}
public class Test {
    void main(String[] args) {
        Child c= new Child();
    }
}
```

Output

```
Assigning values
Name: Usharani, Age: 25
```

This program works in java22; for other versions it will throw an error because we used super() in the child class constructor after the println() statement. In this program, we demonstrate constructor chaining where values are passed from the child class to the parent class constructor. The `Base` class has a constructor that takes a `String` (representing a name) and an `int` (representing an age). When invoked, the `Base` class constructor prints the name and age in the format "Name: [name], Age: [age]". In the `Child` class constructor, two local variables `name` and `age` are initialized with the values "Usharani" and 25, respectively. The program first prints "Assigning values" before calling the parent class constructor using `super(name, age)`. This call passes the `name` and `age` to the `Base` constructor, which then prints "Name: Usharani, Age: 25". When the `Test` class creates an instance of `Child`, the sequence begins with the `Child` constructor printing "Assigning values". After that, the `super(name, age)` call transfers control to the `Base` constructor, which prints "Name: Usharani, Age: 25".

7.8 SUPER

The `super` keyword in Java is primarily used in inheritance to refer to the immediate parent class. Its usage can be categorized into three main scenarios:

1. Accessing Superclass Variables: When a subclass overrides a variable of the superclass, you can use the `super` keyword to access the superclass's version of that variable.
2. Invoking Superclass Methods: Similarly, if a subclass overrides a method of the superclass, you can use `super` to call the superclass's version of that method from within the subclass.
3. Invoking Superclass Constructor: In the subclass constructor, you can use `super` to call the superclass's constructor. This is typically used to initialize the superclass's state before initializing the subclass's state.

By using the `super` keyword, users can achieve better code organization and leverage the features provided by the superclass within the subclass.

7.8.1 Accessing Super Class Variables

In Java, when a subclass inherits from a superclass, it can access the superclass's variables using the super keyword. This keyword helps distinguish between the variables of the subclass and the superclass, especially when they share the same name. This feature is vital for maintaining clear and unambiguous code, particularly in complex inheritance structures.

Program

```
// Superclass (Base)
class Base {
  int num = 10;
  void display() {
    System.out.println("Base Class num: " + this.num);
  }
}
// Subclass (Child)
class Child extends Base {
  int num = 20; // Shadowing the superclass variable
  void display() {
      System.out.println("Child Class num: " + this.num);
    System.out.println("Accessing Super Class num: " + super.num);
super.display(); // Invoking superclass method
  }
}
public class Main {
  void main(String[] args) {
    // Creating an object of subclass
    Child myChild = new Child();
    // Calling the display method of subclass
    myChild.display();
  }
}
Output:
Child Class num: 20
Accessing Super Class num: 10
Base Class num: 10
```

In this program, we demonstrate the concept of variable shadowing and method overriding in Java. The `Base` class defines an integer variable `num` with a value of 10 and a method `display()` that prints "Base Class num: " followed by the value of `num`. The `Child` class extends the `Base` class and also declares a variable `num`, which shadows the variable from the `Base` class, setting its value to 20. The `Child` class overrides the `display()` method to print both the local `num` (from the `Child` class) and the `num` from the `Base` class using the `super.num` reference. In the `Main` class, an object of the `Child` class is created, and the overridden `display()` method is called. The output begins with "Child Class num: 20," showing the value of the `num` variable in the `Child` class. Then, "Accessing Super Class num: 10" is printed, demonstrating how the `super.num` accesses the `Base` class's `num` variable. Finally, the `super.display()` method is invoked, which calls the `Base` class's `display()` method, printing "Base Class num: 10."

7.8.2 Accessing Super Class Methods

In Java, when a subclass inherits from a superclass, it often needs to call or reuse the methods defined in the superclass. This is where the `super` keyword comes into play. The `super` keyword in Java provides a reference to the immediate parent class object. It is used to access methods and constructors of the superclass that are overridden or hidden in the subclass. Using `super`, a subclass can invoke a method defined in its superclass even if it has overridden that method. This allows for method reuse and code clarity, ensuring that the functionality provided by the superclass can be leveraged and extended in the subclass without redundancy. This mechanism plays a critical role in achieving polymorphism, maintaining code organization, and enabling clean, manageable inheritance hierarchies.

Program

```
// Superclass (Base)
class Base {
  void display() {
    System.out.println("Method in Base class");
  }
}
// Subclass (Child)
class Child extends Base {
  @Override
  void display() {
    System.out.println("Method in Child class");
    super.display(); // Invoking superclass method
  }
}
public class Main {
  void main(String[] args) {
    // Creating an object of subclass
    Child myChild = new Child();
    // Calling the display method of subclass
    myChild.display();
  }
}
Output:
Method in Child class
Method in Base class
```

In this program, we demonstrate method overriding and the use of the `super` keyword to call a superclass method in Java. The `Base` class contains a method `display()` that prints "Method in Base class." The `Child` class, which extends `Base`, overrides the `display()` method and provides its own implementation, printing "Method in Child class." After printing its own message, the overridden method in the `Child` class calls the `super.display()` method to invoke the `display()` method from the `Base` class. In the `Main` class, an object of the `Child` class is created, and the `display()` method is called on this object. The output starts with "Method in Child class," showing the overridden method from the `Child` class. Afterward, "Method in Base class" is printed, as the `super.display()` call invokes the method from the `Base` class.

7.8.3 Invoking Superclass Constructor

In Java, the super keyword can be used to invoke a superclass's constructor from a subclass. This is particularly useful when you want to initialize the superclass part of the subclass object. When a subclass constructor calls super, it can pass arguments to the constructor of the superclass, allowing for the initialization of fields in the superclass.

Program

```
// Base class
```

```
class Base {
  private int baseValue;
  // Constructor with parameter
  public Base(int baseValue) {
    this.baseValue = baseValue;
    System.out.println("Base class constructor called with baseValue: "
       + baseValue);
  }
  // Getter method
  public int getBaseValue() {
    return baseValue;
  }
}
// Child class inheriting from Base
class Child extends Base {
  private int childValue;
  // Constructor with parameters for both Base and Child
  public Child(int baseValue, int childValue) {
    super(baseValue); // Invoking superclass constructor
    this.childValue = childValue;
    System.out.println("Child class constructor called with childValue: "
       + childValue);
  }
  // Getter method
  public int getChildValue() {
    return childValue;
  }
}
// Main class to demonstrate superclass constructor invocation
public class Main {
  void main(String[] args) {
    // Creating an object of Child class
    Child childObj = new Child(10, 20);
    // Accessing values using getters
    System.out.println("Base value: " + childObj.getBaseValue());
    System.out.println("Child value: " + childObj.getChildValue());
  }
}
```

Output:

```
Base class constructor called with baseValue: 10
Child class constructor called with childValue: 20
Base value: 10
Child value: 20
```

The `Base` class contains a constructor that takes an integer parameter `baseValue` and sets it to the class's private variable `baseValue`. It also includes a getter method `getBaseValue()` to access this variable. When the constructor is invoked, it prints the message "Base class constructor called with baseValue: " followed by the value. The `Child` class inherits from the `Base` class and has its own constructor that takes two parameters: `baseValue` (to be passed to the `Base` class) and `childValue`. The `super(baseValue)` call invokes the `Base` class constructor, passing the value for `baseValue`. Additionally, the `Child` constructor initializes its own `childValue` and prints "Child class constructor called with childValue: " followed by the `childValue`. A getter method `getChildValue()` is provided to access the `childValue`.In the `Main` class, we create an instance of the `Child` class by passing `10` and `20` as arguments for `baseValue` and `childValue`, respectively. The output begins with "Base class constructor called with baseValue: 10," indicating that the `Base` class constructor was executed first. Next, "Child class constructor called with childValue: 20" confirms that the `Child` class constructor was executed. The values are then accessed through the getter methods, printing "Base value: 10" and "Child value: 20."

7.9 STATIC KEYWORD IN INHERITANCE

In Java, the static keyword is used to declare members (fields, methods, and nested classes) that belong to the class itself rather than to instances of the class. It indicates that the member is shared among all instances of the class and can be accessed directly through the class name without needing to create an instance of the class.

Key Uses of the static Keyword

- Static Fields: Static fields are class-level variables shared by all instances of the class. They are initialized only once when the class is loaded into memory and remain in memory until the program exits.
- Static Methods: Static methods belong to the class rather than to instances of the class. They can be invoked directly using the class name without the need for an object instance. Static methods cannot access instance variables directly, but they can access static variables.
- Static Nested Classes: Static nested classes are declared as static within another class. They do not have access to non-static members of the outer class but can be instantiated without an instance of the outer class.
- Static Initialization Blocks: Static initialization blocks are used to initialize static fields of a class. They are executed only once when the class is loaded into memory.

7.9.1 Static Field

In Java, static fields belong to the class rather than any specific instance. When a static field is inherited, it is shared across all instances of both the base and derived classes.

Program

```
public class Main {
  static class Base {
    protected static String staticField = "Base static field";
    public static void staticMethod() {
      System.out.println("Base static method");
    }
  }
  static class Child extends Base {
    // Static field in the child class
    protected static String childStaticField = "Child static field";
    public static void childStaticMethod() {
      System.out.println("Child static method");
    }
  }
    void main(String[] args) {
      // Accessing the static field from the base class
      System.out.println("Base static field accessed from child class: "
        + Base.staticField);
```

```
        System.out.println("Base static field accessed directly from child
            class: " + Child.staticField);
        // Accessing the static method from the base class
        Base.staticMethod();
        Child.staticMethod();
        // Accessing the child class's static field
        System.out.println("Child static field: " + Child.childStaticField);
          // Accessing the child class's static method
        Child.childStaticMethod();
    }
}
```

Output:

```
Base static field accessed from child class: Base static field
Base static field accessed directly from child class: Base static field
Base static method
Base static method
Child static field: Child static field
Child static method
```

In this program, the `Base` class contains a protected static field named `staticField` initialized to "Base static field" and a public static method called `staticMethod()`, which prints "Base static method." The `Child` class extends the `Base` class and introduces its own static field, `childStaticField`, initialized to "Child static field," along with a static method `childStaticMethod()` that prints "Child static method." In the `Main` class, the `main` method contains various statements to demonstrate the access of these static members. It first accesses the static field `staticField` from the `Base` class directly, printing "Base static field accessed from child class: Base static field." It then shows that the static field can also be accessed directly through the `Child` class, displaying "Base static field accessed directly from child class: Base static field." Next, the program calls the static method from the `Base` class, confirming its accessibility by printing "Base static method" twice: once via `Base.staticMethod()` and again via `Child.staticMethod()`. Then, it accesses the `childStaticField` from the `Child` class and prints "Child static field: Child static field." Finally, it invokes the static method `childStaticMethod()` from the `Child` class, resulting in the output "Child static method."

Program

Program for static variables can be inherited in java

```
// Base class with a static variable
class Base {
  static int i = 10;
}
// Child class extending Base
class Child extends Base {
  int i = 100;
  void display() {
    // Print the instance variable of Child
    System.out.println("Instance variable i in Child: " + i);
    // Print the static variable of Base using the class name
    System.out.println("Static variable i in Base: " + Base.i);
  }
}
// Main class containing the main method
public class Sample {
```

```
  void main(String[] args) {
    // Create an instance of Child
    Child c = new Child();
    // Call the display method
    c.display();
  }
}
```

Output:

```
Instance variable i in Child: 100
Static variable i in Base: 10
```

The Java program consists of three classes: `base`, `child`, and `sample`. In the `base` class, there is a static variable `i` initialized to the value 10. The `child` class extends the `base` class and declares its own instance variable `i` initialized to 100. It also contains a method `display()`, which prints the values of both the instance variable `i` defined in the `child` class and the static variable `i` inherited from the `base` class. Inside the `display()` method, the keyword `super` is used to access the static variable `i` of the superclass. The `sample` class contains the `main` method where an instance of the `child` class is created, and its `display()` method is called to print the values of the instance variables. When executed, the program will print the values of both the instance variable `i` of the `child` class and the static variable `i` of the `base` class, demonstrating the use of the `super` keyword to access superclass members.

Program

```
// Base class with static variable and method
class Test {
  static String name = "parent";
  void display() {
    System.out.println("Parent class method");
  }
}
// Child class extending Test
class Sample extends Test {
  static String name1 = "sub";
  void put() {
    System.out.println("child class method");
    System.out.println("name in Test: " + name);
    System.out.println("name1 in Sample: " + name1);
  }
}
// Main class extending Sample
public class Main extends Sample {
void main(String[] args) {
    // Create an instance of Sample
    Sample s = new Sample();
    // Call methods from Test and Sample
    s.display();
    s.put();
    // Update static variables
    Test.name = "superclass";
    Sample.name1 = "childclass";
    // Print updated static variables
    System.out.println("Updated name in Test: " + Test.name);
    System.out.println("Updated name1 in Sample: " + Sample.name1);
```

```
  }
}
```

Output:

```
Parent class method
child class method
name in Test: parent
name1 in Sample: sub
Updated name in Test: superclass
Updated name1 in Sample: childclass
```

The Java program consists of four classes: “test”, “sample”, “Main”, and a public class named “Main”. The “test” class defines a static string variable “name” with the value “parent” and a method named “display()”. The “display()” method prints “Parent class method” to the console when called. The “sample” class extends the “test” class, inheriting the static variable “name” and the “display()” method. Additionally, it declares a new static string variable “name1” with the value “sub” and defines a method named “put()”. The “put()” method prints “child class method” to the console and accesses both the “name” and “name1” variables, printing their values along with respective messages. The “Main” class extends the “sample” class, inheriting all its static variables and methods. Within the main method of the “Main” class, an instance of the “sample” class is created using the statement “sample s = new sample();”. This object is used to call the “display()” method inherited from the “test” class and the “put()” method defined in the “sample” class.Additionally, within the main method, the values of the static variables “name” and “name1” are changed to “superclass” and “childclass” respectively. When the program is executed, the “display()” method prints “Parent class method” to the console, followed by the “put()” method printing “child class method”. Additionally, it accesses and prints the values of both “name” and “name1” variables. Finally, within the main method, the updated values of “name” and “name1” are accessed and printed, demonstrating the visibility and modification of static variables across classes in the inheritance hierarchy.

7.9.2 Static Method

In Java, a static method is a method that belongs to the class itself rather than to instances of the class. Static methods can be called without creating an instance of the class. They are defined using the static keyword.

Program

Program for inheriting static methods in java

```
// Base class with a static method
class Base {
  static void show() {
    System.out.println("static method in parent");
  }
}
// Derived class extending Base with a non-static method
class Derived extends Base {
  void display() {
    System.out.println("non static method in child");
  }
}
// Main class to test method calls
public class Main {
  void main(String[] args) {
```

```
    // Create an instance of Derived and call its non-static method
    new Derived().display();
    // Call the static method of Base class using the subclass name
    Derived.show();
  }
}
```

Output:

```
non static method in child
static method in parent
```

This Java program comprises two classes: "base" and "derived". The "base" class contains a static method named "show()", which prints "static method in parent" to the console. The "derived" class extends the "base" class and defines a non-static method named "display()", which prints "non static method in child" to the console. In the "Main" class's main method, an object of the "derived" class is created using the statement "new derived().display();". This creates an instance of the "derived" class and immediately calls its "display()" method. As a result, "non static method in child" is printed to the console. Additionally, the static method "show()" from the "base" class is called using the syntax "derived.show();". Since static methods are inherited in Java, the static method "show()" from the "base" class can be directly accessed using the subclass name. Thus, "static method in parent" is printed to the console.

Program

Program for same static method in both parent and child class in java

```
// Base class with a static method
class Base {
  static void show() {
    System.out.println("static method in parent");
  }
}
// Derived class extending Base with its own static method and non-
static method
class Derived extends Base {
  // Static method in Derived class, hiding the static method in Base class
  static void show() {
    System.out.println("static method in child");
  }
  // Non-static method in Derived class
  void display() {
    // Prints message for the non-static method
    System.out.println("non static method in child");
    // Calls the static method from the superclass
    super.show();
  }
}
// Main class to test method calls
public class Main {
  void main(String[] args) {
    // Create an instance of Derived and call its non-static method
    new Derived().display();
    // Call the static method of Derived class
    Derived.show();
  }
}
```

Output:
```
non static method in child
static method in parent
static method in child
```

This Java program consists of two classes: “base” and “derived”. The “base” class contains a static method named “show()”, which prints “static method in parent” to the console. The “derived” class extends the “base” class and defines its own static method named “show()”, which prints “static method in child” to the console. Additionally, the “derived” class defines a non-static method named “display()”, which calls the static method “show()” from its superclass using the “super” keyword and prints “non static method in child” to the console.

In the “Main” class’s main method, an object of the “derived” class is created using the statement “new derived().display();”. This creates an instance of the “derived” class and immediately calls its “display()” method. Inside the “display()” method, the static method “show()” from the superclass is called using the “super” keyword, resulting in the message “static method in parent” being printed to the console. Subsequently, “non static method in child” is printed to the console.Additionally, the static method “show()” from the “derived” class is called directly using the syntax “derived. show();”. Since static methods are not overridden in Java, the static method “show()” from the “derived” class is invoked, and “static method in child” is printed to the console.

7.9.3 Static Block

In Java, a static block (also known as a static initialization block) is used to initialize static variables. It is executed when the class is loaded into memory, before any objects of the class are created and before any static methods are accessed.

Program

```
// Base class with a static block
class Base {
  static {
    System.out.println("Static block in Base class");
  }
}
// Child class inheriting from Base
class Main extends Base {
  static {
    System.out.println("Static block in Child class");
  }
  void main(String[] args) {
    // Main method of Child class
    System.out.println("Main method of Child class");
  }
}
```
Output:
```
Static block in Base class
Static block in Child class
Main method of Child class
```

In this program, the `Base` class includes a static block, which executes when the class is loaded, printing “Static block in Base class.” The `Main` class extends the `Base` class and also contains a static block that prints “Static block in Child class.” Both static blocks are executed when their respective classes are loaded into memory, before any object creation or method invocation. When the program runs, the static block in the `Base` class is executed first since the parent class is loaded before the child class. Then, the static block in the `Main` class (the child class) is executed. Following this, the `main` method in the `Main` class is called, printing "Main method of Child class."

7.10 THIS KEYWORD IN INHERITANCE

In Java, the `this` keyword refers to the current instance of the class in which it appears. It is primarily used within class methods and constructors to refer to the instance variables and methods of the current object. Key uses of the `this` keyword include:

- Accessing Instance Variables: It can be used to access instance variables of the current object, especially when there is a local variable with the same name, to disambiguate between the two.
- Invoking Current Class Constructors: It can be used to invoke another constructor of the same class. This is known as constructor chaining and is often used to reuse initialization code.
- Passing Current Object as a Parameter: It can be used to pass the current object as a parameter to another method.
- Returning Current Object: It can be used to return the current object from a method, enabling method chaining.
- Referring to Inner Class: Within an inner class, `this` refers to the current instance of the inner class, while `OuterClassName.this` refers to the current instance of the outer class.

7.10.1 Accessing Variables

In Java, the keyword "this" is used to refer to the current instance of a class. When used in inheritance, this can be particularly useful for distinguishing between instance variables of the superclass and subclass, especially when they have the same name.

Program

```
// Superclass (Base)
class Base {
  int num;
  // Parameterized constructor
  public Base(int num) {
    this.num = num; // 'this' refers to the current instance of the class
  }
  void display() {
    System.out.println("Base Class: " + this.num);
  }
}
// Subclass (Child)
class Child extends Base {
  int num; // Shadowing the superclass variable
  // Parameterized constructor
  public Child(int baseNum, int childNum) {
    super(baseNum); // Invoking superclass constructor
    this.num = childNum; // 'this' refers to the current instance of
                         the class
  }
    void display() {
       System.out.println("Child Class: " + this.num);
```

```
super.display(); // Invoking superclass method
  }
}
public class Main {
  void main(String[] args) {
    // Creating an object of subclass
    Child myChild = new Child(10, 20);
    // Calling the display method of subclass
    myChild.display();
  }
}
```

Output:

```
Child Class: 20
Base Class: 10
```

This program demonstrates inheritance in Java, with a superclass named `Base` and a subclass named `Child`. The `Base` class contains an instance variable `num` and a parameterized constructor to initialize it. It also has a `display()` method to print the value of `num`. The `Child` class extends `Base` and adds another instance variable `num`, shadowing the one in the superclass. Its constructor initializes both superclass and subclass variables using `super` and `this` respectively. The `display()` method in `Child` invokes the superclass method using `super.display()` and prints the value of both superclass and subclass variables. In the `Main` class, an object of `Child` is created, and its `display()` method is called to demonstrate the functionality of inheritance and variable shadowing.

7.10.2 Accessing Constructors

In Java, the "this" keyword is used to refer to the current instance of a class. When used in the context of constructors, "this" can be employed to call other constructors within the same class or to invoke constructors of the superclass in inheritance scenarios.

Program

Program for invoking the private constructor from the overloaded constructor

```
class Base {
  // Private constructor
  private Base() {
    System.out.println("private base constructor");
  }
  // Public constructor
  public Base(boolean usePrivateConstructor) {
    if (usePrivateConstructor) {
      throw new IllegalArgumentException("Use static factory method to
        create instance.");
    }
    System.out.println("public base constructor");
  }
  // Static factory method to use private constructor
  public static Base createBaseWithPrivateConstructor() {
    return new Base();
  }
}
// Child class extending Base
class Child extends Base {
```

```
  // Constructor for Child class
  public Child(boolean usePrivateConstructor) {
    // Call the public constructor of the Base class
    System.out.println("public child constructor");
super(usePrivateConstructor);
  }
}
// Test class with the main method
public class Test {
  void main(String[] args) {
    // Creating an instance of Base using the static factory method
    Base base1 = Base.createBaseWithPrivateConstructor();
    // This will use the private constructor
    // Creating an instance of Child class using the public constructor
    of Base
    Child child1 = new Child(false); // This will use the public constructor
                                        of Base
  }
}
Output:
private base constructor
public child constructor
public base constructor
```

This program demonstrates using private constructors in Java. The `Base` class has a private constructor, accessible only through a static factory method (`createBaseWithPrivate Constructor`) that creates instances of `Base`. The `Child` class inherits from `Base` and uses the public constructor of `Base` to initialize itself. In the `Test` class, `Base` is instantiated via the static factory method, and `Child` is instantiated using its public constructor.

Program

Program for invoking the private constructor from the overloaded constructor and crating object for private constructor class

```
// Base class with constructor chaining and a method
class Base {
  // Private constructor
  private Base(int i) {
    System.out.println("private base constructor");
  }
  // Public constructor
  public Base() {
    this(10); // Calls the private constructor with an argument
    System.out.println("public base constructor");
  }
  // Method to be inherited
  public void display() {
    System.out.println("method in base");
  }
}
// Child class extending Base class
class Child extends Base {
  // Constructor for Child class
  public Child() {
```

```
        System.out.println("public child constructor");
    }
}
// Test class with main method
public class Test {
  void main(String[] args) {
    // Create an instance of Child class
    Child c = new Child();
    // Call the inherited display method
    c.display();
  }
}
```

Output:

```
private base constructor
public base constructor
public child constructor
method in base
```

This Java program demonstrates constructor chaining and method inheritance in a class hierarchy consisting of "base", "child", and "test" classes. The "base" class has two constructors: a public constructor and a private constructor. The public constructor calls the private constructor with an argument of 10 using the "this" keyword before printing "public base constructor" to the console. The private constructor, in turn, prints "private base constructor" to the console. Additionally, the "base" class defines a method named "display()" that prints "method in base" to the console. The "child" class extends the "base" class and defines a constructor that prints "public child constructor" to the console. In the "test" class, the main method creates an object of the "child" class. Upon object creation, the constructors of both the superclass ("base") and the subclass ("child") are invoked due to inheritance. The object "c" then calls the "display()" method, which is inherited from the "base" class. When the program is executed, the constructor chaining mechanism is observed. Firstly, the private constructor of the "base" class is called, printing "private base constructor". Then, the public constructor of the "base" class is executed, printing "public base constructor". After that, the constructor of the "child" class is invoked, printing "public child constructor" to the console. Finally, the "display()" method is called, printing "method in base" to the console.

7.10.3 Passing Current Object as Parameter

In Java, the `this` keyword is used to reference the current object within a class. We can pass the current object as a parameter to methods using `this`.

Program

```
public class InheritanceExample {
  static class Base {
    protected static String staticField;
    // Static block in the base class
    static {
      staticField = "Base static field initialized";
      System.out.println("Base static block executed");
    }
    protected static void staticMethod() {
      System.out.println("Base static method");
    }
    protected String instanceField;
```

```
    public Base() {
      this.instanceField = "Base instance field";
    }
    public void instanceMethod(Base obj) {
      System.out.println("Base instance method called with instanceField: "
         + obj.instanceField);
    }
  }
  static class Child extends Base {
    // Static block in the child class
    static {
      System.out.println("Child static block executed");
    }
    public Child() {
      super(); // Call to the constructor of the base class
    }
    public void childInstanceMethod() {
      // Passing `this` to the base class's instance method
      instanceMethod(this);
    }
    protected static void childStaticMethod() {
      System.out.println("Child static method");
    }
}
    void main(String[] args) {
      // Static field and static methods demonstration
      System.out.println("Static field from base class: " + Base.staticField);
      Base.staticMethod();
      Child.childStaticMethod();
      // Instance method and passing `this` demonstration
      Child childInstance = new Child();
      childInstance.childInstanceMethod();
  }
}
```

Output:

```
Base static block executed
Static field from base class: Base static field initialized
Base static method
Child static block executed
Child static method
```

Base instance method called with instanceField: Base instance field

In this program, the `Base` class contains a static block that is executed when the class is loaded, initializing a static field and printing a message indicating that the static block has been executed. The class also includes a static method, `staticMethod()`, which can be called without creating an object and prints a message to indicate its invocation. Additionally, the `Base` class has an instance field, `instanceField`, which is initialized in the constructor, and an instance method, `instanceMethod()`, that accepts an object of the `Base` class and prints the value of `instanceField`, showing how instance methods can interact with object attributes. The `Child` class, which extends the `Base` class, also contains a static block that is executed when the class is loaded, showcasing the execution order of static blocks in an inheritance chain. The `Child` class inherits the static and instance methods of the `Base` class and introduces its own static method, `childStaticMethod()`. It also has an instance method, `childInstanceMethod()`, which calls the inherited `instanceMethod()` using the `this` reference to pass the current instance of the `Child` class.

7.10.4 Returing `this` from Method

In Java, the `this` keyword is used within a method to refer to the current object instance. This can be particularly useful when you want to return the current object from a method, enabling method chaining.

Program

```
class Main {
  private int value;
Main(){}
Main (int value) {
    this.value = value;
  }
  public Main setValue(int value) {
    this.value = value;
    return this; // Returning the current object
  }
  public Main incrementValue() {
    this.value++;
    return this; // Returning the current object
  }
  public void displayValue() {
    System.out.println("Value: " + this.value);
  }
  void main(String[] args) {
Mainm = new Main (5);
    // Method chaining using the returned 'this' keyword
m.setValue(10).incrementValue().displayValue();
  }
}
```

Output:

```
Value: 11
```

In this program, the `Main` class has a private integer field `value` and two constructors: a parameterless constructor and another that initializes the `value` field. The class provides a setter method `setValue(int value)` that sets the `value` and returns the current object using `this`. Another method, `incrementValue()`, increments the `value` by 1 and also returns the current object. By returning the object itself in each method, we enable method chaining. This allows multiple methods to be called in a single statement, where each method modifies the object and passes it to the next. For example, the chain `m.setValue(10). incrementValue().displayValue()` first sets the value to 10, increments it by 1 (making it 11), and then prints the updated value.

7.11 INITIALIZATION BLOCK IN INHERITANCE

In Java, an initialization block is a block of code within a class that is executed when an instance of the class is created or when the class is loaded into memory, depending on whether it's a static or instance initialization block.

- Static Initialization Block: It's declared using the static keyword and is executed only once when the class is loaded into memory. It's primarily used to initialize static variables of the class.

- Instance Initialization Block: It's not marked with any keyword and is executed each time an instance of the class is created, before the constructor is invoked. It's useful for performing common initialization tasks across multiple constructors.

Initialization blocks provide a way to initialize class variables or perform common initialization tasks regardless of which constructor is called. They are especially useful when you have multiple constructors that need to perform the same initialization logic.

Program

Program for initialize blocks in child class

```
// Base class
class Base {
  // Constructor of Base class
  Base() {
    System.out.println("parent class constructor invoked");
  }
}
// Child class extending Base
class Child extends Base {
  // Instance initializer block in Child class
  {
    System.out.println("instance initializer block is invoked");
  }
  // Constructor of Child class
  Child() {
      System.out.println("child class constructor invoked");
super(); // Explicitly call the superclass constructor
  }
}
// Main class with the main method
public class Main {
void main(String[] args) {
    // Create an instance of Child class
    Child b = new Child();
  }
}
```

Output:

```
child class constructor invoked
parent class constructor invoked
instance initializer block is invoked
```

This Java program consists of two classes: "base" and "child". The "base" class defines a constructor that prints "parent class constructor invoked" to the console when invoked. The "child" class extends the "base" class and defines its own constructor. In the constructor of the "child" class, the "super()" keyword is used to explicitly invoke the constructor of the superclass, and then "child class constructor invoked" is printed to the console. Additionally, an instance initializer block is included within the "child" class, which prints "instance initializer block is invoked" to the console when an object of the "child" class is created. In the "main" method of the "Main" class, an object of the "child" class is created using the statement "child b=new child();". When this object is created, the constructor of the "child" class is invoked, which in turn invokes the constructor of the superclass "base" due to the "super()" keyword. As a result, the messages "parent class constructor invoked", "child class constructor invoked", and "instance initializer block is invoked" are printed to the console in that order.

Program

Program for initialize blocks with constructoroverloading

```
// Base class
class Base {
  // Constructor of Base class
  Base() {
    System.out.println("parent class constructor invoked");
  }
}
// Child class extending Base
class Child extends Base {
  // Instance initializer block in Child class
  {
    System.out.println("instance initializer block is invoked");
  }
  // Parameterless constructor of Child class
  Child() {
        System.out.println("child class constructor invoked");
  super(); // Call the superclass constructor
  }
  // Parameterized constructor of Child class
  Child(int a) {
         System.out.println("child class constructor invoked " + a);
  super(); // Call the superclass constructor
  }
}
// Main class with the main method
public class Main {
  void main(String[] args) {
    // Create an instance of Child class using the parameterless constructor
    Child c1 = new Child();
    // Create an instance of Child class using the parameterized constructor
    Child c2 = new Child(10);
  }
}
```

Output

```
child class constructor invoked
parent class constructor invoked
instance initializer block is invoked
child class constructor invoked 10
parent class constructor invoked
instance initializer block is invoked
```

This Java program defines two classes: "base" and "child". The "base" class contains a constructor that prints "parent class constructor invoked" when invoked. The "child" class extends the "base" class and defines two constructors: one parameterless constructor and one parameterized constructor. Both constructors call the superclass constructor using the "super()" keyword. The parameterized constructor also prints "child class constructor invoked" followed by the value of the parameter "a" when invoked. In addition to constructors, an instance initializer block is included within the "child" class, which prints "instance initializer block is invoked" whenever an object of the "child" class is created.In the "main" method of the "Main" class, two objects of the "child" class are created: "c1" using the parameterless constructor and "c2" using the parameterized constructor with the argument "10".When the program is executed, the constructors and instance initializer block are invoked as follows:

- Upon creating the object "c1" using the parameterless constructor, the constructor of the superclass ("base") is invoked first, printing "parent class constructor invoked", followed by the instance initializer block, printing "instance initializer block is invoked", and then the constructor of the subclass ("child"), printing "child class constructor invoked".
- Upon creating the object "c2" using the parameterized constructor, the same sequence of invocations occurs, with the addition of printing "child class constructor invoked 10" to account for the parameter passed to the constructor.

Program

Program for static and initialize blocks in inheritance

```
// Base class
class Base {
  // Static initializer block of Base class
  static {
    System.out.println("parent class static initializer invoked");
  }
  // Instance initializer block of Base class
  {
    System.out.println("parent class initializer invoked");
  }
  // Constructor of Base class
  Base() {
    System.out.println("parent class constructor invoked");
  }
}
// Child class extending Base
class Child extends Base {
  // Static initializer block of Child class
  static {
    System.out.println("child class static initializer invoked");
  }
  // Instance initializer block of Child class
  {
    System.out.println("child class initializer block is invoked");
  }
  // Constructor of Child class
  Child() {
    System.out.println("child class constructor invoked");
super(); // Call the superclass constructor
  }
}
// Main class with the main method
public class Main {
  void main(String[] args) {
    // Create an instance of Child class
    Child c = new Child();
  }
}
```

Output:

```
parent class static initializer invoked
```

```
child class static initializer invoked
child class constructor invoked
parent class initializer invoked
parent class constructor invoked
child class initializer block is invoked
```

This Java program consists of two classes: "base" and "child". The "base" class contains a static initializer block, an instance initializer block, and a constructor. The static initializer block prints "parent class static initializer invoked", the instance initializer block prints "parent class initializer invoked", and the constructor prints "parent class constructor invoked".The "child" class extends the "base" class and contains its own static initializer block, instance initializer block, and constructor. The static initializer block of the "child" class prints "child class static initializer invoked", the instance initializer block prints "child class initializer block is invoked", and the constructor invokes the superclass constructor using "super()" and prints "child class constructor invoked".In the "main" method, an object of the "child" class is created, triggering the execution of its constructors and initializer blocks. The sequence of execution is as follows:

- The static initializer block of the "base" class is executed first, printing "parent class static initializer invoked".
- Next, the instance initializer block of the "base" class is executed, printing "parent class initializer invoked".
- Then, the constructor of the "base" class is invoked, printing "parent class constructor invoked".
- Following this, the static initializer block of the "child" class is executed, printing "child class static initializer invoked".
- The instance initializer block of the "child" class is executed next, printing "child class initializer block is invoked".
- Finally, the constructor of the "child" class is invoked, which first invokes the superclass constructor, printing "parent class constructor invoked", and then prints "child class constructor invoked".

7.12 METHOD OVERRIDING

When a method in a child class shares the same name, return type, and parameter list as a method in its parent class, it's termed as method overriding in Java. Method overriding allows a subclass to provide a specific implementation for a method that is already defined in its superclass. The primary purpose of method overriding is to enable runtime polymorphism, where the appropriate method implementation is determined dynamically based on the object's actual type at runtime.
Key rules for method overriding include:

- The method in the subclass must have the same name and signature (parameter list) as the method in the superclass.
- The return type of the overridden method can be a subtype of the return type of the method in the superclass, but it must be compatible with it.
- The access modifier of the overriding method should be the same or more accessible than the method it overrides.
- The overriding method cannot throw a checked exception broader than the exception thrown by the overridden method, but it can throw unchecked exceptions or narrower checked exceptions.

By adhering to these rules, developers can ensure proper method overriding, allowing subclasses to customize behavior while retaining the original method signature and functionality from the superclass.

Program

Program for covariant return type with private specifier for base method and protected specifier for child class

```
// Base class
class Base {
  // Private method in Base class
  private void display() {
    System.out.println("private method in base");
  }
  // Method in Base class that calls the private method
  void show() {
    display();
  }
}
// Child class extending Base class
class Child extends Base {
    protected void display() {
    // Call the show() method from Base class
    // Print the message from Child class
    System.out.println("protected method in child");
super.show();
  }
}
// Test class with main method
public class Test {
  void main(String[] args) {
    // Create an instance of Child class
    Child c = new Child();
    // Call the display() method of Child class
    c.display();
  }
}
```

Output:

```
protected method in child
private method in base
```

In this Java program, there are three classes: "base", "child", and "Test". The "base" class contains a private method named "display()" that prints "private method in base" when invoked. Additionally, it includes a method named "show()", which calls the private "display()" method. The "child" class extends the "base" class and overrides the private "display()" method with a protected version. Within this overridden method, it first invokes the "show()" method of the superclass using "super.show()", which in turn calls the private "display()" method of the "base" class. After that, it prints "protected method in child". In the "Test" class's main method, an instance of the "child" class is created, and its "display()" method is called. As a result, the overridden "display()" method in the "child" class is invoked due to dynamic method dispatch.

Program

Program for covariant return type with private specifier for base method and public specifier for child class

```
// Base class
class Base {
  // Private method in Base class
```

```
  private void display() {
    System.out.println("private method in base");
  }
  // Public method to access the private display() method within Base
  public void show() {
    display(); // Calls the private display() method in Base
  }
}
// Child class extending Base class
class Child extends Base {
  // Public method with the same name in Child class (method hiding)
  public void display() {
    System.out.println("public method in child");
show();
  }
}
// Test class with the main method
public class Main {
  void main(String[] args) {
    // Create an instance of Child class
    Child c = new Child();
    // Call the display() method of Child class
    c.display(); // This will call the Child's display() method
  }
}
```

Output:

```
public method in child
private method in base
```

In this Java program, there are three classes: "base", "child", and "Test". The "base" class contains a private method named "display()", which prints "private method in base" when invoked, and a method named "show()", which calls the private "display()" method. The "child" class extends the "base" class and overrides the private "display()" method with a public version. The overridden "display()" method in the "child" class prints "public method in child" and then calls the "show()" method of its superclass. As "show()" method is inherited by the "child" class from its superclass, it can be accessed within the "child" class. In the "Test" class's main method, an instance of the "child" class is created, and its "display()" method is called. As a result, the overridden "display()" method in the "child" class is invoked due to dynamic method dispatch.

Program

Program for covariant return type with private specifier for base method and public specifier for child class

```
// Base class
class Base {
  // Protected method in Base class
  protected void display() {
    System.out.println("protected method in base");
  }
}
// Child class extending Base class
class Child extends Base {
  // Public method in Child class overriding the protected method
  @Override
```

```
  public void display() {
    // Print the message from Child class
    System.out.println("public method in child");
// Call the display() method from Base class
    super.display();
  }
}
// Test class with main method
public class Test {
  void main(String[] args) {
    // Create an instance of Child class
    Child c = new Child();
    // Call the display() method of Child class
    c.display();
  }
}
```

Output:

```
public method in child
protected method in base
```

In this Java program, there are two classes: "base" and "child", along with a main class named "Test". The "base" class contains a protected method named "display()", which prints "protected method in base" when invoked. The "child" class extends the "base" class and overrides the "display()" method with a public version. The overridden "display()" method in the "child" class first calls the "display()" method of its superclass using the "super" keyword to access the superclass method. After that, it prints "public method in child". In the "Test" class's main method, an instance of the "child" class is created, and its "display()" method is called. Due to dynamic method dispatch, the overridden "display()" method in the "child" class is invoked.

Program

Program for covariant return type with default specifier for base method and public specifier for child class

```
// Base class
class Base {
  // Default (package-private) method in Base class
  void display() {
    System.out.println("default method in base");
  }
}
// Child class extending Base class
class Child extends Base {
  // Protected method in Child class overriding the default method
  @Override
  protected void display() {
      // Print the message from Child class
    System.out.println("protected method in child");
// Call the display() method from Base class
    super.display();
  }
}
// Test class with main method
public class Test {
  void main(String[] args) {
```

```
    // Create an instance of Child class
    Child c = new Child();
    // Call the display() method of Child class
    c.display();
  }
}
```

Output:

```
protected method in child
default method in base
```

In this Java program, there are two classes: "base" and "child", along with a main class named "Test". The "base" class contains a default method named "display()", which prints "default method in base" when invoked. The "child" class extends the "base" class and overrides the "display()" method with a protected version. The overridden "display()" method in the "child" class first calls the "display()" method of its superclass using the "super" keyword to access the superclass method. After that, it prints "protected method in child".In the "Test" class's main method, an instance of the "child" class is created, and its "display()" method is called. Due to dynamic method dispatch, the overridden "display()" method in the "child" class is invoked.

Program

Program for covariant return type by returning user-defined classes.

```
// Base class with a constructor initializing a string variable
class Base {
  String s;
  // Constructor for Base class
  Base(String s) {
    this.s = s;
  }
}
// Child class extending Base class
class Child extends Base {
  // Constructor for Child class
  Child(String s) {
    super(s); // Call the constructor of Base class
  }
}
// Sample class with a protected method returning an instance of Base
class Sample {
  // Protected method returning an instance of Base
  protected Base get() {
    return new Base("base");
  }
}
// Testing class extending Sample and overriding the get() method
class Testing extends Sample {
  // Overridden method returning an instance of Child
  @Override
  protected Base get() {
    return new Child("child");
  }
}
// Main class with the main method
public class Test {
```

```
  void main(String[] args) {
    // Create an instance of Sample class
    Sample sample = new Sample();
    // Call the get() method and print the value of s
    System.out.println(sample.get().s);
    // Create an instance of Testing class
    Testing testing = new Testing();
    // Call the get() method and print the value of s
    System.out.println(testing.get().s);
  }
}
```

Output:

```
base
child
```

This Java program defines several classes: "base", "child", "sample", "testing", and "Test". The "base" class has a constructor that initializes a string variable "s" with the provided argument. The "child" class extends the "base" class and has its constructor that calls the superclass constructor using the "super" keyword. The "sample" class has a method named "get()" that returns an instance of the "base" class with the string "base" passed to its constructor. The method is declared as "protected". The "testing" class extends the "sample" class and overrides the "get()" method. The overridden method returns an instance of the "child" class with the string "child" passed to its constructor. In the "Test" class's main method, an instance of the "sample" class is created, and its "get()" method is called, returning an instance of the "base" class with the string "base" assigned to its "s" variable. This instance's "s" value is then printed. Next, an instance of the "testing" class is created, and its "get()" method is called, returning an instance of the "child" class with the string "child" assigned to its "s" variable. This instance's "s" value is printed.

7.13 THE FINAL KEYWORD

The final keyword in Java can be used in several contexts to define entities that cannot be changed or extended. It can be applied to variables, methods, and classes, each with specific implications.

Advantages of Using Final

- Immutability: When applied to variables, final ensures that the value assigned cannot be changed, which can be crucial for defining constants.
- Security: Final methods cannot be overridden, which can help prevent unintended behavior or misuse of critical methods in a class.
- Performance: The use of final can lead to optimizations by the compiler, as it can make certain assumptions about the code that wouldn't be possible otherwise.
- Simplicity and Safety: Using final can make the code easier to understand and maintain, by clearly signaling which parts of the code are intended to remain unchanged.

Limitations of Using Final

- Lack of Flexibility: Final classes cannot be extended, which may limit reuse and flexibility in some situations.
- Inheritance Constraints: Final methods cannot be overridden, which might be restrictive in scenarios where behavior modification in subclasses is required.

- Initialization Requirement: Final variables must be initialized when they are declared or within a constructor, which might not always be convenient.

Use Cases for Final

- Constants: Define constants that should not change.
- Immutable Objects: Create immutable objects where none of the fields can be modified after creation.
- Preventing Inheritance: Secure classes from being extended, especially utility or helper classes.
- Preventing Method Overriding: Ensure critical methods are not overridden by subclasses to maintain their original behavior.

7.13.1 Final Class

A class declared as final cannot be subclassed. This prevents other classes from inheriting from it.

Program

```
final class FinalClass {
  public void display() {
    System.out.println("This is a final class.");
  }
}
// The following line would cause a compile-time error
// class SubClass extends FinalClass {
// }
public class FinalClassExample {
void main(String[] args) {
    FinalClass finalClass = new FinalClass();
    finalClass.display();
  }
}
Output:
This is a final class.
```

In this program, the `FinalClass` is marked as `final`, which means it cannot be inherited by any other class. This is useful when you want to prevent further subclassing or modification of the class. The `display()` method in the `FinalClass` simply prints a message indicating that it is part of a final class. In the `FinalClassExample` class, we create an instance of `FinalClass` and call its `display()` method, which prints the message.

7.13.2 Method Overloading in Final Class

Method overloading in a final class in Java is a concept where multiple methods with the same name coexist in a single class but differ in parameters (type, number, or both). The final keyword, when applied to a class, prevents the class from being subclassed, but it does not affect the ability to overload methods within the class itself.

Program

Program for final class method overloading in java

```
// Define a final class named test
final class Test {
  // Method with no parameters
  void display() {
    System.out.println("0 parameter display()");
  }
  // Method with one int parameter
  void display(int i) {
    System.out.println("1 int parameter display()" + i);
  }
  // Method with one String parameter
  void display(String s) {
    System.out.println("1 string parameter display()" + s);
  }
  // Method with two int parameters
  void display(int i, int j) {
    System.out.println("2 int parameter display()" + i + " " + j);
  }
}
// Sample class with the main method
public class Sample {
  void main(String[] args) {
    // Create an instance of Test class
    Test test = new Test();
    // Call the overloaded display methods with different parameters
    test.display();          // Calls display() with no parameters
    test.display(10);          // Calls display(int i) with one integer
parameter
    test.display("testing");      // Calls display(String s) with one string
parameter
    test.display(100, 200);       // Calls display(int i, int j) with two
integer parameters
  }
}
```

Output:

```
0 parameter display()
1 int parameter display()10
1 string parameter display()testing
2 int parameter display()100 200
```

The program defines a `final` class named `test` with multiple overloaded methods named `display`. Each `display` method accepts different parameter types, including no parameters, one integer, one string, or two integers. Inside each `display` method, a message is printed indicating the number and type of parameters passed to the method. In the `sample` class's `main` method, an instance of the `test` class is created, and the `display` methods of the `test` class are invoked with different parameter combinations. Each method call results in the corresponding `display` method being executed, printing a message indicating the parameters passed to it.

7.13.3 FINAL METHOD

A method declared as final cannot be overridden by subclasses. This ensures that the implementation of the method remains unchanged in any subclass.

Program

```
class Parent {
  public final void display() {
    System.out.println("This is a final method.");
  }
}
class Child extends Parent {
  public void display () {
    System.out.println("Trying to override final method.");
    }
}
public class FinalMethodExample {
  void main(String[] args) {
    Child child = new Child();
    child.display();
child.func()
  }
}
```

Output:

```
Main.java:7: error: display() in Child cannot override display() in Parent
  public void display () {
        ^
  overridden method is final
Main.java:16: error: cannot find symbol
child.func();
    ^
  symbol:   method func()
  location: variable child of type Child
2 errors
error: compilation failed
```

7.13.3.1 Final Parameters

In Java, the `final` keyword can be used with parameters in methods. When a parameter is declared as `final`, it means that the parameter cannot be reassigned within the method or block where it is used. This ensures that the value of the parameter remains constant throughout the method's execution.

Need for Final Parameters

- Immutability: By making parameters final, you can ensure that they are not modified within the method, enhancing the method's robustness and predictability.
- Readability and Maintenance: It improves code readability by clearly indicating that the parameter should not be reassigned. This can be particularly useful in long methods where the parameter might be passed to multiple helper methods.
- Thread Safety: Final parameters can help in creating thread-safe code, as their immutability ensures that their values cannot be changed inadvertently, which is crucial in concurrent programming.
- Avoiding Errors: Using final parameters can help prevent errors that occur due to unintended reassignment of variables, leading to fewer bugs and more reliable code.

Advantages of Final Parameters

- Prevents Reassignment: Final parameters prevent accidental reassignment, which can lead to fewer bugs and more stable code.
- Improves Clarity: It makes the intention of the code clearer, signaling to other developers that the parameter should remain constant.
- Enhanced Optimization: The Java compiler can optimize code better when it knows certain values will not change.
- Consistency: Using final parameters promotes consistent use of values within methods, which can improve overall code quality and maintainability.

Limitations of Final Parameters

- Rigidity: Once a parameter is declared as final, it cannot be changed, which can be restrictive in cases where reassignment within the method might be necessary.
- Verbosity: Declaring parameters as final can add verbosity to the code, especially in methods with multiple parameters.
- imited Use Case: Final parameters are mainly useful for ensuring immutability within a method, which might not be necessary for all method parameters.

Program

Program for final parameters

```
public class Test {
  // Method that takes two parameters: n (regular) and m (final)
  void display(int n, final int m) {
    n = n * m; // Compute the product of n and m
    System.out.println("n*m=" + n + "\tm="+m); // Print the result along
                                                   with the value of m
  }
void main(String[] args) {
    Test test = new Test(); // Create an instance of the Test class
    test.display(10, 20); // Call the display method with arguments 10 and 20
  }
}
Output:
n*m=200 m=20
```

The above program defines a class named `test` containing a `main` method. Inside the `main` method, an instance of the `test` class is created. Then, the `display` method of the `test` class is called with two integer arguments: `10` and `20`. The `display` method takes two parameters: `n` and `m`, where `n` is a regular integer parameter and `m` is a final integer parameter. Inside the `display` method, the value of `n` is assigned the product of `m` and `n`, and then the result is printed along with the value of `m`.

7.13.4 Final Variable

The final variable is a constant whose value cannot be changed once it has been assigned. To declare a final variable in Java, you use the `final` keyword followed by the data type and the variable name. Then, you initialize it with a value. Once assigned, the value of a final variable remains constant throughout the program's execution. Here's the syntax:

```
final dataType variableName = value;
```

For example

```
final int MAX_VALUE = 100;
final String MESSAGE = "Hello";
```

7.13.4.1 Blank Variable

In Java, a "blank final" variable refers to a final variable that is not assigned a value at the time of declaration, but rather is initialized in the constructor of the class. Once initialized, the value of a blank final variable cannot be changed.

Program

Program for final blank variable

```
class Sample {
  final int i; // Final instance variable
  // Constructor to initialize the final variable
  Sample(int val) {
    i = val; // Initialize the final variable
  }
}
public class Test {
  void main(String[] args) {
    Sample s = new Sample(10); // Create an instance of Sample with value 10
    System.out.println("final blank value is " + s.i); // Print the value of
                                                            the final variable
  }
}
Output:
final blank value is 10
```

The program defines a class named `sample`, which contains a final instance variable `i` of type integer. The `sample` class also has a constructor that takes an integer parameter `val` and assigns it to the final variable `i`. The constructor initializes the final variable `i` with the value passed as an argument. In the `test` class's `main` method, an instance of the `sample` class is created by passing the value `10` to its constructor. Then, the value of the final variable `i` is printed using the statement `System.out.println("final blank value is " + s.i);`.Since the variable `i` is declared as final, it must be initialized before it is accessed. Therefore, initializing `i` in the constructor ensures that it has a value when accessed, and the program prints the value of `i` as `10`.

Program

Program for final blank variable initialization incase if there is more than one constructor in a class.

```
class Sample {
  final int i; // Final instance variable
  // Constructor with an integer parameter
  Sample(int val) {
    i = val; // Initialize the final variable
  }
  // Parameterless constructor
  Sample() {
```

```
    this(150); // Delegate to the constructor with the integer parameter
  }
}
public class Test {
void main(String[] args) {
    Sample s = new Sample(); // Create an instance of Sample using the
                                parameterless constructor
    System.out.println("final blank value is " + s.i); // Print the value of
                                                          the final variable
  }
}
```

Output:

```
final blank value is 150
```

The above program defines a class named `sample`, which contains a final instance variable `i` of type integer. The `sample` class has two constructors: one that takes an integer parameter `val` and another constructor with no parameters. In the constructor with the integer parameter, the final variable `i` is initialized with the value passed as an argument. In the parameterless constructor, `this(150);` is used to call the constructor with the integer parameter and pass `150` as the argument. In the `test` class's `main` method, an instance of the `sample` class is created using the parameterless constructor `new sample();`. Since the parameterless constructor delegates to the other constructor passing `150`, the final variable `i` is initialized with this value. Then, the value of the final variable `i` is printed using the statement `System.out.println("final blank value is " + s.i);`, which prints `150` as the output.

Program

Program for final blank variable for multiple objects

```
class Sample {
  final int i; // Final instance variable
  // Constructor that initializes the final variable with the given value
  Sample(int val) {
    i = val; // Set the final variable i
  }
  // Default constructor that initializes the final variable with a
  default value
  Sample() {
    this(100); // Calls the parameterized constructor with a default
               value of 100
  }
}
public class Test {
  void main(String[] args) {
    Sample s = new Sample(10); // Create an instance of Sample with value 10
    Sample s1 = new Sample(); // Create an instance of Sample with default
                                value 100
    System.out.println("final blank value for s object is " + s.i);
    // Print value of i for s
    System.out.println("final blank value for s1 object is " + s1.i);
    // Print value of i for s1
  }
}
```

Output:

```
final blank value for s object is 10
final blank value for s1 object is 100
```

The program defines a class `sample` with a final integer variable `i`. Two constructors are provided: one that initializes `i` with a given value and another that initializes it to a default value of `100`. In the `test` class's `main` method, two `sample` objects, `s` and `s1`, are created using different constructors. For `s`, the constructor with a parameter is invoked, setting `i` to `10`, while for `s1`, the default constructor is invoked, setting `i` to `100`.Finally, the values of `i` for both `s` and `s1` are printed. As `i` is final, its value cannot be modified after initialization, ensuring that it retains the assigned value throughout the object's lifetime.

7.13.4.2 Final Static Variable Initialization

In Java, static initialization blocks are used to initialize static variables or perform other tasks that need to be executed once when the class is loaded into memory. Using a static initialization block with final variable initialization allows for the initialization of constants within a class.

Program

```
Program for static final blank variable
class Test {
  static final int i; // Final static variable
  // Static initialization block
  static {
    i = 100; // Initialize the final static variable
  }
  void main(String[] args) {
    Test t = new Test(); // Create an instance of the Test class
    System.out.println("static final blank value is " + t.i);
    // Access and print the static final variable
  }
}
Output:
static final blank value  is 100
```

The program defines a class named `test`, which contains a final static integer variable `i`. Inside the class, there is a static initialization block that initializes the final static variable `i` with the value `100`. In the `main` method of the `test` class, an instance of the `test` class is created. Then, the value of the static final variable `i` is accessed using the instance `t` and printed to the console using `System.out.println("static final blank value is " + t.i);`. Since `i` is a static variable, it can be accessed using the class name or an instance of the class. Thus, the output will be "static final blank value is 100".

7.13.4.3 Final Initialization Block

In Java, a final initialization block refers to a block of code within a class that is executed when an instance of the class is created. Initialization blocks are used to initialize instance variables and perform other initialization tasks when an object is instantiated. They can be either static or non-static. A final initialization block would be structured similarly to a regular initialization block, but with the addition of the final keyword, which does not have any significant effect.

Program

```
Program for final blank variable initialization in instance block
class Test {
  final int i = 5; // Final variable initialized to 5
  final int k; // Final variable, not initialized here
  // Instance initializer block
```

```
  {
    k = i * i; // Initialize k to the square of i
    display(); // Call the display method
  }
  // Method to display the message and the value of k
  void display() {
    System.out.println("changing final variable in initializer block");
    System.out.println("k=" + k);
  }
  void main(String[] args) {
    new Test(); // Create an instance of Test
  }
}
```

Output:

```
changing final variable in initializer block
k=25
changing final variable in initializer block
k=25
```

The above program defines a class `test` with two final integer variables: `i` and `k`. Variable `i` is initialized with a value of `5`, while variable `k` is left uninitialized, making it a "final blank variable". Inside an instance initializer block, the value of `k` is assigned as the square of `i`, and the `display()` method is invoked. The `display()` method prints a message indicating that it's changing the final variable in the initializer block, followed by the value of `k`. In the `main` method, an instance of the `test` class is created using the constructor. Upon object creation, the instance initializer block is executed, which initializes `k` and invokes the `display()` method. The output will display the value of `k`, which is the square of `i` (25).

7.13.4.4 Final Variable in Lambda Expression

In lambda expressions, variables used must be either `final` or effectively final. This ensures that the value of the variable doesn't change after its initialization, maintaining consistency in the lambda's behavior.

Program

```
import java.util.function.Consumer;
public class LambdaExample {
  void main(String[] args) {
    // Final and effectively final variables
    final String title = "Dr. ";
    String name = "Usharani Bhimavarapu";
    // Lambda expression that uses the final and effectively final variables
    Consumer<String> printFullName = suffix -> {
      // Concatenate and print the variables
      System.out.println(title + name + suffix);
    };
    // Execute the lambda expression with the argument "!"
    printFullName.accept("!");
  }
}
```

Output:

```
Dr. Usharani Bhimavarapu!
```

The above Java program demonstrates the use of lambda expressions with final and effectively final variables. The `title` variable is declared as `final` and the `name` variable is effectively final because it is not modified after assignment. A `Consumer<String>` lambda expression is created to concatenate and print the `title`, `name`, and a suffix. The lambda expression is then executed with the argument `"!"`, resulting in the output "Dr. Usharani Bhimavarapu!".

7.13.5 Final Object Instantiation

In Java, the final keyword can be used with object references to ensure that the reference cannot be changed to point to another object after it is assigned. However, the state of the object itself can still be modified unless the fields within the object are also declared as final. This allows for the creation of immutable objects.

Program

```
Program for final objects
public class Test {
  int i;
  int j;
  void main(String[] args) {
    // Create an instance of the Test class
    Test t = new Test();
    t.i = 10;
    t.j = 20;
    // Create another instance of the Test class and declare it as final
    final Test t1 = new Test();
    t1.i = 100;
    t1.j = 200;
    // Print values for t
    System.out.println("i=" + t.i + " j= " + t.j);
    // Print values for t1
    System.out.println("i=" + t1.i + " j= " + t1.j);
    // Assign t1 to t
    t = t1;
    // Print values for t after reassignment
    System.out.println("i=" + t.i + " j= " + t.j);
  }
}
Output:
i=10 j= 20
i=100 j= 200
i=100 j= 200
```

The above program defines a class named `test` with two integer variables `i` and `j`. In the `main` method, an instance of the `test` class named `t` is created, and its `i` and `j` variables are set to `10` and `20`, respectively. Another instance of the `test` class named `t1` is created, and it is declared as `final`, meaning its reference cannot be changed once assigned. The `i` and `j` variables of `t1` are then set to `100` and `200`, respectively. The values of `i` and `j` for both `t` and `t1` are printed. Then, the reference variable `t` is reassigned to refer to the same object as `t1`. Consequently, both `t` and `t1` now refer to the same object, and their `i` and `j` values are the same.

7.14 ABSTRACT KEYWORD

In Java, the `abstract` keyword is used to declare abstract classes and abstract methods. An abstract class is a class that cannot be instantiated on its own but can be subclassed. Abstract methods are methods declared without an implementation, leaving it to the subclasses to provide their own implementation.

Advantages of Using Abstract Classes and Methods

- Abstraction: Allows for the definition of common behavior without specifying implementation details.
- Encapsulation: Helps in organizing and structuring code by grouping related methods together.
- Inheritance: Facilitates code reuse and promotes hierarchical relationships between classes.

Limitations

- Limited Instantiation: Abstract classes cannot be directly instantiated, which can sometimes add complexity when designing class hierarchies.
- Complexity: Overuse of abstract classes and methods can lead to complex class hierarchies and harder-to-understand code.

7.14.1 Abstract Classes

Abstract classes in Java serve the purpose of providing a blueprint for other classes to inherit from. When a class is declared as abstract, it means that it may contain abstract methods—methods without a body— that must be implemented by any concrete subclass. Abstract classes cannot be instantiated directly; they exist solely to serve as a template for other classes.

In situations where not all methods in the superclass need to be implemented, declaring the superclass as abstract allows for this flexibility. Any subclass extending an abstract class must either implement all abstract methods declared in the superclass or be declared as abstract itself.

Abstract classes can also contain non-abstract methods with a body, providing default behavior that can be overridden by subclasses if necessary. Conversely, non-abstract classes cannot have abstract methods, as they must provide concrete implementations for all methods defined in the class.

Syntax

```
abstract class ClassName {
  // Abstract method (does not have a body)
  abstract void abstractMethod();
  // Regular method (with a body)
  void regularMethod() {
    // method implementation
  }
}
```

The syntax for declaring an abstract class in Java involves using the `abstract` keyword before the class definition. Within the abstract class, abstract methods can be declared by using the `abstract` keyword before the method signature, followed by a semicolon. Abstract methods are methods without a body, serving as placeholders for methods that must be implemented by concrete subclasses.

Additionally, abstract classes can contain concrete methods with a body, providing default behavior that can be inherited by subclasses. These concrete methods are defined in the usual manner, without the `abstract` keyword, and include the method signature followed by curly braces containing the method's implementation. Here's a breakdown of the syntax:

- `abstract class classname`: Declares an abstract class with the name `classname`.
- `abstract void MethodName();`: Declares an abstract method named `MethodName()`.

Abstract methods end with a semicolon and do not include a method body.

- `void anotherMethodName() {// Method implementation}`: Defines a concrete method named `anotherMethodName()` with a body. Concrete methods provide default behavior that can be inherited by subclasses.

Note: The child class, which is extending abstract class must override all the abstract methods in the parent class.

An abstract class is a restricted class that cannot be instantiated directly, meaning objects cannot be created from it.

Program

```
Program for main method in abstract class
abstract class Sample {
  // Abstract class with a static main method
  void main(String[] args) {
System.out.println("abstract main");
    System.out.println(args);
  }
}
public class Test extends Sample {
  public Test() {
String[] s = {"main", "in", "abstract", "class"};
    // Constructor in subclass
    System.out.println("Constructor in child");
    // Invoking the static main method of the abstract class
super.main(s); // Direct call to static method
  }
  void main(String[] args) {
    System.out.println("in main");
    // Create an instance of Test
    new Test();
  }
}
Output:
abstract main
[Ljava.lang.String;@23986957
```

The above Java code exemplifies the use of an abstract class and method. In Java, an abstract class is marked by the `abstract` keyword, indicating that it cannot be instantiated directly and may contain abstract methods. Although the `sample` class doesn't include any abstract methods, it's still designated as abstract due to the presence of the `abstract` keyword in its declaration. Typically, abstract classes serve as blueprints for other classes to inherit from, providing a structure for subclasses to implement specific functionalities. The `Test` class extends the abstract class `sample`, denoting that `Test` inherits its properties and methods. Here, `Test` includes a `main` method, which serves as the entry point of the program. However, it's important to note that the `main` method within the `sample` class cannot be directly executed because it's part of an abstract class. Instead, it's invoked indirectly through inheritance. Within the `Test` class, an instance of `Test` is created, triggering its constructor. Inside the constructor, the `main` method of the `sample` class is invoked using `super.main(s)`, where `s` represents an array of strings. Consequently, the output of the program would display "in main" followed by the elements of the string array `s`.

7.14.1.1 Constructors in Abstract Class

In Java, constructors in abstract classes play a crucial role in initializing the state of objects created from concrete subclasses. Although abstract classes cannot be instantiated directly, their constructors are invoked implicitly when concrete subclasses are instantiated. Constructors in abstract classes are similar to constructors in regular classes but with some differences and restrictions.

Characteristics of Constructors in Abstract Classes

- Initialization of Abstract Class Fields: Constructors in abstract classes can initialize fields defined within the abstract class just like constructors in regular classes. This allows for the initialization of a common state shared by all subclasses.
- Invocation from Subclasses: Constructors in abstract classes are invoked implicitly by constructors of concrete subclasses. When a concrete subclass is instantiated, the constructor of the abstract superclass is called automatically to initialize the inherited state.
- Access Modifiers: Constructors in abstract classes can have different access modifiers (public, protected, default, or private), depending on the design requirements. However, if a constructor in an abstract class is declared private, it cannot be accessed by subclasses.

Program

```
Program for invoking constructor in abstract class in java
abstract class Base {
  // Constructor in the abstract class
  Base() {
    System.out.println("abstract parent constructor");
  }
}
class Child extends Base {
  // Constructor in the subclass
  Child() {
        System.out.println("child constructor");
  super(); // Calls the constructor of Base
  }
}
public class Sample {
  void main(String[] args) {
    // Creating an instance of Child
    new Child();
  }
}
Output:
child constructor
abstract  parent constructor
```

The above Java code demonstrates the usage of an abstract class along with its interaction with a subclass. In Java, an abstract class is declared using the `abstract` keyword, as seen in the `base` class. Abstract classes cannot be instantiated directly but can be extended by other classes. The `base` class in this example contains a constructor, implying that constructors can exist in abstract classes. However, since the `base` class is abstract, it cannot be instantiated on its own. The `child` class extends the `base` abstract class, indicating that it inherits the properties and methods defined in `base`. Inside the `child` class, a constructor is implemented. When an instance of `child` is created, its constructor is invoked. The `super()` keyword is used within the constructor to call the constructor of the superclass, `base`, allowing for initialization of the superclass's state before executing the code within the `child` constructor. In the `main` method of the `sample` class, an object of type `child` is created. Upon instantiation, the constructor of `child` is invoked, which in turn invokes the constructor of the abstract class `base` using `super()`. This sequence of constructor calls results in the output displaying "abstract parent constructor" followed by "child constructor", illustrating the execution flow when working with abstract classes and subclasses in Java.

7.14.2 Abstract Method

An abstract method is a method declared without an implementation (body). It's meant to be implemented by subclasses. Abstract methods are declared using the `abstract` keyword in abstract classes. Subclasses extending an abstract class must provide implementations for all abstract methods defined in the superclass.

Program

```
// Abstract base class
abstract class Base {
  // Abstract method (no implementation)
  abstract void display();
  // Constructor of the abstract class
  Base() {
    System.out.println("Base class constructor");
  }
}
// Concrete child class
class Child extends Base {
  // Constructor of the child class
  Child() {
    System.out.println("Child class constructor");
  }
  // Providing concrete implementation for the abstract method
  @Override
  void display() {
    System.out.println("Child class method");
  }
}
public class Main {
  void main(String[] args) {
    // Creating an instance of Child class
    Child obj = new Child();
    // Calling the display method
    obj.display();
  }
}
```

Output:

```
Base class constructor
Child class constructor
Child class method
```

In this Java program the `base` class serves as an abstraction, containing an abstract method `display()` without implementation. In contrast, the `child` class extends the `base` class, inheriting its abstract method while providing a concrete implementation for it. Upon instantiation of an object of type `child`, the constructor of the child class is invoked, printing "child class constructor". Subsequently, invoking the `display()` method on this object triggers the execution of the overridden method in the child class, which outputs "child class method".

7.15 ARRAY OF OBJECTS IN INHERITANCE

Arrays can be declared to hold objects of a specific class or its subclasses, initialized with objects of varying types, and accessed to invoke overridden methods and access inherited members uniformly. Iterating over the array allows for operations to be performed on each object, providing flexibility in managing collections of related objects while leveraging polymorphism and code reusability.

Program

```
// Base class
class Test {
  // Method to be called from derived classes
  void display() {
    System.out.println("Parent class method");
  }
}
// Intermediate class
class Sample extends Test {
  // Method specific to Sample class
  void put() {
    System.out.println("Child class method");
  }
}
// Main class that extends Sample
public class Main extends Sample {
  void main(String[] args) {
    // Creating an array of Sample objects
    Sample[] s = new Sample[4];
    // Loop to initialize each element of the array
    for (int i = 0; i < s.length; i++) {
      s[i] = new Sample(); // Initializing the array with Sample objects
      System.out.println("Iteration number: " + i);
      s[i].display(); // Calling method from Test class
      s[i].put();    // Calling method from Sample class
    }
  }
}
```

Output:

```
Iteration number: 0
Parent class method
Child class method
Iteration number: 1
Parent class method
Child class method
Iteration number: 2
Parent class method
Child class method
Iteration number: 3
Parent class method
Child class method
```

The above Java program includes three classes: "test", "sample", and "Main". The "test" class defines a method named "display()" that prints "Parent class method" to the console. The "sample" class extends the "test" class and defines a method named "put()" that prints "child class method" to the console. The "Main" class extends the "sample" class. Within its main method, an array of "sample" objects named "s" is created with a size of 4. Then, a loop iterates over the array, initializing each element with a new "sample" object. During each iteration, the iteration number is printed to the console. Then, both the "display()" and "put()" methods are called on the current "sample" object in the array. When the program is executed, for each iteration of the loop, the iteration number is printed to the console. Additionally, the "display()" method from the "test" class and the "put()" method from the "sample" class are called on each "sample" object in the array, resulting in the corresponding messages being printed to the console.

Program

```
Array of class objects and multi level inheritance
// Base class
class Test {
  // Method in the base class
  void display() {
    System.out.println("Parent class method");
  }
}
// Intermediate class extending Test
class Sample extends Test {
  // Method in the Sample class
  void put() {
    System.out.println("Child class method");
  }
}
// Further extension of Sample
class Test1 extends Sample {
  // Method in Test1 class
  void printing() {
    System.out.println("Subchild class method");
  }
}
// Further extension of Test1
class Test2 extends Test1 {
  // Method in Test2 class
  void method() {
    System.out.println("Subsubchild class method");
  }
}
// Main class that extends Sample
public class Main extends Sample {
  void main(String[] args) {
    // Creating an array of Test2 objects
    Test2[] t = new Test2[2];
    // Loop to initialize each element of the array
    for (int i = 0; i < t.length; i++) {
      t[i] = new Test2(); // Initializing the array with Test2 objects
      System.out.println("Iteration number: " + i);
      t[i].display(); // Method from Test
      t[i].put();    // Method from Sample
```

```
      t[i].printing();    // Method from Test1
      t[i].method();    // Method from Test2
    }
  }
}
```

Output:

```
Iteration number: 0
Parent class method
Child class method
Subchild class method
Subsubchild class method
Iteration number: 1
Parent class method
Child class method
Subchild class method
Subsubchild class method
```

The above Java program demonstrates multilevel inheritance through a hierarchy of classes: “test”, “sample”, “test1”, “test2”, and a public class named “Main”. The “test” class defines a method named “display()” that prints “Parent class method” to the console. The “sample” class extends the “test” class and defines a method named “put()” that prints “child class method” to the console. The “test1” class extends the “sample” class and defines a method named “printing()” that prints “subchild class method” to the console. The “test2” class extends the “test1” class and defines a method named “method()” that prints “subsubchild class method” to the console. The “Main” class extends the “sample” class. Within its main method, an array of “test2” objects named “t” is created with a size of 2. Then, a loop iterates over the array, initializing each element with a new “test2” object. During each iteration, the iteration number is printed to the console. Then, the “display()”, “put()”, “printing()”, and “method()” methods are called on the current “test2” object in the array.

7.16 MEDICAL APPLICATIONS

7.16.1 Case Study 1

Fatty liver cancer refers to the development of liver cancer in individuals with fatty liver disease, also known as non-alcoholic fatty liver disease (NAFLD). This condition occurs when excess fat accumulates in the liver cells, which can lead to inflammation (steatohepatitis) and eventually progress to fibrosis, cirrhosis, and in some cases, liver cancer. The parameters considered are:

- **Fatigue**: Whether the patient experiences persistent tiredness or lack of energy.
- **Abdominal Pain**: Any discomfort or pain in the abdominal region, which can be indicative of liver issues.
- **Swelling**: Any abnormal swelling or enlargement, particularly in the abdominal area, which could suggest fluid retention or liver dysfunction.
- **Weight Loss**: Significant and unintentional weight loss, which may accompany liver diseases.

```
import java.util.Scanner;
class Person {
  private String name;
  private int age;
  private String gender;
  public Person(String name, int age, String gender) {
```

```
    this.name = name;
    this.age = age;
    this.gender = gender;
  }
  public String getName() {
    return name;
  }
  public int getAge() {
    return age;
  }
  public String getGender() {
    return gender;
  }
  @Override
  public String toString() {
    return "Person{" +
        "name='" + name + '\'' +
        ", age=" + age +
        ", gender='" + gender + '\'' +
        '}';
  }
}
class Patient extends Person {
  private String medicalHistory;
  private boolean hasFatigue;
  private boolean hasJaundice;
  public Patient(String name, int age, String gender, String medicalHistory,
     boolean hasFatigue, boolean hasJaundice) {
    super(name, age, gender);
    this.medicalHistory = medicalHistory;
    this.hasFatigue = hasFatigue;
    this.hasJaundice = hasJaundice;
  }
  public String getMedicalHistory() {
    return medicalHistory;
  }
  public boolean hasFatigue() {
    return hasFatigue;
  }
  public boolean hasJaundice() {
    return hasJaundice;
  }
  @Override
  public String toString() {
    return "Patient{" +
        "name='" + getName() + '\'' +
        ", age=" + getAge() +
        ", gender='" + getGender() + '\'' +
        ", medicalHistory='" + medicalHistory + '\'' +
        ", hasFatigue=" + hasFatigue +
        ", hasJaundice=" + hasJaundice +
        '}';
  }
}
```

```
class LiverPatient extends Patient {
  private boolean hasAbdominalPain;
  private boolean hasSwelling;
  private boolean hasWeightLoss;
  public LiverPatient(String name, int age, String gender, String
     medicalHistory, boolean hasFatigue, boolean hasJaundice,
     boolean hasAbdominalPain, boolean hasSwelling, boolean hasWeightLoss) {
    super(name, age, gender, medicalHistory, hasFatigue, hasJaundice);
    this.hasAbdominalPain = hasAbdominalPain;
    this.hasSwelling = hasSwelling;
    this.hasWeightLoss = hasWeightLoss;
  }
  public boolean hasAbdominalPain() {
    return hasAbdominalPain;
  }
  public boolean hasSwelling() {
    return hasSwelling;
  }
  public boolean hasWeightLoss() {
    return hasWeightLoss;
  }
  public boolean isSuspectedOfFattyLiverCancer() {
    return hasFatigue() && hasJaundice() && hasAbdominalPain && hasSwelling
    && hasWeightLoss;
  }
  @Override
  public String toString() {
    return "LiverPatient{" +
        "name='" + getName() + '\'' +
        ", age=" + getAge() +
        ", gender='" + getGender() + '\'' +
        ", medicalHistory='" + getMedicalHistory() + '\'' +
        ", hasFatigue=" + hasFatigue() +
        ", hasJaundice=" + hasJaundice() +
        ", hasAbdominalPain=" + hasAbdominalPain +
        ", hasSwelling=" + hasSwelling +
        ", hasWeightLoss=" + hasWeightLoss +
        '}';
  }
}
public class FattyLiverCancerDetection {
  void main(String[] args) {
    Scanner scanner = new Scanner(System.in);
    System.out.print("Enter name: ");
    String name = scanner.nextLine();
    System.out.print("Enter age: ");
    int age = scanner.nextInt();
    scanner.nextLine(); // Consume newline
    System.out.print("Enter gender: ");
    String gender = scanner.nextLine();
    System.out.print("Enter medical history: ");
    String medicalHistory = scanner.nextLine();
    System.out.print("Has fatigue (true/false): ");
    boolean hasFatigue = scanner.nextBoolean();
    System.out.print("Has jaundice (true/false): ");
```

```
    boolean hasJaundice = scanner.nextBoolean();
    System.out.print("Has abdominal pain (true/false): ");
    boolean hasAbdominalPain = scanner.nextBoolean();
    System.out.print("Has swelling (true/false): ");
    boolean hasSwelling = scanner.nextBoolean();
    System.out.print("Has weight loss (true/false): ");
    boolean hasWeightLoss = scanner.nextBoolean();
    LiverPatient patient = new LiverPatient(name, age, gender, medicalHistory,
    hasFatigue, hasJaundice, hasAbdominalPain, hasSwelling, hasWeightLoss);
    System.out.println(patient);
    if (patient.isSuspectedOfFattyLiverCancer()) {
      System.out.println("The patient is suspected of having fatty liver
cancer.");
    } else {
      System.out.println("The patient is not suspected of having fatty liver
cancer.");
    }
  }
}
```

The above Java program begins by prompting the user to input personal information such as name, age, and gender, followed by medical history details. It then queries the user for the presence of specific symptoms like fatigue, jaundice, abdominal pain, swelling, and weight loss, capturing these as boolean values. Based on these inputs, an instance of the `LiverPatient` class is created, inheriting from `Patient`, which in turn extends the `Person` class to maintain a structured hierarchy of personal and medical information. Finally, the program evaluates whether the collected symptoms indicate a suspicion of fatty liver cancer and outputs a diagnostic message accordingly, demonstrating its role in medical data collection and preliminary assessment.

7.16.2 Case Study 2

Jaundice is a medical condition characterized by the yellowing of the skin and eyes due to elevated levels of bilirubin in the blood. Bilirubin is a yellow pigment produced during the normal breakdown of red blood cells in the liver. When the liver is unable to metabolize bilirubin effectively or when there is an obstruction in the bile ducts, bilirubin builds up in the bloodstream, leading to jaundice. The parameters considered are:

- **Yellow Eyes:** Check whether the patient has yellow eyes.
- **Yellow Skin:** Check whether the patient has yellow skin.

```
import java.util.Scanner;
public class JaundiceDetection {
    static class Patient {
    private String name;
    private int age;
    private String gender;
    public Patient(String name, int age, String gender) {
      this.name = name;
      this.age = age;
      this.gender = gender;
    }
```

```
  public String getName() {
    return name;
  }
  public int getAge() {
    return age;
  }
  public String getGender() {
    return gender;
  }
  @Override
  public String toString() {
    return "Patient{" +
        "name='" + name + '\'' +
        ", age=" + age +
        ", gender='" + gender + '\'' +
        '}';
  }
    class JaundiceDetector {
    private boolean hasYellowEyes;
    private boolean hasYellowSkin;
    public JaundiceDetector(boolean hasYellowEyes, boolean hasYellowSkin) {
      this.hasYellowEyes = hasYellowEyes;
      this.hasYellowSkin = hasYellowSkin;      }
    public boolean isJaundiceDetected() {
      return hasYellowEyes || hasYellowSkin;
    }
    @Override
    public String toString() {
      return "JaundiceDetector{" +
          "hasYellowEyes=" + hasYellowEyes +
          ", hasYellowSkin=" + hasYellowSkin +
          '}';
    }
  }
}
void main(String[] args) {
  Scanner scanner = new Scanner(System.in);
  System.out.print("Enter patient name: ");
  String name = scanner.nextLine();
  System.out.print("Enter patient age: ");
  int age = scanner.nextInt();
  scanner.nextLine(); // Consume newline
  System.out.print("Enter patient gender: ");
  String gender = scanner.nextLine();
  System.out.println("Jaundice symptoms:");
  System.out.print("Has yellow eyes (true/false): ");
  boolean hasYellowEyes = scanner.nextBoolean();
  System.out.print("Has yellow skin (true/false): ");
  boolean hasYellowSkin = scanner.nextBoolean();
  // Create Patient instance
  Patient patient = new Patient(name, age, gender);
  // Create JaundiceDetector instance using inner class
  Patient.JaundiceDetector jaundiceDetector = patient.new
  JaundiceDetector(hasYellowEyes, hasYellowSkin);
  // Print patient details
```

```
    System.out.println("Patient details: " + patient);
    // Print jaundice detection result
    System.out.println("Jaundice detection result: " + (jaundiceDetector.
    isJaundiceDetected() ? "Jaundice detected" : "No jaundice detected"));
  }
}
```

The above Java program `JaundiceDetection` models a system to detect jaundice based on user-provided information. It begins by prompting the user to input patient details such as name, age, and gender. Following this, it asks for specific symptoms related to jaundice, including whether the patient has yellow eyes and yellow skin. Using an inner class structure, the program defines a `Patient` class to encapsulate basic personal information and a nested `JaundiceDetector` class to evaluate jaundice symptoms. Upon instantiation, the `JaundiceDetector` checks if either symptom is present and determines if jaundice is detected. Finally, the program outputs both the patient's details and the result of the jaundice detection, providing a straightforward tool for preliminary medical assessment.

8 Interfaces

8.1 INTRODUCTION

Abstraction in Java refers to the process of hiding certain details and showing only essential features of an object or system to the outside world. It involves defining a set of methods and properties that provide a simplified view of entities or operations, focusing on what an object does rather than how it does it.

Key Aspects of Abstraction

- Abstract Classes and Interfaces: Abstraction is typically achieved in Java through abstract classes and interfaces. Abstract classes may contain abstract methods (methods without a body) that subclasses must implement, while interfaces define a contract that classes must adhere to by implementing its methods.
- Hiding Implementation Details: Abstraction allows developers to focus on the essential aspects of an object or system by hiding unnecessary implementation details. This improves code readability, reduces complexity, and enhances maintainability.

Need for Abstraction

- Simplicity and Manageability: By abstracting away complex implementation details, abstraction simplifies the understanding and management of software systems, making them easier to design, implement, and modify.
- Encapsulation: Abstraction complements encapsulation by providing a clear separation between a class's internal implementation and its external interface. This separation promotes modular design and reduces dependencies between components.

Benefits of Abstraction

- Enhanced Modularity: Encourages modular design by defining clear boundaries between different components of a system. This facilitates code reuse and promotes scalability.
- Code Reusability: Abstraction enables the creation of reusable components (through abstract classes and interfaces) that can be implemented by different classes without altering their external behavior.
- Flexibility and Extensibility: Allows software systems to evolve over time by modifying or extending abstract components without affecting the functionality provided to other parts of the program.

DOI: 10.1201/9781003544319-8

Limitations of Abstraction

- Increased Complexity: Designing effective abstractions requires careful consideration of which details to hide and which to expose. Over-abstracting can lead to overly complex designs that are difficult to understand and maintain.
- Performance Overhead: Indirectly accessing abstracted components (e.g., through interfaces) may introduce a slight performance overhead compared to direct access. However, this impact is usually negligible in modern applications.

Program

```
// Abstract class for Course Registration
abstract class CourseRegistration {
  // Fields for student and course information
  protected String studentName;
  protected String courseName;
  // Constructor to initialize the student and course details
  public CourseRegistration(String studentName, String courseName) {
    this.studentName = studentName;
    this.courseName = courseName;
  }
  // Abstract method to register for the course
  public abstract void register();
  // Method to display registration details (implemented, not abstract)
  public void displayDetails() {
    System.out.println("Student: " + studentName);
    System.out.println("Course: " + courseName);
  }
}
// Concrete class implementing the abstract methods
class OnlineCourseRegistration extends CourseRegistration {
  public OnlineCourseRegistration(String studentName, String courseName) {
    super(studentName, courseName);
  }
  // Implement the abstract method
  @Override
  public void register() {
    System.out.println(studentName + " has been registered for the online
       course: " + courseName);
  }
}
// Interface for additional operations like canceling a course
interface CourseManagement {
  void cancelRegistration();
}
// Class implementing both abstract class and interface
class AdvancedCourseRegistration extends CourseRegistration implements
CourseManagement {
  public AdvancedCourseRegistration(String studentName, String courseName) {
    super(studentName, courseName);
  }
```

```
  // Implement the abstract method from CourseRegistration
  @Override
  public void register() {
    System.out.println(studentName + " has been registered for the
       advanced course: " + courseName);
  }
  // Implement the method from CourseManagement interface
  @Override
  public void cancelRegistration() {
    System.out.println("Registration  for  "  +  studentName  +  "  in  "  +
courseName + " has been canceled.");
  }
}
// Main class to demonstrate the registration process
public class Main {
void main(String[] args) {
    // Register for an online course
    CourseRegistration onlineCourse = new OnlineCourseRegistration("Usha",
        "Java Programming");
    onlineCourse.register();
    onlineCourse.displayDetails();
    System.out.println(); // Line break for readability
    // Register for an advanced course and cancel it
    AdvancedCourseRegistration advancedCourse = new AdvancedCourseRegistr
       ation("Rani", "Advanced Algorithms");
    advancedCourse.register();
    advancedCourse.displayDetails();
    advancedCourse.cancelRegistration();
  }
}
```

Output:

```
Usha has been registered for the online course: Java Programming
Student: Usha
Course: Java Programming
Rani has been registered for the advanced course: Advanced Algorithms
Student: Rani
Course: Advanced Algorithms
Registration for Rani in Advanced Algorithms has been canceled.
```

This program demonstrates abstraction in Java by using an abstract class `CourseRegistration` for student course registration, with concrete classes implementing the specific registration logic. It also uses an interface `CourseManagement` for additional functionalities like canceling a registration. The `Main` class creates instances to showcase the registration and cancelation process.

8.2 INTERFACE

An interface in Java is a reference type, similar to a class, that can contain only constants, method signatures, default methods, static methods, and nested types. Interfaces cannot contain instance fields or constructors. They are used to define a contract that other classes can implement. An interface specifies what a class must do, but not how it does it.

8.2.1 Importance of Interfaces

Interfaces are crucial in Java for several reasons:

- Abstraction: Interfaces provide a way to abstract the behavior of classes. They allow you to define methods that must be implemented by the classes, without specifying the exact implementation.
- Multiple Inheritance: Java does not support multiple inheritance (a class inheriting from more than one class), but a class can implement multiple interfaces. This allows for a form of multiple inheritance.
- Loose Coupling: Interfaces promote loose coupling by defining a set of methods that can be implemented by any class. This allows for the interchangeability of objects.
- Standardization: They provide a standard form of interaction. Different classes can implement the same interface, ensuring that they provide specific methods.

8.2.2 Need for Interfaces

The need for interfaces arises from several scenarios in software development:

- Multiple Inheritance: As Java does not support multiple inheritance, interfaces provide a way to implement multiple sets of behaviors.
- Code Reusability: Interfaces allow for the creation of generic methods and classes that can operate on any class that implements a specific interface.
- Frameworks and APIs: Interfaces are widely used in frameworks and APIs to provide a common structure and ensure that different components can interact with each other.

8.2.3 Advantages of Interfaces

- Flexibility: Interfaces allow a class to become more flexible by implementing multiple interfaces.
- Decoupling: By using interfaces, you can decouple the implementation of methods from their declaration, which helps in changing the implementation without affecting the classes that use the interface.
- Testability: Interfaces make it easier to test code because you can provide mock implementations of the interfaces for testing purposes.
- Interoperability: They allow for different classes to work together more easily, facilitating communication between disparate parts of a program.
- Code Organization: Interfaces help in organizing code by defining a clear set of methods that must be implemented, making the code easier to understand and maintain.

8.2.4 Limitations of Interfaces

- No Implementation: Interfaces cannot contain any implementation logic in their methods (except default and static methods), which means that every implementing class must provide its own implementation.
- Rigid Contracts: Once an interface is published, changing it can break all the implementations. This makes the design of interfaces very critical.
- Complexity: Using too many interfaces can make the design complex and hard to manage, especially when there are many interdependencies.
- Performance Overhead: Interface method calls have a slight performance overhead compared to direct method calls due to the additional level of indirection.

8.3 INTERFACE

In Java, an interface is a reference type, similar to a class, that can contain only constants, method signatures, default methods, static methods, and nested types. Interfaces cannot contain instance fields or constructors. They are used to specify a set of methods that a class must implement, providing a way to achieve abstraction and multiple inheritance in Java.

Interfaces address the issue of multiple inheritance by allowing a class to implement multiple interfaces. When a class implements an interface, it agrees to provide implementations for all the methods declared in that interface. Since Java does not support multiple inheritance through class extension, implementing interfaces provides a way for classes to inherit behavior from multiple sources.

Methods declared in an interface are by default abstract, meaning they do not have a body and must be implemented by the implementing class. Variables declared in an interface are implicitly public, static, and final, making them constants that can be accessed using the interface name. This allows interfaces to define constants that implementing classes can use without having to redefine them.

Note: We cannot create objects to interfaces.

Note: To use an interface, classes must implement it. We have to use the implements keyword to implement an interface.

Syntax

```
// Define an interface
public interface InterfaceName {
  // Constants (implicitly public, static, and final)
  Type CONSTANT_NAME = value;
  // Abstract method declaration (no body)
  ReturnType methodName(ParameterType parameterName);
  // Default method with an implementation
  default ReturnType defaultMethodName(ParameterType parameterName) {
    // method body
  }
  // Static method with an implementation
  static ReturnType staticMethodName(ParameterType parameterName) {
    // method body
  }
  // Nested interface (optional)
  interface NestedInterfaceName {
    ReturnType nestedMethodName(ParameterType parameterName);
  }
}
```

The syntax for defining an interface in Java involves using the `interface` keyword followed by the name of the interface. Within the interface body, method signatures are declared, which specify the methods that classes implementing the interface must provide implementations for. By default, all methods declared in an interface are public and abstract, meaning they do not have a body and must be implemented by the implementing classes. Additionally, interfaces can contain variables, which are implicitly public, static, and final. These variables act as constants and must be initialized when declared. Since they are static and final, they are effectively constants shared among all classes implementing the interface. Therefore, the syntax for declaring variables within an interface involves specifying the access modifier (`public`), followed by the modifiers `static` and `final`, and then the data type and variable name. These variables are constants that can be accessed using the interface name.

8.3.1 Default Methods

Default methods in Java are methods defined within an interface with the `default` keyword, providing a default implementation. They allow interfaces to evolve by adding new methods without breaking existing implementations. This feature helps achieve backward compatibility and supports the creation of more flexible and reusable interfaces. Default methods can be overridden by implementing classes if specific behavior is required.

Program

```
Program for default methods in java interface
// Define an interface with a constant, abstract method, and default method
interface definterface {
  // Constant variable
  int i = 10;
  // Abstract method
  void display();
  // Default method
  default void cube(int x) {
    System.out.println(x * x * x);
  }
}
// Class implementing the interface
class sample implements definterface {
  // Implement the display method
  public void display() {
    System.out.println(i);
  }
}
// Main class
public class test {
void main(String[] args) {
    // Create an instance of sample and call methods
    definterface obj = new sample();
    obj.display();      // Prints value of i (10)
    obj.cube(10);      // Prints cube of 10 (1000)
  }
}
Output:
10
1000
```

Firstly, an interface named `definterface` is declared using the `interface` keyword, which includes the declaration of a constant integer variable `i` initialized with a value of 10. Additionally, a method signature for the `display()` method is specified without a body, indicating that classes implementing this interface must provide an implementation for this method. Moreover, a default method named `cube()` is defined, which includes a body and provides a default implementation for computing the cube of a given integer parameter. Next, a class named `sample` implements the `definterface` interface using the `implements` keyword. Within the `sample` class, the `display()` method is implemented to print the value of the constant `i` declared in the interface. Finally, a class named `test` is defined, which contains the `main()` method. Inside the `main()` method, an instance of the `sample` class is created and assigned to a reference variable of the `definterface` type.

8.3.2 Static Methods

Static methods in Java are methods defined in a class with the `static` keyword, meaning they belong to the class itself rather than any instance of the class. These methods can be called without creating an object of the class and are used for operations that don't require data from instance variables. Static methods can access static variables and other static methods directly but cannot access instance variables or methods. They are commonly used for utility or helper methods.

Program

```
Program on static methods in java interface
// Define the interface with a constant, static method, and abstract method
interface itest {
  // Constant variable
  int i = 10;
  // Static method to calculate cube
  static int cube(int x) {
    return x * x * x;
  }
  // Abstract method
  void display();
}
// Class implementing the interface
class sample implements itest {
  // Implement the display method
  public void display() {
    System.out.println(i); // Prints the constant i
  }
  // Method that uses the static cube method from the interface
  public void fcube() {
    int result = itest.cube(i); // Call the static cube method from the
                                   interface
    System.out.println(result); // Prints the cube of i
  }
}
// Main class
public class test {
void main(String[] args) {
    // Create an instance of sample and call methods
    sample obj = new sample();
    obj.display();       // Prints value of i (10)
    obj.fcube();         // Prints cube of i (1000)
  }
}
Output:
10
1000
```

The `itest` interface is declared using the `interface` keyword. It includes the declaration of an integer constant `i` initialized with a value of 10. Additionally, a static method `cube()` is defined within the interface, which calculates and returns the cube of a given integer parameter. The `display()` method signature is also specified, indicating that classes implementing this interface must provide an implementation for this method. Next, a class named `sample` implements the `itest` interface using the `implements` keyword. Within the `sample` class, the `display()` method is implemented to print the value of the constant `i` declared in the interface. Additionally, a method named `fcube()` is defined in the `sample` class, which calculates the cube of a given integer parameter using the static `cube()` method defined in the `itest` interface. Finally, a class named `test` contains the `main()` method. Inside the `main()` method, an instance of the `sample` class is created, and its `display()` and `fcube()` methods are invoked.

8.4 IMPLEMENTS INTERFACE

In Java, when a class implements an interface, it agrees to perform the specific behaviors defined by that interface. This means the class must provide concrete implementations for all the abstract methods declared in the interface. Implementing an interface allows a class to be more flexible and decoupled from specific implementations, promoting better design principles such as abstraction and polymorphism.

Syntax for Implementing an Interface:

```
class classname implements interface
{
}
```

To implement an interface, a class uses the `implements` keyword followed by the interface name. Here is the basic syntax:

```
Syntax
interface MyInterface {
  void method1();
  void method2();
}
class MyClass implements MyInterface {
  @Override
  public void method1() {
    // Implementation of method1
  }
  @Override
  public void method2() {
    // Implementation of method2
  }
}
```

Program

```
// Define an interface
interface sample {
  void data();
}
// Class Test implementing the sample interface
class Test implements sample {
  @Override
  public void data() {
    System.out.println("Implementing interface in class.");
  }
void main(String[] args) {
    Test test = new Test();
    test.data(); // Calling the data() method
  }
```

```
}
Output:
Implementing interface in class
```

The above Java program showcases the implementation of an interface called `sample` and its integration within the `Test` class. The interface `sample` declares a single method `data()` without providing its implementation details. In the `Test` class, which implements the `sample` interface, the `data()` method is overridden to specify its behavior, which in this case is to print the message "Implementing interface in class." In the `main` method of the `Test` class, an object `test` of type `Test` is instantiated using the `new` keyword. Through this object, the `data()` method defined in the `sample` interface is invoked using the dot operator (`test.data()`).

8.5 EXTENDS INTERFACE

In Java, an interface can extend one or more other interfaces, allowing it to inherit their abstract methods. This capability enables the creation of more specialized interfaces based on general ones. When an interface extends another, it inherits all the methods declared in the parent interface, thus promoting reusability and modularity in the design of the application. This mechanism allows developers to build flexible and scalable systems by breaking down complex behaviors into smaller, manageable, and reusable pieces of functionality, which can be combined and extended as needed. However, an interface extending another cannot provide implementations for the inherited methods; it simply declares that any implementing class must provide the concrete behavior for these methods. This design principle is a cornerstone of interface-based programming in Java, supporting the development of loosely coupled and easily maintainable codebases.

Program

```
Program for Implementing multiple interfaces in a class
// Define the first interface with a constant and an abstract method
interface myinterface {
  int i = 10;  // Constant variable
  void display();  // Abstract method
}
// Define the second interface with a constant and an abstract method
interface myinterface1 {
  int j = 50;  // Constant variable
  void put();  // Abstract method
}
// Class implementing both interfaces
class sample implements myinterface, myinterface1 {
  // Implement display method from myinterface
  public void display() {
    System.out.println(i);  // Prints the constant i
  }
  // Implement put method from myinterface1
  public void put() {
    System.out.println(j);  // Prints the constant j
  }
}
// Main class
public class test {
void main(String[] args) {
    // Create an instance of sample and call methods
```

```
    sample obj = new sample();
    obj.display();  // Prints value of i (10)
    obj.put();    // Prints value of j (50)
  }
}
```

Output:

```
10
50
```

This Java program demonstrates the use of multiple interfaces and their implementation in a class. Two interfaces, `myinterface` and `myinterface1`, are defined, each containing a constant field and an abstract method. The `myinterface` interface declares an integer constant `i` and an abstract method `display()`. Similarly, the `myinterface1` interface declares an integer constant `j` and an abstract method `put()`. The `sample` class implements both interfaces `myinterface` and `myinterface1`. It provides implementations for the abstract methods `display()` and `put()`. In the `display()` method, the value of the constant `i` from the `myinterface` interface is printed, while in the `put()` method, the value of the constant `j` from the `myinterface1` interface is printed. In the `main()` method of the `test` class, an instance of the `sample` class is created, and its `display()` and `put()` methods are called to demonstrate the implementation of both interfaces.

Program

```
Program for interface extends another interface
// Define the first interface with a constant and an abstract method
interface myinterface {
  int i = 10;  // Constant variable
  void display();  // Abstract method
}
// Define the second interface that extends the first one
interface myinterface1 extends myinterface {
  int j = 50;  // Constant variable
  void put();  // Abstract method
}
// Class implementing the extended interface
class sample implements myinterface1 {
  // Implement the display method inherited from myinterface
  public void display() {
    System.out.println(i);  // Prints the constant i
  }
  // Implement the put method from myinterface1
  public void put() {
    System.out.println(j);  // Prints the constant j
  }
}
// Main class
public class test {
void main(String[] args) {
    // Create an instance of sample and call methods
    sample obj = new sample();
    obj.display();  // Prints value of i (10)
    obj.put();    // Prints value of j (50)
  }
}
```

```
Output:
10
50
```

This Java program demonstrates interface inheritance and implementation. Two interfaces, `myinterface` and `myinterface1`, are defined. `myinterface` contains a constant `i` and an abstract method `display()`, while `myinterface1` extends `myinterface` and adds a constant `j` and an abstract method `put()`. The `sample` class implements the `myinterface1` interface. It provides implementations for the `display()` and `put()` methods inherited from `myinterface1`. In the `display()` method, the constant `i` from `myinterface` is printed, and in the `put()` method, the constant `j` from `myinterface1` is printed. In the `main()` method of the `test` class, an instance of the `sample` class is created and used to call its `display()` and `put()` methods.

8.5.1 Interface Inside Class

In Java, it is possible to define an interface inside a class, which is referred to as an inner interface. This approach is useful when you want to encapsulate related behaviors or contract definitions within the scope of a specific class.

Program

```
Program for inner interface of a class extends outside interface in java
// Define the interface with an abstract method
interface testing {
  void put();  // Abstract method
}
// Outer class
class outer {
  // Inner interface extending the testing interface
  interface inner extends testing {
    void display();  // Abstract method
  }
}
// Class implementing the outer.inner interface
class sample implements outer.inner {
  // Implement the display method
  public void display() {
    System.out.println("interface implemented method");
  }
  // Implement the put method
  public void put() {
    System.out.println("inner interface extends anonymous interface");
  }
}
// Main class
public class Test {
void main(String[] args) {
    // Create an instance of the sample class
    sample obj = new sample();
    // Call the implemented methods
    obj.display();  // Prints "interface implemented method"
    obj.put();    // Prints "inner interface extends anonymous interface"
  }
```

```
}
Output:
interface implemented method
inner interface extends anonymous interface
```

In the above program, an interface named `testing` is declared with an abstract method `put()`, indicating that any class implementing this interface must provide an implementation for the `put()` method. Next, a class named `outer` is defined, which contains an inner interface named `inner`. This `inner` interface extends the `testing` interface, inheriting its abstract method `put()` while also declaring its own abstract method `display()`. This approach allows for the extension of an interface within another interface, enabling hierarchical structuring of interface types. Then, a class named `sample` implements the `outer.inner` interface, providing concrete implementations for both the `display()` and `put()` methods. The `display()` method prints a message indicating that it implements a method defined in the interface, while the `put()` method prints a message specific to the functionality it provides. Finally, in the `Test` class, an instance of the `sample` class is created, and its `display()` and `put()` methods are invoked, demonstrating the usage of the implemented interface methods.

Program

```
Program for implementing interface method of class inside interface in java
// Define an interface with a nested class and an abstract method
interface Outer {
  // Nested class inside the interface
  class Inner {
    public void show() {
      System.out.println("class inside interface");
    }
  }
  // Abstract method in the interface
  void put();
}
// Class extending the nested class and implementing the interface
class Sample extends Outer.Inner implements Outer {
  // Override the abstract method from the interface
  public void put() {
    System.out.println("implementing interface method");
  }
  // Empty display method (optional)
  public void display() {
    // Empty display method does nothing
  }
}
// Main class
public class Test {
void main(String[] args) {
    // Create an instance of Sample class
    Sample obj = new Sample();
    // Call methods from the Sample class
    obj.display();  // Calls empty display method (does nothing)
    obj.show();    // Prints "class inside interface"
    obj.put();    // Prints "imlementing interface method"
  }
}
```

```
Output:
class inside interface
implementing interface method
```

This Java program showcases the concept of nested classes within interfaces and the implementation of abstract methods. The `Outer` interface contains a nested class `Inner`, which has a method `show()` to display a message indicating it's a class inside an interface. Additionally, the `Outer` interface declares an abstract method `put()`, which is meant to be implemented by classes that implement the interface. The `Sample` class extends the `Outer.Inner` class and implements the `Outer` interface. It provides an implementation for the `put()` method, as required by the interface. However, it also defines a method `display()`, which is not present in the `Outer` interface or its nested class. This is permissible as long as `Sample` provides the necessary implementation for the methods declared in the interface. In the `main()` method of the `Test` class, an instance of `Sample` is created. First, the `display()` method of the `Sample` class is invoked, which doesn't print any message because the method is empty. Then, the `show()` method inherited from the `Outer.Inner` class is called, printing the message indicating it's a class inside an interface. Finally, the `put()` method implemented by the `Sample` class is invoked, printing the message indicating the implementation of the interface method.

Program

```
Program on private inner  class implements interface
// Define an interface with an abstract method
interface sample {
  void put();  // Abstract method
}
// Outer class containing a private inner class
class outer {
  // Private inner class implementing the sample interface
  private class inner implements sample {
    public void put() {
      System.out.println("This is an inner class");
    }
  }
  // Method to instantiate inner class and invoke its put method
  public void display() {
    inner obj = new inner();  // Create an instance of the inner class
    obj.put();  // Call the put method from the inner class
  }
}
// Main class
public class test {
void main(String[] args) {
    outer obj = new outer();  // Create an instance of the outer class
    obj.display();  // Call the display method, which invokes the inner
                       class's method
  }
}
Output:
This is an inner class
```

An interface named `sample` is declared using the `interface` keyword. Within the interface, a method named `put()` is abstractly defined using the `abstract` and `public` modifiers. This method serves as a contract that any class implementing the `sample` interface must implement. Next, a class named `outer` is defined. Inside the `outer` class, a private inner class named `inner` is declared, which implements the `sample` interface. The `put()` method is implemented within the `inner` class according to the requirements of the `sample` interface. The `outer` class also contains a method named `display()`, which instantiates an object of the `inner` class and invokes its `put()` method. This method serves as a way to access the functionality provided by the `inner` class. Lastly, a class named `test` contains the `main()` method, which serves as the entry point of the program. Inside the `main()` method, an instance of the `outer` class is created, and its `display()` method is invoked.

Program

```
Program for invoking main method in interface in java
// Define an interface with a static main method
interface test {
  // Static main method inside the interface
  static void main(String[] args) {
    System.out.println("main in interface");
    for (String arg : args) {
      System.out.println(arg);
    }
  }
  // Abstract method to be implemented
  void display();
}
// Class implementing the test interface
class Main implements test {
  // Implement the display method from the interface
  public void display() {
    System.out.println("display() of interface");
  }
  // Main method of the class, entry point of the program
void main(String[] args) {
    System.out.println("main in class");
    // Create an instance of the class and call display method
    Main obj = new Main();
    obj.display();
    // Simulate passing command-line arguments
    String[] interfaceArgs = {"test","ing"};
    // Call the main method of the test interface with arguments
    test.main(interfaceArgs);
  }
}
Output:
main in interface
```

An interface named `test` is defined. This interface contains a `main()` method, which defies the conventional usage of the `main()` method as the entry point of a Java program. Inside this `main()` method, a message is printed to the console, followed by a loop that iterates through the command-line arguments passed to the program. Next, a class named `Main` implements the `test` interface. Within this class, a `display()` method is defined to fulfill the contract specified by the `test` interface. Additionally, the conventional `main()` method is implemented in this class, serving as the entry point of the program. Inside the `main()` method, messages are printed to the console to indicate its execution. Furthermore, an instance of `Main` is created to invoke its `display()` method.

Additionally, an array of strings is created to mimic command-line arguments, and the `main()` method of the `test` interface is invoked with this array.

Program

```
Program for private inner interface inside class in java
// Outer class with a private interface and a public interface extending
the private one
class Outer {
  // Private interface Inner with an abstract method
  private interface Inner {
    void show();
  }
  // Public interface Sub extending Inner and declaring another abstract method
  public interface Sub extends Inner {
    void put();
  }
}
// Sample class implementing the Outer.Sub interface
class Sample implements Outer.Sub {
  // Implementing the show() method from the Inner interface
  public void show() {
    System.out.println("implementing private interface method");
  }
  // Implementing the put() method from the Sub interface
  public void put() {
    System.out.println("extending private interface");
  }
  // A display method specific to this class
  public void display() {
    System.out.println("interface implemented method");
  }
}
// Test class with the main method
public class Test {
void main(String[] args) {
    // Creating an instance of Sample
    Sample obj = new Sample();
    // Invoking methods of Sample
    obj.display(); // Calls display() to show "interface implemented
                   method"
    obj.put();    // Calls put() to show "extending private interface"
    obj.show();    // Calls show() to show "implementing private interface
                   method"
  }
}
Output:
interface implemented method
extending private interface
implementing private interface method
```

The `Outer` class contains a private interface `Inner`, which declares an abstract method `show()`. Additionally, there's another interface `Sub`, which extends the `Inner` interface and declares another abstract method `put()`. The `Sample` class implements the `Outer.Sub` interface, which includes the methods `show()` and `put()`. However, since `Inner` is a private interface, it cannot be directly implemented by classes outside of the `Outer` class. Therefore, `Sample` only implements `Outer.Sub`, not `Outer.Inner`. In the `main()` method of the `Test` class, an instance of `Sample` is created. The `display()`, `put()`, and `show()` methods of the `Sample` class are then invoked. The `display()` method prints a message indicating it's an interface-implemented method, while the `put()` method prints a message indicating it's extending a private interface. Finally, the `show()` method prints a message indicating it's implementing a private interface method.

Program

```
Program for static inner interface in java
// Outer class containing a static nested interface
class Outer {
  // Static nested interface with an abstract method
  static interface Inner {
    void display();
  }
}
// Sample class implementing the Outer.Inner interface
class Sample implements Outer.Inner {
  // Providing implementation for the display() method
  public void display() {
    System.out.println("static interface implemented method");
  }
}
// Test class with the main method
public class Test {
void main(String[] args) {
    // Creating an instance of Sample and referencing it as Outer.Inner
    Outer.Inner obj = new Sample();
    // Calling the display() method
    obj.display();  // Prints: static interface implemented method
  }
}
Output:
static interface implemented method
```

This Java program illustrates the usage of a static nested interface and its implementation in a separate class. The `Outer` class contains a static nested interface named `Inner`, which declares an abstract method `display()`. The `Sample` class implements the `Outer.Inner` interface, providing an implementation for the `display()` method. In the `display()` method of the `Sample` class, a message "static interface implemented method" is printed to the console.In the `main()` method of the `Test` class, an instance of the `Sample` class is created and assigned to a reference of type `Outer.Inner`. This is possible because nested interfaces can be accessed using the enclosing class name. Finally, the `display()` method of the `Sample` instance is invoked, resulting in the message being printed to the console.

Program

```
Program for static class inside interface in java
// Interface containing a static nested class
interface Outer {
  // Static nested class
```

```
  static class Inner {
    // Method of the static nested class
    void show() {
      System.out.println("static class inside interface");
    }
  }
}
// Test class with the main method
public class Test {
void main(String[] args) {
    // Creating an instance of the static nested class
    Outer.Inner obj = new Outer.Inner();
    // Calling the show() method
    obj.show();  // Prints: static class inside interface
  }
}
```

Output:

```
static class inside interface
```

This Java program demonstrates the usage of a static nested class inside an interface. The `Outer` interface contains a static nested class named `Inner`, which defines a method `show()` that prints "static class inside interface" to the console. In the `main()` method of the `Test` class, an instance of the `Outer.Inner` class is created using the syntax `outer.inner o = new outer.inner();`. Since `Inner` is a static nested class, it can be accessed directly using the enclosing interface name `Outer`. Then, the `show()` method of the `Inner` instance `o` is invoked, resulting in the message being printed to the console.

Program

```
Program for static class implements outside interface in java
// Interface declaring an abstract method
interface testing {
  void display();
}
// Interface containing a static nested class
interface outer {
  // Static nested class implementing the testing interface
  static class inner implements testing {
    // Method of the static nested class
    void show() {
      System.out.println("static class inside interface");
    }
    // Implementing the display() method from the testing interface
    public void display() {
      System.out.println("static   class   implements   outside   interface
         method");
    }
  }
}
// Test class with the main method
public class Test {
void main(String[] args) {
    // Creating an instance of the static nested class
    outer.inner o = new outer.inner();
```

```
    // Calling methods of the static nested class
    o.show();  // Prints: static class inside interface
    o.display(); // Prints: static class implements outside interface method
  }
}
```

Output:

```
static class inside interface
static class implements outside interface method
```

This Java program illustrates the usage of a static nested class implementing an interface inside another interface. There are two interfaces defined: `testing` and `outer`. The `testing` interface declares an abstract method `display()`. Within the `outer` interface, there's a static nested class `inner` that implements the `testing` interface. The `inner` class also defines its own method `show()`, which prints "static class inside interface" to the console, and implements the `display()` method from the `testing` interface, printing "static class implements outside interface method" when called. In the `main()` method of the `Test` class, an instance of the `outer.inner` class is created using the syntax `outer.inner o = new outer.inner();`. Then, both the `show()` and `display()` methods of the `inner` instance `o` are invoked.

8.6 OVERRIDING METHODS IN INTERFACE

Overriding methods in an interface in Java involves providing a new implementation of a method that is defined in a parent interface or class. This allows the implementing class to offer a specific behavior for the method. When a class implements an interface, it must override all the abstract methods of the interface. Default methods in interfaces can also be overridden if a specific implementation is needed. Overriding methods ensure that the class fulfills the contract defined by the interface while potentially adding or modifying functionality.

Program

```
Program on overriding main method by using interface and java class in java
// Interface containing a main method
interface test {
  // Method inside the interface
  static void main(String[] args) {
    System.out.println("main in interface");
  }
  // Abstract method to be implemented by classes
  void display();
}
// Class implementing the test interface
public class Main implements test {
  // Implementation of the display() method
  public void display() {
    System.out.println("display() of interface");
  }
  // Conventional main method
void main(String[] args) {
    System.out.println("main in class");
    // Creating an instance of Main
    Main obj = new Main();
    // Calling the display() method
    obj.display();
  }
```

```
}
```

Output:

```
main in interface
```

The code illustrates the syntax for defining an interface with a `main()` method and then implementing that interface in a class in Java. Firstly, the `test` interface is declared. This interface includes a `main()` method, which deviates from the typical usage of the `main()` method as the entry point of a Java program. Inside this `main()` method, a message is printed to the console. Next, a class named `Main` implements the `test` interface. Within this class, a `display()` method is defined to fulfill the contract specified by the `test` interface. Additionally, the conventional `main()` method is implemented in this class, serving as the entry point of the program. Inside the `main()` method, a message is printed to the console to indicate its execution. Furthermore, an instance of `Main` is created to invoke its `display()` method.

Program

```
Program for overriding default method of interface in class in java
interface definterface
{
  int i=10;
  public void display();
  public default int cube(int x)
  {
    return(x*x*x);
  }
}
class sample implements definterface
{
  public void display()
  {
  System.out.println(i);
  }
  public int cube(int x)
  {
  System.out.println("inside cube");
    return definterface.super.cube(x);
  }
}
class test
{
  void main(String a[])
  {
    definterface t=new sample();
    t.display();
    int n=t.cube(10);
    System.out.println(n);
  }
}
```

Output:

```
10
inside cube
1000
```

In this program, we have defined an interface named `definterface` that declares a constant `i` and includes two methods: an abstract method `display()` and a default method `cube(int x)` that returns the cube of a given integer. The default method provides a way to implement functionality directly within the interface, allowing implementing classes to either use the provided method or override it. The `sample` class implements `definterface` and provides its own implementation for the `display()` method, printing the value of `i`. It also overrides the `cube(int x)` method but still calls the interface's default implementation using `definterface.super.cube(x)` to maintain the original cube calculation. In the `test` class, we create an instance of `sample` using the `definterface` reference and call the `display()` and `cube()` methods.

8.7 MULTIPLE INHERITANCE

Multiple Inheritance is a feature in object-oriented programming where a class can inherit behaviors and properties from more than one parent class. While many languages, like C++, support multiple inheritance, Java does not due to its complexity and the potential for ambiguity, known as the "diamond problem."

8.7.1 Advantages

- Enhanced Functionality: Combines behaviors of multiple classes, providing richer functionality in derived classes.
- Code Reusability: Promotes the reuse of existing classes without rewriting code, reducing redundancy.
- Expressive Design: Allows for more natural modeling of certain problems where multiple inheritance better represents the domain.
- Reusability: Allows a class to use functionalities of multiple parent classes, promoting code reuse.
- Flexibility: Enables the creation of more complex class structures and relationships, allowing for more flexible and dynamic designs.
- Modularity: Helps in separating concerns and organizing code into smaller, manageable units.

8.7.2 Limitations

- Complexity: Increases the complexity of the class hierarchy, making it harder to understand and maintain.
- Ambiguity: Can lead to the diamond problem, where the same base class is inherited multiple times through different paths, causing ambiguity in method resolution.
- Conflict Resolution: Requires mechanisms to resolve conflicts when the same method is inherited from multiple parent classes, adding to the complexity.

In Java, multiple inheritance is achieved using interfaces, which allow a class to implement multiple interfaces and inherit their abstract methods, avoiding the pitfalls of traditional multiple inheritance.

Program

```
Program for Multiple inheritance through interfaces
// Interface with a constant and an abstract method
interface myinterface {
  int i = 10;
  void display();
}
// Interface with a different constant and abstract method
```

```
interface myinterface1 {
  int j = 50;
  void put();
}
// Interface extending the previous interfaces and adding more functionality
interface myinterface2 extends myinterface, myinterface1 {
  int k = 50;
  void printing();
}
// Class implementing the myinterface2 interface
class sample implements myinterface2 {
  // Implementing the display() method
  public void display() {
    System.out.println(i);
  }
  // Implementing the put() method
  public void put() {
    System.out.println(j);
  }
  // Implementing the printing() method
  public void printing() {
    System.out.println(k);
  }
}
// Test class with the main method
public class test {
void main(String[] args) {
    // Creating an instance of sample
    sample obj = new sample();
    // Calling the implemented methods
    obj.display();  // Prints: 10
    obj.put();    // Prints: 50
    obj.printing();  // Prints: 50
  }
}
```

Output:

```
10
50
50
```

In this Java program there are three interfaces: `myinterface`, `myinterface1`, and `myinterface2`. The `myinterface` interface declares a constant `i` and an abstract method `display()`, while `myinterface1` declares a constant `j` and an abstract method `put()`. The `myinterface2` interface extends both `myinterface` and `myinterface1`, and introduces a constant `k` and an abstract method `printing()`. The `sample` class implements the `myinterface2` interface, providing implementations for the `display()`, `put()`, and `printing()` methods inherited from the interfaces it implements. In the `main()` method of the `test` class, an instance of the `sample` class is created, and its `display()`, `put()`, and `printing()` methods are invoked.

Program

```
Program for multiple inheritance by using implements interface
// Interface with a constant and an abstract method
interface myinterface {
```

```
  int i = 10;
  void display();
}
// Interface with a different constant and abstract method
interface myinterface1 {
  int j = 50;
  void put();
}
// Class implementing both interfaces
class sample implements myinterface, myinterface1 {
  // Implementing the display() method from myinterface
  public void display() {
    System.out.println("i=" + i);
  }
  // Implementing the put() method from myinterface1
  public void put() {
    System.out.println("j=" + j);
  }
}
// Test class with the main method
public class test {
void main(String[] args) {
    // Creating an instance of sample
    sample obj = new sample();
    // Calling the implemented methods
    obj.display();  // Prints: i=10
    obj.put();     // Prints: j=50
  }
}
```

Output:

```
i=10
j=50
```

In this Java program we defined two interfaces: `myinterface` and `myinterface1`. The `myinterface` interface declares a constant `i` and an abstract method `display()`, while `myinterface1` declares a constant `j` and an abstract method `put()`. The `sample` class implements both `myinterface` and `myinterface1`, providing concrete implementations for the `display()` and `put()` methods. In the `display()` method, it prints the value of the constant `i`, and in the `put()` method, it prints the value of the constant `j`. In the `main()` method of the `test` class, an instance of the `sample` class is created, and its `display()` and `put()` methods are invoked.

8.8 HYBRID INHERITANCE

Hybrid Inheritance is a combination of two or more types of inheritance (such as single, multiple, hierarchical, and multilevel inheritance) in a single program. This allows a class to inherit properties and behaviors from multiple sources, creating a more complex and flexible inheritance structure.

8.8.1 Advantages

- Rich Class Hierarchies: Enables the creation of intricate class structures that can encapsulate a wide range of functionalities.
- Code Reuse: Facilitates the reuse of existing code by allowing classes to inherit features from multiple parent classes.

- Modularity: Supports the development of modular code, where different parts of the system can be developed and maintained independently.
- Complex Modeling: Allows for the representation of more complex real-world scenarios where an entity might need to inherit features from multiple sources.
- Enhanced Flexibility: Provides the ability to create highly flexible and dynamic class hierarchies that can adapt to changing requirements.

8.8.2 Limitations

- Increased Complexity: Leads to more complex class hierarchies, which can be difficult to understand, debug, and maintain.
- Potential for Ambiguity: In languages that support multiple inheritance, hybrid inheritance can introduce ambiguity, especially regarding method resolution and inheritance conflicts.
- Maintenance Challenges: Requires careful design to avoid issues like the diamond problem and to ensure that changes in parent classes do not inadvertently affect derived classes.

In Java, hybrid inheritance is typically achieved through a combination of classes and interfaces. Java does not support multiple inheritance of classes directly but allows a class to implement multiple interfaces, which can be used to simulate hybrid inheritance while avoiding many of its pitfalls.

Program

```
// Base class
class Base {
  void displayBase() {
    System.out.println("This is the Base class.");
  }
}
// First intermediate class
class Child1 extends Base {
  void displayChild1() {
    System.out.println("This is Child1 class, inheriting from Base.");
  }
}
// Second intermediate class
class Child2 extends Base {
  void displayChild2() {
    System.out.println("This is Child2 class, inheriting from Base.");
  }
}
// Interface for running capability
interface Runnable {
  void run();
}
// First sub class inheriting from Child1
class SubChild1 extends Child1 {
  void displaySubChild1() {
    System.out.println("This is SubChild1 class, inheriting from Child1.");
  }
}
// Second sub class inheriting from Child2 and implementing Runnable
class SubChild2 extends Child2 implements Runnable {
```

```
  void displaySubChild2() {
    System.out.println("This is SubChild2 class, inheriting from Child2.");
  }
  @Override
  public void run() {
    System.out.println("SubChild2 can run.");
  }
}
// Main class to test the functionality
public class HybridInheritanceExample {
void main(String[] args) {
    SubChild1 subChild1 = new SubChild1();
    subChild1.displayBase();  // From Base class
    subChild1.displayChild1();  // From Child1 class
    subChild1.displaySubChild1();  // From SubChild1 class
    SubChild2 subChild2 = new SubChild2();
    subChild2.displayBase();  // From Base class
    subChild2.displayChild2();  // From Child2 class
    subChild2.displaySubChild2();  // From SubChild2 class
    subChild2.run();  // From Runnable interface
  }
}
```

Output:

```
This is the Base class.
This is Child1 class, inheriting from Base.
This is SubChild1 class, inheriting from Child1.
This is the Base class.
This is Child2 class, inheriting from Base.
This is SubChild2 class, inheriting from Child2.
SubChild2 can run.
```

In the above Java program the `Base` class defines a basic method. Two intermediate classes, `Child1` and `Child2`, inherit from `Base` and add their own methods. The `Runnable` interface declares a `run` method. `SubChild1` extends `Child1`, and `SubChild2` extends `Child2` and implements `Runnable`. In the `main` method, objects of `SubChild1` and `SubChild2` are created.

8.9 NESTED INTERFACE

A nested interface is an interface defined within another class or interface. This means that the interface is encapsulated within the scope of its containing class or interface, and it can be accessed using the containing class or interface's name.

8.9.1 Need for Nested Interfaces

- Logical Grouping: Nested interfaces are used to group related interfaces or classes, providing better organization and modularity in large programs.
- Encapsulation: They encapsulate the interface within the outer class, providing a clear relationship and restricting access, which enhances encapsulation.
- Namespace Management: Helps in avoiding namespace pollution by keeping the nested interface within the scope of the containing class or interface, making the codebase cleaner.
- Better Abstraction: When an interface is closely related to its containing class, it makes sense to nest it to reflect this relationship, enhancing readability and abstraction.

- Implementation Specifics: If an interface is meant to be implemented by the enclosing class or is very specific to the enclosing class, it can be nested to indicate this relationship.

8.9.2 Limitations of Nested Interfaces

- Accessibility: A nested interface is less accessible from outside the containing class or interface. This restriction can sometimes make it harder to use, especially if broader access is later required.
- Complexity: Nesting interfaces can add complexity to the code, making it harder to understand, especially for developers who are new to the codebase.
- Maintenance: As the number of nested interfaces grows, maintaining the code can become challenging due to increased depth and hierarchy.
- Confusion with Nested Classes: Developers might confuse nested interfaces with nested classes, leading to misunderstandings and incorrect implementations.
- Limited Scope: The nested interface is tightly coupled with its enclosing class, which might limit its reusability outside the specific context it was created for.

Program

```
Program for default method in nested interface in java
// Outer interface containing an inner interface
interface outer {
  // Inner interface with default and abstract methods
  interface inner {
    // Default method with implementation
    default void display() {
      System.out.println("inner interface method");
    }
    // Abstract method that must be implemented
    void show();
  }
}
// Class implementing the inner interface
class sample implements outer.inner {
  // Providing implementation for the abstract method
  public void show() {
    System.out.println("implemented inner interface method");
  }
}
// Test class with the main method
public class Test {
void main(String[] args) {
    // Creating an instance of the sample class
    outer.inner obj = new sample();
    // Calling the implemented methods
    obj.show();  // Prints: implemented inner interface method
    obj.display(); // Prints: inner interface method
  }
}
```

Output:

```
implemented inner interface method
inner interface method
```

In the above code, Firstly, an interface named `outer` is declared, containing an inner interface named `inner`. The `inner` interface includes a default method `display()` and an abstract method `show()`. The `display()` method has a default implementation provided within the interface, while the `show()` method is left abstract, requiring concrete implementations in classes that implement the `inner` interface. Next, a class named `sample` implements the `outer.inner` interface, providing a concrete implementation for the `show()` method. The implementation simply prints a message indicating that it has implemented the inner interface method. In the `Test` class, an instance of `sample` is created and assigned to a variable of type `outer.inner`. The `show()` method of the `sample` object is then invoked. Additionally, the `display()` method, which is a default method from the inner interface, is also invoked. Since it has a default implementation provided within the interface, it prints a message indicating it is from the inner interface.

Program

```
Program for default and static methods in nested interface in java
interface outer {
  interface inner {
    // Default method with implementation
    default void display() {
      System.out.println("inner interface default method");
    }
    // Static method with implementation
    static void show() {
      System.out.println("inner interface static method");
    }
  }
}
// Class implementing the inner interface
class sample implements outer.inner {
  // Overriding the default method
  @Override
  public void display() {
    // Calling the static method from the inner interface
    outer.inner.show();
    // Calling the default method from the inner interface using outer.
    inner.super
    outer.inner.super.display(); // This calls the default method of the
    inner interface
    System.out.println("implemented default inner interface method in
    class");
  }
}
// Test class with the main method
public class Main {
void main(String[] args) {
    // Creating an instance of the sample class
    outer.inner obj = new sample();
    // Calling the display method of the sample class
    obj.display();
  }
}
```

Output:

```
inner interface static method
```

```
inner interface default method
implemented default inner interface method in class
```

In the above Java program, the `outer` interface declares an inner interface `inner`, which contains a default method `display()` and a static method `show()`. The `sample` class implements the `inner` interface. First the static method `show()` of the `inner` interface was called using the syntax `outer.inner.show()`, demonstrating how to access a static method of the inner interface. Then, the default `display()` method of the `inner` interface was called using the `super` keyword. In the `Test` class, an instance of the `sample` class is created and assigned to a reference of type `outer.inner`. The `display()` method is then invoked on this instance, which triggers the overridden `display()` method in the `sample` class. The output of the program will display the messages printed by both the `display()` method in the `sample` class and the default `display()` method in the `inner` interface. Additionally, the static method `show()` is invoked, which will print the corresponding message from the `inner` interface.

Program

```
Program for static methods in inner interfaces in java
// Outer interface with nested interfaces
interface Outer {
  interface Inner {
    interface Sub {
      // Static method in Sub interface
      static void show() {
        System.out.println("inner sub interface static method");
      }
    }
    // Static method in Inner interface
    static void show() {
      System.out.println("inner interface static method");
    }
  }
  // Static method in Outer interface
  static void show() {
    System.out.println("outer interface static method");
  }
}
// Sample class implementing all interfaces
class Sample implements Outer, Outer.Inner, Outer.Inner.Sub {
  // Static method in Sample class
  public static void show() {
    // Print message from Sample class
    System.out.println("same static interface method in class");
    // Call static methods from the interfaces
    Outer.show();
    Outer.Inner.show();
    Outer.Inner.Sub.show();
  }
}
// Test class with main method
public class Test {
void main(String[] args) {
    // Call the static show method of Sample class
    Sample.show();
```

```
  }
}
```

Output:

```
same static interface method in class
outer interface static method
inner interface static method
inner sub interface static method
```

In the Java program an `Outer` interface contains a nested interface called `Inner`, which, in turn, contains another nested interface called `Sub`. Each interface defines its own static `show()` method, displaying a specific message when invoked. The `Sample` class implements all three interfaces: `Outer`, `Outer.Inner`, and `Outer.Inner.Sub`. Within the `Sample` class, a static `show()` method is defined, which first prints a message specific to the class itself. Then, invoke the static `show()` methods of each interface using the interface names as qualifiers, resulting in the display of messages defined in the respective interfaces. In the `main()` method of the `Test` class, the `show()` method of the `Sample` class is called, initiating the chain of method invocations and printing the messages defined in the interfaces and the `Sample` class.

Program

```
Program for default and static methods in outer and inner interface in java
// Outer interface with default and static methods
interface outer {
  // Default method in outer interface
  default void display() {
    System.out.println("outer interface default method");
  }
  // Static method in outer interface
  static void show() {
    System.out.println("outer interface static method");
  }
  // Inner interface
  interface inner {
    // Default method in inner interface
    default void display() {
      System.out.println("inner interface default method");
    }
    // Static method in inner interface
    static void show() {
      System.out.println("inner interface static method");
    }
  }
}
// Sample class implementing both outer and outer.inner interfaces
class sample implements outer, outer.inner {
  // Override default method from outer and inner interfaces
  @Override
  public void display() {
    System.out.println("implemented default inner interface method in
       class");
    // Invoke default methods from both interfaces
    outer.super.display();
    outer.inner.super.display();
    // Invoke static methods from both interfaces
```

```
    outer.show();
    outer.inner.show();
  }
}
// Test class with main method
public class Test {
void main(String[] args) {
    // Create instance of sample class
    outer.inner obj = new sample();
    // Invoke the display method
    obj.display();
  }
}
```

Output:

```
implemented default inner interface method in class
outer interface default method
inner interface default method
outer interface static method
inner interface static method
```

In the above Java program the `outer` interface contains another interface `inner`, which itself contains a default method `display()` and a static method `show()`. Additionally, the `outer` interface declares its own default method `display()` and a static method `show()`. The `sample` class implements both the `outer` interface and the `outer.inner` interface. It provides an implementation for the `display()` method, where it first prints a custom message. Then, it invokes the default `display()` method of the `outer` interface using `outer.super.display()`, the default `display()` method of the `outer.inner` interface using `outer.inner.super.display()`, and the static `show()` methods of both interfaces using `outer.inner. show()` and `outer.show()`.In the `Test` class, an instance of the `sample` class is created and assigned to a reference of type `outer.inner`. The `display()` method is then invoked on this instance, which triggers the overridden `display()` method in the `sample` class. As a result, the custom message is printed along with the default method implementations of both the `outer` and `outer.inner` interfaces. Additionally, the static methods `show()` of both interfaces are invoked, printing the corresponding messages.

Program

Program for interface inside class in java

```
// Outer class containing the inner interface
class Outer {
  // Inner interface
  interface Inner {
    // Static method in inner interface
    static void show() {
      System.out.println("inner interface static method");
    }
    // Abstract method in inner interface
    void display();
  }
}
// Sample class implementing the Inner interface
class Sample implements Outer.Inner {
```

```
  // Implementing the abstract method from Inner interface
  @Override
  public void display() {
    System.out.println("interface implemented method");
    // Calling the static method of the Inner interface
    Outer.Inner.show();
  }
}
// Test class with the main method
public class Test {
void main(String[] args) {
    // Create an instance of Sample
    Outer.Inner obj = new Sample();
    // Call the display method
    obj.display();
  }
}
```

Output:

```
interface implemented method
inner interface  static method
```

In the above Java program the `Outer` class contains an interface named `Inner`, which declares both a static method `show()` and an abstract method `display()`. The `show()` method simply prints a message indicating it's a static method of the interface, while `display()` is an abstract method that does not provide an implementation within the interface. The `Sample` class implements the `outer.inner` interface. It provides an implementation for the `display()` method, which prints a message indicating it's the method implemented by the interface. Additionally, within the `display()` method, it invokes the static `show()` method of the `outer. inner` interface. In the `main()` method of the `Test` class, an instance of `Sample` is created, and its `display()` method is called. This triggers the execution of the implemented `display()` method in the `Sample` class, which in turn invokes the static `show()` method of the `outer. inner` interface, resulting in the display of both messages.

Program

```
Program for class inside interface in java
// Outer interface containing an inner class
interface Outer {
  // Inner class
  class Inner {
    // Method of the inner class
    void show() {
      System.out.println("class inside interface");
    }
  }
}
// Sample class extending the inner class of Outer interface
class Sample extends Outer.Inner {
  // Constructor to create an instance of Sample
  Sample() {
    super(); // Call the constructor of Outer.Inner
  }
  // Method to demonstrate functionality
```

```
  void display() {
    System.out.println("class extending class inside interface");
  }
}
// Test class with the main method
public class Test {
void main(String[] args) {
    // Create an instance of Sample
    Sample sample = new Sample();
    // Call the display method of Sample
    sample.display();
    // Call the show method inherited from Outer.Inner
    sample.show();
  }
}
```

Output:

```
class extending class inside interface
class inside interface
```

The Java program demonstrates a unique scenario where an interface `Outer` contains an inner class `Inner`. This inner class `Inner` has a non-static method `show()` that simply prints a message indicating it's a method of a class inside an interface. The `Sample` class extends the inner class `Outer.inner`. However, `Sample` does not implement any interfaces but inherits from the inner class of the `Outer` interface. In the `main()` method of the `Test` class, an instance of `Sample` is created. When the `display()` method of `Sample` is invoked, it prints a message indicating that it's from a class extending another class inside an interface. Additionally, the `show()` method inherited from `Outer.inner` is invoked, printing a message indicating it's from the inner class of the interface.

Program

```
Program for protected inner interface in java
// Outer class containing an inner interface
class Outer {
  // Protected inner interface
  protected interface Inner {
    // Static method in the inner interface
    static void show() {
      System.out.println("inner interface static method");
    }
    // Abstract method in the inner interface
    void display();
  }
}
// Sample class implementing the Outer.Inner interface
class Sample implements Outer.Inner {
  @Override
  public void display() {
    System.out.println("interface implemented method");
    // Call the static method of the Outer.Inner interface
    Outer.Inner.show();
  }
}
```

```
// Test class with the main method
public class Test {
void main(String[] args) {
    // Create an instance of Sample
    Sample sample = new Sample();
    // Call the display method of Sample
    sample.display();
  }
}
```

Output:

```
interface implemented method
inner interface  static method
```

The Java program demonstrates the use of a protected interface `Inner` within the `Outer` class. This interface `Inner` contains a static method `show()` and an abstract method `display()`. The `show()` method prints a message indicating it's a static method of the inner interface. The `Sample` class implements the `Outer.inner` interface. It overrides the `display()` method, which prints a message indicating it's the method implemented by the interface. Additionally, it invokes the `show()` method of the `Outer.inner` interface within its `display()` method. In the `main()` method of the `Test` class, an instance of `Sample` is created and its `display()` method is invoked. This triggers the execution of the overridden `display()` method in `Sample`, which in turn calls the static `show()` method of the `Outer.inner` interface. Consequently, both messages are printed to the console.

Program

```
Program for default method in interface with inner class in interface
in java
// Outer interface containing a nested class and a default method
interface Outer {
  // Nested class inside the Outer interface
  class Inner {
    void show() {
      System.out.println("class inside interface");
    }
  }
  // Default method in the Outer interface
  default void put() {
    System.out.println("default method of interface");
  }
}
// Sample class extending the Outer.Inner class and implementing the Outer
interface
class Sample extends Outer.Inner implements Outer {
  // Constructor for Sample
  Sample() {
    super();
  }
  // Overriding the put() method from the Outer interface
  @Override
  public void put() {
    // Call the default put() method from the Outer interface using Outer.
super
    Outer.super.put();  // This calls the default method of the interface
```

```
    System.out.println("class extending class inside interface");
  }
  // Adding a display() method for demonstration
  public void display() {
    // Calling the show() method inherited from Outer.Inner
    show();
    // Calling the put() method from the Outer interface
    put();
  }
}
// Test class with the main method
public class Main {
void main(String[] args) {
    // Create an instance of Sample
    Sample sample = new Sample();
    // Call the display method of Sample
    sample.display();
  }
}
```

Output:

```
class inside interface
default method of interface
class extending class inside interface
```

In the above Java program an `Outer` interface contains a nested class `Inner`, which has a method `show()` that prints a message indicating it's a class inside the interface. Additionally, the interface `Outer` includes a default method `put()`, which prints a message indicating it's a default method of the interface. The `Sample` class extends the `Outer.Inner` class and implements the `Outer` interface. Additionally, the `Sample` class extends `Outer.Inner`, it inherits the `show()` method from the nested class `Inner`. In the `main()` method of the `Test` class, an instance of `Sample` is created, and its `display()` method is invoked. Additionally, the `show()` method of the `Sample` class is invoked, which calls the `show()` method of the `Outer.Inner` class, printing the message indicating it's a class inside the interface. Finally, the `put()` method of the `Outer` interface is invoked, printing the message indicating it's a default method of the interface.

8.10 FUNCTIONAL INTERFACE

In Java, a functional interface is an interface that contains exactly one abstract method. A functional interface can have multiple default or static methods but only one abstract method.

8.10.1 Key Characteristics of a Functional Interface

- Single Abstract Method: It must have exactly one abstract method.
- Annotations: The `@FunctionalInterface` annotation can be used to explicitly declare that the interface is intended to be a functional interface. This annotation is not mandatory but provides a compile-time check.
- Lambda Expressions: Functional interfaces are the target types for lambda expressions and method references.

8.10.2 Common Functional Interfaces in Java

Java provides several built-in functional interfaces in the `java.util.function` package, which are widely used in the standard library and Java Streams API. Some common examples include:

- `Predicate<T>`: Represents a boolean-valued function of one argument.
- `Function<T, R>`: Represents a function that takes one argument and produces a result.
- `Supplier<T>`: Represents a supplier of results.
- `Consumer<T>`: Represents an operation that takes a single input argument and returns no result.
- `BiFunction<T, U, R>`: Represents a function that takes two arguments and produces a result.

8.10.3 Benefits of Functional Interfaces

- Concise Code: Lambda expressions and method references allow for more concise and readable code.
- Parallelism: Simplifies parallel processing by using streams and functional operations.
- Higher-Order Functions: Enables passing behavior as parameters, returning functions from methods, and composing functions.

8.10.4 Limitations of Functional Interfaces

- Single Abstract Method: Only one abstract method is allowed, limiting the interface's complexity.
- Readability: Overuse of lambda expressions can make code harder to read and understand.
- Debugging: Debugging lambda expressions can be more challenging compared to traditional anonymous inner classes.

Program

```
Program for functional interface in java
// Define a functional interface
@FunctionalInterface
interface Sample {
  // Abstract method
  void display();
}
// Implementing the functional interface
class Test implements Sample {
  // Providing implementation for the abstract method
  @Override
  public void display() {
    System.out.println("functional interface method”);
  }
}
// Main class to test the implementation
public class Main {
void main(String[] args) {
    // Creating an instance of Test
    Test test = new Test();
    // Invoking the display() method
    test.display();
  }
}
```

```
Output:
functional interface method
```

In the above Java program the `sample` interface is annotated with `@FunctionalInterface`, indicating that it is intended to be used as a functional interface. It declares a single abstract method `display()`. The `test` class implements the `sample` interface and provides the implementation for the `display()` method. In the `main()` method, an instance of the `test` class is created, and its `display()` method is invoked. When executed, the program will print "functional interface method" to the console, indicating that the implementation of the `display()` method defined in the `test` class is executed successfully.

Program

```
// Define a functional interface with default and static methods
@FunctionalInterface
interface Sample {
  // Abstract method
  void display();
  // Default method
  default void put() {
    System.out.println("default method in interface");
  }
  // Static method
  static void func() {
    System.out.println("static method in interface");
  }
}
// Implementing the functional interface
class Test implements Sample {
  // Providing implementation for the abstract method
  @Override
  public void display() {
    System.out.println("functional interface method");
    // Call default method of the interface
    this.put();
    // Call static method of the interface
    Sample.func();
  }
}
// Main class to test the implementation
public class Main {
void main(String[] args) {
    // Creating an instance of Test
    Test test = new Test();
    // Invoking the display() method
    test.display();
  }
}
Output:
functional interface method
default method in interface
static method in interface
```

This Java program illustrates the usage of a functional interface along with default and static methods. The `sample` interface is annotated with `@FunctionalInterface`, indicating that it's intended to be used as a functional interface. It declares a single abstract method `display()` along with a default method `put()` and a static method `func()`. The `test` class implements the `sample` interface and provides an implementation for the `display()` method. In the `main()` method, an instance of the `test` class is created, and its `display()` method is invoked. Within the `display()` method implementation of the `test` class, the `put()` method (a default method of the `sample` interface) is called using the `this` reference, and the `func()` method (a static method of the `sample` interface) is called directly.

Program

```
Program for two abstract methods in functional interface reports error
@FunctionalInterface
interface sample
  {
    public abstract void display();
    public abstract void put();
  }
public class test implements sample
{
void main(String a[])
  {
    test t=new test();
t.display();
  }
  public void display()
  {
System.out.println("functional interface method2");
  }
    public void put()
  {
System.out.println("functional interface method2");
  }
}
Output:
test.java:1: error: Unexpected @FunctionalInterface annotation
@FunctionalInterface
^
  sample is not a functional interface
  multiple non-overriding abstract methods found in interface sample
1 error
```

Program

```
Program for writing any number of default and static methods in functional
interface in java
// Define a functional interface with default and static methods
@FunctionalInterface
interface Sample {
  // Abstract method
  void display();
  // Default method
  default void put() {
    System.out.println("default method in interface");
  }
  // Static method
```

```
  static void func() {
    System.out.println("static method in interface");
  }
  // Default method with a parameter
  default void square(int x) {
    System.out.println("default method,square of " + x + " is " + (x * x));
  }
  // Static method with a parameter
  static void cube(int x) {
    System.out.println("static method,cube of " + x + " is " + (x * x * x));
  }
}
// Implementing the functional interface
class Test implements Sample {
  // Providing implementation for the abstract method
  @Override
  public void display() {
    System.out.println("functional interface method");
    // Call default method of the interface
    this.put();
    // Call static method of the interface
    Sample.func();
    // Call default method with parameter
    this.square(5);
    // Call static method with parameter
    Sample.cube(5);
  }
}
// Main class to test the implementation
public class Main {
void main(String[] args) {
    // Creating an instance of Test
    Test test = new Test();
    // Invoking the display() method
    test.display();
  }
}
```

Output:

```
functional interface method
default method in interface
static method in interface
default method,square of 5 is 25
static method,cube of 5 is 125
```

In the above Java program the `sample` interface is annotated with `@FunctionalInterface` and declares an abstract method `display()`, along with default methods `put()` and `square(int x)`, and a static method `func()`. Additionally, it defines a static method `cube(int x)` to calculate the cube of a given number. The `test` class implements the `sample` interface and provides an implementation for the `display()` method. Within the `display()` method implementation, it invokes the `put()` method (a default method of the interface), calls the `func()` method (a static method of the interface), and utilizes both the `square(int x)` and `cube(int x)` methods.

8.10.5 Functional Interface and Inheritance

Inheritance in functional interfaces allows a functional interface to extend another interface, including another functional interface. When a functional interface inherits from another interface, it must ensure that it still only has a single abstract method, either by not declaring any new abstract methods or by inheriting an abstract method from the parent interface. This inherited method becomes the functional method for the derived interface. This mechanism allows for the extension and reuse of functionality while maintaining the functional interface's requirement of having exactly one abstract method, enabling the use of lambda expressions and method references with the derived interface.

Program

```
Program for non functional interface extends functional interface in java
// Define the functional interface
@FunctionalInterface
interface Sample {
  // Abstract method
  void display();
}
// Define another interface that extends the functional interface
interface Change extends Sample {
  // Another abstract method
  void put();
}
// Implementing the Change interface
class Test implements Change {
  // Providing implementation for the display() method from Sample interface
  @Override
  public void display() {
    System.out.println("functional interface method of sample interface");
  }
  // Providing implementation for the put() method from Change interface
  @Override
  public void put() {
    System.out.println("functional interface method of change interface");
  }
}
// Main class to test the implementation
public class Main {
void main(String[] args) {
    // Creating an instance of Test
    Test test = new Test();
    // Invoking the display() method
    test.display();
    // Invoking the put() method
    test.put();
  }
}
```

Output:

```
functional interface method of sample interface
functional interface method of change interface
```

In the above Java program the `sample` interface is annotated with `@FunctionalInterface` and declares a single abstract method `display()`. The `change` interface extends the `sample` interface and adds another abstract method `put()`. The `test` class implements the `change` interface, which indirectly implements the `sample` interface due to inheritance. In the `test` class, the `main()` method creates an instance of the `test` class and calls both the `display()` and `put()` methods.

Program

Program on a functional interface extends non-functional interface (contains abstract method) reports error in java.

```
interface sample
  {
    public abstract void display();
  }
@FunctionalInterface
interface change extends sample
{
    public abstract void put();
}
public class test implements change
{
void main(String a[])
  {
    test t=new test();
t.display();
t.put();
  }
  public void display()
  {
System.out.println("functional interface method of sample interface");
  }
  public void put()
  {
System.out.println("functional interface method of change interface");
  }
}
Output:
test.java:5: error: Unexpected @FunctionalInterface annotation
@FunctionalInterface
^
  change is not a functional interface
  multiple non-overriding abstract methods found in interface change
1 error
```

Program

```
Program for functional interface extends non-functional interface(does not
consists of abstract method)
// Define the interface with a default method and a static method
interface Sample {
  // Default method
  default void func() {
```

```
    System.out.println("default method in interface");
  }
  // Static method
  static void display() {
    System.out.println("static method in interface");
  }
}
// Define a functional interface that extends the Sample interface
@FunctionalInterface
interface Change extends Sample {
  // Abstract method
  void put();
}
// Implementing the Change interface
class Test implements Change {
  // Providing implementation for the put() method
  @Override
  public void put() {
    System.out.println("functional interface method of change interface");
  }
  // Main method to test the implementation
void main(String[] args) {
    // Creating an instance of Test
    Test test = new Test();
    // Invoking the put() method
    test.put();
    // Invoking the default method func() from the Sample interface
    test.func();
    // Invoking the static method display() from the Sample interface
    Sample.display();
  }
}
```

Output:

```
functional interface method of change interface
default method in interfaace
static method in interface
```

In the above Java program the `sample` interface defines a default method `func()` and a static method `display()`. The `change` interface, annotated with `@FunctionalInterface`, extends the `sample` interface and declares an abstract method `put()`.The `test` class implements the `change` interface, providing an implementation for the `put()` method. In the `main()` method of the `test` class, an instance of `test` is created, and its `put()` method is called to demonstrate the implementation of the `change` interface method. Additionally, the `func()` method inherited from the `sample` interface is invoked to illustrate the usage of default methods. Finally, the static method `display()` from the `sample` interface is called directly using the interface name to demonstrate static method access in interfaces.

8.11 METHOD REFERENCE

Method reference is a technique in Java that provides a shorthand syntax for defining a lambda expression that only calls an existing method. Method references come in four main types:

- Reference to a static method: `ClassName::staticMethodName`
- Reference to an instance method of a particular object: `instance::instanceMethodName`

- Reference to an instance method of an arbitrary object of a particular type: `ClassName::instanceMethodName`
- Reference to a constructor: `ClassName::new`

Using method references makes the code cleaner and often more readable compared to equivalent lambda expressions. They are particularly useful when the lambda expression simply calls a method and does not perform any additional processing. This technique leverages existing methods and constructors to be used as functional interfaces, thus promoting code reusability and simplification.

Program

```
Program for method reference to a static method in java
// Define an interface with a single abstract method
interface Test {
  void display();
}
// Define a class with a static method
class Main {
  // Static method to be referenced
  public static void show() {
    System.out.println("testing method references");
  }
  // Main method to execute the program
void main(String[] args) {
    // Create an instance of the Test interface, initialized with a method
    reference
    Test t = Main::show;
    // Invoke the display() method using the interface instance
    t.display();
  }
}
Output:
testing method references
```

The above Java program defines an interface named `test` with a single method `display()`, which does not take any arguments and does not return any value. Following this, a class named `Main` is declared. Within this class, there is a static method named `show()` that prints the message "testing method references" to the console. In the `main()` method of the `Main` class, an instance of the `test` interface named `t` is created, initialized with a reference to the `show()` method of the `Main` class using method references. Finally, the `display()` method of the `test` interface is invoked using the `t` reference, resulting in the message "testing method references" being printed to the console.

Program

```
Program for invoking instance method by using method reference technique
// Define a functional interface with a single abstract method
interface Test {
  void display();
}
// Define a class with a method to be referenced
```

```
class Main {
  // Method to be referenced
  public void show() {
    System.out.println("testing method reference");
  }
  // Main method to execute the program
void main(String[] args) {
    // Create an instance of Main
    Main j = new Main();
    / Create an instance of Test using method reference to show() of
    instance j
    Test t = j::show;
    // Create another instance of Test using method reference to show() of
    a new Main instance
    Test t1 = new Main()::show;
    // Invoke the display() method using both instances
    t.display(); // Prints: testing method reference
    t1.display(); // Prints: testing method reference
  }
};
```

Output

```
testing method reference
testing method reference
```

The Java program defines an interface named `test` with a single abstract method `display()`, representing a functional interface. Within the `Main` class, there's a method `show()` responsible for printing "testing method reference" when invoked. In the `main` method, two instances of the `test` interface are created using method references. The first instance, `t`, is instantiated by referencing the `show()` method of the current `Main` instance (`j::show`). The second instance, `t1`, is created by referencing the `show()` method of a new `Main` instance (`new Main()::show`). Both instances of `test` interface are then invoked using the `display()` method. This method call internally executes the `show()` method, resulting in "testing method reference" being printed twice.

Program

Program for invoking the constructor using method reference technique

```
// Define a functional interface with a single abstract method that takes
a string parameter
interface Test {
  void display(String m);
}
// Define a class with a constructor that takes a string parameter
class Sample {
  // Constructor method that prints the string passed to it
  public Sample(String m) {
    System.out.println(m);
  }
}
// Main class to run the program
public class Main {
void main(String[] args) {
    // Create a method reference to the constructor of the Sample class
    Test t = Sample::new;
```

```
    // Invoke the display() method using the method reference
    t.display("testing method reference constructor");
  }
}
```

Output:

```
testing method reference constructor
```

The above Java program defines an interface named `test` with a single method `display(String m)`, which takes a string parameter `m` but does not return any value. Additionally, there is a class named `sample` that includes a constructor method, which prints the string passed to it as an argument. Within the `main()` method of the `Main` class, an instance of the `test` interface named `t` is created, initialized with a reference to the constructor of the `sample` class using method references. This allows the `display()` method of the `test` interface to create a new instance of the `sample` class and pass the string "testing method reference constructor" to its constructor. Consequently, this message is printed to the console when the `display()` method is invoked.

8.12 STRICTF KEYWORD

The `strictfp` keyword in Java is used to restrict floating-point calculations to ensure portability and predictability across different platforms. When a class, method, or interface is declared with `strictfp`, it enforces strict IEEE 754 compliance on all floating-point operations, ensuring that the results are consistent and predictable regardless of the underlying hardware or JVM implementation.

8.12.1 Need for `strictfp`

In Java, floating-point arithmetic can sometimes yield different results on different platforms due to variations in hardware architectures and optimizations. The `strictfp` keyword ensures that floating-point calculations produce the same results on all platforms by adhering strictly to the IEEE 754 standard. This is particularly important for scientific and financial applications where consistent numerical results are crucial.

8.12.2 Advantages of `strictfp`

- Portability: Ensures consistent floating-point behavior across different platforms.
- Predictability: Provides predictable results in floating-point operations, aiding in debugging and testing.
- Standards Compliance: Enforces adherence to the IEEE 754 floating-point standard, which is a widely recognized standard for floating-point computation.

8.12.3 Limitations of `strictfp`

- Performance: Enforcing strict IEEE 754 compliance can lead to performance overheads because certain hardware-specific optimizations may be disabled.
- Limited Scope: Only affects floating-point arithmetic and does not extend to other numerical operations or types.
- Less Flexibility: Restricts the use of some hardware-specific enhancements and optimizations that could potentially provide faster calculations.

8.12.4 STRICTFP CLASS

A `strictfp` class in Java is one in which all floating-point operations are performed strictly according to the IEEE 754 standard. This ensures that floating-point calculations yield consistent results across different platforms and JVM implementations. The `strictfp` keyword can be applied to classes, interfaces, and methods.

Program

```
Program for strictfp class
// Define a class with the strictfp keyword to enforce IEEE 754 floating-
point operations
strictfp class Test {
  // Method to perform floating-point operations
  void display() {
    // Define float variables
    float f = Float.MIN_VALUE; // Minimum positive value for float
    float g = Float.MAX_VALUE; // Maximum positive value for float
    // Calculate the product of the minimum and maximum values of float, and
    assign to a double variable
    double d = f * g;
    // Print the result
    System.out.println("Value of d: " + d); // Output the value of d
    System.out.println("Result of f * g: " + (f * g));
    // Output the result of the multiplication
  }
}
// Main class to run the program
public class Main {
void main(String[] args) {
    // Create an instance of the Test class
    Test t = new Test();
    // Call the display() method
    t.display();
  }
}
Output:
Value of d: 4.7683712978141557E-7
Result of f * g: 4.7683713E-7
```

The above Java program begins by defining a class named `test`, which is declared with the `strictfp` keyword. This keyword ensures that all floating-point operations within the class adhere to the IEEE 754 standard, thereby guaranteeing consistent results across different platforms. Inside the `test` class, there is a method named `display()`, which calculates the product of the minimum and maximum values of the `float` data type and assigns the result to a `double` variable `d`. This calculation is performed using floating-point multiplication. Subsequently, the program prints the value of `d` followed by the result of the floating-point multiplication operation `(f * g)` to the console. In the `main` method of the `Main` class, an instance of the `test` class is created, and the `display()` method is invoked on this instance. As a result, the calculated value of `d` and the result of the floating-point multiplication operation are displayed on the console.

8.12.5 STRICTFP INTERFACE

In Java, a `strictfp` interface ensures that all floating-point operations within any methods declared in the interface adhere to strict floating-point semantics. This means that all calculations involving floating-point numbers will follow the IEEE 754 standard for floating-point arithmetic consistently across different platforms, ensuring predictability and portability of the floating-point computations.

Program

```
Program for strictfp interface
// Define an interface with the strictfp keyword to enforce IEEE 754
floating-point operations
strictfp interface Sample {
  // Define double constants with large exponential values
  double num1 = 10e+102;
  double num2 = 6e+08;
  // Declare an abstract method
  double calculate();
}
// Implement the Sample interface in the Test class
class Test implements Sample {
  // Provide implementation for the calculate() method
  @Override
  public double calculate() {
    return num1 + num2; // Return the sum of num1 and num2
  }
}
// Main class to run the program
public class Main {
void main(String[] args) {
    // Create an instance of the Test class
    Test t = new Test();
    // Call the calculate() method and print the result
    System.out.println("Result of calculation: " + t.calculate());
  }
}
Output:
Result of calculation: 1.0E103
```

The above Java program consists of an interface named `sample` declared with the `strictfp` keyword. This ensures that all floating-point operations inside the interface adhere to the IEEE 754 standard for consistent precision. Within the `sample` interface, two `double` constants `num1` and `num2` are defined, initialized with large exponential values. Additionally, an abstract method `calculate()` is declared, which must be implemented by classes that implement the `sample` interface. The `test` class implements the `sample` interface and provides an implementation for the `calculate()` method, which returns the sum of `num1` and `num2`. In the `main` method of the `Main` class, an instance of the `test` class is created, and the `calculate()` method is invoked on this instance. The result of the calculation is then printed to the console.

8.13 INNER CLASS

Inner classes, also known as nested classes, are classes that are defined within the scope of another class in Java. These classes are declared within the body of another class and have access to all members of the enclosing class, including private members. There are several types of inner classes:

- Member Inner Class: Defined at the member level of a class, just like any other member variable or method. It can access both static and non-static members of the outer class.
- Local Inner Class: Defined within a block of code, typically within a method. Its scope is restricted to the block in which it is defined.
- Anonymous Inner Class: A type of local inner class that does not have a name and is instantiated at the point of use. It is often used for implementing interfaces or extending classes in a concise manner.
- Static Nested Class: Similar to a regular class but declared with the `static` keyword. It cannot access non-static members of the outer class directly but can access them through an object reference.

Inner classes provide several benefits, including encapsulation, improved code organization, and increased readability. They are commonly used to implement callbacks, event handling, and other design patterns in Java programming.

Syntax

```
public class OuterClass {
// Non-static inner class
public class InnerClass {
}
}
```

The syntax for defining inner classes, also known as nested classes, in Java. In Java, inner classes are classes declared within the scope of another class. In this example, the outer class, named `OuterClass`, encapsulates the inner class, named `innerClass`.

The outer class declaration is denoted by the `public class OuterClass{...}` syntax, where the outer code resides within the curly braces. Within the outer class scope, the inner class is declared using the syntax `public class innerClass{...}`. The inner class declaration is nested within the outer class and is referred to as the inner class or nested class.

Following the declaration of the inner class, the code block within the curly braces of the inner class defines the members, methods, and fields specific to the inner class. These members are accessible within the inner class and can interact with the outer class's members if needed.

8.13.1 Nested Inner Class in Java

Nesting a class inside another class, also known as inner class or nested class, refers to the practice of defining a class within the scope of another class. In Java, inner classes have the unique ability to access private variables and methods of their enclosing outer class. This allows for tighter encapsulation and more modular code organization.

To modify the access to the inner class itself, access modifier keywords such as private, protected, and default (also known as package-private) can be used. These modifiers control the visibility of the inner class from outside its enclosing class.

8.13.1.1 Private Inner Class

Declaring an inner class as private restricts its access only to the enclosing outer class. It cannot be accessed from outside the outer class.

```
public class OuterClass {
  private class InnerClass {
    // Inner class code
  }
}
```

8.13.1.2 Protected Inner Class

Declaring an inner class as protected allows it to be accessed within the same package and by subclasses of the enclosing outer class, regardless of whether they are in the same package or not.

```
public class OuterClass {
  protected class InnerClass {
    // Inner class code
  }
}
```

8.13.1.3 Default (Package-Private) Inner Class

If no access modifier is specified for an inner class, it defaults to package-private. This means the inner class can be accessed by other classes in the same package, but not from classes outside the package.

```
public class OuterClass {
  class InnerClass {
    // Inner class code
  }
}
```

By using these access modifiers, the visibility and accessibility of the inner class can be precisely controlled, allowing for better encapsulation and more secure code design.

Program

```
Java program to illustrate the usage of Nested Inner class:
// Outer class
class Outer {
  // Inner class
  class Inner {
    // Method in the inner class
    void display() {
      System.out.println("inner class");
    }
  }
}
// Entry point of the program
public class Nested {
void main(String[] args) {
    // Create an instance of the outer class
    Outer outer = new Outer();
    // Create an instance of the inner class using the outer class instance
    Outer.Inner inner = outer.new Inner();
    // Call the display method of the inner class
```

```
    inner.display();
  }
}
```

Output:
```
inner class
```

In the above Java program there are two classes: `Outer` and `Nested`. The `Outer` class contains an inner class named `Inner`. Within the `Inner` class, there is a method called `display()`, which prints "inner class" to the console when called. In the `Nested` class, which serves as the entry point of the program, the `main()` method is defined. Inside `main()`, an instance of the `Inner` class is created using the syntax `Outer.Inner`, indicating that `Inner` is a member of `Outer`. To instantiate the inner class, first, an instance of the outer class `Outer` is created using `new Outer()`, and then `new Inner()` is called on it. Finally, the `display()` method of the inner class instance `in` is invoked using the dot operator (`.`), resulting in the output "inner class" being printed to the console when the program is executed.

8.13.2 Method Local Inner Classes in Java

In Java, an inner class can indeed access variables of the outer class, even if they are not declared as `final`. However, if the inner class is accessing non-static members (instance variables or methods) of the outer class, and if the inner class is defined within a method of the outer class, then the variables accessed by the inner class must be effectively final.

Effectively final means that the variables are not explicitly declared as `final`, but they are treated as if they were. This restriction ensures that the variables accessed by the inner class maintain a consistent value throughout their lifetime, as modifying them after the inner class instance is created could lead to unexpected behavior.

Program

```
public class Outer {
  // Instance variable of the outer class
  int o = 10;
  void method() {
    // Local variable in the enclosing method
    final int l = 20;
    // Inner class
    class Inner {
      void display() {
        // Accessing instance variable of the outer class
        System.out.println("Outer instance variable o: " + o);
        // Accessing local variable from the enclosing method
        System.out.println("Local variable l: " + l);
      }
    }
    // Create an instance of the inner class and call its method
    Inner inner = new Inner();
    inner.display();
  }
void main(String[] args) {
    // Create an instance of the outer class
    Outer outer = new Outer();
    // Call the method that contains the inner class
```

```
    outer.method();
  }
}
```

Output:

```
Outer instance variable o: 10
Local variable l: 20
```

In the above program, the inner class `Inner` is accessing both the `o` and `l` variables. `o` is an instance variable of the outer class, while `l` is a local variable of the `method()` method. `l` is effectively final because it is not modified after being initialized. If `l` were to be modified after the inner class instance is created, it would result in a compilation error. However, `o` can be accessed without any such restrictions.

Program

```
Java program to illustrate the use of Method Local Inner Classes:
class Outer {
  void display() {
    final String s = "testing";  // Final string variable
    // Inner class definition
    class Inner {
      void fun() {
        // Accesses the final string variable from the outer class method
        System.out.println("Inner class " + s);
      }
    }
    // Create an instance of the inner class and call its method
    Inner inner = new Inner();
    inner.fun();
  }
}
public class test {
void main(String[] args) {
    // Create an instance of the outer class
    Outer outer = new Outer();
    // Invoke the display() method of the outer class
    outer.display();
  }
}
```

Output:

```
Inner class testing
```

The above Java program consists of an outer class named `Outer` and a separate class named `test` with a `main` method. Within the `Outer` class, there's a method named `display()`, which initializes a final string variable `s` with the value "testing". This method also contains an inner class named `Inner`, which has a method named `fun()`. Inside the `fun()` method of the `Inner` class, it prints the message "Inner class" concatenated with the value of the string `s`. In the `main` method of the `test` class, an instance of the `Outer` class is created, and its `display()` method is invoked, leading to the execution of the inner class's `fun()` method, printing "Inner class testing".

8.13.3 Anonymous Inner Classes in Java

Anonymous inner classes are a type of inner class in Java that have no name. They are primarily used when there is a need to implement an interface or override a method without explicitly creating a separate class. These classes are particularly useful for providing implementations for abstract methods of interfaces or for extending abstract classes. There are two main types of anonymous inner classes:

- Subclass of a specified type: In this type, an anonymous inner class extends a specific class. It is created using the `new` keyword followed by the class definition or an expression that evaluates to an instance of a class.
- Implementer of a specified interface: In this type, an anonymous inner class implements a particular interface. Similar to the first type, it is created using the `new` keyword followed by the interface definition or an expression that evaluates to an instance of an interface.

These anonymous inner classes are often used to provide concise and localized implementations of functionality without the need for creating separate named classes. They are especially handy for event handling and callback mechanisms in GUI programming and other scenarios where a single-use implementation is required.

8.13.3.1 Subclass of the Specified Type

In Java, an anonymous inner class can indeed be put inside a subclass of the outer class. This allows for the creation of a class with no name, directly within the scope of another class, typically for the purpose of overriding methods or providing implementations for interfaces.

Here's a general structure of how an anonymous inner class can be defined inside a subclass of an outer class:

```
class outer{
class inner{}
void method(){
inner inn=new inner();};
}
}
```

In the above code, the `method()` of the `Outer` class contains the definition of an anonymous inner class that extends the `Inner` class. This anonymous inner class can override methods from the `Inner` class or provide implementations for interfaces. It is instantiated and used within the `method()` of the `Outer` class.

Program

```
class Outer {
  // Method in the Outer class
  void display() {
    System.out.println("outer class");
  }
}
public class Main {
void main(String[] args) {
    // Create an instance of Outer with an anonymous inner class
    Outer out = new Outer() {
      // Override the display method
      @Override
```

```
      void display() {
        super.display(); // Call the display method of the Outer class
        System.out.println("Anonymous class"); // Additional behavior
      }
    };
    // Call the overridden display method
    out.display();
  }
}
```

Output:

```
outer class
Anonymous class
```

This Java program illustrates the use of an anonymous inner class within another class. The `Outer` class contains a method `display()` responsible for printing "outer class" when invoked. Inside the `Main` class, an instance of `Outer` named `out` is declared as static and instantiated. However, this instantiation incorporates an anonymous inner class. Within this anonymous inner class, the `display()` method undergoes overriding to append "Anonymous class" after invoking the `super.display()` method. When `out.display()` is invoked in the `main()` method, the program prints "outer class" followed by "Anonymous class".

8.13.3.2 The Implementer of Specified Interface

An anonymous class in Java can either extend a class or implement an interface, but it cannot do both simultaneously. This means that when creating an anonymous class, you have the option to either extend a class or implement an interface, depending on your requirements. When extending a class, the anonymous class inherits the properties and methods of the parent class, and you can override methods or add new functionality as needed. On the other hand, when implementing an interface, the anonymous class must provide implementations for all the abstract methods declared in that interface. This feature of anonymous classes provides flexibility in Java programming, allowing developers to create concise and specialized implementations on-the-fly without the need to define a separate named class.

Program

```
// Define an interface with a single abstract method
interface Test {
  void display();
}
public class Anonymous {
  // Declare a static field of type Test and initialize it with an
  anonymous class
  static Test t = new Test() {
    @Override
    public void display() {
      System.out.println("Anonymous");
    }
  };
void main(String[] args) {
    // Call the display method on the anonymous class instance
    t.display();
  }
}
```

Output

```
Anonymous
```

In the above Java program an interface named `test` is declared, which contains a single abstract method `display()`. Then, within the `Anonymous` class, a static field named `t` is declared of type `test`. This field is initialized with an anonymous class instance that implements the `test` interface. Inside the anonymous class definition, the `display()` method is overridden to print "Anonymous" to the console. In the `main` method of the `Anonymous` class, an attempt is made to invoke the `display()` method on the `t` object, which prints "Anonymous" to the console.

8.13.4 Static Nested Classes

In Java, a static nested class is a class defined within another class, known as the outer class. Unlike inner classes, static nested classes do not have access to the instance variables and methods of the outer class directly. They are essentially a static member of the outer class and can be accessed using the outer class name.

Program

```
public class OuterClass {
  private static String outerStaticVariable = "Outer static variable";
  // Static nested class
  public static class StaticNestedClass {
    private String nestedVariable = "Nested variable";
    public void display() {
      // Accessing static variable of outer class
System.out.println("Outer static variable: " + outerStaticVariable);
      // Accessing instance variable of nested class
System.out.println("Nested variable: " + nestedVariable);
    }
  }
void main(String[] args) {
    // Accessing static nested class
OuterClass.StaticNestedClassnestedObject = new OuterClass.
    StaticNestedClass();
nestedObject.display();
  }
}
Output:
Outer static variable: Outer static variable
Nested variable: Nested variable
```

In this program, we have an outer class `OuterClass` with a static variable `outerStaticVariable`. Inside the outer class, there's a static nested class `StaticNestedClass` that has an instance variable `nestedVariable` and a method `display()` to print both the outer class's static variable and its own instance variable. In the `main` method, an instance of the static nested class is created using `OuterClass.StaticNestedClass`, and its `display()` method is called to demonstrate accessing the outer class's static variable from within the nested class.

Static nested classes are primarily used for grouping classes that are closely related to the outer class but do not require access to its instance members. They are similar to regular top-level classes but provide a way to logically group classes together within the same source file.

8.14 LAMBDA EXPRESSIONS

Lambda expressions are a concise way to represent anonymous functions (functions without a name) in programming languages such as Java, Python, and C#. They allow the creation of simple function definitions on-the-fly, often used to pass a function as a parameter to higher-order functions.

8.14.1 Need for Lambda Expressions

- Conciseness: Lambda expressions reduce the verbosity of code by enabling the definition of small functions in a single line, which is especially useful for operations like filtering, mapping, and reducing collections.
- Functional Programming: They support functional programming paradigms by allowing functions to be treated as first-class citizens, enabling higher-order functions and more expressive code.
- Event Handling and Callbacks: In GUI applications and asynchronous programming, lambda expressions simplify the creation of event handlers and callbacks.

8.14.2 Advantages of Lambda Expressions

- Readability: By reducing code, lambda expressions make the code more readable and easier to understand, especially for small, simple functions.
- Flexibility: They enable the creation of inline functions that can be passed around and used where traditional named methods would be cumbersome.
- Parallel Processing: Lambda expressions are well-suited for parallel operations on collections, such as those provided by the Stream API in Java, allowing for more concise and expressive parallel processing.
- Reduced Code Size: By allowing the definition of functions directly where they are used, lambda expressions help in reducing the overall code size.

8.14.3 Limitations of Lambda Expressions

- Debugging Difficulty: Since lambda expressions are often anonymous and inline, they can be harder to debug compared to traditional named functions.
- Complexity in Overuse: Overuse of lambda expressions can lead to complex and less maintainable code, especially when combined with other functional programming constructs.
- Limited to Single Expressions or Statements: Lambda expressions are generally limited to single expressions or statements, making them unsuitable for more complex function definitions.
- Performance Overhead: In some cases, the use of lambda expressions can introduce performance overhead due to the creation of additional function objects and potential impacts on optimization by the compiler or runtime.

Program

```
Program for lambda expressions for single parameter
// Define a functional interface with a single abstract method
@FunctionalInterface
interface Sample {
  int display(int a);
}
public class Test {
void main(String[] args) {
```

```
    // Lambda expressions implementing the display method of the Sample
interface
    Sample s1 = (a) -> a;        // Returns the input integer a
    Sample s2 = (a) -> a + 10;    // Returns the input integer a plus 10
    Sample s3 = (a) -> a * 2;    // Returns the input integer a multi-
                                  plied by 2
    Sample s4 = (a) -> {
      System.out.println("Input integer: " + a); // Prints the input integer
      return a * a;              // Returns the square of the input integer
    };
    // Test the lambda expressions with different inputs
    int result1 = s1.display(5);  // Calls s1 with input 5
    int result2 = s2.display(10);  // Calls s2 with input 10
    int result3 = s3.display(15);  // Calls s3 with input 15
    int result4 = s4.display(20);  // Calls s4 with input 20
    // Print the results
    System.out.println("Result from s1: " + result1);
    System.out.println("Result from s2: " + result2);
    System.out.println("Result from s3: " + result3);
    System.out.println("Result from s4: " + result4);
  }
}
```

Output:

```
Input integer: 20
Result from s1: 5
Result from s2: 20
Result from s3: 30
Result from s4: 400
```

The Java program demonstrates the usage of lambda expressions with a functional interface. The `sample` interface is annotated with `@FunctionalInterface`, indicating that it contains a single abstract method. This interface declares a method `display` that takes an integer parameter and returns an integer. The `test` class contains the `main` method where lambda expressions are used to implement the `display` method of the `sample` interface. In the `main` method, four instances of the `sample` interface are created using lambda expressions. Each lambda expression represents an implementation of the `display` method. The first three instances simply return the input integer `a`. The fourth instance includes a block of code within curly braces, printing the input integer `a` before returning a constant value. The program then invokes the `display` method on each instance of the `sample` interface, passing different integer values as arguments. Finally, the program prints the result returned by each invocation of the `display` method.

Program

```
Program for lambda expressions for zero parameter
// Define a functional interface with a single abstract method
@FunctionalInterface
interface Sample {
  int display();
}
public class Test {
void main(String[] args) {
    // Lambda expressions implementing the display method of the Sample
    interface
    Sample s1 = () -> 100;    // Returns the constant integer value 100
```

```
    Sample s2 = () -> {
      return 150;          // Returns the integer value 150
    };
    Sample s3 = () -> {
      int a = 200;        // Local variable a with value 200
      return a;         // Returns the value of a
    };
    Sample s4 = () -> {
      System.out.println("testing lambda"); // Prints the string
      return 1;            // Returns the integer value 1
    };
    // Invoke the display method on each instance and print the result
    int result1 = s1.display();  // Calls s1
    int result2 = s2.display();  // Calls s2
    int result3 = s3.display();  // Calls s3
    int result4 = s4.display();  // Calls s4
    // Print the results
    System.out.println("Result from s1: " + result1);
    System.out.println("Result from s2: " + result2);
    System.out.println("Result from s3: " + result3);
    System.out.println("Result from s4: " + result4);
  }
}
```

Output:

```
testing lambda
Result from s1: 100
Result from s2: 150
Result from s3: 200
Result from s4: 1
```

The Java program illustrates the usage of lambda expressions with a functional interface. The `sample` interface, annotated with `@FunctionalInterface`, declares a single abstract method `display` with no parameters and returning an integer. In the `test` class's `main` method, lambda expressions are utilized to implement the `display` method for different instances of the `sample` interface. Four instances of the `sample` interface were created using lambda expressions. Each lambda expression defines the behavior of the `display` method. The first lambda expression simply returns the constant integer value `100`. The second lambda expression includes a block of code within curly braces, returning the integer value `150`. The third lambda expression declares a local variable `a` with the value `200` and returns it. The fourth lambda expression contains a block of code that prints the string "testing lambda" before returning the integer value `1`.

Program

```
Program for lambda expressions using user defined interface
// Define a functional interface with a single abstract method
@FunctionalInterface
interface Sample {
  void display();
}
public class Test {
  // Static method that takes a Sample object and invokes its display method
  public static void put(Sample s) {
    s.display();
  }
```

```
void main(String[] args) {
    // Call the put method with a lambda expression
    put(() -> System.out.println("testing lambda expression"));
  }
}
```

Output:

```
testing lambda expression
```

In the above Java program an interface named `sample` is defined as a functional interface using the `@FunctionalInterface` annotation. This interface contains a single abstract method `display()`. Within the `test` class, a static method `put()` is defined, which takes an object of type `sample` as an argument and invokes its `display()` method. In the `main` method, the `put()` method is called with a lambda expression as an argument. The lambda expression `() ->System.out.println("testing lambda expression")` represents an implementation of the `display()` method. It simply prints the string "testing lambda expression" to the console. When the `put()` method is invoked with this lambda expression, it is treated as an instance of the `sample` interface, and its `display()` method is executed. As a result, the message "testing lambda expression" is printed to the console.

Program

```
Program for lambda expressions using  2 interface
// Define the first functional interface with a single abstract method
display()
@FunctionalInterface
interface One {
  void display();
}
// Define the second functional interface with a single abstract method put()
@FunctionalInterface
interface Two {
  void put();
}
public class Test {
  // Method that accepts a One interface implementation and prints a message
  public void first(One o) {
    System.out.println("Invoking first.");
    o.display();
  }
  // Method that accepts a Two interface implementation and prints a message
  public void second(Two t) {
    System.out.println("Invoking second.");
    t.put();
  }
  // Method that demonstrates lambda expressions with functional interfaces
  public void invoke() {
    // Lambda expression for the display() method of the One interface
    first(() -> System.out.println("Lambda expression for display()"));
    // Lambda expression for the put() method of the Two interface
    second(() -> System.out.println("Lambda expression for put()"));
  }
void main(String[] args) {
    Test test = new Test();
    test.invoke();
  }
}
```

```
Output:
Invoking first.
Lambda expression for display()
Invoking second.
Lambda expression for put()
```

The Java program defines two functional interfaces named `one` and `two`, each containing a single abstract method `display()` and `put()`, respectively, marked with the `@FunctionalInterface` annotation. Additionally, a class named `test` is defined, which contains two methods: `first()` and `second()`. The `first()` method accepts an object of type `one` as an argument, while the `second()` method accepts an object of type `two`. Both methods simply print messages to the console indicating their invocation. In the `invoke()` method of the `test` class, lambda expressions are used to provide implementations for the `display()` and `put()` methods defined in the `one` and `two` interfaces, respectively. When the `invoke()` method is called within the `main()` method, it invokes the `first()` and `second()` methods of the `test` class, passing lambda expressions as arguments. These lambda expressions represent implementations of the `display()` and `put()` methods and print messages indicating their invocation. Finally, when the program is executed, the `invoke()` method is called, causing the messages "Invoking first." and "Invoking second." to be printed to the console.

Program

```
Program for lambda expressions with multiple operations
// Define the functional interface with a single abstract method for arith-
metic operations
@FunctionalInterface
interface Calculate {
  int op(int a, int b);
}
public class Test {
  // Method to perform an arithmetic operation using the provided Calculate
  interface object
  public int operate(int a, int b, Calculate calc) {
    return calc.op(a, b);  // Call the op() method of the Calculate instance
  }
void main(String[] args) {
    // Create an instance of the Test class
    Test test = new Test();
    // Define lambda expressions for addition, subtraction, multiplication,
    and division
    Calculate addition = (a, b) -> a + b;
    Calculate subtraction = (a, b) -> a - b;
    Calculate multiplication = (a, b) -> a * b;
    Calculate division = (a, b) -> b != 0 ? a / b : 0; // Handle division
    by zero
    // Perform operations using the operate() method and lambda expressions
    int a = 100;
    int b = 20;
    // Perform and print the results of different operations
    System.out.println("Addition: " + test.operate(a, b, addition));      //
       10 + 5 = 15
    System.out.println("Subtraction:  "  +  test.operate(a,  b,  subtrac-
       tion)); // 10 - 5 = 5
```

```
    System.out.println("Multiplication: " + test.operate(a, b, multiplica-
       tion)); // 10 * 5 = 50
    System.out.println("Division: " + test.operate(a, b, division));
// 10 / 5 = 2
  }
}
```

Output:

```
Addition: 120
Subtraction: 80
Multiplication: 2000
Division: 5
```

The above Java program defines a functional interface named `calculate`, which contains a single abstract method `op(int a, int b)` for performing arithmetic operations on two integers.

In the `test` class, the `main()` method instantiates the `test` class and defines four lambda expressions for addition, subtraction, multiplication, and division operations. Each lambda expression implements the `calculate` interface's `op` method to perform the respective arithmetic operation. Subsequently, the `operate()` method is called four times with different arithmetic operations: addition, subtraction, multiplication, and division. This method takes two integer operands and a functional interface object representing the desired arithmetic operation. It then invokes the `op` method of the provided functional interface object, passing the operands, and returns the result of the operation. When the program is executed, the `main()` method invokes the `operate()` method four times with different arithmetic operations, and the results are printed to the console.

Program

```
Program for lambda expressions by creating object for interface in a
different way
// Define the class containing the main method
public class Main {
  // Define the functional interface with a single abstract method
  @FunctionalInterface
  interface Test {
    String display(String s);
  }
void main(String[] args) {
    // Create an instance of the Test interface using a lambda expression
    Test t = s -> "lambda " + s;
    // Use the instance to call the display method with a string argument
    String result = t.display("expressions");
    // Print the result to the console
    System.out.println(result);
  }
}
```

Output:

```
lambda expressions
```

The above Java program defines a class named `Main`, which contains an interface named `test`. This interface declares a single abstract method `display(String s)` that takes a string parameter and returns a string. In the `main()` method of the `Main` class, a lambda expression is used to implement the `display` method of the `test` interface. The lambda expression takes a string parameter `s` and returns a string concatenation of "lambda" and the input string `s`. After defining the lambda expression, an instance of the `test` interface is created and initialized with the lambda expression.

This instance `t` is then used to call the `display` method, passing the string "expressions" as an argument. Finally, the result returned by the `display` method is printed to the console.

Program

```
Program for accessing local and class variables using lambda expressions
public class Main {
  // Public instance variable
  public String s = "testing";
  // Method to create and start a new thread
  public void display() {
    // Local variable
    String ss = "lambda";
    // Create and start a new thread with a lambda expression as the
Runnable implementation
    new Thread(() -> {
      // Print the values of instance variable `s` and local variable `ss`
      System.out.println("Instance variable s: " + s);
      System.out.println("Local variable ss: " + ss);
    }).start();
  }
void main(String[] args) {
    // Create an instance of Main and call the display method
    new Main().display();
  }
}
Output:
Instance variable s: testing
Local variable ss: lambda
```

The above Java program defines a class named `Main`, which contains a public instance variable `s` initialized with the string "testing". In the `main()` method of the `Main` class, a new instance of `Main` is created using an anonymous object, and its `display()` method is invoked. The`display()` method initializes a local variable `ss` with the string "lambda". Inside the `display()` method, a new thread is created using a lambda expression as the `Runnable` implementation. The lambda expression prints the values of the instance variable `s` and the local variable `ss` to the console. Since the lambda expression is defined within the context of the `display()` method, it has access to both the instance variable `s` and the local variable `ss`. When the program is executed, a new thread is started, and the lambda expression is executed concurrently with the main thread. As a result, the output may not appear in the same order as the statements are written, but it will include the values of `s` and `ss` from the enclosing scope.

Program

```
Program for anonymous class implementation as function argument using
lambda technique.
public class Main {
    // Define the functional interface with a single abstract method `get`
  @FunctionalInterface
  interface test {
    double get(double radius);
  }
  // Method to perform operations using the provided `test` interface
instance
```

```
  public double testop(double radius, test operation) {
    return operation.get(radius);
  }
void main(String[] args) {
    // Create an instance of Main
    Main m = new Main();
    // Lambda expression to calculate the area of a circle
    test c = radius -> Math.PI * radius * radius;
    // Lambda expression to calculate the circumference of a circle
    test cc = radius -> 2 * Math.PI * radius;
    // Radius of the circle
    double radius = 10;
    // Calculate area and circumference using the lambda expressions
    double a = m.testop(radius, c);
    double cr = m.testop(radius, cc);
    // Print the results
    System.out.println("Area of the circle with radius " + radius + "
       is: " + a);
    System.out.println("Circumference of the circle with radius " + radius
       + " is: " + cr);
  }
}
```

Output:

```
Area of the circle with radius 10.0 is: 314.1592653589793
Circumference of the circle with radius 10.0 is: 62.83185307179586
```

The above Java program defines a class named `Main`, which includes an interface named `test`. This interface declares a single abstract method `get()` that takes a double parameter representing the radius of a circle and returns a double value. Within the `Main` class, there's a method named `testop()` that takes a double radius and an instance of the `test` interface as parameters. This method invokes the `get()` method of the provided `test` interface instance, passing the radius as an argument, and returns the result. In the `main()` method of the `Main` class, an instance of `Main` is created named `m`. Two lambda expressions are then used to create instances of the `test` interface: `c` calculates the area of a circle using the formula πr^2, and `cc` calculates the circumference using the formula $2\pi r$. The `testop()` method is invoked twice with `reference` as the instance and the lambda expressions `c` and `cc` as arguments to calculate the area and circumference of a circle with a radius of 10, respectively. The results are stored in variables `a` and `cr`, and then printed to the console. Upon execution, the program calculates and displays the area and circumference of a circle with a radius of 10 using the lambda expressions provided for the calculations.

Program

```
Program for lambda initialization
import java.util.concurrent.Callable;
public class Main {
void main(String[] args) throws Exception {
    // Create an array of Callable objects using lambda expressions
    Callable<String>[] callables = new Callable[] {
      () -> "lambda",  // First Callable lambda expression
      () -> "expressions" // Second Callable lambda expression
    };
    // Call the call method on the first Callable object and print the result
    String result = callables[0].call();
```

```
    System.out.println(result);  // Output: lambda
  }
}
```

Output:

```
Lambda
```

The above Java program showcases the usage of the `Callable` interface along with lambda expressions. In the `Main` class, the `main` method is defined to throw `Exception`, accommodating any checked exceptions thrown by the `Callable`'s `call` method. Within the `main` method, an array of `Callable` objects is created using lambda expressions. The first lambda expression returns the string "lambda", while the second returns "expressions". The program then calls the `call` method on the first `Callable` object in the array and prints its result, which is "lambda".

Program

```
Program for sorting the lambda expressions
import java.util.Arrays;
import java.util.concurrent.Callable;
public class Main {
  // Define the Test class as a member of Main class
  static class Test {
    String name;
    Test(String name) {
      this.name = name;
    }
    @Override
    public String toString() {
      return name;
    }
  }
  // Static method for comparing Test objects
  public static int tc(Test t1, Test t2) {
    return t1.name.compareTo(t2.name);
  }
void main(String[] args) throws Exception {
    // Part 1: Using Callable with lambda expressions
    @SuppressWarnings("unchecked")
    Callable<String>[] c = (Callable<String>[]) new Callable[] {
      () -> "lambda",
      () -> "expressions"
    };
    // Call the call method on the first Callable object and print the result
    String result = c[0].call();
    System.out.println(result);  // Output: lambda
    // Part 2: Sorting custom objects using method references
    // Create and initialize an array of Test objects
    Test[] t = {
      new Test("Dr."),
      new Test("Usha"),
      new Test("Rani"),
      new Test("Bhimavarapu")
    };
    // Print the array before sorting
    System.out.println("Before sorting:");
```

```
    for (Test test : t) {
      System.out.println(test);
    }
    // Sort the array using the static method tc as a comparator
    Arrays.sort(t, Main::tc);
    // Print the array after sorting
    System.out.println("After sorting:");
    for (Test test : t) {
      System.out.println(test);
    }
  }
}
```

Output:

```
lambda
Before sorting:
Dr.
Usha
Rani
Bhimavarapu
After sorting:
Bhimavarapu
Dr.
Rani
Usha
```

The above Java program consists of two separate parts. The first part utilizes the `java.util.concurrent.Callable` interface to create an array `c` of `Callable` instances using lambda expressions. Each lambda expression returns a string value when invoked. In the `main` method, the first element of the `c` array is called using the `call()` method, and its result is printed to the console. The output of the program displays "lambda" as expected, indicating that the first lambda expression in the array was invoked successfully. The second part of the program demonstrates sorting of custom objects using lambda expressions. It defines a `test` class with a `name` attribute and a static method `tc` for comparing `test` objects based on their `name` attribute. Additionally, the `toString()` method is overridden to provide a string representation of the `test` objects. In the `main` method of the `Main` class, an array `t` of `test` objects is created and initialized with instances of the `test` class. The array is then sorted using `Arrays.sort()` method, passing a reference to the `tc` method as a comparator. This is achieved using a method reference `test::tc`, which specifies that the `tc` method of the `test` class should be used for comparison during sorting. The program first prints the contents of the array `t` before sorting, and then prints the array again after sorting. The output displays the array elements sorted alphabetically by their names, confirming that the sorting operation was successful.

8.15 MEDICAL APPLICATIONS

8.15.1 Case Study 1

A cough is a reflex action to clear your airways of mucus, irritants, foreign particles, and microbes. It is a common respiratory response that involves a sudden, forceful expulsion of air from the lungs, typically resulting in a distinctive sound. Coughing helps to protect the respiratory system by preventing the inhalation of harmful substances and clearing out secretions or debris.

- **Body Temperature**:
  Higher temperatures can indicate the presence of an infection or inflammation.

- **Medical History**:
  This includes information about the patient's past health conditions, which can be crucial for diagnosing chronic illnesses or conditions that might cause coughing.
- **White Blood Cell Count**:
  An elevated white blood cell count can indicate an infection or inflammation in the body, which could be a potential cause of a cough.

```
import java.util.Random;
interfaceDataSource
{
voidcollectData();
}
interface PredictionAlgorithm {
  void predict();
}
class TemperatureSensor implements DataSource {
  private double temperature;
  public void setTemperature(double temperature) {
    this.temperature = temperature;
  }
  public double getTemperature() {
    return temperature;
  }
  @Override
  public void collectData() {
    temperature = new Random().nextDouble() * 10 + 36;
    System.out.println("Collecting temperature data from sensor: " + tem-
       perature + " °C");
  }
}
class MedicalHistory implements DataSource {
  private String history;
  public void setMedicalHistory(String history) {
    this.history = history;
  }
  public String getMedicalHistory() {
    return history;
  }
  @Override
  public void collectData() {
    history = "No significant medical history.";
    System.out.println("Collecting medical history data: " + history);
  }
}
class BloodTest implements DataSource {
  private double whiteBloodCellCount;
  public void setWhiteBloodCellCount(double whiteBloodCellCount) {
    this.whiteBloodCellCount = whiteBloodCellCount;
  }
  public double getWhiteBloodCellCount() {
    return whiteBloodCellCount;
  }
  @Override
  public void collectData() {
```

```
    // Simulate collecting blood test data
    whiteBloodCellCount = new Random().nextDouble() * 5 + 4;
    System.out.println("Collecting blood test data: White blood cell
       count = " + whiteBloodCellCount + " x10^9/L");
  }
}
class SimplePredictionAlgorithm implements PredictionAlgorithm {
  private TemperatureSensor temperatureSensor;
  private MedicalHistory medicalHistory;
  private BloodTest bloodTest;
  public SimplePredictionAlgorithm(TemperatureSensor temperatureSensor,
     MedicalHistory medicalHistory, BloodTest bloodTest) {
    this.temperatureSensor = temperatureSensor;
    this.medicalHistory = medicalHistory;
    this.bloodTest = bloodTest;
  }
  @Override
  public void predict() {
       double temperature = temperatureSensor.getTemperature();
    String history = medicalHistory.getMedicalHistory();
    double whiteBloodCellCount = bloodTest.getWhiteBloodCellCount();
    if (temperature > 38.0 && whiteBloodCellCount > 7.0) {
      System.out.println("Prediction: The patient might have an infection
         or inflammation causing cough.");
    } else if (temperature > 37.0 && history.contains("chronic")) {
      System.out.println("Prediction: The patient might have chronic bron-
         chitis or other chronic respiratory conditions.");
    } else {
      System.out.println("Prediction: The patient's cough might be due to a
         mild cause or an unknown factor.");
    }
  }
}
class CoughPredictionSystem {
  private final TemperatureSensor temperatureSensor;
  private final MedicalHistory medicalHistory;
  private final BloodTest bloodTest;
  private final SimplePredictionAlgorithm predictionAlgorithm;
  public CoughPredictionSystem() {
    this.temperatureSensor = new TemperatureSensor();
    this.medicalHistory = new MedicalHistory();
    this.bloodTest = new BloodTest();
    this.predictionAlgorithm = new SimplePredictionAlgorithm(temperatureSe
      nsor, medicalHistory, bloodTest);
  }
  public void collectAllData() {
    temperatureSensor.collectData();
    medicalHistory.collectData();
    bloodTest.collectData();
  }
  public void runPrediction() {
    System.out.println("Collecting all necessary data:");
    collectAllData();
    System.out.println("Data collection complete. Running prediction:");
    predictionAlgorithm.predict();
```

```
  }
}
public class CoughPredictionInChildren {
void main(String[] args) {
    CoughPredictionSystem predictionSystem = new CoughPredictionSystem();
    predictionSystem.runPrediction();
  }
}
```

The program implements a simple cough prediction system using various data sources and a prediction algorithm. It defines classes for collecting temperature data from sensors, medical history data, each implementing the `DataSource` interface. The `SimplePredictionAlgorithm` class uses these data sources to predict potential causes of cough based on predefined conditions. The `CoughPredictionSystem` class aggregates these components, facilitating the collection of data and running the prediction. Finally, the main class `CoughPredictionInChildren` creates an instance of the prediction system and triggers the data collection and prediction process, simulating a basic diagnostic tool for assessing cough causes.

8.15.2 Case Study 2

Osteoporosis is a medical condition characterized by weakened bones that are more susceptible to fractures. It occurs when the body loses too much bone, makes too little bone, or both. This leads to a decrease in bone density and bone quality, making bones fragile and prone to fractures, especially in the hip, spine, and wrist. Osteoporosis often progresses silently without symptoms until a fracture occurs, making early detection and management crucial for prevention and treatment. The parameters considered here are:

- **Bone Density Data (g/cm^2)**: This is the primary parameter used to assess osteoporosis risk.
- **Threshold for Osteoporosis**: Typically, a threshold value for bone density below which osteoporosis is diagnosed.

```
import java.util.Scanner;
interface BoneDensityTest {
  void collectData(); // Method to collect bone density data
  boolean predictOsteoporosis(); // Method to predict osteoporosis
}
class DEXA implements BoneDensityTest {
  private double boneDensity;
  @Override
  public void collectData() {
    Scanner scanner = new Scanner(System.in);
    System.out.print("Enter bone density value (g/cm^2) measured by DEXA: ");
    boneDensity = scanner.nextDouble();
  }
  @Override
  public boolean predictOsteoporosis() {
    return boneDensity < 0.8; // Threshold for osteoporosis (example value)
  }
}
class QuantitativeUltrasound implements BoneDensityTest {
  private int Tscore;
  @Override
```

```
  public void collectData() {
    Scanner scanner = new Scanner(System.in);
    System.out.print("Enter T-score measured by Quantitative Ultrasound: ");
    Tscore = scanner.nextInt();
  }
  @Override
  public boolean predictOsteoporosis() {
    return Tscore <= -2.5;
  }
}
public class OsteoporosisDetection {
void main(String[] args) {
    BoneDensityTest dexaTest = new DEXA();
    BoneDensityTest ultrasoundTest = new QuantitativeUltrasound();
    dexaTest.collectData();
    boolean osteoporosisPredicted = dexaTest.predictOsteoporosis();
    System.out.println("Predicted osteoporosis (DEXA): " +
       osteoporosisPredicted);
    ultrasoundTest.collectData();
    osteoporosisPredicted = ultrasoundTest.predictOsteoporosis();
    System.out.println("Predicted osteoporosis (Quantitative Ultrasound): "
       + osteoporosisPredicted);
  }
}
```

The `OsteoporosisDetection` includes an interface `BoneDensityDataSource` for data collection methods and a class `DEXAScan` implementing this interface to collect bone density measurements at runtime. The `OsteoporosisDetection` class contains a method `predictOsteoporosis()` that evaluates if the collected bone density falls below a threshold indicative of osteoporosis.

9 Exception Handling

9.1 INTRODUCTION

Exception handling in Java is a mechanism to handle runtime errors, allowing a program to continue or gracefully terminate instead of crashing unexpectedly. It involves using specific constructs to detect, manage, and respond to exceptional conditions (errors) that occur during program execution.

9.1.1 Need for Exception Handling

Exception handling is crucial in programming for several reasons:

- Robustness: It ensures that a program can handle unexpected situations or errors gracefully without crashing.
- Error Propagation: It provides a mechanism to propagate errors up the call stack, allowing higher-level parts of the application to handle them appropriately.
- Code Readability and Maintenance: Separating error-handling code from regular code improves readability and maintainability.
- Resource Management: It ensures that resources (like files, network connections, and memory) are properly managed and released even when errors occur.
- Custom Error Handling: It allows developers to define custom error responses for specific situations, providing better user feedback and debugging information.

9.1.2 Advantages of Exception Handling

- Separates Error-Handling Code: Exception handling separates the regular code from the error-handling code, making programs more readable and maintainable.
- Propagates Errors: Exceptions can be propagated up the call stack, allowing higher-level methods to handle errors appropriately.
- Consistent Error Management: It provides a consistent approach to handling different types of errors and exceptions in a program.
- Improves Program Reliability: By catching and handling exceptions, programs can prevent crashes and continue running, thus improving reliability.
- Facilitates Debugging: Exception handling can provide detailed error messages and stack traces, which help in debugging and identifying the root cause of issues.
- Automatic Resource Management: With features like try-with-resources in Java, exception handling ensures that resources are automatically closed, avoiding resource leaks.

DOI: 10.1201/9781003544319-9

9.1.3 Limitations of Exception Handling

- Performance Overhead: The process of throwing and catching exceptions involves performance overhead, which can impact the efficiency of the program, especially if exceptions are used for regular control flow.
- Overuse: Overuse of exceptions can lead to complex and hard-to-maintain code. Exceptions should be used for exceptional conditions, not for regular control flow.
- Complexity: Writing robust exception-handling code can be complex, especially when dealing with multiple exceptions and ensuring that all resources are properly managed.
- Error Masking: Improper handling of exceptions can lead to error masking, where the real cause of the issue is hidden, making it difficult to debug and fix the problem.
- Unexpected Exceptions: Unhandled exceptions can still occur, potentially causing the program to terminate abruptly if not properly anticipated.
- Dependency on Language Features: Exception handling mechanisms vary across programming languages, so developers must understand the specific features and best practices for the language they are using.

Program

```
public class DivisionByZeroExample {
  void main(String[] args) {
    try {
      int numerator = 10;
      int denominator = 0;
      int result = numerator / denominator; // This will throw
ArithmeticException
System.out.println("Result: " + result);
    } catch (ArithmeticException e) {
System.out.println("Error: Division by zero is not allowed.");
    }
    // Example of floating-point division
    double numerator = 5.0;
    double denominator = 0.0;
    double result = numerator / denominator;  // This will result in Infinity
System.out.println("Result: " + result);
  }
}
Output:
Error: Division by zero is not allowed.
Result: Infinity
```

The above program is not handling any exceptions, so the compiler will handle those exceptions.

9.2 EXCEPTION

In Java, an exception is an event that occurs during the execution of a program, disrupting the normal flow of instructions. Exceptions can be caused by a variety of factors, including user error, programmer error, or failure of physical resources. Examples of exceptions include trying to open a file that doesn't exist, dividing by zero, or attempting to access an index that is out of bounds in an array.

There are many predefined exception classes in Java, each serving different purposes. These exceptions are part of the Java standard library and are organized in a class hierarchy that stems from java.lang.Throwable. All predefined exception classes in Java are subclasses of the java.lang. Exception class, which itself is a subclass of the Throwable class.

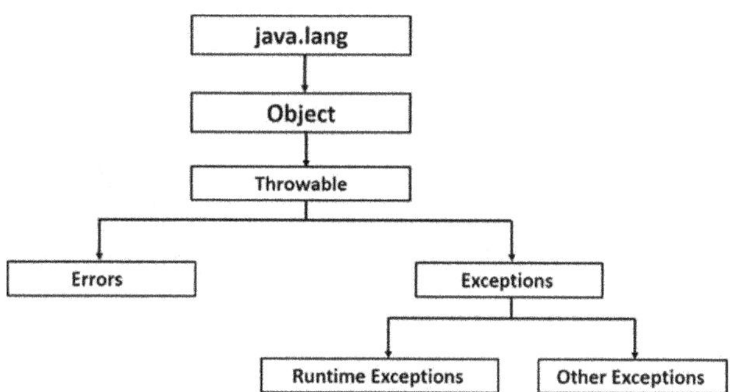

FIGURE 9.1 Hierarchy of the exception.

On the other hand, errors represent severe failures that occur in the Java Virtual Machine (JVM) or system environment. Examples of errors include OutOfMemoryError, StackOverflowError, and VirtualMachineError. Errors are typically irrecoverable and usually result in termination of the program. Unlike exceptions, errors are not usually caught and handled by the program.

Actually, while both IOException and RuntimeException are important subclasses of the exception class in Java, they serve different purposes:

- IOException: This subclass of Exception represents an input/output (I/O) exception that occurs during reading from or writing to external sources such as files, network connections, or streams. IOExceptions typically occur due to factors such as file not found, invalid file permissions, network errors, or disk space issues. Examples of IOExceptions include FileNotFoundException, SocketException, and EOFException.
- RuntimeException: This subclass of Exception represents exceptions that occur due to programming errors or logic flaws within the application code. Unlike checked exceptions (such as IOExceptions), RuntimeExceptions are unchecked, meaning they do not need to be declared in method signatures or caught by the calling code. They can occur at any time during program execution and are usually indicative of bugs or unexpected conditions in the code. Examples of RuntimeExceptions include NullPointerException, ArrayIndexOutOfBoundsException, and ArithmeticException.

While both IOException and RuntimeException are subclasses of exception, they serve distinct purposes and are typically handled differently in Java programs. IOExceptions are often caught and handled explicitly, as they represent expected and recoverable errors in I/O operations. In contrast, RuntimeExceptions are often indicative of more serious issues in the code and may require debugging and fixing to ensure the correctness and stability of the program. Figure 9.1 shows the hierarchy of the exceptions.

9.3 EXCEPTION TYPES

Java supports three types of exceptions:

- Checked Exception
- Unchecked Exception
- Error

9.3.1 Checked Exceptions

Checked exceptions are exceptions that are checked by the compiler at compile time. Also known as compile-time exceptions, checked exceptions must be either caught by the code or declared to be thrown by the method using the `throws` keyword. This ensures that the programmer explicitly handles or acknowledges the possibility of the exception occurring.

Checked exceptions are typically caused by external factors or conditions that may prevent the normal execution of the program. Examples of checked exceptions include file not found (FileNotFoundException), invalid user input (IOException), and network errors (SocketException). The characteristics of checked exceptions:

- Checked exceptions are tested by the compiler at compile time.
- Programmers are required to handle or declare checked exceptions.
- All exceptions in Java, except those belonging to the Error and RuntimeException classes and their subclasses, are checked exceptions.
- Checked exceptions are typically caused by external factors or conditions outside the control of the program.

Handling checked exceptions is an essential aspect of writing robust and reliable Java programs, as it ensures that potential issues are addressed and the program behaves predictably in various scenarios. Table 9.1 tabulates the checked exceptions.

Program

```
import java.io.*;
class Main
{
   void main(String a[])
  {
   FileInputStream fis=null;
fis=new FileInputStream("f.txt");
int n;
while((n=fis.read())!=-1){
System.out.println((char)n);
  }
fis.close();
}
}
Output:
Main.java:7: error: unreported exception FileNotFoundException; must be
caught or declared to be thrown
```

TABLE 9.1
Checked exceptions

Name	Description
IOException	File input/output stream related exception.
SQLException	Database related exceptions.
DataAccessException	Related to accessing data/database.
ClassNotFoundException	When the JVM can't find a class.
InstantiationException	Attempt to create an object of an abstract class or interface.

```
fis=new FileInputStream("aa.txt");
  ^
Main.java:9: error: unreported exception IOException; must be caught or
declared to be thrown
while((n=fis.read())!=-1){
        ^
Main.java:12: error: unreported exception IOException; must be caught or
declared to be thrown
fis.close();
      ^
3 errors
error: compilation failed
```

When a program throws exceptions during the compilation process, they are not visible in the output. Instead, they are reported as compilation errors or warnings by the compiler. These errors or warnings indicate that there are issues in the code that need to be resolved before the program can be successfully compiled and executed. There are two common approaches to resolving such compilation issues:

- Fixing Compilation Errors: Compilation errors occur when the code does not conform to the syntax and semantics of the programming language. To resolve compilation errors, you need to identify and fix the issues in the code. This may involve correcting syntax errors, resolving type mismatches, adding missing import statements, or addressing other issues reported by the compiler.
- Handling Compilation Warnings: Compilation warnings are issued by the compiler when it detects potential issues in the code that may cause problems during runtime, even though the code is syntactically correct. While warnings do not prevent the program from being compiled and executed, they indicate areas of the code that may need attention to ensure correct behavior. To handle compilation warnings, you should review the warnings reported by the compiler, understand their implications, and take appropriate actions to address them, such as making code modifications or adding annotations to suppress specific warnings.

By addressing compilation errors and handling compilation warnings effectively, you can ensure that your code compiles successfully and runs without unexpected issues. This contributes to the overall quality and reliability of your software.

9.3.1.1 Throws Keyword

In Java, the `throws` keyword is used in method declarations to indicate that a particular method may throw one or more exceptions during its execution. By using the `throws` keyword, the programmer declares that the method may potentially propagate the specified exceptions to its caller, rather than handling them within the method itself.

Here's the basic syntax of using the `throws` keyword:

```
returnTypemethodName(parameters) throws ExceptionType1, ExceptionType2 {
  // Method implementation
}
```

In this syntax:

- `returnType` specifies the data type of the value returned by the method (or `void` if the method does not return a value).
- `methodName` is the name of the method.

- `parameters` are the parameters accepted by the method, if any.
- `throws ExceptionType1, ExceptionType2, ...` is an optional clause that specifies the exceptions that the method may throw during its execution.

For example:

```
public void readFile(String fileName)throwsFileNotFoundException {{
  // Method implementation
}
```

In the above code, the `readFile` method is declared to potentially throw a `FileNotFoundException` when attempting to read from the specified file. By using the `throws` keyword, the method indicates to its caller that it does not handle the `FileNotFoundException` internally and that the caller is responsible for handling or propagating the exception further.

Using the `throws` keyword allows for more flexibility in exception handling, as it enables exceptions to be handled at higher levels of the program's execution hierarchy, such as in calling methods or in the application's main method. However, it's important for callers of the method to be aware of the exceptions it may throw and handle them appropriately to ensure the robustness and reliability of the program.

Syntax

```
returntype  functionname(parameters list) throws exceptionname
```

Program

```
import java.io.File;
import java.io.FileReader;
import java.io.IOException;
import java.io.BufferedReader;
public class FileReaderExample {
  // Method that declares it can throw IOException
  public void readFile(String fileName) throws IOException {
    File file = new File(fileName);
    try (BufferedReader br = new BufferedReader(new FileReader(file))) {
      String line;
      while ((line = br.readLine()) != null) {
System.out.println(line);
      }
    }
  }
  void main(String[] args) {
FileReaderExample example = new FileReaderExample();
    try {
example.readFile("example.txt"); // Call method that can throw an exception
    } catch (IOException e) {
System.out.println("An  error  occurred  while  reading  the  file:  "  +
e.getMessage()); // Handle the exception
    }
  }
}
example.txt
```

```
Dr. Usharani Bhimavarapu
```
Output:
```
Dr. Usharani Bhimavarapu
```

The method which is calling main method must handle the exceptions. The above program demonstrates reading a file using `BufferedReader`. The `readFile` method reads each line from the file "example.txt" and prints it to the console. If an `IOException` occurs, it is caught and handled by printing an error message.

9.3.1.2 Try-Catch Block

In Java, the try-catch block is used for exception handling. It allows you to catch and handle exceptions that occur during the execution of a block of code. Here's the basic syntax of the try-catch block:

```
try {
  // Code that may throw exceptions
} catch (ExceptionType1 e1) {
  // Code to handle ExceptionType1
} catch (ExceptionType2 e2) {
  // Code to handle ExceptionType2
} catch (ExceptionType3 e3) {
  // Code to handle ExceptionType3
} finally {
  // Optional block that always executes
}
```

Here's what each part of the try-catch block does:

- `try`: The try block contains the code that may throw an exception. If an exception occurs within this block, it is thrown and control is transferred to the appropriate catch block.
- `catch`: The catch block catches and handles the exception. It specifies the type of exception it can handle, denoted by `ExceptionType`. When an exception of the specified type (or one of its subclasses) is thrown within the try block, control is transferred to the corresponding catch block. You can have multiple catch blocks to handle different types of exceptions.
- `finally` (optional): The finally block contains code that is always executed, regardless of whether an exception occurred or not. It is typically used for cleanup code, such as closing resources (e.g., files, database connections) or releasing locks. The finally block is executed even if an exception is thrown and caught, or if the try block completes normally without throwing any exceptions.

Program

```
import java.io.BufferedReader;
import java.io.FileReader;
import java.io.FileNotFoundException;
import java.io.IOException;
public class FileReadExample {
  void main(String[] args) {
BufferedReader reader = null;
    try {
      // Attempt to open and read from the file
```

```
      reader = new BufferedReader(new FileReader("test.txt"));
      String line = reader.readLine(); // Read the first line of the file
System.out.println("First line of the file: " + line);
    } catch (FileNotFoundException e) {
      // Handle the case where the file is not found
System.out.println("Error: File not found - " + e.getMessage());
    } catch (IOException e) {
      // Handle other I/O errors
System.out.println("Error: An I/O error occurred - " + e.getMessage());
    } finally {
      // Cleanup code, executed regardless of whether an exception occurred
      try {
        if (reader != null) {
reader.close(); // Close the file reader
        }
      } catch (IOException e) {
System.out.println("Error: Failed to close the file reader - " +
    e.getMessage());
      }
    }
  }
}
test.txt
Dr. Usharani Bhimavarapu
```

Output:

```
First line of the file: Dr. Usharani Bhimavarapu
```

In this example:

- The try block attempts to read the first line of a file named "test.txt". If the file is not found or an IO error occurs during reading, exceptions of type `FileNotFoundException` or `IOException` may be thrown.
- The catch blocks handle these exceptions. The first catch block handles `FileNotFoundException`, while the second catch block handles `IOException`. Each catch block contains code to handle the specific exception, such as printing an error message.
- The finally block contains cleanup code to close the file reader and perform any necessary cleanup tasks. This block is executed regardless of whether an exception occurred or not.

9.3.2 Unchecked Exceptions

Unchecked exceptions, also known as runtime exceptions, are exceptions that occur at runtime during the execution of a program. Unlike checked exceptions, which must be either caught or declared by the method using the `throws` keyword, unchecked exceptions are not required to be caught or declared. Instead, they are typically ignored during compilation time.

Unchecked exceptions often occur due to logic errors or misuse of an API, such as passing null or incorrect arguments to a method, dividing by zero, or accessing an invalid index in an array. These exceptions are not detected by the compiler at compile time, but they can cause the program to terminate abnormally if not handled properly.

Handling unchecked exceptions is important for ensuring the robustness and reliability of Java programs. While they may not be explicitly caught or declared, it's good practice to anticipate and handle potential runtime exceptions to prevent unexpected program behavior or crashes. Table 9.2 tabulates the unchecked exception.

TABLE 9.2
Unchecked exceptions

Name	Description
NullPointerException	When attempting to access an object with a reference variable whose current value is null.
ArrayIndexOutOfBound	When attempting to access an array with an invalid index value i.e. generally beyond the length of the array.
IllegalArgumentException	When a method receives an argument formatted differently than the method expects.
NumberFormatException	When a method that converts a String to a number.
ArithmaticException	Arithmetic error, such as divide-by-zero.

9.3.3 Error

Errors represent severe issues that occur at runtime and typically result in the termination of the program. Unlike exceptions, which can often be caught and handled by the program, errors usually indicate critical problems that cannot be recovered from.

Here are some key points about errors in Java:

- Errors illustrate situations that cannot be handled gracefully and result in program crashes or abnormal termination.
- The Error class is a subclass of the Throwable class, similar to exceptions.
- Examples of errors include OutOfMemoryError, AssertionError, and VirtualMachineError, among others.
- OutOfMemoryError occurs when the Java Virtual Machine (JVM) cannot allocate more memory to create objects, typically due to insufficient heap space.
- AssertionErrors occur when assertions fail, indicating a violation of the program's internal consistency.
- VirtualMachineError represents errors that occur within the Java Virtual Machine itself, such as stack overflow or inability to create a new thread.

Errors are typically not caught or handled by the program because they often indicate severe failures in the runtime environment or in the execution of the program itself. Instead, they signal the need for investigation and resolution at the system level to address underlying issues and ensure the stability and reliability of the application.

9.4 EXCEPTION HANDLING TECHNIQUES

The try-catch block is a fundamental construct in Java used for exception handling.

- The try block contains the code that may potentially throw an exception.
- If an exception occurs within the try block, control is transferred to the catch block.
- The catch block catches the exception and contains code to handle it.
- Each catch block specifies the type of exception it can handle, allowing for different exception handling logic based on the type of exception thrown.
- If no exceptions occur within the try block, the catch block is skipped, and execution continues after the try-catch block.
- The catch block cannot be used without a corresponding try block.

- Additionally, multiple catch blocks can be used to handle different types of exceptions that may occur within the try block.
- The finally block (optional) can be used to execute cleanup code that should be run regardless of whether an exception occurred or not. The finally block is executed even if an exception is caught or if the try block completes normally without throwing any exceptions.

9.4.1 Try Block

- The try block contains a set of statements where an exception may occur during execution.
- It is always followed by one or more catch blocks, which handle the exceptions that occur within the associated try block.
- A try block must be followed by one or more catch blocks or a finally block, or both.
- The catch blocks specify the type of exceptions they can handle and contain code to handle those exceptions.
- If an exception occurs within the try block, control is transferred to the appropriate catch block based on the type of exception thrown.
- If no exceptions occur within the try block, the catch blocks are skipped, and execution continues after the try-catch block.
- The finally block (optional) contains cleanup code that should be executed regardless of whether an exception occurred or not. The finally block is executed even if an exception is caught or if the try block completes normally without throwing any exceptions.

By using the try-catch block, you can gracefully handle exceptions that may occur during the execution of your Java programs, ensuring proper error recovery and robustness.

Syntax

```
try {
  // Code that may throw an exception
} catch (ExceptionType1 e1) {
  // Code to handle ExceptionType1
}
```

9.4.2 The Catch Block

- A catch block handles exceptions that are thrown within the associated try block.
- The catch block must follow the try block, and a single try block can have multiple catch blocks associated with it.
- Each catch block specifies the type of exception it can handle, allowing for different exception handling logic based on the type of exception thrown.
- When an exception occurs within the try block, control is transferred to the corresponding catch block that matches the type of the thrown exception.
- The catch block contains code to handle the exception, such as logging an error message, performing cleanup operations, or taking appropriate corrective actions.

Program

```
public class MultipleCatchExample {
  void main(String[] args) {
```

```
    try {
      int numerator = 100;
      int denominator = 0; // This will cause division by zero
      // Attempt to perform division
      int result = numerator / denominator;
      // Potentially other code that might throw different exceptions
      String[] array = new String[5];
      array[10] = "Out of bounds"; // This will cause
                                   ArrayIndexOutOfBoundsException
    } catch (ArithmeticException e) {
      // Handle division by zero
System.out.println("Error: Division by zero is not allowed.");
    } catch (ArrayIndexOutOfBoundsException e) {
      // Handle array index out of bounds
System.out.println("Error: Array index is out of bounds.");
    } catch (Exception e) {
      // Handle any other exceptions
System.out.println("An unexpected error occurred: " + e.getMessage());
    } finally {
      // Code that will always be executed
System.out.println("This will always be executed.");
    }
  }
}
```

Output:

```
Error: Division by zero is not allowed.
This will always be executed.
```

The above program illustrates multiple `catch` blocks to handle different types of exceptions. A division by zero is attempted, triggering an `ArithmeticException`, and an array access is performed that would result in an `ArrayIndexOutOfBoundsException`. If any other exceptions occur, they are caught in the generic `Exception` block. The `finally` block ensures that a message is printed regardless of whether an exception occurs.

By using multiple catch blocks with different exception types, you can handle various types of exceptions in a more granular and specific manner, improving the robustness and reliability of your Java programs.

9.4.2.1 Multi-Catch Block

In Java, the multi-catch block allows a programmer to handle multiple types of exceptions in a single catch block. This is useful when the programmer needs to perform similar tasks or logic for different types of exeptions. Here's the syntax of the multi-catch block:

```
try {
  // Code that may throw exceptions
} catch (ExceptionType1 | ExceptionType2 | ExceptionType3 e) {
  // Handle all listed exceptions
}
```

In this syntax:

- The `|` (pipe) symbol is used to separate multiple exception types in the catch block.
- When an exception occurs within the try block, if it matches any of the specified exception types in the multi-catch block, control is transferred to the catch block, and the appropriate exception variable (`e` in this case) is initialized with the caught exception.

- The catch block contains code to handle the caught exceptions, which can be the same for all specified exception types or can vary based on the specific exception type.

Program

```
import java.io.FileNotFoundException;
import java.io.FileReader;
import java.io.IOException;
public class MultiCatchExample {
  void main(String[] args) {
    try {
FileReader file = new FileReader("nonexistentfile.txt");
      // Code that might throw exceptions
    } catch (FileNotFoundException | ArithmeticException e) {
      // Handle both FileNotFoundException and IOException
System.out.println("An error occurred: " + e.getMessage());
    } finally {
      // Code that will always be executed
System.out.println("Execution completed.");
    }
  }
}
Output:
Execution completed.
```

In the above program, the catch block handles both `FileNotFoundException` and `ArithmeticException` exceptions. The same error-handling logic is applied for both types of exceptions, such as printing an error message. Using the multi-catch block can help simplify exception handling code and make it more concise, especially when dealing with multiple related exception types that require similar handling.

NOTE: The exception types specified in the multi-catch block must be disjoint, meaning they cannot have a common subclass.

Program

```
Program for Handling multiple exceptions using single catch statement
import java.io.FileReader;
import java.io.IOException;
public class MultiCatchExample {
  void main(String[] args) {
    try {
      // Attempting to perform division
      int result = divide(10, 0); // This will throw ArithmeticException
      // Attempting to read from a file
FileReader file = new FileReader("nonexistentfile.txt"); // This might throw
FileNotFoundException
      int data = file.read(); // This might throw IOException
System.out.println("Data read: " + data);
    } catch (ArithmeticException | IOException e) {
      // Handle both ArithmeticException and IOException
System.out.println("Error: " + e.getMessage());
    } finally {
```

```
      // Cleanup code that always executes
System.out.println("Execution completed.");
    }
  }
  // Method to perform division
  public static int divide(int a, int b) {
    return a / b; // This can throw ArithmeticException if b is zero
  }
}
```

Output:

```
Error: / by zero
Execution completed.
```

In the above program, a division by zero is attempted, leading to an `ArithmeticException`. Additionally, an attempt is made to read from a nonexistent file, which may result in a `FileNotFoundException` or `IOException` being triggered. Both exceptions are handled together in a multi-catch block, printing the error message. The `finally` block ensures that the cleanup code is always executed. The `divide` method is responsible for performing the division, which may throw an `ArithmeticException`.

9.4.3 The Finally Block

- A finally block contains a set of statements that will always execute, regardless of whether an exception occurs within the associated try block or not.
- The statements within the finally block are guaranteed to be executed, even if an exception is thrown and caught, or if the try block completes normally without throwing any exceptions.
- The finally block is typically used for cleanup code, such as closing resources like connections, streams, or releasing locks, that should be executed regardless of the outcome of the try block.
- If a try block is followed by a catch block, the finally block executes after the catch block, once the catch block's code has completed execution.
- If a try block is not followed by a catch block (i.e., if there is only a finally block), the finally block executes after the try block's code has completed execution, regardless of whether an exception occurred.
- The finally block is optional, and it can be used in conjunction with a try-catch block or independently.

By using the finally block, you can ensure that critical cleanup tasks are performed reliably, even in the presence of exceptions, improving the robustness and reliability of your Java programs.

Syntax

```
try {
  // Code that may throw exceptions
} catch (ExceptionType1 e1) {
  // Code to handle ExceptionType1
} catch (ExceptionType2 e2) {
  // Code to handle ExceptionType2
} finally {
  // Code that always executes, regardless of exceptions
}
```

In Java, the `try-catch-finally` syntax is used to handle exceptions that may occur during program execution. The `try` block contains the code that might throw exceptions, allowing it to be monitored for errors. If an exception occurs, the `catch` blocks handle specific types of exceptions, such as `ExceptionType1` or `ExceptionType2`. Each `catch` block contains code that responds to a particular exception type. For example, if an exception of type `ExceptionType1` is thrown, the corresponding `catch` block executes. Following the `catch` blocks, the `finally` block contains code that will always run, regardless of whether an exception was thrown or not. This is useful for tasks like cleaning up resources or closing files to ensure the system operates smoothly.

Program

```
public class DivisionByZeroExample {
  void main(String[] args) {
    int numerator = 10;
    int denominator = 0;
    try {
      // Attempt to divide by zero
      int result = numerator / denominator;
System.out.println("Result: " + result);
    } catch (ArithmeticException e) {
      // Handle division by zero exception
System.out.println("Exception caught: Division by zero is not allowed.");
    } finally {
      // Cleanup code, executed regardless of exception
System.out.println("Finally block executed: Cleaning up resources.");
    }
  }
}
Output:
Exception caught: Division by zero is not allowed.
Finally block executed: Cleaning up resources.
```

The above program demonstrates handling a division by zero error. The `try` block attempts to divide a numerator by a denominator, but since the denominator is zero, an `ArithmeticException` is thrown. The `catch` block catches this exception and displays an error message, indicating that division by zero is not allowed. Regardless of whether an exception occurs, the `finally` block always executes, which in this case prints a message about resource cleanup.

The finally block gets executed after executing the catch block.

- The finally block is indeed optional, but if it's present, it will execute whether an exception occurs or not.
- For each try block, there can only be one finally block. This ensures that cleanup code is executed exactly once after the try block completes, regardless of whether an exception occurs.
- If an exception occurs and is caught by a catch block, the finally block will be executed after the catch block completes its execution.
- If no exception occurs within the try block, the finally block will still be executed after the try block completes its execution.
- The finally block is commonly used for cleanup tasks such as closing resources (e.g., files, database connections) or releasing locks, ensuring that these tasks are performed reliably even in the presence of exceptions.

By adhering to these rules, Java developers can ensure proper exception handling and resource management in their programs, leading to more robust and reliable software.

Note: It is a good practice to use the finally block because it includes cleanup codes

Program

```
Program for not executing the finally block
public class FinallyBlockExample {
  void main(String[] args) {
    try {
System.out.println("inside try");
      // Terminate the JVM
System.exit(0);
    } catch (Exception e) {
System.out.println("In catch block.");
    } finally {
      // This block will not be executed
System.out.println("In finally block.");
    }
  }
}
Output:
inside try
```

In the above Java program, the main method demonstrates the behavior of the try-catch-finally blocks when System.exit(0) is called within the try block.Inside the try block, "inside try" is printed, indicating the start of execution within the try block. The System.exit(0) statement is then executed, which immediately terminates the Java Virtual Machine (JVM) with a status code of 0. Since the JVM is terminated, the catch block is skipped entirely, and the finally block is also not executed. As a result, "inside finally block" is not printed because the finally block is not reached due to the JVM termination.

9.4.4 Java Throw

- The throw keyword in Java is used to explicitly throw a single exception.
- When an exception is thrown using the throw keyword, the normal flow of the program is disrupted, and the control is transferred to the nearest catch block that can handle the thrown exception.
- This allows for the deliberate triggering of exceptions based on certain conditions or criteria within the program.
- The throw statement can be used to throw any exception object, including predefined exceptions provided by Java or custom exceptions defined by the programmer.

By using the throw keyword, developers can control the flow of their programs and handle exceptional conditions in a structured and predictable manner, improving the robustness and reliability of their Java applications.

Syntax

```
throw exceptionname;
```

Program

```
public class FinallyBlockExample {
  void main(String[] args) {
    try {
```

```
System.out.println("In try block.");
      // Explicitly throw an ArithmeticException
      throw new ArithmeticException("Explicitly thrown ArithmeticException");
    } catch (ArithmeticException e) {
System.out.println("Caught exception: " + e.getMessage());
    } finally {
      // This block will be executed
System.out.println("In finally block.");
    }
  }
}
```

Output

```
In try block.
Caught exception: Explicitly thrown ArithmeticException
In finally block.
```

The above program demonstrates the use of the `finally` block in exception handling. Inside the `try` block, an `ArithmeticException` is explicitly thrown. The `catch` block handles this exception, printing the message associated with the exception. Regardless of the exception, the `finally` block is executed, ensuring that certain cleanup actions or code run after the try-catch block. In this case, it prints a message indicating that the `finally` block has been executed.

9.4.5 Java Throws Keyword

- The throws keyword is used in method declarations to indicate the types of exceptions that the method might throw during its execution.
- It is followed by a list of exception types separated by commas.
- By declaring the exceptions that a method may throw using the throws keyword, the method signature provides information to callers about the potential exceptions that they need to handle or propagate.
- If a method declares that it throws a checked exception using the throws keyword, the calling code must handle the exception by using a try-catch block or propagate it by declaring the exception in its own throws clause.

Using the throws keyword helps to document the exception behavior of methods and promotes better error handling and propagation in Java programs.

Syntax

```
returnTypemethodName(parameters) throws ExceptionType1, ExceptionType2 {
  // Method body
}
```

Program

```
import java.io.FileInputStream;
import java.io.FileNotFoundException;
import java.io.IOException;
public class ExceptionDemo {
  // Method that specifies it might throw IOException
  public static void fun() throws IOException {
FileInputStreamfis = null;
```

```
    try {
fis = new FileInputStream("test.txt");
      // Perform file operations
    } catch (FileNotFoundException e) {
System.out.println("File not found: " + e.getMessage());
      // Handle the FileNotFoundException specifically
    } finally {
      if (fis != null) {
        try {
fis.close(); // Ensure the file is closed properly
        } catch (IOException e) {
System.out.println("Error closing the file: " + e.getMessage());
        }
      }
    }
  }
  void main(String[] args) {
    try {
      fun(); // Call the method that may throw IOException
    } catch (IOException e) {
System.out.println("IOException caught in main: " + e.getMessage());
      // Handle the IOException from fun() method
    }
  }
}
```

In the above program, if the file test.txt does not exist, FileInputStream throws a FileNotFoundException which extends the IOExceptionclass.The fun() method specifies that an IOException can be thrown. The main() method calls this method and handles the exception if it is thrown. If a method does not handle exceptions, the type of exceptions that may occur within it must be specified in the throws clause.

9.5 USER-DEFINED EXCEPTION

In Java, programmers can create their own exception classes to represent specific types of errors or exceptional conditions that may occur within their applications. These custom exceptions are known as user-defined or custom exceptions.

To create a custom exception class, developers typically extend one of the existing exception classes provided by Java, such as Exception or RuntimeException. They can then add custom behavior or properties to the exception class as needed.

Once the custom exception class is defined, developers can throw instances of this exception using the throw keyword, just like any other exception. This allows them to handle specific error scenarios in their code and provide meaningful error messages or context to the caller.

By creating custom exceptions, developers can improve the clarity and maintainability of their code by clearly defining and handling different types of exceptional conditions that may arise during program execution. This promotes better error-handling practices and helps to make Java applications more robust and reliable.

Syntax

```
// Define a custom checked exception by extending Exception
public class CustomException extends Exception {
```

```
  // Constructor with no arguments
  public CustomException() {
    super();
  }
  // Constructor that accepts a message
  public CustomException(String message) {
    super(message);
  }
  // Constructor that accepts a message and a cause
  public CustomException(String message, Throwable cause) {
    super(message, cause);
  }
  // Constructor that accepts a cause
  public CustomException(Throwable cause) {
    super(cause);
  }
}
```

While creating a user-defined exception class, it needs to be extended from Java. lang.Exception. The above syntax defines a custom-checked exception in Java by extending the `Exception` class. The class `CustomException` provides four constructors, each serving a different purpose:

1. Default Constructor: `public CustomException()` calls the parent class's constructor without any arguments, creating a generic exception with no specific message or cause.
2. Constructor with Message: `public CustomException(String message)` allows a custom message to be passed, which can describe the error more clearly.
3. Constructor with Message and Cause: `public CustomException(String message, Throwable cause)` allows passing both a custom message and the underlying cause of the exception, providing more context about what caused the exception.
4. Constructor with Cause: `public CustomException(Throwable cause)` allows passing only the cause of the exception, which might be another exception that triggered this custom exception.

Program

```
// Custom exception class
class TestException extends Exception {
  private int statusCode; // Field to store status code
  // Constructor to initialize status code
  public TestException(int statusCode) {
this.statusCode = statusCode;
  }
  // Overridden toString() method to provide custom output
  @Override
  public String toString() {
    return "Custom Exception with status code: " + statusCode;
  }
}
// Main class to demonstrate exception handling
public class Main {
  void main(String[] args) {
    try {
      // Throwing an instance of custom exception with status code 400
      throw new TestException(400);
```

```
    } catch (TestException e) {
      // Catching the custom exception and printing status code
System.out.println(e.toString());
    }
  }
}
```

Output:

```
Custom Exception with status code: 400
```

The above demonstrates the use of a custom exception class, `TestException`, which includes a status code field. The custom exception's constructor initializes this status code. The `toString()` method is overridden to return a custom message, including the status code. In the main class, an instance of `TestException` is thrown with a status code of 400. The `catch` block catches the exception and prints the custom message provided by the `toString()` method.

Program

```
// Custom exception class
class TestException extends Exception {
  // Constructor that accepts a string message
  public TestException(String message) {
    super(message); // Pass the message to the superclass constructor
  }
}
// Sample class with a method that throws the custom exception
class Sample {
  // Method that throws TestException if the input number is invalid
  public void check(int n) throws TestException {
    if (n <= 0 || n > 99) {
      throw new TestException("Invalid number"); // Throw custom exception
                                                    with a message
    }
    // Optionally, add other logic here
  }
}
// Main class to demonstrate exception handling
public class Main {
  void main(String[] args) {
    Sample sample = new Sample();
    try {
      // Calling the check method with a valid number (90)
sample.check(90);
System.out.println("Number is valid"); // Message indicating valid number
    } catch (TestException e) {
      // Handle the custom exception
System.out.println("Exception handled");
System.out.println("Error message: " + e.getMessage());
// Print the message from the exception
    }
  }
}
```

Output:

```
Number is valid
```

The above program defines a custom exception class, `TestException`, which accepts a string message during initialization. The `Sample` class contains a method, `check()`, that throws a `TestException` if the input number is less than or equal to 0 or greater than 99. In the `Main` class, an instance of `Sample` is created, and the `check()` method is called with a valid number (90). If the number is valid, a message indicating this is printed; otherwise, the exception is caught, and the error message is displayed.

Program

```
// Custom exception class
class TestException extends Exception {
  private int e; // Field to store integer value
  // Constructor to initialize field
  public TestException(int n1) {
this.e = n1;
  }
  // Overridden toString() method
  @Override
  public String toString() {
    return "Value of e (" + e + ") is less than 10";
  }
}
// Sample class with static method
class Sample {
  // Static method that throws TestException if n2 is less than 10
  public static void sum(int n1, int n2) throws TestException {
    if (n2 < 10) {
      throw new TestException(n2); // Throw custom exception with n2 as
                                   parameter
    } else {
      // Print the sum if n2 is not less than 10
System.out.println("Sum: " + (n1 + n2));
    }
  }
}
// Main class to demonstrate exception handling
public class Main {
  void main(String[] args) {
    try {
      // Calling sum method with arguments -5 and 4
      Sample.sum(-5, 4);
    } catch (TestException e) {
      // Handle the custom exception
System.out.println("Exception caught: " + e);
    }
  }
}
Output:
Exception caught: Value of e (4) is less than 10
```

The above program defines a custom exception class, `TestException`, which stores an integer value and overrides the `toString()` method to provide a specific error message. The `Sample` class contains a static method, `sum()`, that throws a `TestException` if the second parameter (`n2`) is less than 10. If `n2` is 10 or greater, it calculates and prints the sum of `n1` and `n2`. In the `Main` class, the `sum()` method is called with the arguments -5 and 4, triggering the exception since 4 is less than 10. The exception is caught in the `try-catch` block, and the custom error message is printed.

Program

```
// Custom exception class
class TestException extends Exception {
  // Constructor that initializes the exception message
  public TestException(String message) {
    super(message); // Pass the message to the superclass constructor
  }
}
// Sample class with a static method
class Sample {
  // Static method that checks if id exists in the array
  public static void fun(int[] a, int id) throws TestException {
boolean found = false;
    for (int num : a) {
      if (num == id) {
        found = true;
        break;
      }
    }
    if (!found) {
      // Throw custom exception if id is not found
      throw new TestException("num is not Valid!");
    } else {
      // Print message if id is found
System.out.println("num is Valid!");
    }
  }
  // Main method to demonstrate exception handling
  void main(String[] args) {
    int[] array = {1, 2, 3, 4, 5, 6}; // Array containing integers 1
through 6
    int id = 8; // ID to search for
    try {
      // Call the fun method with the array and id
Sample.fun(array, id);
    } catch (TestException e) {
      // Handle the custom exception and print its message
System.out.println("Exception caught: " + e.getMessage());
    }
  }
}
```

Output:

```
Exception caught: num is not Valid!
```

This program defines a custom exception class, `TestException`, which is initialized with an error message passed to its constructor. The `Sample` class contains a static method, `fun()`, that checks if a specified `id` exists within an integer array. It iterates through the array, and if the `id` is not found, it throws a `TestException` with the message "num is not Valid!" If the `id` is found, it prints "num is Valid!" In the `main` method, an array of integers is defined, and the `fun()` method is called with an `id` of 8, which is not present in the array. The exception is caught in the `try-catch` block, and the custom error message is printed, demonstrating effective error handling for invalid input.

Program

```
Example of User defined exception in Java
// Custom exception class
class MyException extends Exception {
  // Constructor to initialize the exception message
  public MyException(String message) {
    super(message); // Pass the message to the superclass constructor
  }
  // Override the toString() method to provide a custom string representation
  @Override
  public String toString() {
    return "Custom Exception: " + getMessage();
  }
}
// Main class to demonstrate exception handling
public class Main {
  void main(String[] args) {
    try {
      // Throwing an instance of MyException with a custom message
      throw new MyException("This is a custom exception message.");
    } catch (MyException e) {
      // Catching the custom exception and printing it
System.out.println(e); // Calls e.toString() implicitly
    }
  }
}
Output:
Custom Exception: This is a custom exception message.
```

The above code defines a custom exception class MyException that extends Exception. This class has a constructor to initialize the exception message and overrides the toString method to provide a custom string representation of the exception. The main method throws an instance of MyException with the message "This is a custom exception message."The thrown exception is caught using a catch block that handles MyException objects. Inside the catch block, the exception is printed using System.out.println(e).

9.6 NESTED TRY

Using nested `try-catch` blocks in Java is a technique to handle multiple layers of exceptions, where an exception caught in an inner block can be handled separately from exceptions caught in an outer block. This structure allows for more granular error handling and can be useful in complex operations where different types of errors need distinct handling strategies.

Benefits of Nested Try-Catch Blocks

- Granular Error Handling
  Allows different types of exceptions to be handled at different levels of the code. This means you can handle specific exceptions close to where they occur and more general exceptions at a higher level.
- Specific Error Recovery
  Enables recovery from specific exceptions without interrupting the overall program flow. For example, you can attempt an alternative operation if a particular exception occurs.

- Code Clarity and Maintainability
  Helps in organizing complex error-handling logic, making the code easier to read and maintain. By separating concerns, you avoid having a single, large `try-catch` block that handles multiple types of exceptions in one place.
- Readability
  While nested `try-catch` blocks can improve error handling specificity, they can also make the code harder to read if overused or nested too deeply. It's important to balance the depth of nesting with readability.
- Exception Propagation
  Exceptions not caught by an inner `catch` block will propagate to the outer `try-catch` block. Ensure that exceptions are either handled appropriately at the level they occur or allowed to propagate intentionally.
- Resource Management
  Properly manage resources within nested `try-catch` blocks. Use `finally` blocks or try-with-resources statements to ensure resources are closed properly, even when exceptions occur.

9.6.1 Outer Try-Catch Block

The outer `try` block encompasses a larger section of code or multiple operations that might throw exceptions. The outer `catch` block catches any exceptions that are not handled by the inner `catch` blocks or exceptions thrown by the inner `catch` blocks themselves.

Program

```
Program for nested try ,exception is caught  in outer catch block
public class NestedTryCatchExample {
  void main(String[] args) {
    try {
      // Outer try block
      int[] a = new int[1]; // Array with one element
      try {
        // Inner try block
        int result = a[1] / 0; // Attempt to access array out of bounds and
                                  divide by zero
      } catch (ArrayIndexOutOfBoundsException e) {
        // Inner catch block for ArrayIndexOutOfBoundsException
System.out.println("array out of bounds error");
      }
    } catch (ArithmeticException e) {
      // Outer catch block for ArithmeticException
System.out.println("division by zero error");
    }
  }
}
Output:
array out of bounds error
```

In this program, a nested try-catch structure is used to handle multiple exceptions. The outer try block initializes an integer array with one element, and the inner try block attempts to access an out-of-bounds index and perform a division by zero. When the out-of-bounds access occurs, it triggers an `ArrayIndexOutOfBoundsException`, which is caught by the inner catch block, printing "array out of bounds error." The outer catch block is designed to catch `ArithmeticException`, but in this case, it is not executed because the inner exception is handled first. The program demonstrates how nested try-catch blocks can effectively manage different levels of error handling. Since no arithmetic exception occurs, only the message from the inner catch block is displayed.

Program

```
public class NestedTryCatchExample {
  void main(String[] args) {
    try {
      // Outer try block
System.out.println("Outer try block started.");
      // Array with one element
      int[] a = new int[1];
      try {
        // Inner try block
        // Attempt to access array out of bounds and divide by zero
System.out.println("Inner try block started.");
        // This line will throw ArrayIndexOutOfBoundsException
        int value = a[1];
        // This line will throw ArithmeticException
        int result = value / 0;
      } catch (ArrayIndexOutOfBoundsException e) {
        // Inner catch block
System.out.println("Caught ArrayIndexOutOfBoundsException: " +
   e.getMessage());
      }
      // Additional statement in the outer try block
System.out.println("Statement after inner try-catch.");
    } catch (ArithmeticException e) {
      // Outer catch block
System.out.println("Caught ArithmeticException: " + e.getMessage());
    } catch (Exception e) {
      // Generic catch block for any other exceptions
System.out.println("Caught Exception: " + e.getMessage());
    } finally {
      // Finally block always executes
System.out.println("Finally block executed.");
    }
  }
}
```

Output:

```
Outer try block started.
Inner try block started.
Caught ArrayIndexOutOfBoundsException: Index 1 out of bounds for length 1
Statement after inner try-catch.
Finally block executed.
```

In the above program, a nested try-catch structure is implemented to handle exceptions arising from array access and arithmetic operations. The outer try block begins by printing a message and initializing an array with a single element. Inside the inner try block, the program attempts to access an out-of-bounds index, which triggers an `ArrayIndexOutOfBoundsException`. This exception is caught in the inner catch block, which prints an appropriate message. Following this, the program executes an additional statement in the outer try block. If any `ArithmeticException` occurs, it is caught by the outer catch block, while a generic catch block handles any other exceptions. The finally block executes regardless of whether an exception occurred, ensuring that cleanup or final statements are always run.

9.6.2 Inner Try-Catch Block

The inner `try` block is nested within the outer `try` block and surrounds specific operations that might throw exceptions. The inner `catch` block handles exceptions that occur within the inner `try` block, allowing for targeted error handling specific to that segment of code.

Program

```
Program for nested try ,exception  caught in inner catch block
public class NestedTryCatchFinallyExample {
  void main(String[] args) {
    try {
      // Outer try block
System.out.println("outer try block");
      // Array with one element
      int[] a = new int[1];
System.out.println("Value of a[0]: " + a[0]);
      try {
        // Nested try block
System.out.println("nested try block");
        // This will throw ArithmeticException
        int result = a[0] / 0;
      } catch (ArithmeticException e) {
        // Inner catch block
System.out.println("exception caught inside nested catch");
System.out.println("division by zero error");
      } finally {
        // Inner finally block
System.out.println("nested finally block");
      }
    } catch (ArrayIndexOutOfBoundsException e) {
      // Outer catch block
System.out.println("exception caught inside outer catch");
System.out.println("array out of bound error");
    } finally {
      // Outer finally block
System.out.println("outer finally block");
    }
  }
}
Output:
outer try block
Value of a[0]: 0
nested try block
exception caught inside nested catch
division by zero error
nested finally block
outer finally block
```

The above Java program illustrates the usage of nested try-catch-finally blocks for exception handling. The outer try block contains the main logic, where an array with one element is initialized. Within this block, "outer try block" is printed, followed by accessing and printing the value of a[0]. Inside the outer try block, there's a nested try block. "nested try block" is printed before an attempt to perform an invalid division operation a[0]/0. If an ArithmeticException occurs within the nested try block, it's caught by the inner catch block, which prints "exception caught inside nested catch" followed by "division by zero error". The inner finally block executes regardless of whether an exception occurs, printing "nested finally block". If an ArrayIndexOutOfBoundsException occurs in the outer try block, it's caught by the outer catch block, which prints "exception caught inside outer catch" followed by "array out of bound error". The outer finally block executes after the outer try block or catch block, printing "outer finally block".

9.7 RETURN STATEMENT IN EXCEPTION HANDLING

Using a `return` statement in either a `catch` or `finally` block in Java can significantly impact the control flow of your program.

9.7.1 Return in a Catch Block

When a `return` statement is used within a `catch` block, the method exits immediately after handling the exception. However, before the method returns, the `finally` block (if present) is executed. This approach allows the method to handle exceptions and provide a return value based on the error condition. The `catch` block thus serves to catch specific exceptions, perform necessary actions (such as logging or cleanup), and then return a value indicative of the error condition.

Program

```
Program for catch with return statement
public class Test {
  void main(String[] args) {
    // Create an instance of the Test class
    Test test = new Test();
    // Invoke the display method and store the returned value
    int i = test.display();
    // Print the returned value
System.out.println("i value is " + i);
  }
  public int display() {
    try {
      // Print message inside the try block
System.out.println("inside try block");
      // Attempt to perform division by zero, which will cause
      ArithmeticException
      int result = 10 / 0;
      return 1; // This line will not be executed due to the exception
    } catch (ArithmeticException e) {
      // Catch block for handling ArithmeticException
System.out.println("inside exception block");
      return 2; // Return value if an exception occurs
    } finally {
      // Finally block that will always execute
System.out.println("finally block");
    }
```

```
  }
}
```

Output:

```
inside try block
inside exception block
finally block
i value is 2
```

The above Java program demonstrates the behavior of the try-catch-finally blocks and return statements within a method. The display method attempts to perform a division operation (10/0) inside the try block. "inside try block" is printed before the division operation is attempted. Since division by zero results in an ArithmeticException, the catch block is executed. "inside exception block" is printed, and the method returns 2. Regardless of whether an exception occurs or not, the finally block is always executed. "finally block" is printed. In the main method, an instance of the test class is created, and the display method is invoked. The returned value (2) is stored in the variable i, and "i value is 2" is printed.

9.7.2 Return in a Finally Block

Using a `return` statement within a `finally` block is more complex and often not recommended. The reason is that it can override any return value from the `try` or `catch` blocks, making the code harder to understand and maintain. When a `return` statement is present in the `finally` block, it will override any return value that was set in the `try` or `catch` blocks, effectively making it the final return value of the method. This behavior can lead to unexpected results and can make debugging more difficult, as the final outcome is determined by the `finally` block regardless of the logic in the `try` or `catch` blocks.

Program

```
Program for finally with return statement
public class Test {
  void main(String[] args) {
    // Create an instance of the Test class
    Test test = new Test();
    // Invoke the display method and store the returned value
    int i = test.display();
    // Print the returned value
System.out.println("i value is " + i);
  }
  public int display() {
    try {
      // Print message inside the try block
System.out.println("inside try block");
      // Attempt to perform division by zero, which will cause
ArithmeticException
      int result = 10 / 0;
      return 1; // This line will not be executed due to the exception
    } catch (ArithmeticException e) {
      // Catch block for handling ArithmeticException
System.out.println("inside exception block");
      return 2; // Return value if an exception occurs
    } finally {
      // Finally block that will always execute
System.out.println("finally block");
      // Return value from finally block
```

```
        return 3; // This will override any return value from try or catch
      }
    }
}
```

Output:

```
inside try block
inside exception block
finally block
i value is 3
```

In this Java program, the display method demonstrates the behavior of try-catch-finally blocks with return statements. Inside the try block, "inside try block" is printed, followed by an attempt to perform an invalid division operation (10/0).Since division by zero throws an ArithmeticException, the catch block is executed. "inside exception block" is printed, and the method returns 2. The finally block is always executed regardless of whether an exception occurs. "finally block" is printed, and the method returns 3. In the main method, an instance of the test class is created, and the display method is invoked. The returned value (3) is stored in the variable i, and "i value is 3" is printed.

9.8 CALL STACK

In Java programming, using `try-catch-finally` blocks is a fundamental approach to managing exceptions and ensuring the robustness of code. Within this structure, the `catch` block is responsible for handling exceptions that occur in the `try` block, while the `finally` block is used to execute code that must run regardless of whether an exception was thrown or not, such as releasing resources.

When it comes to throwing exceptions within these blocks, developers have the flexibility to rethrow the caught exception or throw a new one. In the `catch` block, rethrowing the exception can be useful for passing the exception up the call stack after logging it or performing specific error-handling actions. This approach ensures that the exception is not silently ignored and can be dealt with at a higher level if necessary. For example:

```
try {
  // Code that may throw an exception
} catch (Exception e) {
  // Handle the exception
  // Rethrow the exception
  throw e;
}
```

In the `finally` block, although it is less common, throwing an exception is also possible. However, doing so should be approached with caution, as it can obscure exceptions thrown in the `try` or `catch` blocks, leading to potentially hard-to-debug scenarios. The `finally` block is typically reserved for cleanup code, and throwing exceptions here can disrupt this purpose. For example:

```
try {
  // Code that may throw an exception
} catch (Exception e) {
  // Handle the exception
} finally {
  // Clean up code
  if (someCondition) {
    throw new RuntimeException("Exception in finally");
  }
}
```

While it is technically feasible to throw exceptions from both `catch` and `finally` blocks, it is crucial to carefully consider the implications for program flow and exception visibility, ensuring that error handling remains clear and effective.

The `throw` statement in Java is used to explicitly throw an exception from a method or any block of code. This statement can be used to throw both checked and unchecked exceptions. The `throw` statement allows you to handle error conditions gracefully and control the flow of your program when exceptional conditions arise.

9.8.1 Categories of Exceptions Thrown by the `throw` Statement

9.8.1.1 Throwing Checked Exceptions

Checked exceptions must be handled or declared by the method that throws them. These exceptions are checked at compile time and represent conditions that a reasonable application might want to catch.

Program

```
import java.io.IOException;
class Base {
  void readFile() throws IOException {
    // Simulating an I/O exception
    throw new IOException("File not found");
  }
}
public class Main {
  void main(String[] args) {
    Base base = new Base();
    try {
base.readFile();
    } catch (IOException e) {
System.out.println("Caught an IOException: " + e.getMessage());
    }
  }
}
Output:
Caught an IOException:File not found
```

In the above program, a custom exception handling mechanism is demonstrated using the `IOException`. The `Base` class has a method called `readFile`, which simulates throwing an `IOException` with the message "File not found." In the `Main` class, an instance of `Base` is created, and the `readFile` method is called within a try block. If the `IOException` is thrown, it is caught in the corresponding catch block, which prints a message indicating that the exception was caught along with the error message.

Program

```
Program for throwing checked exception in method and caught in main method.
import java.io.IOException;
public class ExceptionHandlingExample {
  void main(String[] args) {
    try {
```

```
      // Call the display method, which can throw an IOException
      display();
    } catch (IOException e) {
      // Catch block to handle IOException
System.out.println("catched in main method");
    }
  }
  // Method that declares it can throw an IOException
  public static void display() throws IOException {
    // Print message inside the display method
System.out.println("inside display method");
    // Throw an IOException
    throw new IOException("Custom IOException message");
  }
}
```

Output:

```
inside display method
catched in main method
```

The above Java program demonstrates exception handling using a try-catch block. In the main method, the display method is called within a try block. The display method declares that it can throw an IOException. Inside the display method, "inside display method" is printed, followed by throwing an IOException. Since the IOException is thrown, it's caught by the catch block in the main method, which prints "catched in main method".

Program

```
Program for user defined exceptions for checked exceptions
// Custom exception class
class ex extends Exception {
  // Constructor that accepts a string message
  public ex(String message) {
    // Pass the message to the superclass constructor
    super(message);
  }
}
public class Test {
  void main(String[] args) {
    try {
      // Throw an instance of the custom exception with a message
      throw new ex("user defined exception");
    } catch (ex e) {
      // Catch the custom exception
      // Print "Caught" along with the exception message
System.out.println("Caught: " + e.getMessage());
    }
  }
}
```

Output:

```
Caught: user defined exception
```

The above Java program defines a custom exception class ex, which extends exception. The constructor of the ex class takes a string argument and passes it to the superclass constructor using super(s). In the Test class, the main method throws an instance of ex with the message "user defined exception" inside a try block. It catches this exception type using a catch block specified for ex. When caught, it prints "Caught" along with the message associated with the exception using e.getMessage().

9.8.1.2 Throwing Unchecked Exceptions

Unchecked exceptions do not need to be declared or handled. Include runtime exceptions and errors. They represent conditions that typically reflect programming errors, such as logic errors or improper use of an API.

Program

```
class Base {
  void divide(int a, int b) {
    if (b == 0) {
      throw new ArithmeticException("Division by zero");
    }
System.out.println("Result: " + a / b);
  }
}
public class Main {
  void main(String[] args) {
    Base base = new Base();
    try {
base.divide(10, 0);
    } catch (ArithmeticException e) {
System.out.println("Caught an ArithmeticException: " + e.getMessage());
    }
  }
}
Output:
Caught an ArithmeticException: Division by zero
```

In the above program, a custom method for division is defined in the `Base` class. The `divide` method takes two integers as parameters and checks if the denominator (`b`) is zero. If `b` is zero, it throws an `ArithmeticException` with the message "Division by zero." In the `Main` class, an instance of `Base` is created, and the `divide` method is called within a try block with the arguments `10` and `0`. When the division by zero occurs, the exception is caught in the corresponding catch block, which prints a message indicating that the exception was caught along with the error message.

```
unchecked exceptions
```

Program

```
Program for throwing the exception using throw statement
public class ExceptionHandlingExample {
  void main(String[] args) {
    try {
      // Try block where exceptions are anticipated
System.out.println("try block");
      // Throwing a NullPointerException
      String str = null;
str.length(); // This will throw NullPointerException
```

```
    } catch (NullPointerException e) {
      // Catch block to handle NullPointerException
System.out.println("exception caught in catch block");
    }
    // Continue with the rest of the program
System.out.println("Program continues after catch block");
  }
}
```

Output:

```
try block
exception caught in catch block
Program continues after catch block
```

This Java program showcases exception handling through a try-catch block. Within the try block, "try block" is printed, followed by throwing a NullPointerException. The catch block catches this exception type, and "exception caught in catch block" is printed.

Program

```
Program for throwing the object of the exception using throw statement
public class CustomNullPointerExceptionExample {
  void main(String[] args) {
    try {
      // Print message inside the try block
System.out.println("try block");
      // Create and throw a custom NullPointerException with a message
      throw new NullPointerException("Custom NullPointerException message");
    } catch (NullPointerException e) {
      // Catch block to handle NullPointerException
      // Print the exception message
System.out.println(e.getMessage());
    }
  }
}
```

Output:

```
try block
Custom NullPointerException message
```

In the above Java program, a custom NullPointerException is created and thrown explicitly within a try block in the main method. Inside the try block, the message "try block" is printed before the exception is thrown. The catch block then catches the thrown NullPointerException, and its message is printed using e.getMessage().

9.9 EXCEPTION HANDLING IN INHERITANCE

In Java, exception handling in inheritance involves how exceptions are managed in a class hierarchy, particularly when methods are overridden. When overriding methods in a subclass, it's essential to understand the rules regarding the exceptions that these methods can throw. These rules ensure consistency and predictability in exception handling across the hierarchy.

- Checked Exceptions:
  If a superclass method declares a checked exception, the overriding method in the subclass can declare the same exception or its subclass.

The overriding method cannot declare new or broader checked exceptions than those declared by the superclass method.

- Unchecked Exceptions:
  Unchecked exceptions (subclasses of `RuntimeException`) are not subject to these rules and can be declared freely in the subclass methods.
- No Exception Declaration:
  If the superclass method does not declare any exceptions, the subclass overriding method cannot declare any checked exceptions. However, it can declare unchecked exceptions.

Advantages

- Consistency in Exception Handling: Ensuring that overridden methods do not throw broader checked exceptions than the methods they override maintains consistency and predictability.
- Flexibility with Unchecked Exceptions: Since unchecked exceptions are not subject to these rules, they offer more flexibility but should be used judiciously to avoid runtime surprises.
- Encapsulation of Exception Handling: By following these principles, exception handling can be effectively encapsulated and managed within the class hierarchy, leading to more maintainable and robust code.

9.9.1 Checked Exceptions

Checked exceptions in Java enforce strict rules at compile time to ensure they are properly handled or declared. When working with inheritance, the overriding methods in subclasses must adhere to the exception declarations of the superclass methods. This ensures consistency and predictability in how exceptions are managed across the inheritance hierarchy, preserving the robustness and reliability of the code.

Program

Program for parent and child class throwing same exception.

```
import java.io.IOException;
import java.io.IOException;
// Base class
class Base {
  // Method that declares it can throw IOException
  public void msg() throws IOException {
System.out.println("Base class method");
    // Optionally throw IOException here
  }
}
// Child class that overrides the msg method
class Child extends Base {
  // Overriding method that also declares it can throw IOException
  @Override
  public void msg() throws IOException {
System.out.println("Child class method");
    // Optionally throw IOException here
  }
}
public class Test {
  void main(String[] args) {
    Base obj = new Child();
```

```
    try {
      // Call the overridden msg method
      obj.msg();
    } catch (IOException e) {
      // Handle IOException if thrown
System.out.println("Caught in main: " + e.getMessage());
    }
  }
}
```

Output:

```
Child class method
```

In the above Java program, method overriding is demonstrated in inheritance. The base class has a method msg that declares it can throw IOException. The child class overrides the msg method and specifies that it throws IOException as well. This is valid because overridden methods in Java can declare the same exceptions as the parent class method or narrower exceptions. In the main method, an instance of child is created using a base reference, and the overridden msg method is called, printing " Child class method" to the console.

Program

```
Program for child class throwing subtype checked exception of parent class
exception
import java.io.FileNotFoundException;
import java.io.IOException;
// Base class
class Base {
  // Method that declares it can throw IOException
  public void msg() throws IOException {
    System.out.println("Base class method");
    // Optionally throw IOException here
  }
}
// Child class that overrides the msg method
class Child extends Base {
  // Overriding method that throws FileNotFoundException
  @Override
  public void msg() throws FileNotFoundException {
    System.out.println("Child class method");
    // Optionally throw FileNotFoundException here
  }
}
public class Test {
  void main(String[] args) {
    Base obj = new Child();
    try {
      // Call the overridden msg method
      obj.msg();
    } catch (FileNotFoundException e) {
      // Handle FileNotFoundException if thrown
      System.out.println("Caught in main (FileNotFoundException): " +
e.getMessage());
    } catch (IOException e) {
```

```
      // Handle other IOExceptions if thrown
      System.out.println("Caught in main (IOException): " + e.getMessage());
    }
  }
}
```

Output

```
Child class method
```

In the above Java program, method overriding is demonstrated in inheritance. The base class has a method msg that declares it can throw IOException. The child class overrides the msg method and specifies that it throws FileNotFoundException. This is valid because overridden methods in Java can throw fewer or no exceptions compared to the parent class method. In the main method, an instance of child is created using a base reference, and the overridden msg method is called, printing " Child class method" to the console.

Program

```
Program for child class throwing no exception
import java.io.IOException;
// Base class
import java.io.IOException;
class Base {
  // Method that declares it can throw IOException
  public void msg() throws IOException {
    System.out.println("Base class method");
    // Optionally throw IOException here
    // throw new IOException("Base class exception");
  }
}
// Child class that overrides the msg method
class Child extends Base {
  // Overriding method that does not specify any exceptions
  @Override
  public void msg() {
    System.out.println("Child class method");
    // No exception thrown here
  }
}
public class Test {
  void main(String[] args) {
    Base obj = new Child();
    try {
      // Call the overridden msg method
      obj.msg();
    } catch (IOException e) {
      // Handle IOException if thrown
      System.out.println("Caught in main: " + e.getMessage());
    }
  }
}
```

Output:

```
Child class method
```

In the above Java program, method overriding is demonstrated in inheritance. The base class has a method msg that declares it can throw IOException. The child class overrides the msg method without specifying any exceptions. This is allowed since overridden methods in Java can throw fewer or no exceptions compared to the parent class method. In the main method, an instance of child is created using a base reference, and the overridden msg method is called, printing " Child class method " to the console.

Program

```
Program for parent class throwing multiple exceptions & child class throwing
sub class single exception
// Base class
import java.io.FileNotFoundException;
import java.io.IOException;
class Base {
  // Method that declares it can throw IOException and ClassNotFoundException
  public void msg() throws IOException, ClassNotFoundException {
    System.out.println("Base class method");
    // Optionally throw exceptions here
  }
}
// Child class that overrides the msg method
class Child extends Base {
  // Overriding method that declares it can throw FileNotFoundException
  @Override
  public void msg() throws FileNotFoundException {
    System.out.println("Child class method");
    throw new FileNotFoundException("Exception from child class");
  }
}
public class Test {
  void main(String[] args) {
    Base obj = new Child();
    try {
      // Call the overridden msg method
      obj.msg();
    } catch (FileNotFoundException e) {
      // Handle FileNotFoundException if thrown
      System.out.println("Caught in main: " + e.getMessage());
    } catch (IOException e) {
      // Handle IOException if thrown
      System.out.println("Caught in main: " + e.getMessage());
    } catch (ClassNotFoundException e) {
      // Handle ClassNotFoundException if thrown
      System.out.println("Caught in main: " + e.getMessage());
    }
  }
}
Output:
Child class method
Caught in main: Exception from child class
```

The above Java program demonstrates method overriding in inheritance while handling exceptions. The base class has a method msg that declares it can throw IOException and

ClassNotFoundException. The child class overrides the msg method and specifies that it throws FileNotFoundException. This is valid because overridden methods in Java can throw fewer or no exceptions compared to the parent class method, but not more. The main method in the child class creates an instance of child using a base reference and calls the overridden msg method, which outputs " Child class method ".

Program

```
Program for parent class throwing single exception,child class throwing
multiple exceptions(checked exception)
import java.io.FileNotFoundException;
import java.io.IOException;
// Base class
class Base {
  // Method that declares it can throw IOException
  public void msg() throws IOException {
System.out.println("Base class method");
    // Optionally throw IOException here
  }
}
// Child class that overrides the msg method
class Child extends Base {
  //    Overriding    method    that    throws    FileNotFoundException    and
  NumberFormatException
  @Override
  public void msg() throws FileNotFoundException, NumberFormatException {
System.out.println("Child class method");
    // Optionally throw FileNotFoundException and NumberFormatException here
  }
}
public class Test {
  void main(String[] args) {
    Base obj = new Child();
    try {
      // Call the overridden msg method
      obj.msg();
    } catch (IOException e) {
      // Handle IOException if thrown
System.out.println("Caught in main: " + e.getMessage());
    }
  }
}
Output:
Child class method
```

In this program, a base class `Base` defines a method `msg()` that declares it can throw an `IOException`. The `Child` class extends `Base` and overrides the `msg()` method, declaring that it can throw a `FileNotFoundException` (a subclass of `IOException`) and an unchecked `NumberFormatException`. In the `Test` class, an instance of `Child` is assigned to a `Base` reference, and the overridden `msg()` method is called within a try block. If `FileNotFoundException` is thrown, it will be caught by the `IOException` catch block, allowing the program to handle it gracefully. This demonstrates method overriding and the handling of checked exceptions in inheritance.

9.9.2 Unchecked Exception

Unchecked exceptions in Java, which extend RuntimeException, offer more flexibility in inheritance because the Java compiler does not enforce their handling. Subclass methods can freely override methods from the superclass without being constrained by the checked exception rules, allowing for more adaptable and potentially cleaner method signatures. However, the lack of compile-time checks requires careful design and consideration to avoid unexpected runtime errors.

Program

```
Program for parent class throwing unchecked exception child class not
throwing any exception
// Base class
class Base {
  // Method that declares it can throw ArithmeticException
  public void msg() throws ArithmeticException {
System.out.println("Base class method");
    throw new ArithmeticException("Exception from base class");
  }
}
// Child class that overrides the msg method
class Child extends Base {
  // Overriding method does not specify any exceptions
  @Override
  public void msg() {
System.out.println("Child class method");
    // No exception thrown here
  }
}
public class Test {
  void main(String[] args) {
    Base obj = new Child();
    try {
      // Call the overridden msg method
      obj.msg();
    } catch (ArithmeticException e) {
      // Handle ArithmeticException if thrown
System.out.println("Caught in main: " + e.getMessage());
    }
  }
}
Output:
Child class method
```

In the above Java program, method overriding is demonstrated in inheritance. The base class has a method msg that declares it can throw ArithmeticException. The child class overrides the msg method without specifying any exceptions. This is allowed since overridden methods in Java can throw fewer or no exceptions compared to the parent class method. In the main method, an instance of child is created using a base reference, and the overridden msg method is called, printing " Child class method " to the console.

Program

```
Program for child class throwing subtype unchecked exception of parent
class exception
// Base class
class Base {
  // Method that declares it can throw RuntimeException
  public void msg() throws RuntimeException {
System.out.println("Base class method");
    throw new RuntimeException ("RuntimeException from base class");
  }
}
// Child class that overrides the msg method
class Child extends Base {
  // Overriding method that throws NullPointerException
  @Override
  public void msg() {
System.out.println("Child class method");
    throw new NullPointerException("NullPointerException from child class");
  }
}
public class Test {
  void main(String[] args) {
    Base obj = new Child();
    try {
      // Call the overridden msg method
      obj.msg();
    } catch (NullPointerException e) {
      // Handle NullPointerException if thrown
System.out.println("Caught in main: " + e.getMessage());
    } catch (RuntimeException e) {
      // Handle RuntimeException if thrown
System.out.println("Caught in main: " + e.getMessage());
    }
  }
}
Output:
Child class method
Caught in main: NullPointerException from child class
```

The above Java program demonstrates method overriding in inheritance while handling exceptions. The base class has a method msg that declares it can throw RuntimeException. The child class overrides the msg method and specifies that it throws NullPointerException. This is valid because overridden methods in Java can throw fewer or no exceptions compared to the parent class method, but not more. The main method creates an instance of child using a base reference and calls the overridden msg method, which outputs " Child class method ".

Program

```
Program for parent class throwing checked exception child class throwing
unchecked exception
import java.io.IOException;
// Base class
class Base {
```

```
  // Method that declares it can throw a checked exception (IOException)
  public void msg() throws IOException {
System.out.println("Base class method");
    throw new IOException("IOException from base class");
  }
}
// Child class that overrides the msg method
class Child extends Base {
  //Overriding method that throws an unchecked exception (ArithmeticException)
  @Override
  public void msg() {
System.out.println("Child class method");
    throw new ArithmeticException("ArithmeticException from child class");
  }
}
public class Test {
  void main(String[] args) {
    Base obj = new Child();
    try {
      // Call the overridden msg method
      obj.msg();
    } catch (ArithmeticException e) {
      // Handle ArithmeticException if thrown
System.out.println("Caught in main: " + e.getMessage());
    } catch (IOException e) {
      // Handle IOException if thrown
System.out.println("Caught in main: " + e.getMessage());
    }
  }
}
```

Output:

```
Child class method
Caught in main: ArithmeticException from child class
```

The above Java program demonstrates method overriding in inheritance while handling exceptions. The base class has a method msg that declares it can throw IOException. The child class overrides the msg method and specifies that it throws ArithmeticException. This is valid because overridden methods in Java can throw fewer or no exceptions compared to the parent class method, but not more. The main method in the child class creates an instance of child using a base reference and calls the overridden msg method, which outputs "Child".

Program

```
Program for parent class throwing single exception,child class throwing
multiple exceptions(unchecked exception)
import java.io.IOException;
// Base class
class Base {
  // Method that declares it can throw RuntimeException
  public void msg() throws RuntimeException {
System.out.println("Base class method");
    // Optionally throw RuntimeException here
  }
}
```

```
// Child class that overrides the msg method
class Child extends Base {
  // Overriding method that throws unchecked exceptions
  @Override
  public void msg() throws NullPointerException, NumberFormatException {
System.out.println("Child class method");
    // Optionally throw unchecked exceptions here
  }
}
public class Test {
  void main(String[] args) {
    Base obj = new Child();
    try {
      // Call the overridden msg method
      obj.msg();
    } catch (RuntimeException e) {
      // Handle IOException if thrown
System.out.println("Caught in main: " + e.getMessage());
    }
  }
}
```

Output:

```
Child class method
```

In this program, a base class `Base` defines a method `msg()` that declares it can throw an ` 'RuntimeException `. The `Child` class extends `Base` and overrides the `msg()` method, throwing unchecked exceptions (`NullPointerException` and `NumberFormatException`) instead of the checked exception. In the `Test` class, an instance of `Child` is assigned to a `Base` reference. The overridden `msg()` method is invoked within a try block, but since it throws unchecked exceptions, these are not caught by the ` RuntimeException ` catch block. The program illustrates method overriding and the behavior of checked versus unchecked exceptions in inheritance.

Program

```
// Base class
class Base {
  // Method that throws unchecked exceptions
  public void msg() {
    System.out.println("Base class method");
    throw new IllegalArgumentException("Illegal argument exception thrown");
  }
}
// Child class that overrides the msg method
class Child extends Base {
  // Overriding method that can also throw unchecked exceptions
  @Override
  public void msg() {
    System.out.println("Child class method");
    throw new IndexOutOfBoundsException("Index out of bounds exception
    thrown");
  }
}
public class Test {
  void main(String[] args) {
```

```
    Base obj = new Child();
    try {
      // Call the overridden msg method
      obj.msg();
    } catch (IllegalArgumentException e) {
      // Handle exception thrown by the base class
      System.out.println("Caught in main from Base: " + e.getMessage());
    } catch (IndexOutOfBoundsException e) {
      // Handle exception thrown by the child class
      System.out.println("Caught in main from Child: " + e.getMessage());
    }
  }
}
```

Output:

```
Child class method
Caught in main from Child: Index out of bounds exception thrown
```

In this program, the `Base` class has a method `msg()` that throws an `IllegalArgumentException`. The `Child` class overrides this method, throwing an `IndexOutOfBoundsException`. In the `main` method, an instance of `Child` is created, and `msg()` is called. The program handles both exceptions with separate catch blocks. If an `IllegalArgumentException` is thrown, it is caught and printed from the base class. If an `IndexOutOfBoundsException` is thrown, it is caught and printed from the child class, demonstrating how to manage unchecked exceptions in an inheritance hierarchy.

9.9.3 No Exception Declaration

When a superclass method or constructor does not declare any exceptions, it restricts the subclass methods or constructors from declaring new checked exceptions. Subclass methods can still throw unchecked exceptions, but these do not need to be declared. This design choice simplifies the method signature and client code by not requiring explicit handling of exceptions, but it requires careful documentation and handling of potential unchecked exceptions to ensure runtime reliability.

Program

```
Program for parent class method not throwing any exception  but child class
can throw unchecked exception
// Base class
class Base {
  // Method without any declared exceptions
  public void msg() {
System.out.println("Base class method");
  }
}
// Child class that overrides the msg method
class Child extends Base {
  // Overriding method that throws RuntimeException (an unchecked exception)
  @Override
  public void msg() throws RuntimeException {
System.out.println("Child class method");
    // Optionally throw RuntimeException here
  }
}
```

```
public class Test {
  void main(String[] args) {
    Base obj = new Child();
    // Call the overridden msg method
    obj.msg();
  }
}
```

Output:

```
Child class method
```

In the above Java program, method overriding is demonstrated in inheritance. The base class has a method msg without any declared exceptions. The child class overrides the msg method and specifies that it throws RuntimeException. This is valid because overridden methods in Java can throw fewer or no exceptions compared to the parent class method, but not more. In the main method, an instance of child is created using a base reference, and the overridden msg method is called, printing "Child" to the console.

Program

```
Program for parent class throwing (checked &unchecked exception) child does
not throw anything
import java.io.IOException;
class Base {
  // Method that declares it can throw IOException and NumberFormatException
  public void msg() throws IOException, NumberFormatException {
    System.out.println("Base class method");
  }
}
class Child extends Base {
  // Overriding method that does not declare any exceptions
  @Override
  public void msg() {
    System.out.println("Child");
  }
}
public class Test {
  void main(String[] args) {
    Base obj = new Child();
    try {
      // Call the overridden msg method
      obj.msg();
    } catch (IOException e) {
      // Handle IOException if thrown by the Base class
      System.out.println("Caught IOException: " + e.getMessage());
    } catch (NumberFormatException e) {
      // Handle NumberFormatException if thrown
      System.out.println("Caught NumberFormatException: " + e.getMessage());
    }
  }
}
```

Output:

```
Child
```

The above Java program demonstrates method overriding in inheritance while handling exceptions. The base class has a method msg that declares it can throw IOException and NumberFormatException. The child class overrides the msg method without declaring any exceptions. This is valid because overridden methods in Java can throw fewer or no exceptions compared to the parent class method. The main method in the child class creates an instance of child using a base reference and calls the overridden msg method, which outputs "Child".

9.10 EXCEPTION PROPAGATION

Exception propagation in Java refers to the process by which an exception is passed up the call stack from the point where it occurred to higher levels of the program, until it is caught by an appropriate exception handler or causes the program to terminate. This mechanism allows a method to defer the responsibility of handling an exception to its caller, rather than handling it within the method itself.

9.10.1 How Exception Propagation Works

Exception propagation in Java is the mechanism by which an exception is passed from the point where it occurs to higher levels of the call stack until it is caught by an appropriate handler or causes the program to terminate. When an exception is thrown, if the method where it occurred does not handle it with a try-catch block, the exception is passed to the calling method. This calling method can either handle the exception or let it propagate further up the call stack to its caller. This process continues until an exception handler is found or the exception reaches the top of the call stack, typically the `main` method. If no handler is found, the program terminates and the Java runtime system prints the exception's stack trace.

Figure 9.2 illustrates exception propagation.

In this example, `Method3` throws an `ArithmeticException`. Since `Method3` does not catch the exception, it propagates to `Method2`, which also does not handle it. The exception then moves to `Method1`, which similarly does not catch it. Finally, the exception reaches the `main` method, which contains a try-catch block that catches and handles the exception, preventing the program from terminating unexpectedly.

9.10.2 Advantages of Exception Propagation

- Simplifies Error Handling: By allowing exceptions to propagate up the call stack, methods can remain focused on their primary functionality and leave error handling to higher-level methods.
- Promotes Code Reusability: Methods can be reused without needing to include repetitive error-handling code, making the code cleaner and easier to maintain.
- Separation of Concerns: Higher-level methods can take on the responsibility of handling errors in a centralized way, making the error-handling strategy more consistent and manageable.

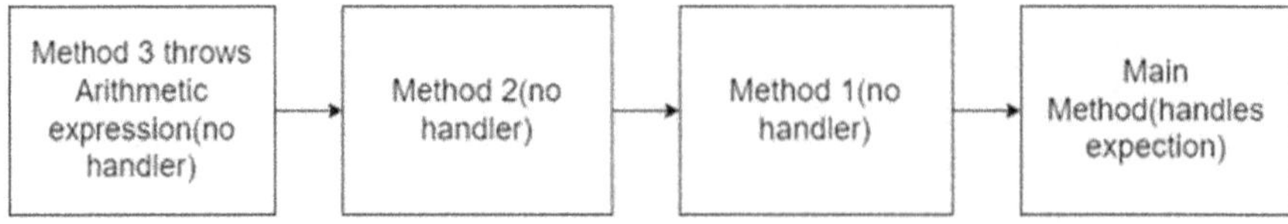

FIGURE 9.2 Exception propagation.

9.10.3 Limitations of Exception Propagation

- Uncaught Exceptions: If no appropriate exception handler is found in the call stack, the program will terminate, which may not be desirable for robust applications.
- Debugging Complexity: Exception propagation can make it harder to trace the origin of an error, especially in large and complex applications with deep call stacks.
- Performance Overhead: Excessive use of exception propagation can lead to performance overhead, as exceptions are computationally expensive.

Program

```
Program for Exception propagation for unchecked exception
public class ExceptionPropagation {
  // Method m3 throws a NullPointerException
  public static void m3() {
System.out.println("Inside m3");
    throw new NullPointerException("Exception from m3");
  }
  // Method m2 calls m3
  public static void m2() {
System.out.println("Inside m2");
    m3();
  }
  // Method m1 calls m2
  public static void m1() {
System.out.println("Inside m1");
    m2();
  }
  void main(String[] args) {
    try {
      // Call m1, which propagates the exception up the call stack
      m1();
    } catch (NullPointerException e) {
      // Handle the exception here
System.out.println("Exception caught in main: " + e.getMessage());
    }
  }
}
Output:
Inside m1
Inside m2
Inside m3
Exception caught in main: Exception from m3
```

The above Java program demonstrates exception propagation and handling. The main method calls m1, which calls m2, which in turn calls m3. The m3 method throws a NullPointerException, which propagates back through m2 and m1 to the main method. The exception is caught in the main method, where a message is printed indicating that the exception has been handled. This process shows how exceptions can be thrown and propagated up the call stack and then managed at a higher level.

Program

```
Program for Exception propagation for checked exception
import java.io.IOException;
public class ExceptionPropagationDemo {
  // Method m3 throws an IOException
  public static void m3() throws IOException {
System.out.println("Inside m3");
    throw new IOException("Exception from m3");
  }
  // Method m2 calls m3
  public static void m2() throws IOException {
System.out.println("Inside m2");
    m3();
  }
  // Method m1 calls m2
  public static void m1() throws IOException {
System.out.println("Inside m1");
    m2();
  }
  void main(String[] args) {
    try {
      // Call m1, which propagates the exception up the call stack
      m1();
    } catch (IOException e) {
      // Handle the exception here
System.out.println("Exception caught in main: " + e.getMessage());
    }
  }
}
Output:
Inside m1
Inside m2
Inside m3
Exception caught in main: Exception from m3
```

The above Java program demonstrates exception propagation and handling. In the test class, the main method calls m1, which calls m2, which in turn calls m3. The m3 method throws an IOException, which is propagated back through m2 and m1 to the main method. The exception is caught in the main method, where a message is printed indicating the exception has been handled.

9.11 RETHROWING EXCEPTIONS

Rethrowing exceptions in Java is useful when a method catches an exception but cannot fully handle it, allowing it to pass the exception up the call stack for higher-level handling. It preserves the original exception's context, aiding in debugging. However, rethrowing can lead to longer call stacks and more complex error handling, making the code harder to maintain if overused.

9.11.1 Rethrowing Predefined Exceptions

Rethrowing predefined exceptions in Java refers to catching an exception within a method, performing some processing or logging, and then throwing the same exception again or throwing a different exception based on the context. This technique is often used to handle exceptions gracefully while providing additional context or information to aid in debugging or error recovery.

Benefits of Rethrowing Predefined Exceptions

- Error Propagation: Rethrowing exceptions allows errors to propagate up the call stack, ensuring that higher-level components or client code can handle or log exceptions appropriately.
- Contextual Information: It enables adding contextual information, such as logging details or custom error messages, before propagating the exception. This helps in diagnosing issues and understanding the cause of the exception.
- Consistent Exception Handling: By rethrowing predefined exceptions, you maintain consistency in error handling across different layers of the application. This promotes cleaner and more maintainable code.
- Exception Wrapping: It allows wrapping checked exceptions into unchecked exceptions or vice versa, depending on the needs of the application or framework being used.

Limitations of Rethrowing Predefined Exceptions

- Loss of Stack Trace: If not handled properly, rethrowing exceptions can lead to loss of valuable stack trace information. This makes it harder to trace the origin and cause of the exception.
- Overhead: Rethrowing exceptions with additional logging or processing can introduce overhead, impacting performance, especially in critical or frequently executed code paths.
- Complexity: Handling and rethrowing exceptions can increase the complexity of code, especially when dealing with multiple exceptions or layers of exception handling.
- Potential for Obscured Errors: Incorrect handling or rethrowing of exceptions can obscure the original error message or cause misleading error handling logic, leading to harder debugging and maintenance.

Program

```
Program for rethrowing same type of exception
public class ExceptionRethrowingDemo {
  // Method that triggers and rethrows an ArithmeticException
  public static void display() {
    try {
System.out.println("Inside display method");
      int result = 10 / 0;  // This will throw ArithmeticException
    } catch (ArithmeticException e) {
System.out.println("Exception caught in display method: " + e.getMessage());
      throw e;  // Rethrow the exception
    }
  }
  void main(String[] args) {
    try {
      // Call display method which will rethrow the exception
      display();
    } catch (ArithmeticException e) {
      // Handle the rethrown exception
System.out.println("Exception caught in main method: " + e.getMessage());
    }
  }
}
```

```
Output:
Inside display method
Exception caught in display method: / by zero
Exception caught in main method: / by zero
```

The above Java program demonstrates rethrowing exceptions within a try-catch block. The main method calls the display method, which deliberately triggers an ArithmeticException by dividing by zero. This exception is caught in the display method, where a message is printed, and then the exception is rethrown. The main method catches the rethrown ArithmeticException and prints a message indicating that the exception was handled. This process shows how an exception can be caught, rethrown, and then handled at a higher level in the program.

Program

```
Program for rethrowing different type of exception
public class ExceptionHandlingDemo {
  // Method that triggers and rethrows an exception as RuntimeException
  public static void display() {
    try {
System.out.println("Inside display method");
      int result = 10 / 0;  // This will throw ArithmeticException
    } catch (ArithmeticException e) {
System.out.println("Exception caught in display method: " + e.getMessage());
      throw new RuntimeException("Exception rethrown as RuntimeException",
      e);  // Rethrow as RuntimeException
    }
  }
  void main(String[] args) {
    try {
      // Call display method which will rethrow the exception as
      RuntimeException
      display();
    } catch (RuntimeException e) {
      // Handle the rethrown RuntimeException
System.out.println("Exception caught in main method: " + e.getMessage());
    }
  }
}
Output:
Inside display method
Exception caught in display method: / by zero
Exception caught in main method: Exception rethrown as RuntimeException
```

The above Java program demonstrates exception handling and rethrowing of exceptions. The `main` method invokes the `display` method, which deliberately triggers an `ArithmeticException` by dividing by zero. This exception is caught within the `display` method, where a message is printed before rethrowing it as a `RuntimeException`. The `main` method then catches this rethrown exception and prints a message indicating it has been handled.

9.11.2 Rethrowing User-Defined Exceptions

Rethrowing user-defined exceptions in Java involves catching a custom exception within a method, performing additional processing or logging, and then throwing the same exception again or throwing a different exception based on the context. This approach allows developers to handle custom exceptions gracefully while providing additional context or information for debugging or error recovery.

Program

```
Program for rethrowing user defined exception
public class CustomExceptionDemo {
  // Define a custom exception as a nested static class
  public static class Ex extends Exception {
    public Ex(String message) {
      super(message);
    }
  }
  // Method that throws an ArithmeticException and rethrows it as custom
exception Ex
  public static void msg() throws Ex {
    try {
System.out.println("Inside msg method");
      int result = 10 / 0;  // This will throw ArithmeticException
    } catch (ArithmeticException e) {
System.out.println("Caught ArithmeticException in msg method");
      throw new Ex("Custom exception after ArithmeticException");
      // Rethrow as custom exception
    }
  }
  void main(String[] args) {
    try {
      // Call the method that throws the custom exception
msg();
    } catch (Ex e) {
      // Handle the custom exception
System.out.println("Caught custom exception: " + e.getMessage());
    }
  }
}
Output:
Inside msg method
Caught ArithmeticException in msg method
Caught custom exception: Custom exception after ArithmeticException
```

The above Java program demonstrates custom exception handling. The `main` method that calls the `msg` method, which intentionally causes an `ArithmeticException` by dividing by zero. This exception is caught and rethrown as a custom exception `ex`, defined as a nested static class extending `Exception`. The `main` method catches this custom exception and prints its message. The program effectively shows how to create and handle user-defined exceptions in Java.

9.12 UNUSED VARIABLES IN TRY CATCH

In Java 22, try-with-resources statements can use unnamed variables (using `_`) for resource specification. This feature allows you to create and use resources without explicitly naming them, which can be particularly useful for concise and readable code.

Program

```
import java.io.BufferedReader;
import java.io.FileReader;
import java.io.IOException;
public class UnnamedVariableInCatchBlock {
  void main(String[] args) {
    try {
BufferedReader reader = new BufferedReader(new FileReader("test.txt"));
      String line;
      while ((line = reader.readLine()) != null) {
System.out.println(line);
      }
    } catch (IOException _) {
System.err.println("Error reading file: File not found or could not be
   read.");
    }
  }
}
test.txt
This is to test
Output
This is to test
```

In the above program, a `BufferedReader` is created to read from a file named "test.txt." The program attempts to read each line of the file within a try block, printing each line to the console. If an `IOException` occurs, such as if the file is not found, the catch block is executed, using an unnamed variable `_` to handle the exception. This approach allows for concise code without the need to name the exception variable explicitly. The program outputs the content of "test.txt," and if an error occurs, it prints an error message. This feature in Java 22 enhances code readability while managing exceptions effectively.

9.13 MEDICAL APPLICATIONS

Medical Application manages a patient database through console input, allowing users to add patients with validated data and search for patients by name, using custom exceptions to handle invalid data scenarios, manages patient records and throws exceptions when operations fail.

9.13.1 Case Study 1

```
Case study-1
import java.util.ArrayList;
import java.util.List;
import java.util.Scanner;
class InvalidPatientDataException extends Exception {
  public InvalidPatientDataException(String message) {
    super(message);
  }
}
class Patient {
  private String name;
  private int age;
```

```
  private String diagnosis;
  public  Patient(String  name,  int  age,  String  diagnosis)  throws
InvalidPatientDataException {
    if (name == null || name.isEmpty() || age <= 0 || diagnosis == null ||
diagnosis.isEmpty()) {
      throw new InvalidPatientDataException("Invalid patient data.");
    }
    this.name = name;
this.age = age;
this.diagnosis = diagnosis;
  }
  @Override
  public String toString() {
    return "Patient{" +
        "name='" + name + '\'' +
        ", age=" + age +
        ", diagnosis='" + diagnosis + '\'' +
        '}';
  }
}
class PatientDatabase {
  private List<Patient> patients;
  public PatientDatabase() {
this.patients = new ArrayList<>();
  }
  public void addPatient(Patient patient) throws InvalidPatientDataException {
    if (patient == null) {
      throw new InvalidPatientDataException("Cannot add a null patient.");
    }
patients.add(patient);
  }
  public   Patient   findPatientByName(String   name)   throws
InvalidPatientDataException {
    for (Patient patient : patients) {
      if (patient.toString().contains(name)) {
        return patient;
      }
    }
    throw new InvalidPatientDataException("Patient not found.");
  }
  @Override
  public String toString() {
    return "PatientDatabase{" +
        "patients=" + patients +
        '}';
  }
}
public class MedicalApplication {
  void main(String[] args) {
PatientDatabase database = new PatientDatabase();
    Scanner scanner = new Scanner(System.in);
    while (true) {
System.out.println("1. Add Patient");
System.out.println("2. Find Patient by Name");
System.out.println("3. Exit");
```

```
System.out.print("Choose an option: ");
     int option = scanner.nextInt();
scanner.nextLine();
     switch (option) {
       case 1:
         try {
System.out.print("Enter name: ");
           String name = scanner.nextLine();
System.out.print("Enter age: ");
           int age = scanner.nextInt();
scanner.nextLine(); // Consume newline
System.out.print("Enter diagnosis: ");
           String diagnosis = scanner.nextLine();
           Patient patient = new Patient(name, age, diagnosis);
database.addPatient(patient);
System.out.println("Patient added successfully.");
         } catch (InvalidPatientDataException e) {
System.out.println("Error: " + e.getMessage());
         }
         break;
       case 2:
         try {
System.out.print("Enter name to search: ");
           String name = scanner.nextLine();
           Patient patient = database.findPatientByName(name);
System.out.println("Patient found: " + patient);
         } catch (InvalidPatientDataException e) {
System.out.println("Error: " + e.getMessage());
         }
         break;
       case 3:
System.out.println("Exiting...");
         return;
       default:
System.out.println("Invalid option. Please try again.");
     }
    }
  }
}
```

The program defines a custom-checked exception `InvalidPatientDataException` to handle invalid patient data entries. The `Patient` class encapsulates patient information such as name, age, and diagnosis, ensuring data validity upon instantiation and throwing exceptions when data is invalid. The `PatientDatabase` class manages a list of patients and provides methods to add a patient (`addPatient`) and find a patient by name (`findPatientByName`). Both methods throw `InvalidPatientDataException` when appropriate conditions are met, such as adding a null patient or when a patient is not found in the database. The `MedicalApplication` class serves as the main application driver, providing a console-based user interface with options to add a patient, find a patient by name, or exit the program. Input validation is implemented using try-catch blocks to handle exceptions thrown during data entry and retrieval operations, ensuring robust error handling and user feedback.

9.13.2 Case Study 2

Psoriasis is a chronic autoimmune condition that causes the rapid buildup of skin cells. This buildup of cells causes scaling on the skin's surface. Inflammation and redness around the scales are fairly common. Typical psoriatic scales are whitish-silver and develop in thick, red patches. The parameters considered in this study are

- **Itchy Scalp**: whether the patient has an itchy scalp.
- **Red Patches**: whether the patient has red patches on their skin.
- **Dry Skin**: whether the patient has dry skin.
- **Joint Pain**: whether the patient has joint pain).

```
import java.util.ArrayList;
import java.util.List;
import java.util.Scanner;
class PsoriasisException extends RuntimeException {
  public PsoriasisException(String message) {
    super(message);
  }
}
class Patient {
  private String name;
  private int age;
  private booleanitchyScalp;
  private booleanredPatches;
  private booleandrySkin;
  private booleanjointPain;
  public Patient(String name, int age, booleanitchyScalp, booleanredPatches,
booleandrySkin, booleanjointPain) {
    if (name == null || name.isEmpty() || age <= 0) {
      throw new PsoriasisException("Invalid patient data.");
    }
    this.name = name;
this.age = age;
this.itchyScalp = itchyScalp;
this.redPatches = redPatches;
this.drySkin = drySkin;
this.jointPain = jointPain;
  }
  public booleanhasPsoriasis() {
    return itchyScalp&&redPatches&&drySkin;
  }
  @Override
  public String toString() {
    return "Patient{" +
        "name='" + name + '\'' +
        ", age=" + age +
        ", itchyScalp=" + itchyScalp +
        ", redPatches=" + redPatches +
        ", drySkin=" + drySkin +
        ", jointPain=" + jointPain +
        '}';
  }
}
```

```
class PatientDatabase {
  private List<Patient> patients;
  public PatientDatabase() {
this.patients = new ArrayList<>();
  }
  public void addPatient(Patient patient) {
    if (patient == null) {
      throw new PsoriasisException("Cannot add a null patient.");
    }
patients.add(patient);
  }
  public Patient findPatientByName(String name) {
    for (Patient patient : patients) {
      if (patient.toString().contains(name)) {
        return patient;
      }
    }
    throw new PsoriasisException("Patient not found.");
  }
  @Override
  public String toString() {
    return "PatientDatabase{" +
       "patients=" + patients +
       '}';
  }
}
public class PsoriasisDetection {
  void main(String[] args) {
PatientDatabase database = new PatientDatabase();
    Scanner scanner = new Scanner(System.in);
    while (true) {
System.out.println("1. Add Patient");
System.out.println("2. Find Patient by Name");
System.out.println("3. Exit");
System.out.print("Choose an option: ");
      int option = scanner.nextInt();
scanner.nextLine();
      switch (option) {
        case 1:
          try {
System.out.print("Enter name: ");
            String name = scanner.nextLine();
System.out.print("Enter age: ");
            int age = scanner.nextInt();
System.out.print("Itchy Scalp (true/false): ");
booleanitchyScalp = scanner.nextBoolean();
System.out.print("Red Patches (true/false): ");
booleanredPatches = scanner.nextBoolean();
System.out.print("Dry Skin (true/false): ");
booleandrySkin = scanner.nextBoolean();
System.out.print("Joint Pain (true/false): ");
booleanjointPain = scanner.nextBoolean();
scanner.nextLine(); // Consume newline
            Patient patient = new Patient(name, age, itchyScalp, redPatches,
drySkin, jointPain);
```

```
database.addPatient(patient);
System.out.println("Patient added successfully.");
        } catch (PsoriasisException e) {
System.out.println("Error: " + e.getMessage());
        }
        break;
      case 2:
        try {
System.out.print("Enter name to search: ");
          String name = scanner.nextLine();
          Patient patient = database.findPatientByName(name);
System.out.println("Patient found: " + patient);
          if (patient.hasPsoriasis()) {
System.out.println("This patient has symptoms of psoriasis.");
          } else {
System.out.println("This patient does not have symptoms of psoriasis.");
          }
        } catch (PsoriasisException e) {
System.out.println("Error: " + e.getMessage());
        }
        break;
      case 3:
System.out.println("Exiting...");
        return;
      default:
System.out.println("Invalid option. Please try again.");
     }
    }
  }
}
```

This, `PsoriasisDetection`, application manages patient data related to psoriasis symptoms using exception handling and user input. It includes a `PsoriasisException` for invalid data, a `Patient` class with attributes for patient details and psoriasis symptoms, and a `PatientDatabase` class to store and retrieve patient records. The main method (`main`) allows users to add patients with their symptoms and retrieve patient details by name. Exception handling ensures robust data validation and error management, enhancing the program's reliability in handling patient data interactions.

10 Multithreading

10.1 INTRODUCTION

A "thread" can be conceptualized as the smallest unit of execution in a computer program. Threads allow for concurrent execution, enabling software to perform multiple tasks simultaneously. The lightweight nature of threads makes them particularly useful for managing parallel processes efficiently.

In the context of server-side programming, threads play a crucial role. Servers often adopt a multi-threaded approach to handle numerous client requests concurrently. This enhances the server's ability to serve multiple clients simultaneously, improving overall system responsiveness.

Java, being a versatile programming language, supports multithreading, a paradigm that involves executing multiple threads concurrently. This capability is leveraged to enhance the performance of applications, especially those with graphics, animations, or other computationally intensive tasks.

In Java, a "single thread" is the most basic unit of processing. It is implemented using the "Thread Class." There are two main types of threads: "user threads" and "daemon threads." User threads are created by the application and continue to run until their assigned task is completed or the application terminates. On the other hand, daemon threads are designed for background tasks, such as application cleanup, and are automatically terminated when no more user threads are running.

Program

```
    void main(String[] args) {
    System.out.println("Single Thread");
  }
Output:
Single Thread
```

The above Java program is a minimalist implementation that serves as an introduction to the structure of a basic Java application. The program is encapsulated within a class named "Main," adhering to Java conventions. The primary entry point for the execution of the program is the `main` method, declared as ` void main(String args[])`. This method is invoked when the program is run and is responsible for initiating the program's execution. Within the `main` method, a single statement is present: `System.out.println("Single Thread");`. This statement utilizes the `System.out.println` method to print the text "Single Thread" to the standard output, typically the console. The `println` method is used for printing a line, and in this context, it outputs the specified message, creating a line break afterward.

DOI: 10.1201/9781003544319-10

Advantages of employing a single thread in Java include reduced overhead in the application and decreased maintenance costs. This simplicity is beneficial for scenarios where parallel execution is not a primary concern.

Java's support for "multithreading" is facilitated through built-in features for creating and managing threads. The language provides a "Thread class," which can be extended to create custom threads, or the "Runnable interface," which defines tasks for threads. Threads are started using the "start()" method, initiating their concurrent execution in the Java Virtual Machine (JVM).

10.2 MULTITHREADING

Multithreading is the concept of executing multiple threads concurrently within a single process. A thread is a lightweight process that can perform a specific task independently. In a multithreaded program, multiple threads run independently and share the same memory space, allowing them to interact and coordinate with each other.

The need for multithreading arises from several factors:

- Improved Performance: Multithreading can enhance the performance of applications by utilizing available CPU resources more efficiently. By running multiple threads concurrently, tasks can be executed in parallel, reducing overall execution time.
- Responsiveness: Multithreading enables responsive user interfaces in applications. Long-running tasks, such as file I/O or network operations, can be executed in background threads, preventing the user interface from becoming unresponsive.
- Concurrency: Multithreading allows applications to handle multiple tasks simultaneously. This is particularly important in applications that require concurrent processing, such as web servers handling multiple client requests simultaneously.
- Resource Utilization: Multithreading allows efficient utilization of system resources, such as CPU cores. By dividing tasks into multiple threads, a multithreaded application can fully utilize available hardware resources.
- Scalability: Multithreading enables applications to scale with increasing workloads. By adding more threads to handle additional tasks, a multithreaded application can accommodate higher levels of concurrency without sacrificing performance.
- Asynchronous Programming: Multithreading facilitates asynchronous programming, where tasks can execute independently of each other and notify the main thread upon completion. This is commonly used in event-driven and reactive programming models.

The importance of multithreading lies in its ability to optimize resource usage, improve performance, and enhance responsiveness in modern software applications. It allows developers to design efficient, scalable, and concurrent systems capable of handling complex tasks effectively.

Program

```
public class Main implements Runnable {

  @Override
  public void run() {
    // The run method is currently empty.
  }
    void main(String[] args) {
    // Create two threads, each associated with the Main class instance.
    Thread t1 = new Thread(new Main(), "usha");
    Thread t2 = new Thread(new Main(), "rani");
```

```
    // Start the threads.
    t1.start();
    t2.start();

    // Print the names of the threads.
    System.out.println("Thread names are following:");
    System.out.println(t1.getName());
    System.out.println(t2.getName());
  }
}
```

Output:

```
Thread names are following:
usha
rani
```

The above Java program illustrates the introduction of multithreading by implementing the `Runnable` interface within the `Main` class. The `Runnable` interface is employed to define a task that can be executed concurrently by multiple threads. However, in this initial example, the `run` method within the `Main` class is currently empty, indicating that specific tasks for the threads are yet to be defined. Within the `main` method, two threads (`t1` and `t2`) are created using the `Thread` class constructor. Each thread is assigned a distinct name, "usha" and "rani," respectively. The `start` method is then invoked on each thread, initiating their concurrent execution. Following the thread starts, we printed the names of the threads using the `getName` method, displaying the assigned names of the threads.

In Java, there are two primary types of threads: "user threads" and "daemon threads." User threads, created by the application, persist until their task is complete or the application terminates. On the contrary, daemon threads are background threads automatically terminated when no more user threads are active. Daemon threads are often utilized for tasks like garbage collection.

Multithreading in Java finds application in scenarios where tasks can be divided into smaller units, allowing for concurrent execution and efficient utilization of the CPU. This concurrency prevents blocking, saves time by performing multiple operations simultaneously, and ensures that exceptions in one thread do not impact others.

The "life cycle of a thread" in Java involves five states: "New," "Runnable," "Running," "Non-Runnable (Blocked)," and "Terminated." These states are managed by the Java Virtual Machine (JVM), with each state representing a different phase in the thread's existence.

Creating a thread in Java can be achieved through two main approaches. The first involves extending the "Thread class" and overriding its "run()" method. The second method involves implementing the "Runnable interface" and passing an instance of the class to the "Thread constructor." Subsequently, the "start()" method is called to commence the execution of the thread, allowing it to run concurrently with other threads in the JVM.

Java's support for multithreading provides developers with the tools to create efficient, concurrent, and responsive applications by managing the execution of multiple threads. This capability is particularly valuable in scenarios such as server-side programming, graphics processing, and other tasks where parallelism enhances overall performance.

10.3 LIFE CYCLE OF THREAD

The life cycle of a thread, controlled by the Java Virtual Machine (JVM), unfolds through a series of distinct states, each marked by specific activities and characteristics.

The life cycle of a thread comprises several stages, as depicted in the diagram:

- New:
  In the initial stage, a thread is created using the "Thread class." It remains in the "New" state until the program initiates the thread. This phase is also known as the birth of the thread.
- Runnable:
  Upon invoking the start method on the instance of the thread, it enters the "Runnable" state. Control is passed to the scheduler, which decides when the thread will be executed. The thread is ready to run, but the actual execution depends on the scheduler's decision.
- Running:
  The "Running" state is reached when the thread starts executing its assigned tasks. The scheduler selects a thread from the pool, and it begins its execution within the application. During this phase, the thread actively contributes to the program's operation.
- Waiting:
  The "Waiting" state occurs when a thread must pause its execution. In situations where multiple threads are running concurrently, synchronization is required between them. Consequently, a thread may need to wait until another thread completes its execution. This state is appropriately termed the "Waiting" state.
- Dead:
  The final stage in the thread's life cycle is the "Dead" state. This occurs when the thread has completed its processing and is terminated. A thread transitions into the "Dead" state from the "Running" state as soon as it finishes its tasks. In this state, the thread has concluded its execution and is no longer active.

10.4 THREAD METHODS

In Java, the Thread class provides several methods for managing and controlling threads. These methods allow developers to create, start, pause, resume, and manipulate threads within a Java program.

10.4.1 START()

This method is used to start the execution of a thread. When called, the run() method of the thread is invoked, and the thread begins execution.

Program

```
public class Main extends Thread {
  @Override
  public void run() {
    // Task to be executed by the thread
    System.out.println("Thread is running...");
  }
    void main(String[] args) {
    // Create an instance of the Main class, which extends Thread
    Main t = new Main();

    // Start the thread
    t.start();
  }
}
Output:
Thread is running...
```

The above Java program exemplifies multithreading by extending the `Thread` class. The `Main` class extends `Thread` and overrides its `run` method, which contains the specific tasks to be executed when the thread runs. In this case, the `run` method prints the message "Thread is running..." In the `main` method, an instance of the `Main` class is created with `Main t = new Main();`, and then the `start` method is called on this instance (`t.start();`). The `start` method initiates the execution of the `run` method in a separate thread of control. Consequently, the output displays the message "Thread is running..." to signify that the thread has started and is executing the tasks specified in the `run` method.

10.4.2 SLEEP(LONG MILLIS)

This method pauses the execution of the current thread for the specified number of milliseconds. It can be used for introducing delays or implementing timeouts in a thread.

Program

```
public class Main extends Thread {
  @Override
  public void run() {
    // Loop to simulate a task with a delay
    for (int i = 1; i <= 4; i++) {
      try {
        // Pause for 500 milliseconds
        Thread.sleep(500);
      } catch (InterruptedException e) {
        e.printStackTrace();
      }
      // Print the current value of i
      System.out.println(i);
    }
  }
    void main(String[] args) {
    // Create an instance of the Main class
    Main t = new Main();

    // Start the thread
    t.start();
  }
}
```

Output:

```
1
2
3
4
```

The above Java program extends the `Thread` class to implement multithreading with a specific task in the overridden `run` method. In this program, the `run` method contains a loop that iterates from 1 to 4. Within each iteration, the thread is programmed to pause for 500 milliseconds using the `Thread.sleep(500)` method. This pause simulates a delay in the execution of each iteration. In the `main` method, an instance of the `Main` class is created with `Main t = new Main();`, and the `start` method is invoked on this instance (`t.start();`). This initiates the concurrent execution of the thread, and the overridden `run` method is executed asynchronously. During execution, the values of i are printed within the loop, separated by 500-millisecond pauses. The output illustrates the interleaved nature of thread execution, showcasing how the main thread and the newly started thread execute concurrently. Due to the sleep intervals, the output displays the values 1 through 4 with a delay between each value.

10.4.3 GET() AND SET()

The getName() method is a method provided by the Thread class in Java, and it is used to retrieve the name of a thread. When you create a thread object, you can optionally assign it a name using the setName() method. Later, you can retrieve this name using the getName() method.

Program

```
public class Main extends Thread {
  @Override
  public void run() {
    // Print the name of the currently executing thread
    System.out.println(Thread.currentThread().getName());
  }
    void main(String[] args) {
    // Create two instances of the Main class
    Main t1 = new Main();
    Main t2 = new Main();

    // Start both threads
    t1.start();
    t2.start();
  }
}
```

Output

```
Thread-1
Thread-2
```

The above Java program extends the `Thread` class to demonstrate multithreading with a focus on retrieving and printing the names of the executing threads. In the `Main` class, the overridden `run` method contains a single line that prints the name of the currently executing thread using `Thread.currentThread().getName()`.In the `main` method, two instances of the `Main` class, namely `t1` and `t2`, are created. These instances represent two separate threads. The `start` method is then invoked on each instance, initiating the concurrent execution of both threads. Upon execution, the names of the concurrently running threads are printed. The `Thread.currentThread().getName()` method retrieves the name of the thread executing the `run` method. Since the `start` method initiates the execution of the `run` method in separate threads, the output displays the names of `t1` and `t2` in an interleaved manner, reflecting the concurrent execution of the two threads.

Program

```
public class Main extends Thread {
  @Override
  public void run() {
    // Print a message to signify thread execution
    System.out.println("running...");
  }
    void main(String[] args) {
```

```
    // Create two instances of the Main class, representing two threads
    Main t1 = new Main();
    Main t2 = new Main();

    // Start both threads
    t1.start();
    t2.start();

    // Print default names of threads before changing them
    System.out.println("Before changing name of t1: " + t1.getName());
    System.out.println("Before changing name of t2: " + t2.getName());
    // Change the names of the threads
    t1.setName("Usha");
    t2.setName("Rani");

    // Print updated names of threads after changing them
    System.out.println("After changing name of t1: " + t1.getName());
    System.out.println("After changing name of t2: " + t2.getName());
  }
}
```

Output:

```
running...
running...
Before changing name of t1: Thread-1
Before changing name of t2: Thread-2
After changing name of t1: Usha
After changing name of t2: Rani
```

The above Java program extends the `Thread` class to demonstrate multithreading with a particular focus on changing and retrieving thread names. The `Main` class contains an overridden `run` method that simply prints the message "running..." to signify the execution of the thread. In the `main` method, two instances of the `Main` class, `t1` and `t2`, are created, representing two separate threads. The `start` method is invoked on each instance, initiating the concurrent execution of both threads. Before altering the thread names, default names of `t1` and `t2` use the `getName()` method. After this, it changes the names of the threads using the `setName` method, assigning "Usha" to `t1` and "Rani" to `t2`. Subsequently, updated names of the threads to reflect the changes made are printed.

10.4.4 YIELD()

The yield() method is a static method of the Thread class in Java. It is a hint to the scheduler that the current thread is willing to yield its current use of the processor. It allows other threads with the same priority to be scheduled for execution.

When a thread calls yield(), it temporarily pauses its execution and gives other threads of the same priority a chance to run. However, there's no guarantee that the scheduler will honor the request. It depends on the underlying operating system and the scheduler implementation. The yield() method is primarily used as a hint to improve the efficiency of the thread scheduling process. It's often used in situations where a thread needs to give other threads a chance to execute when it's performing a long-running or CPU-intensive task.

Program

```
public class Main extends Thread {
  @Override
```

```
  public void run() {
    // Loop to print the name of the currently executing thread
    for (int i = 0; i < 3; i++) {
      System.out.println(Thread.currentThread().getName());
    }
  }
    void main(String[] args) {
    // Create two instances of the Main class, representing two threads
    Main t1 = new Main();
    Main t2 = new Main();

    // Start both threads
    t1.start();
    t2.start();
    // Loop in the main thread
    for (int i = 0; i < 3; i++) {
      // Suggest to the scheduler that the main thread is willing to yield
      Thread.yield();
      System.out.println(Thread.currentThread().getName());
    }
  }
}
```

Output:

```
Thread-0
Thread-0
Thread-0
Thread-1
Thread-1
Thread-1
main
main
main
```

The above Java program extends the `Thread` class to demonstrate multithreading, emphasizing the use of the `yield` method for thread control. The `Main` class contains an overridden `run` method, which executes a loop printing the name of the currently executing thread (retrieved using `Thread.currentThread().getName()`). In the `main` method, two instances of the `Main` class, `t1` and `t2`, are created to represent separate threads. The `start` method is invoked on each instance, initiating concurrent execution. As a result, the `run` method of both threads runs concurrently, producing interleaved output of their names. Within the main thread, another loop is executed, where the `yield` method is called on `t1` during each iteration. The `yield` method suggests to the scheduler that the current thread (in this case, `t1`) is willing to relinquish its current use of the processor, allowing other threads, including the main thread, to potentially run. The output of the program demonstrates the interleaved execution of the two child threads (`t1` and `t2`) and the main thread. The `yield` method introduces a level of cooperative multitasking, allowing the main thread and the child threads to share processor time.

10.4.5 SUSPEND() & RESUME()

- suspend(): This method suspends the execution of the thread on which it is called. When a thread is suspended, it stops executing its code but retains all its resources, including locks on critical sections. This can lead to deadlock situations if the suspended thread holds a lock that another thread needs to proceed. Because of this, using suspend() is strongly discouraged.

- resume(): This method resumes the execution of a thread that has been suspended using the suspend() method. It allows the suspended thread to continue its execution from the point where it was suspended. However, using resume() can also lead to problems such as inconsistent program state and race conditions.
- Both suspend() and resume() are deprecated methods. So users may get warnings while running the below program.

Program

```
public class Main extends Thread {
  private static final int SLEEP_DURATION = 400;
  @Override
  public void run() {
    for (int i = 1; i <= 4; i++) {
      try {
        // Pause the thread for 400 milliseconds
        Thread.sleep(SLEEP_DURATION);
        // Print the current thread name and the loop variable
        System.out.println(Thread.currentThread().getName() + "\n" + i);
      } catch (InterruptedException e) {
        // Handle potential interruption
        e.printStackTrace();
      }
    }
  }
    void main(String[] args) {
    // Create three instances of the Main class, representing three threads
    Main t1 = new Main();
    Main t2 = new Main();
    Main t3 = new Main();

    // Start the three threads
    t1.start();
    t2.start();
    t3.start();
    try {
      // Allow the threads to start and run for a bit
      Thread.sleep(500);
      // Suspend the t2 thread
      t2.suspend();

      // Start the t3 thread (already started but ensuring it runs
      concurrently)
      t3.start();

      // Allow the threads to run for a bit
      Thread.sleep(500);
      // Resume the t2 thread
      t2.resume();
    } catch (InterruptedException e) {
      e.printStackTrace();
    }
  }
}
```

Output:
```
Thread-0
1
Thread-2
1
Thread-1
1
Thread-0
2
Thread-2
2
Thread-1
2
Thread-0
3
Thread-2
3
Thread-1
3
Thread-0
4
Thread-2
4
Thread-1
4
```

The above Java program extends the `Thread` class to showcase multithreading with a focus on thread suspension and resumption. The `Main` class contains an overridden `run` method, which includes a loop that iterates from 1 to 4. Within each iteration, the thread is programmed to pause for 400 milliseconds using the `sleep(400)` method and then prints the name of the currently executing thread along with the loop variable `i`. In the `main` method, three instances of the `Main` class, `t1`, `t2`, and `t3`, are created to represent separate threads. The `start` method is invoked on `t1`, `t2`, and `t3`, initiating concurrent execution. First explicitly suspending the `t2` thread using the `suspend` method, which temporarily halts its execution. Subsequently, the `t3` thread is started, running concurrently with `t1`. Finally, the `t2` thread is resumed using the `resume` method, allowing it to continue its execution.

10.4.6 STOP() AND INTERRUPT()

In Java, `stop()` and `interrupt()` are methods used to manage thread execution, but they serve different purposes and have different implications:

stop()

- The `stop()` method is used to abruptly terminate a thread's execution.
- When `stop()` is called on a thread, it immediately stops executing, and its resources are released.
- This method is considered unsafe and deprecated because it can leave objects in an inconsistent state, potentially leading to data corruption or deadlock.
- Due to its unsafe nature, it's generally recommended to avoid using `stop()` in favor of other thread termination mechanisms.

interrupt()

- The `interrupt()` method is used to interrupt a thread's execution by setting its interrupt status.

- When `interrupt()` is called on a thread, it sets the thread's interrupt status to indicate that it has been interrupted.
- The interrupted thread can periodically check its interrupt status using `Thread.interrupted()` or `isInterrupted()` methods and gracefully terminate its execution.
- Unlike `stop()`, `interrupt()` provides a more controlled way of stopping a thread, allowing it to perform cleanup actions or handle the interruption gracefully.
- It's a safer and more recommended way to manage thread interruption and termination compared to `stop()`.

Program

```
public class Main extends Thread {
  @Override
  public void run() {
    try {
      // Simulate a short delay
      Thread.sleep(100);
      System.out.println("testing");
    } catch (InterruptedException e) {
      // Handle interruption
      throw new RuntimeException("Thread interrupted...", e);
    }
  }
    void main(String[] args) {
    Main t = new Main();
    Main t1 = new Main();
    // Start both threads
    t.start();
    t1.start();
    try {
      // Stop the t1 thread forcefully
      t1.stop();
      System.out.println("Thread t1 is stopped");

      // Interrupt the t thread
      t.interrupt();
    } catch (Exception e) {
      e.printStackTrace();
    }
  }
}
```

Output:

```
Thread t1 is stopped
Exception in thread "Thread-0" java.lang.RuntimeException: Thread
interrupted...java.lang.InterruptedException: sleep interrupted
   at Main.run(Main.java:11)
Caused by: java.lang.InterruptedException: sleep interrupted
   at java.base/java.lang.Thread.sleep(Native Method)
   at Main.run(Main.java:7)
testing
testing
```

In the above program, two threads are created by extending the `Thread` class. The `run` method simulates a short delay with `Thread.sleep(100)` before printing "testing." When both threads start, one thread (`t1`) is forcefully stopped using the `stop` method, which is deprecated due to its unsafe behavior. This action triggers an exception in the second thread (`t`), which is interrupted during its sleep, resulting in a `RuntimeException`. The output indicates that `t1` has been stopped, followed by the exception message from the interrupted thread. This highlights issues related to thread management and the potential risks of using deprecated methods for thread control.

10.4.7 JOIN()

In Java multithreading, the join() method is used to wait for a thread to finish its execution before proceeding with the execution of the current thread. When you call join() on a thread object from another thread, the current thread will pause its execution and wait for the specified thread to complete.

How join() works:

- When you call thread.join(), the current thread (let's call it Thread A) will pause its execution and wait for the thread referenced by thread (let's call it Thread B) to finish its execution.
- Thread A will remain in the waiting state until Thread B terminates.
- Once Thread B completes its execution, Thread A will resume its execution.

The join() method also has overloaded versions that allow you to specify a timeout period for waiting. This is useful when you don't want the current thread to wait indefinitely for the other thread to finish.

Program

```
public class Main extends Thread {
  @Override
  public void run() {
    for (int i = 1; i <= 4; i++) {
      try {
        // Simulate a delay
        Thread.sleep(100);
      } catch (InterruptedException e) {
        e.printStackTrace();
      }
      System.out.println(Thread.currentThread().getName() + " : " + i);
    }
  }
    void main(String[] args) {
    Main t1 = new Main();
    Main t2 = new Main();
    Main t3 = new Main();
    // Start thread t1
    t1.start();
    try {
      // Wait for thread t1 to complete
      t1.join();
    } catch (InterruptedException e) {
      e.printStackTrace();
    }
    // Start threads t2 and t3 after t1 has completed
    t2.start();
    t3.start();
  }
}
```

```
Output:
Thread-0 : 1
Thread-0 : 2
Thread-0 : 3
Thread-0 : 4
Thread-1 : 1
Thread-2 : 1
Thread-1 : 2
Thread-2 : 2
Thread-1 : 3
Thread-2 : 3
Thread-1 : 4
Thread-2 : 4
```

The above Java program extends the `Thread` class and showcases multithreading with a specific focus on using the `join` method for thread synchronization. The `Main` class contains an overridden `run` method, which executes a loop that simulates a delay using `Thread.sleep(100)` and prints the name of the currently executing thread along with the loop variable `i`. In the `main` method, three instances of the `Main` class, `t1`, `t2`, and `t3`, are created to represent separate threads. The `start` method is invoked on `t1`, initiating its execution. Following this, the `join` method on `t1`, which causes the main thread to wait until `t1` completes its execution. This ensures that the subsequent threads (`t2` and `t3`) do not start until `t1` has finished. Upon completion of `t1`, the main thread proceeds to start `t2` and `t3` using the `start` method.

10.5 EXTENDS THREAD CLASS

Creating a thread by extending the Thread class in Java involves a two-step process, offering enhanced flexibility in managing multiple threads.

Step 1: Override the run() Method

In the first step, you create a new class that extends the built-in Thread class. This new class serves as the blueprint for your custom thread. Within this class, you need to override the `run()` method provided by the Thread class. The `run()` method acts as the entry point for the thread, and it is where you encapsulate your complete business logic or the specific tasks you want the thread to execute. The syntax for overriding the `run()` method is as follows:

```
public class MyThread extends Thread {
  @Override
  public void run() {
    // Thread execution logic here
  }
}
```

In the example above, `Main` is the custom class that extends the Thread class, and the `run()` method is overridden to contain the specific operations you want the thread to perform.

Step 2: Start the Thread

Once you have created an object of your custom Thread class (`MyThread` in this case), you can start the thread by calling the `start()` method. The `start()` method is responsible for initiating the execution of the thread, and it internally calls the `run()` method that you have overridden with your custom logic. The syntax for starting the thread is as follows:

```
public class Main {
    void main(String[] args) {
    // Create an instance of MyThread
    MyThread myThread = new MyThread();

    // Start the thread
    myThread.start();
  }
}
```

In the above code, an object of the `MyThread` class is created, and the `start()` method is invoked to initiate the execution of the thread. The thread then begins executing the logic defined in the overridden `run()` method.

Program

```
class Threadtest extends Thread {
  private String tName;
  private Thread t;
  // Constructor
  public Threadtest(String name) {
    this.tName = name;
    System.out.println("Creating " + tName);
  }
  @Override
  public void run() {
    try {
      System.out.println("Running " + tName);
      for (int i = 4; i > 0; i--) {
        System.out.println("Thread: " + tName + ", " + i);
        Thread.sleep(50); // Pause for 50 milliseconds
      }
    } catch (InterruptedException e) {
      System.out.println("Thread " + tName + " interrupted.");
    }
    System.out.println("Thread " + tName + " exiting.");
  }
  @Override
  public void start() {
    System.out.println("Starting " + tName);
    if (t == null) {
      t = new Thread(this, tName);
      t.start();
    }
  }
}
public class Main {
    void main(String[] args) {
    // Creating instances of Threadtest
    Threadtest T1 = new Threadtest("Thread-1");
    Threadtest T2 = new Threadtest("Thread-2");
    // Starting threads
    T1.start();
    T2.start();
```

```
  }
}
```

Output:

```
Creating Thread-1
Creating Thread-2
Starting Thread-1
Running Thread-1
Starting Thread-2
Running Thread-2
Thread: Thread-1, 4
Thread: Thread-2, 4
Thread: Thread-1, 3
Thread: Thread-2, 3
Thread: Thread-1, 2
Thread: Thread-2, 2
Thread: Thread-1, 1
Thread: Thread-2, 1
Thread Thread-2 exiting.
Thread Thread-1 exiting.
```

The above Java program demonstrates multithreading using a custom class `Threadtest` that extends the Thread class. This class defines a thread with specific behavior, and creates two instances of this class to run concurrently. In the `Threadtest` class, the constructor initializes the thread name (`tName`) and prints a message indicating the creation of the thread. The `run` method, which is overridden from the Thread class, contains the specific tasks that the thread will execute. In this case, it prints a countdown from 4 to 1 along with the thread name, pausing for 50 milliseconds between each iteration. If the thread is interrupted due to an exception, a corresponding message is printed. Finally, the thread prints an exit message upon completion. The `start` method is also overridden to customize the thread start process. It prints a message indicating the start of the thread, and if the thread has not been initialized yet (`t == null`), it creates a new Thread object and starts it. In the `Main` class, two instances of `Threadtest` are created: `T1` and `T2`. The `start` method is then called on each, initiating the concurrent execution of both threads.

10.6 CREATING THREAD USING RUNNABLE INTERFACE

Creating a thread by implementing the Runnable interface in Java involves a three-step process, offering a flexible way to define tasks for concurrent execution.

Step 1: Define Task Logic

In the initial step, you need to define the logic of the thread by implementing the `run()` method, which acts as the entry point for the thread. This method encapsulates the complete business logic or tasks that you want the thread to execute. The syntax for defining the `run()` method is as follows:

```
public void run() {
  // Your business logic or tasks go here
}
```

Step 2: Create Thread Object

As the second step, you create an instance of the class that implements the Runnable interface, encapsulating the logic of the thread. You then instantiate a Thread object using the provided constructor:

```
Thread myThread = new Thread(myRunnableObject, "ThreadName");
```

Here, `myRunnableObject` is an instance of the class implementing the Runnable interface, and "ThreadName" is the name assigned to the new thread.

Step 3: Start the Thread

The final step involves starting the thread by invoking the `start()` method on the Thread object. This method initiates the execution of the thread and internally calls the `run()` method with the defined logic. The syntax for starting the thread is as follows:

myThread.start();

The process involves defining the task logic within the `run()` method, creating a Thread object by associating it with an instance of the class implementing the Runnable interface, and starting the thread using the `start()` method. This approach provides a versatile way to handle concurrent tasks in Java.

Program

```
class Runnabletest implements Runnable {
  private String tName;
  private Thread t;
  // Constructor
  public Runnabletest(String name) {
    this.tName = name;
    System.out.println("Creating " + tName);
  }
  @Override
  public void run() {
    try {
      System.out.println("Running " + tName);
      for (int i = 4; i > 0; i--) {
        System.out.println("Thread: " + tName + ", " + i);
        Thread.sleep(50); // Pause for 50 milliseconds
      }
    } catch (InterruptedException e) {
      System.out.println("Thread " + tName + " interrupted.");
    }
    System.out.println("Thread " + tName + " exiting.");
  }
  // Start the thread
  public void start() {
    System.out.println("Starting " + tName);
    if (t == null) {
      t = new Thread(this, tName);
      t.start();
    }
  }
}
public class Main {
    void main(String[] args) {
    // Creating instances of Runnabletest
    Runnabletest T1 = new Runnabletest("Thread-1");
    Runnabletest T2 = new Runnabletest("Thread-2");
    // Starting threads
    T1.start();
```

```
    T2.start();
  }
}
```

Output:

```
Creating Thread-1
Starting Thread-1
Creating Thread-2
Starting Thread-2
Running Thread-1
Running Thread-2
Thread: Thread-1, 4
Thread: Thread-2, 4
Thread: Thread-1, 3
Thread: Thread-2, 3
Thread: Thread-1, 2
Thread: Thread-2, 2
Thread: Thread-1, 1
Thread: Thread-2, 1
Thread Thread-2 exiting.
Thread Thread-1 exiting.
```

The above Java program exemplifies multithreading by implementing the `Runnable` interface within the `Runnabletest` class. This class encapsulates the logic of a thread, and the program creates two instances of this class to demonstrate concurrent execution. In the `Runnabletest` class, a constructor initializes the thread name (`tName`) and outputs a message indicating the creation of the thread. The `run` method, required by the `Runnable` interface, contains the specific tasks that the thread will execute. In this case, print a countdown from 4 to 1 along with the thread name, introducing a 50-millisecond pause between each iteration. If an interruption occurs due to an exception, a corresponding message is printed. Finally, the thread outputs an exit message upon completion. The `start` method is overridden to customize the thread start process. Later prints a message indicating the start of the thread, and if the thread has not been initialized yet (`t == null`), it creates a new Thread object and starts it. In the `Main` class, two instances of `Runnabletest` are created: `T1` and `T2`. The `start` method is then called on each, initiating the concurrent execution of both threads.

10.7 THREAD PRIORITIES

Thread priorities play a crucial role in Java concurrency, aiding the operating system in deciding the sequencing of thread scheduling. The priority range for Java threads spans from MIN_PRIORITY (1) to MAX_PRIORITY (10), where the default priority for every thread is set to NORM_PRIORITY (5). In essence, priorities signify the significance of a thread within a program's execution. Threads assigned higher priorities take precedence over lower-priority counterparts, indicating their increased importance in the execution flow. However, it's essential to note that the use of thread priorities doesn't provide a strict guarantee of the execution order, as it is heavily influenced by the underlying platform. Consequently, the prioritization mechanism is platform-dependent, and the same set of priorities might exhibit different behaviors on different systems.

The default priority for a Java thread is set to 5. This default priority is used when a new thread is created. The thread priorities in Java are in the range between `MIN_PRIORITY`, which is a constant with a value of 1, and `MAX_PRIORITY`, another constant with a value of 10.

The three constants defined in the `Thread` class are:

- `public static int NORM_PRIORITY`: This constant represents the normal priority level, which is typically assigned to threads that do not have any specific priority requirements. Its value is set to 5.

- `public static int MIN_PRIORITY`: This constant represents the minimum priority level that a thread can have. Its value is set to 1.
- `public static int MAX_PRIORITY`: This constant represents the maximum priority level that a thread can have. Its value is set to 10.

These constants provide a convenient way to set and compare thread priorities in a Java program. Thread priorities are used by the thread scheduler to determine the order in which threads are scheduled to run when multiple threads are competing for CPU time.

Program

```
public class RunnableExample implements Runnable {
  @Override
  public void run() {
    // This method is executed in the new thread
    System.out.println("Thread Running");
  }
    void main(String[] args) {
    // Create an instance of RunnableExample
    RunnableExample runnableInstance = new RunnableExample();
    // Create a new Thread object, passing the Runnable instance
    Thread t = new Thread(runnableInstance);
    // Start the thread
    t.start();
    // Print the thread's default priority
    System.out.println("Thread Priority: " + t.getPriority());

    //setting the priority
    t.setPriority(10);
    System.out.println("Thread Priority: " + t.getPriority());
  }
}
```

Output:

```
Thread Priority: 5
Thread Priority: 10
Thread Running
```

The above Java program demonstrates basic multithreading functionality using the `Runnable` interface. The `Main` class implements the `Runnable` interface, requiring the implementation of the `run` method, which, in this case, remains empty. In the `main` method, a new `Thread` object named `t` is instantiated. Then invokes the `start()` method on this thread, initiating the execution of the `run` method in a separate thread. Following the thread start, "Thread Running" is printed to indicate that the thread has begun its execution. Subsequently, the default priority of the thread using `t.getPriority()` was retrieved and displayed. By default, the thread inherits the priority of the parent thread, which is usually set to the default priority value, often `NORM_PRIORITY` (5).

10.8 SYNCHRONIZATION

In scenarios where multiple threads operate within the same program, there arises the potential for concurrency issues when accessing shared resources concurrently. These issues can lead to unpredictable outcomes, such as data corruption or conflicts when multiple threads attempt to read from or write to the same resource simultaneously. For instance, if multiple threads attempt to write to the same file concurrently, it can result in data corruption as one thread may overwrite the data while another is closing the file.

To address such concerns, synchronization is employed to ensure that only one thread can access a shared resource at any given time. The concept of monitors is utilized for this purpose. In Java, each object is associated with a monitor, and a thread can lock or unlock this monitor. Only one thread is allowed to hold a lock on a monitor at a time.

In Java, the language provides a convenient mechanism for creating threads and synchronizing their tasks through the use of synchronized blocks. Shared resources are encapsulated within these blocks to ensure controlled access. The general syntax of a synchronized statement is as follows:

```
synchronized (objectIdentifier) {
  // Access shared variables and other shared resources
}
```

Here, `objectIdentifier` is a reference to an object, and the lock associated with this object's monitor is acquired by the synchronized statement. To illustrate, consider two examples where a counter is printed using two different threads. In scenarios where threads are not synchronized, the counter values may appear out of sequence. Conversely, when the counter printing is enclosed within a `synchronized()` block, the output showcases the counter values in a well-defined sequence for both threads. This synchronization ensures that access to shared resources is coordinated, preventing inconsistencies and conflicts in a multithreaded environment.

Synchronization in multithreading is employed for two main purposes:

- Preventing Thread Interference:
  Thread interference occurs when multiple threads access shared resources concurrently, leading to potential data corruption or inconsistent results. Synchronization ensures that only one thread can access a shared resource at any given time, preventing conflicts and maintaining data integrity.
- Preventing Consistency Problems:
  In a multithreaded environment, consistency problems can arise when threads perform operations on shared data concurrently. Synchronization mechanisms help in coordinating access to shared resources, ensuring that operations are executed in a well-defined and predictable manner, thereby avoiding inconsistencies.

10.8.1 Types of Synchronization

- Process Synchronization:
  This type of synchronization deals with coordinating the execution of multiple processes. Processes may need synchronization to ensure proper communication and data sharing.
- Thread Synchronization:
  Thread synchronization focuses on coordinating the execution of multiple threads within the same process. It helps manage access to shared resources and maintain consistency.

10.8.2 Thread Synchronization

Thread synchronization involves two main aspects: mutual exclusion and inter-thread communication.

- Mutual exclusion in multithreading ensures that multiple threads do not access shared resources simultaneously, preventing data inconsistency and race conditions. This is typically achieved using synchronization mechanisms like locks or semaphores.

- Cooperation involves communication and coordination between threads. It allows threads to work together by notifying each other about changes in the shared state. This is typically achieved using methods like `wait()`, `notify()`, and `notifyAll()`.

10.9 MUTUAL EXCLUSION

Mutual exclusion ensures that only one thread can access a shared resource at a time. There are several ways to achieve mutual exclusion in Java:

- Synchronized Method: By declaring a method as synchronized, only one thread can execute that method at a time, preventing interference.
- Synchronized Block: A specific block of code can be synchronized using the `synchronized` keyword, ensuring that only one thread at a time can execute that block.
- Static Synchronization: Synchronization can be applied to static methods, preventing multiple threads from concurrentlyexecuting static synchronized methods of the same class.

10.9.1 Synchronized Block

A synchronized block in Java is a code segment that is locked to a specific object, ensuring that only one thread can execute it at a time for that object. This helps in maintaining thread safety when accessing shared resources.

Program

```
class Display {
  // Synchronized method to ensure thread-safe access
  public synchronized void fun() {
    try {
      for (int i = 5; i > 0; i--) {
        System.out.println("value " + i);
        Thread.sleep(100); // Sleep to simulate time-consuming task
      }
    } catch (InterruptedException e) {
      System.out.println("Thread interrupted.");
    }
  }
}
class ThreadTest extends Thread {
  private Display display;
  private String name;
  // Constructor to initialize the Display object and thread name
  public ThreadTest(Display display, String name) {
    this.display = display;
    this.name = name;
  }
  @Override
  public void run() {
    System.out.println("Starting " + name);
    display.fun(); // Call the synchronized method
    System.out.println("Thread " + name + " exiting.");
  }
}
public class Main {
```

```
    void main(String[] args) {
    // Create a shared Display object
    Display d = new Display();
    // Create two ThreadTest instances, both using the same Display object
    ThreadTest t1 = new ThreadTest(d, "Usha");
    ThreadTest t2 = new ThreadTest(d, "Rani");
    // Start both threads
    t1.start();
    t2.start();
    // Wait for both threads to finish
    try {
      t1.join();
      t2.join();
    } catch (InterruptedException e) {
      System.out.println("Main thread interrupted.");
    }
  }
}
```

Output:

```
Starting Usha
Starting Rani
value 5
value 4
value 3
value 2
value 1
value 5
value 4
value 3
value 2
value 1
Thread Rani  exiting.
Thread Usha  exiting.
```

The above Java program demonstrates the concept of synchronization in multithreading using the `synchronized` keyword. It consists of three classes: `display`, `Threadtest`, and `Main`. The `display` class contains a method named `fun()` that is designed to run in a loop, printing values from 5 to 1. However, the method is enclosed within a try-catch block to catch any potential exceptions, with a message printed if a thread is interrupted during its execution. The `Threadtest` class extends the `Thread` class and is designed to work with an instance of the `display` class. It has a `run` method that, when invoked, acquires a lock on the shared `display` object using the `synchronized` keyword and then calls the `fun` method of the `display` object. This ensures that only one thread can execute the `fun` method at a time, preventing potential conflicts or inconsistencies in the output. In `main` method, an instance of the `display` class (`d`) is created. Subsequently, two instances of the `Threadtest` class (`t1` and `t2`) are created, each associated with the same `display` object. Both threads are then started concurrently using the `start` method. During execution, the `synchronized` block ensures that only one thread at a time can execute the `fun` method of the shared `display` object.

10.9.2 Synchronized Method

A synchronized method in Java is a method that locks the object it belongs to, ensuring that only one thread can execute it at a time.

Program

```
class SyncMethod {
  // Synchronized method to ensure thread-safe access
  public synchronized void display(int n) {
    for (int i = 1; i <= n; i++) {
      try {
        // Print the current number along with the thread name
        System.out.println(Thread.currentThread().getName() + " : " + i);
        // Sleep to simulate processing time
        Thread.sleep(100);
      } catch (InterruptedException e) {
        System.out.println("Thread interrupted.");
      }
    }
  }
}
class Sample extends Thread {
  private SyncMethod syncMethod;
  private int n;
  // Constructor to initialize SyncMethod object and integer parameter
  public Sample(SyncMethod syncMethod, int n) {
    this.syncMethod = syncMethod;
    this.n = n;
  }
  @Override
  public void run() {
    syncMethod.display(n); // Call the synchronized method
  }
}
class Test extends Thread {
  private SyncMethod syncMethod;
  private int n;
  // Constructor to initialize SyncMethod object and integer parameter
  public Test(SyncMethod syncMethod, int n) {
    this.syncMethod = syncMethod;
    this.n = n;
  }
  @Override
  public void run() {
    syncMethod.display(n); // Call the synchronized method
  }
}
public class Main {
    void main(String[] args) {
    // Create a shared SyncMethod object
    SyncMethod syncMethod = new SyncMethod();
    // Create two threads, each associated with the shared SyncMethod object
    Sample t1 = new Sample(syncMethod, 5);
    Test t2 = new Test(syncMethod, 5);
    // Start both threads
    t1.start();
    t2.start();
    // Wait for both threads to finish
    try {
```

```
      t1.join();
      t2.join();
    } catch (InterruptedException e) {
      System.out.println("Main thread interrupted.");
    }
  }
}
```

Output:

```
Thread-0 : 1
Thread-0 : 2
Thread-0 : 3
Thread-0 : 4
Thread-0 : 5
Thread-1 : 1
Thread-1 : 2
Thread-1 : 3
Thread-1 : 4
Thread-1 : 5
```

The above Java program demonstrates the concept of synchronization using a synchronized method in a multithreaded environment. We created three classes: `syncmethod`, `Sample`, and `test`, along with the main class `Main`.The `syncmethod` class contains a method named `display`, which is declared as synchronized. This method takes an integer parameter 'n' and executes a loop that prints sequential numbers along with the name of the currently executing thread. Each iteration of the loop includes a delay to simulate some processing time. The `Sample` and `test` classes both extend the `Thread` class and have a reference to an instance of the `syncmethod` class. They are designed to execute the `display` method of the `syncmethod` class with different integer parameters. In the `Main` class, an instance of the `syncmethod` class (`t`) is created. Subsequently, two threads (`t1` and `t2`) are instantiated, each associated with the same instance of `syncmethod`. Both threads are then started concurrently using the `start` method. Because the `display` method of the `syncmethod` class is synchronized, only one thread can execute it at a time. In this case, the `Sample` and `test` threads take turns executing the synchronized method, ensuring that the sequential numbers are printed in an orderly manner. The synchronization prevents interference, ensuring that one thread's execution of the method is completed before another thread begins its execution.

10.9.3 Static Synchronization

When a static method is marked as synchronized, the lock is applied at the class level rather than on individual objects. Consider the scenario where there are two instances of a shared class, such as object1 and object2. In the case of synchronized methods or synchronized blocks, interference between threads like t1 and t2 or t3 and t4 is prevented because t1 and t2 both reference a common object, which has a single lock. However, interference can still occur between threads like t1 and t3 or t2 and t4, as t1 acquires one lock and t3 acquires another, and the same applies to t2 and t4. To avoid interference between t1 and t3 or t2 and t4, static synchronization is employed. In static synchronization, the lock is applied at the class level, ensuring that only one thread can access the static synchronized method or block at a time, irrespective of the specific object instance. This helps maintain order and prevent potential conflicts when multiple threads are involved.

Program

```
class Test {
  // Synchronized static method to ensure thread-safe access
```

```
  public synchronized static void display(int n) {
    for (int i = 1; i <= n; i++) {
      try {
        // Print the name of the current thread
        System.out.println(Thread.currentThread().getName());
        // Sleep to simulate processing time
        Thread.sleep(100);
      } catch (InterruptedException e) {
        System.out.println("Thread interrupted.");
      }
    }
  }
}
class Test1 extends Thread {
  private int n;
  // Constructor to initialize the integer parameter
  public Test1(int n) {
    this.n = n;
  }
  @Override
  public void run() {
    Test.display(n); // Call the synchronized static method
  }
}
class Test2 extends Thread {
  private int n;
  // Constructor to initialize the integer parameter
  public Test2(int n) {
    this.n = n;
  }
  @Override
  public void run() {
    Test.display(n); // Call the synchronized static method
  }
}
public class Main {
    void main(String[] args) {
    // Create instances of Test1 and Test2 threads
    Test1 t1 = new Test1(5);
    Test2 t2 = new Test2(5);
    // Start both threads
    t1.start();
    t2.start();
    // Wait for both threads to finish
    try {
      t1.join();
      t2.join();
    } catch (InterruptedException e) {
      System.out.println("Main thread interrupted.");
    }
  }
}
```

Output

```
Thread-0
Thread-0
```

```
Thread-0
Thread-0
Thread-0
Thread-1
Thread-1
Thread-1
Thread-1
Thread-1
```

The above Java program involves a class named `test` that contains a synchronized static method named `display`. This method takes an integer parameter `n` and executes a loop printing the current thread's name for a range of values. Inside the loop, there is a brief pause using the `Thread.sleep(100)` statement. Two additional classes, `test1` and `test2`, extend the `Thread` class. Each of these classes has a `run` method that, when invoked, calls the synchronized `display` method of the `test` class with different integer arguments. In the `Main` class, two instances of `Thread` subclasses (`test1` and `test2`), namely `t1` and `t2`, are created. Subsequently, both threads are started concurrently using the `start` method. As a result, the `display` method in the `test` class is executed by both threads simultaneously. The use of the `synchronized` keyword ensures that only one thread at a time can access the critical section of the `display` method, preventing potential interference and ensuring orderly execution. The output of the program will display the names of the concurrently running threads for the specified range of values within the `display` method.

10.10 INTER-THREAD COMMUNICATION

Inter-thread communication, also known as cooperation, refers to the mechanism that allows synchronized threads to communicate with each other in a multithreaded environment.

Cooperation involves the concept of pausing one thread that is currently executing in its critical section, allowing another thread to enter or lock the same critical section and proceed with its execution. This coordination is crucial for synchronization and ensures that threads can work together effectively without interfering with each other.

In Java, inter-thread communication is implemented using three methods of the Object class:

- wait(): The `wait()` method causes the current thread to wait until another thread invokes the `notify()` or `notifyAll()` methods for the same object. The thread enters a waiting state, and it will remain in this state until it is notified by another thread.
- notify(): The `notify()` method wakes up a single thread that is currently waiting on the monitor of the object. It allows one waiting thread to proceed with its execution.
- notifyAll(): The `notifyAll()` method wakes up all threads that are waiting on the monitor of the object. This ensures that multiple waiting threads are notified and can resume their execution.

These methods provide a powerful means for threads to synchronize their actions and communicate effectively. By using `wait()`, `notify()`, and `notifyAll()` within synchronized blocks, Java programmers can design multithreaded applications that coordinate their activities in a controlled and synchronized manner. Threads in Java can establish communication using the `wait()`, `notify()`, and `notifyAll()` methods. These methods are part of the Object class and are declared as final. They can only be invoked within a synchronized context, ensuring proper coordination between threads. The `wait()` method causes the current thread to enter a waiting state until another thread invokes the `notify()` or `notifyAll()` methods on the same object. When the `notify()` method is called, it wakes up a single thread that is currently waiting on the monitor of that object. On the other hand, the `notifyAll()` method wakes up all threads that are waiting on the same object's monitor. Threads enter a waiting state by calling one of the `wait()` methods. It's important to note that these methods may throw an `IllegalMonitorStateException` if the current thread does not own the monitor of the object.

10.10.1 WAIT()

The `wait()` method instructs the calling thread to release its lock and enter a sleeping state until another thread enters the same monitor and invokes `notify()`. While in the waiting state, the thread surrenders the lock and regains it upon returning from the `wait()` method. It's important to note that the `wait()` method is tightly integrated with the synchronization lock and relies on a native implementation not directly accessible through standard Java mechanisms.

In a synchronized block, the general syntax for using the `wait()` method is as follows:

```
synchronized (lockObject) {
  while (!condition) {
    lockObject.wait();
  }
  // Take appropriate action here;
}
```

10.10.2 NOTIFY()

The `notify()` method wakes up a single thread that had previously called `wait()` on the same object. However, it's crucial to understand that invoking `notify()` doesn't immediately release the lock on the resource. The actual release occurs only after the notifier's synchronized block has completed. If the notifier needs additional time for actions within the block, the waiting thread must patiently wait for the lock to be fully released.

In a synchronized block, the general syntax for using the `notify()` method is as follows:

```
synchronized (lockObject) {
  // Establish the condition;
  lockObject.notify();
  // Additional code if needed;
}
```

10.10.3 NOTIFYALL()

The `notifyAll()` method wakes up all threads that had previously called `wait()` on the same object. While it doesn't guarantee the order of awakening, it typically allows the highest-priority thread to run first. Similar to `notify()`, the lock is released only after the synchronized block's completion.

In a synchronized block, the general syntax for using the `notifyAll()` method is as follows:

```
synchronized (lockObject) {
  // Establish the condition;
  lockObject.notifyAll();
}
```

Program

```
class Test {
  // Volatile variable to ensure visibility of changes across threads
  private volatile boolean b = false;
  // Synchronized method to set the flag and notify the waiting thread
  public synchronized void fun1() {
    b = true;
```

```
    System.out.println("Thread-1");
    notify(); // Notify the waiting thread that the condition has been met
  }
  // Synchronized method to wait until the flag is set to true
  public synchronized void fun2() {
    while (!b) {
      try {
        wait(); // Wait until notified
      } catch (InterruptedException e) {
        System.out.println("Thread interrupted.");
      }
    }
    System.out.println("Thread-0");
  }
}
class Test1 extends Thread {
  private Test t;
  // Constructor to initialize the Test object
  public Test1(Test t) {
    this.t = t;
  }
  @Override
  public void run() {
    t.fun1(); // Call the fun1 method
  }
}
class Test2 extends Thread {
  private Test t;
  // Constructor to initialize the Test object
  public Test2(Test t) {
    this.t = t;
  }
  @Override
  public void run() {
    t.fun2(); // Call the fun2 method
  }
}
public class Main {
    void main(String[] args) {
    Test t = new Test(); // Create an instance of the Test class
    Test1 t1 = new Test1(t); // Create a thread to call fun1
    Test2 t2 = new Test2(t); // Create a thread to call fun2
    t2.start(); // Start the thread that calls fun2
    t1.start(); // Start the thread that calls fun1
    // Wait for both threads to finish
    try {
      t1.join();
      t2.join();
    } catch (InterruptedException e) {
      System.out.println("Main thread interrupted.");
    }
  }
}
```

Output

```
Thread-1
Thread-0
```

The above Java program demonstrates the use of synchronization, particularly the `wait()` and `notify()` methods, to achieve communication and coordination between two threads. The program defines a class named `test`, which contains two synchronized methods, `fun1` and `fun2`, and a volatile boolean variable `b`. In the `fun1` method, the boolean variable `b` is set to `true`, and a notification is sent using the `notify()` method. This method is intended to be called by one thread to signal that a specific condition has been met. On the other hand, the `fun2` method is designed to run in another thread. It enters a synchronized block and checks the value of the boolean variable `b`. If the condition is not met (i.e., `b` is `false`), the thread enters a waiting state using the `wait()` method. This waiting state is maintained until the `fun1` method is called, setting `b` to `true` and notifying the waiting thread to resume execution.In the `Main` class, an instance of the `test` class (`t`) is created. Two threads (`t1` and `t2`) are then instantiated, with `t1` invoking the `fun1` method and `t2` invoking the `fun2` method. The order of thread execution is controlled by the `start` method. When the program is executed, the `t2` thread starts executing the `fun2` method and enters a waiting state. Subsequently, the `t1` thread executes the `fun1` method, sets the value of `b` to `true`, and notifies the waiting thread. This causes the `t2` thread to wake up and resume its execution of the `fun2` method.

10.11 STRUCTURED CONCURRENCY

Structured Concurrency, introduced in Java 22, addresses several critical needs in concurrent programming, aiming to simplify development, enhance code reliability, and improve resource management.

10.11.1 Needs for Structured Concurrency

- Simplified Error Handling: Traditional concurrent programming often leads to complex error-handling scenarios, such as thread leaks or incomplete resource cleanup. Structured Concurrency provides a unified approach to managing errors within concurrent tasks, making it easier to handle exceptions and ensure proper cleanup of resources.
- Enhanced Task Coordination: Coordinating tasks in traditional concurrent programming can be challenging, leading to issues like race conditions or deadlock. Structured Concurrency introduces constructs that facilitate task coordination, such as scoped lifetimes and cancellation propagation, ensuring more predictable and manageable task execution.
- Improved Resource Management: Managing resources effectively across multiple concurrent tasks is crucial for application performance and stability. Structured Concurrency promotes better resource management practices by automatically cleaning up resources associated with tasks when they complete or are canceled, reducing memory leaks and improving system reliability.
- Promotion of Best Practices: By enforcing structured approaches to concurrent programming, Structured Concurrency encourages developers to follow best practices consistently. This includes using scoped lifetimes for resources, handling cancellation gracefully, and ensuring tasks complete their execution cleanly, contributing to robust and maintainable codebases.
- Support for Modern Application Requirements: Modern applications often require handling numerous concurrent tasks, such as in web servers, real-time analytics, and event-driven architectures. Structured Concurrency equips developers with tools to manage these complexities efficiently while maintaining code clarity and reducing the risk of errors.

Program

```
import java.util.concurrent.*;
public class StructuredConcurrencyExample {
    void main(String[] args) {
```

```
    ExecutorService executor = Executors.newFixedThreadPool(2);
    try {
      CompletableFuture<Void> task1 = CompletableFuture.runAsync(() -> {
        System.out.println("Task 1: Performing some computation...");
        try {
          Thread.sleep(2000);
        } catch (InterruptedException e) {
          Thread.currentThread().interrupt();
        }
        System.out.println("Task 1: Computation completed.");
      }, executor);
      CompletableFuture<Void> task2 = CompletableFuture.runAsync(() -> {
        System.out.println("Task 2: Performing some computation...");
          try {
          Thread.sleep(3000);
        } catch (InterruptedException e) {
          Thread.currentThread().interrupt();
        }
        System.out.println("Task 2: Computation completed.");
      }, executor);
      CompletableFuture.allOf(task1, task2).join();
    } finally {
      executor.shutdown();
    }
  }
}
```

Output:

```
Task 1: Performing some computation...
Task 2: Performing some computation...
Task 1: Computation completed.
Task 2: Computation completed.
```

In the above program, `CompletableFuture` is used to represent asynchronous tasks (`task1` and `task2`) executed concurrently by an `ExecutorService`. The use of `CompletableFuture` and `ExecutorService` demonstrates structured concurrency principles by managing task execution, ensuring proper resource cleanup (`executor.shutdown()`), and handling exceptions gracefully within the structured environment provided by Java 22.

Program

```
import java.util.Arrays;
import java.util.List;
import java.util.concurrent.CompletableFuture;
import java.util.concurrent.ExecutorService;
import java.util.concurrent.Executors;
import java.util.stream.Collectors;
public class Test {
    void main(String[] args) {
    List<String> urls = Arrays.asList("https://mrcet.com/downloads/digita
l_notes/IT/JAVA%20PROGRAMMING.pdf",  "https://frozennotes.github.io/ICSE_
Resources/ICSE-JavaNotes-V4.7.2.pdf",   "https://mu.ac.in/wp-content/uplo
ads/2022/09/Core-JAVA.pdf");
    // Create a thread pool executor with fixed number of threads
    try (ExecutorService executor = Executors.newFixedThreadPool(3)) {
```

```
      List<CompletableFuture<String>> downloadFutures = urls.stream()
          .map(url -> CompletableFuture.supplyAsync(() -> downloadFile(url),
executor))
          .collect(Collectors.toList());
      CompletableFuture<Void> allDownloads = CompletableFuture.allOf(
          downloadFutures.toArray(new CompletableFuture[0]));
      allDownloads.join();
      // Retrieve results from completed futures
      List<String> downloadedFiles = downloadFutures.stream()
          .map(CompletableFuture::join)
          .collect(Collectors.toList());
           downloadedFiles.forEach(file  ->  System.out.println("Downloaded
file: " + file));
    }
  }
    private static String downloadFile(String url) {
    try {
      Thread.sleep(2000);
    } catch (InterruptedException e) {
      Thread.currentThread().interrupt();
      System.err.println("Thread interrupted while downloading: " + url);
    }
    return "File from " + url;
  }
}
```

Output

```
Downloaded file: File from https://mrcet.com/downloads/digital_notes/IT/
JAVA%20PROGRAMMING.pdf
Downloaded file: File from https://frozennotes.github.io/ICSE_Resources/
ICSE-JavaNotes-V4.7.2.pdf
Downloaded file: File from https://mu.ac.in/wp-content/uploads/2022/09/
Core-JAVA.pdf
```

The above program utilizes a thread pool to concurrently download files from a list of URLs using `CompletableFuture`. Each URL is processed asynchronously, allowing multiple downloads to occur simultaneously, improving efficiency. After all downloads are complete, the results are collected and printed, indicating the successful retrieval of each file.

10.12 SCOPED VALUES

The introduction of Scoped Values in Java 22, as part of Project Loom's ongoing development, addresses several crucial needs in concurrent programming and resource management.

10.12.1 Needs for Scoped Values in Java 22

- Thread-Local Data Management: Traditional Java applications often rely on `ThreadLocal` variables to manage thread-local data. However, managing `ThreadLocal` variables can be error-prone, especially in scenarios involving nested tasks or asynchronous computations. Scoped Values provide a more intuitive and structured approach to managing thread-local data, reducing complexity and potential errors.
- Efficient Context Propagation: In modern applications, propagating context information across asynchronous tasks or threads is essential for maintaining state consistency and ensuring

correct behavior. Scoped Values facilitate efficient and transparent propagation of immutable context data, improving code clarity and reducing the need for explicit parameter passing.
- Concurrency in Microservices and Serverless Architectures: Microservices and serverless applications often handle multiple concurrent requests or events. Scoped Values enable these applications to isolate and manage context data for each request or event efficiently, improving scalability and reducing resource contention.
- Enhanced Resource Sharing: In scenarios where multiple threads or tasks need access to shared, immutable data (such as configuration settings or security credentials), scoped values provide a safe and efficient mechanism for sharing this data across thread boundaries. This reduces the risk of data corruption or unintended modification.
- Support for Reactive Programming: Reactive programming paradigms, which rely heavily on asynchronous and event-driven processing, benefit from scoped values by simplifying the management of reactive state and context across asynchronous boundaries. This improves the robustness and maintainability of reactive applications.

Program

```
import java.util.concurrent.ExecutorService;
import java.util.concurrent.Executors;
class ScopedValue<T> {
  public final T value;
  public ScopedValue(T value) {
    this.value = value;
  }
}
public class ScopedValuesExample {
  public static ScopedValue<String> scopedMessage = new ScopedValue<>("Initial
message");
    void main(String[] args) {
    ExecutorService executor = Executors.newFixedThreadPool(2);
      executor.submit(() -> {
      System.out.println("Parent thread sends: " + scopedMessage.value);
      childThread();
    });
    executor.shutdown();
  }
  private static void childThread() {
    System.out.println("Child thread receives: " + scopedMessage.value);
  }
}
Output:
Parent thread sends: Initial message
Child thread receives: Initial message
```

The above program defines a `ScopedValue` class to hold a value, which is shared between a parent thread and a child thread. A task is submitted using a thread pool that prints a message from the parent thread before `childThread()` is called, which also accesses and prints the same message. The output confirms that both threads can access the shared `scopedMessage`, demonstrating how scoped values can be utilized in concurrent programming.

10.13 MEDICAL APPLICATIONS

10.13.1 Case Study 1

Dengue is a mosquito-borne viral infection that can cause severe flu-like symptoms and potentially lead to serious health complications. The parameters considered for dengue detection are:

- **Fever**: Check whether the patient has a fever.
- **Headache**: Check whether the patient has a headache.
- **Rash**: Check whether the patient has a rash.
- **Joint Pain**: Check whether the patient has joint pain.
- **Nausea**: Check whether the patient experiences nausea.
- **Vomiting**: Check whether the patient experiences vomiting.
- **Positive Test**: Check whether the patient tested positive for dengue.

Program

```
import java.util.ArrayList;
import java.util.List;
import java.util.Scanner;
class DengueRecord {
  private int age;
  private String gender;
  private boolean fever;
  private boolean headache;
  private boolean rash;
  private boolean jointPain;
  private boolean nausea;
  private boolean vomiting;
  private boolean positiveTest;
  public DengueRecord(int age, String gender, boolean fever, boolean head-
ache, boolean rash, boolean jointPain, boolean nausea, boolean vomiting,
boolean positiveTest) {
    this.age = age;
    this.gender = gender;
    this.fever = fever;
    this.headache = headache;
    this.rash = rash;
    this.jointPain = jointPain;
    this.nausea = nausea;
    this.vomiting = vomiting;
    this.positiveTest = positiveTest;
  }
  public boolean isPositiveTest() {
    return positiveTest;
  }
  @Override
  public String toString() {
    return "Age: " + age + ", Gender: " + gender + ", Fever: " + fever + ",
    Headache: " + headache + ", Rash: " + rash + ", Joint Pain: " + jointPain
    + ", Nausea: " + nausea + ", Vomiting: " + vomiting + ", Positive Test: "
    + positiveTest;
  }
}
```

```
class DataCollector implements Runnable {
  private List<DengueRecord> records;
  private Scanner scanner;
  public DataCollector(List<DengueRecord> records, Scanner scanner) {
    this.records = records;
    this.scanner = scanner;
  }
  @Override
  public void run() {
    // Collect data from user input
    synchronized (records) {
      System.out.println("Enter the number of records to input:");
      int numRecords = scanner.nextInt();
      scanner.nextLine();
      for (int i = 0; i < numRecords; i++) {
        System.out.println("Enter details for record " + (i + 1) + ":");
        System.out.print("Age: ");
        int age = scanner.nextInt();
        scanner.nextLine();
        System.out.print("Gender: ");
        String gender = scanner.nextLine();
        System.out.print("Fever (true/false): ");
        boolean fever = scanner.nextBoolean();
        System.out.print("Headache (true/false): ");
        boolean headache = scanner.nextBoolean();
        System.out.print("Rash (true/false): ");
        boolean rash = scanner.nextBoolean();
        System.out.print("Joint Pain (true/false): ");
        boolean jointPain = scanner.nextBoolean();
        System.out.print("Nausea (true/false): ");
        boolean nausea = scanner.nextBoolean();
        System.out.print("Vomiting (true/false): ");
        boolean vomiting = scanner.nextBoolean();
        System.out.print("Positive Test (true/false): ");
        boolean positiveTest = scanner.nextBoolean();
        scanner.nextLine();
        records.add(new DengueRecord(age, gender, fever, headache, rash,
        jointPain, nausea, vomiting, positiveTest));
      }
      System.out.println("Data collection complete.");
    }
  }
}
class Analyzer implements Runnable {
  private List<DengueRecord> records;
  public Analyzer(List<DengueRecord> records) {
    this.records = records;  }
  @Override
  public void run() {
    // Analyze data
    synchronized (records) {
      try {
        Thread.sleep(2000); // Simulate delay in data processing
        int positiveCount = 0;
        for (DengueRecord record : records) {
```

```
        if (record.isPositiveTest()) {
          positiveCount++;
        }
      }
      System.out.println("Data analysis complete. Positive cases: " +
      positiveCount);
    } catch (InterruptedException e) {
      e.printStackTrace();
    }
  }
}
}
public class DengueDetection {
  void main(String[] args) {
  List<DengueRecord> records = new ArrayList<>();
  Scanner scanner = new Scanner(System.in);
  Thread dataCollectorThread = new Thread(new DataCollector(records,
scanner));
  Thread analyzerThread = new Thread(new Analyzer(records));
  dataCollectorThread.start();
  analyzerThread.start();
  try {
    dataCollectorThread.join();
    analyzerThread.join();
  } catch (InterruptedException e) {
    e.printStackTrace();
  }
  System.out.println("Dengue detection process completed.");
  }
}
```

The program defines a `DengueRecord` class to store patient details such as age, gender, and symptoms. The `DataCollector` class implements the `Runnable` interface and collects patient data from user input, adding it to a shared list. The `Analyzer` class, also implementing `Runnable`, processes the collected data to count positive dengue cases. In the `DengueDetection` main class, two threads are created and started: one for data collection and another for data analysis. The threads are synchronized to ensure thread safety during data manipulation.

10.13.2 Case Study 2

Typhoid fever is a bacterial infection caused by the bacterium Salmonella enterica serotype Typhi. It spreads through contaminated food and water and is characterized by symptoms such as prolonged fever, headache, nausea, abdominal pain, and sometimes a rash. Typhoid fever can be serious if not treated promptly with antibiotics. The parameters considered for typhoid fever detection are:

- **Fever**: Check Whether the patient has a fever
- **Headache**: Check Whether the patient has a headache
- **Abdominal Pain**: Check Whether the patient has abdominal pain
- **Diarrhea**: Check Whether the patient has diarrhea
- **Constipation**: Check Whether the patient has constipation
- **Rash**: Check Whether the patient has a rash
- **Positive Test**: Check The result of a typhoid test

Program

```
import java.util.ArrayList;
import java.util.List;
import java.util.Scanner;
class TyphoidFeverRecord {
  private int age;
  private String gender;
  private boolean fever;
  private boolean headache;
  private boolean abdominalPain;
  private boolean diarrhea;
  private boolean constipation;
  private boolean rash;
  private boolean positiveTest;
  public TyphoidFeverRecord(int age, String gender, boolean fever, boolean
headache, boolean abdominalPain, boolean diarrhea, boolean constipation,
boolean rash, boolean positiveTest) {
    this.age = age;
    this.gender = gender;
    this.fever = fever;
    this.headache = headache;
    this.abdominalPain = abdominalPain;
    this.diarrhea = diarrhea;
    this.constipation = constipation;
    this.rash = rash;
    this.positiveTest = positiveTest;
  }
  public boolean isPositiveTest() {
    return positiveTest;
  }
  @Override
  public String toString() {
    return "Age: " + age + ", Gender: " + gender + ", Fever: " + fever +
    ", Headache: " + headache + ", Abdominal Pain: " + abdominalPain + ",
    Diarrhea: " + diarrhea + ", Constipation: " + constipation + ", Rash: "
    + rash + ", Positive Test: " + positiveTest;
  }
}
class DataCollector implements Runnable {
  private final List<TyphoidFeverRecord> records;
  private final Scanner scanner;
  private final Object lock;
  public DataCollector(List<TyphoidFeverRecord> records, Scanner scanner,
Object lock) {
    this.records = records;
    this.scanner = scanner;
    this.lock = lock;
  }
  @Override
  public void run() {
    synchronized (lock) {
      // Collect data from user input
      System.out.println("Enter the number of records to input:");
```

```
      int numRecords = scanner.nextInt();
      scanner.nextLine();
      for (int i = 0; i < numRecords; i++) {
        System.out.println("Enter details for record " + (i + 1) + ":");
        System.out.print("Age: ");
        int age = scanner.nextInt();
        scanner.nextLine();
        System.out.print("Gender: ");
        String gender = scanner.nextLine();
        System.out.print("Fever (true/false): ");
        boolean fever = scanner.nextBoolean();
        System.out.print("Headache (true/false): ");
        boolean headache = scanner.nextBoolean();
        System.out.print("Abdominal Pain (true/false): ");
        boolean abdominalPain = scanner.nextBoolean();
        System.out.print("Diarrhea (true/false): ");
        boolean diarrhea = scanner.nextBoolean();
        System.out.print("Constipation (true/false): ");
        boolean constipation = scanner.nextBoolean();
        System.out.print("Rash (true/false): ");
        boolean rash = scanner.nextBoolean();
        System.out.print("Positive Test (true/false): ");
        boolean positiveTest = scanner.nextBoolean();
        scanner.nextLine();
        records.add(new TyphoidFeverRecord(age, gender, fever, headache,
abdominalPain, diarrhea, constipation, rash, positiveTest));
      }
      System.out.println("Data collection complete.");
      lock.notify();
    }
  }
}
class Analyzer implements Runnable {
  private final List<TyphoidFeverRecord> records;
  private final Object lock;
  public Analyzer(List<TyphoidFeverRecord> records, Object lock) {
    this.records = records;
    this.lock = lock;
  }
  @Override
  public void run() {
    synchronized (lock) {
      try {
        // Wait for the data collection to complete
        lock.wait();
        // Analyze data
        int positiveCount = 0;
        for (TyphoidFeverRecord record : records) {
          if (record.isPositiveTest()) {
            positiveCount++;
          }
        }
        System.out.println("Data analysis complete. Positive cases: " +
        positiveCount);
      } catch (InterruptedException e) {
```

```
        e.printStackTrace();
      }
    }
  }
}
public class TyphoidFeverDetection {
    void main(String[] args) {
    List<TyphoidFeverRecord> records = new ArrayList<>();
    Scanner scanner = new Scanner(System.in);
    Object lock = new Object();
    Thread dataCollectorThread = new Thread(new DataCollector(records,
scanner, lock));
    Thread analyzerThread = new Thread(new Analyzer(records, lock));
    dataCollectorThread.start();
    analyzerThread.start();
    try {
      dataCollectorThread.join();
      analyzerThread.join();
    } catch (InterruptedException e) {
      e.printStackTrace();
    }
    System.out.println("Typhoid fever detection process completed.");
  }
}
```

The `TyphoidFeverRecord` class stores patient data, including symptoms and test results. The `DataCollector` class, running in a separate thread, collects user input to populate the records. The `Analyzer` class, also running in a separate thread, waits for data collection to complete and then analyzes the records to count the number of positive cases. Synchronization is achieved using a shared lock object to ensure thread safety during data collection and analysis.

11 File Handling

11.1 INTRODUCTION

In Java, file handling is a crucial aspect of dealing with data persistence, I/O operations, and communication with external systems. Files in Java can be used to read and write data to various storage mediums such as the local file system, network drives, or databases. The `java.io` and `java.nio` packages provide classes and interfaces for working with files.

Here are some important aspects and functionalities related to files in Java:

1. Reading and Writing Data: Java allows reading data from files using input streams (`FileInputStream`, `BufferedReader`, etc.) and writing data to files using output streams (`FileOutputStream`, `BufferedWriter`, etc.). These streams can be used to read and write different types of data such as text, binary, or serialized objects.
2. File Operations: Java provides classes like `File` and `Path` for working with files and directories. These classes offer methods to perform various file operations such as creating, deleting, renaming, copying, moving files, checking file existence, obtaining file attributes, and navigating directory structures.
3. Serialization: Java Serialization allows converting Java objects into a stream of bytes for storage or transmission. This serialized data can be written to files using output streams and later deserialized back into Java objects using input streams. Serialization is commonly used for saving object states or for inter-process communication.
4. File System Interaction: Java allows interaction with the underlying file system to retrieve information about files and directories, manipulate file properties, and perform file system operations. This interaction is facilitated through classes like `FileSystem`, `FileStore`, `Path`, etc.
5. Resource Management: Java provides constructs like try-with-resources to ensure proper handling and release of file-related resources such as streams. This helps prevent resource leaks and ensures efficient memory management.
6. Network Operations: Java enables file operations over network protocols such as HTTP, FTP, etc., using classes like `URL`, `URLConnection`, `Socket`, `ServerSocket`, etc. This allows reading from and writing to files stored on remote servers.
7. Concurrency: Java provides classes and interfaces for concurrent access to files, allowing multiple threads to read from or write to files simultaneously. Classes like `FileChannel` and `RandomAccessFile` offer support for thread-safe file operations.

One of the primary benefits of utilizing files is to ensure persistent storage of data. File handling encompasses the process of both reading data from and writing data to a file. In Java, file

DOI: 10.1201/9781003544319-11

management is facilitated by the predefined File class, which resides within the java.io package. To interact with files, developers instantiate objects of the File class and specify the file's name or path. This class provides various methods and functionalities to perform operations such as creating, accessing, modifying, and deleting files.

11.1.1 File Operations in Java

A file serves as a named location where data can be stored, while a directory acts as a container for files and other directories. A directory nested within another directory is referred to as a subdirectory.

In Java, there are several operations that can be executed on files, including:

- Creating a File: This operation involves establishing a new file within the file system.
- Reading from a File: Data stored within a file can be retrieved and processed.
- Writing to a File: Information can be added to a file, either appending it to the end or overwriting existing content.
- Deleting a File: Removing a file from the file system, eliminating its stored data and metadata.

Syntax

```
import java.io.File;  // Import the File class
File f = new File("filename.txt"); // Specify the filename
```

Table 11.1 tabulates the File class predefined methods for creating and getting information about files.

11.1.2 Understanding Streams

In Java, Input/Output (I/O) operations are facilitated through streams, which serve as conduits for data flow or communication channels. Streams enable programmers to both write data to a stream and read data from it. Conceptually, streams can be visualized as sequences of bytes that traverse through the program, allowing for efficient handling of data transmission and manipulation. Figure 11.1 shows the stream flow. Table 11.2 and Table 11.3 tabulates the predefined methods for the creation, checking and modification of files and directories.

TABLE 11.1
File methods

Method	Type	Description
canRead()	Boolean	Tests whether the file is readable or not
canWrite()	Boolean	Tests whether the file is writable or not
createNewFile()	Boolean	Creates an empty file
delete()	Boolean	Deletes a file
exists()	Boolean	Tests whether the file exists
getName()	String	Returns the name of the file
getAbsolutePath()	String	Returns the absolute pathname of the file
length()	Long	Returns the size of the file in bytes
list()	String[]	Returns an array of the files in the directory
mkdir()	Boolean	Creates a directory

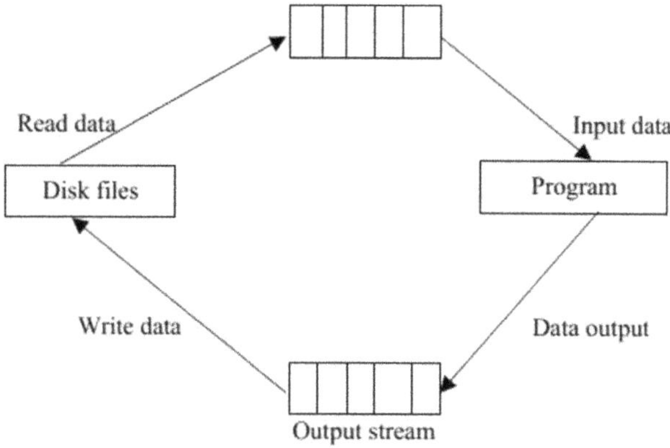

FIGURE 11.1 Stream class flow.

TABLE 11.2
Creating and modifying files and directories directory

METHOD	DESCRIPTION
renameTo(File path)	Current object will be renamed to the path represented by the File object passed as an argument to the method.
setreadonly()	Sets the file represented by the current object as read-only and returns true if the operation is successfully.
mkdir()	Creates a directory with the path specified by the current file object.
mkdirs()	Creates the directory represented by the current file object, including parent directories that are required.
createnewfile()	Create a new empty file with the pathname defined by the current file object as long as the file does exist.
delete()	This will delete the file and directory represented by the current file object and return true if the delete is successful.

TABLE 11.3
Querying files and directories

METHOD	DESCRIPTION
exists()	Returns true if the file or directory referred to by the file object exists and false otherwise.
isfile()	Returns true if the file object refers to an existing file and false otherwise.
canread()	Returns true if you are allowed to read the file referred by the file object.
canwrite()	Returns true if you are allowed to write the file referred by the file object.

11.2 JAVA.IO PACKAGE

The java.io package encompasses classes vital for handling input and output operations in Java. These classes can be categorized into various groups:

- Classes dedicated to reading input from a data stream.
- Classes designed for writing output to a data stream.

- Classes responsible for file manipulation within the local filesystem.
- Classes facilitating object serialization.

The InputStream class serves as the superclass for all Java byte input streams, while the OutputStream class serves as the superclass for all byte output streams. However, it's worth noting that byte streams may not consistently handle Unicode characters correctly.

Since Java 1.1, the java.io package has incorporated character stream classes, which address the limitations of byte streams by properly handling Unicode characters. These character stream classes employ character encoding to ensure accurate conversion between bytes and characters. The Reader class serves as the superclass for all Java character input streams, while the Writer class serves as the superclass for all character output streams.

Note: The Input Stream Reader and Output Stream Writer classes provide a bridge between byte streams and character streams.

Object serialization is a mechanism in Java that allows the entire state of an object to be written to an output stream and subsequently reconstructed by reading the serialized state from an input stream. This enables objects to be saved to a file or transferred over a network.

The ObjectOutputStream and ObjectInputStream classes are responsible for serializing and deserializing objects, respectively. These classes handle the process of converting objects into a stream of bytes for storage or transmission and reconstructing the objects from the byte stream.

On the other hand, RandomAccessFile provides non-sequential access to a file, allowing both reading and writing operations at any position within the file. Unlike other file-related classes that use streams, RandomAccessFile directly interacts with the file system and allows for random access to the data stored in the file.

Figure 11.2 shows the class hierarchy for the java.io package. The java.io package defines a number of standard I/O classes. Table 11.4 tabulates the different streams.

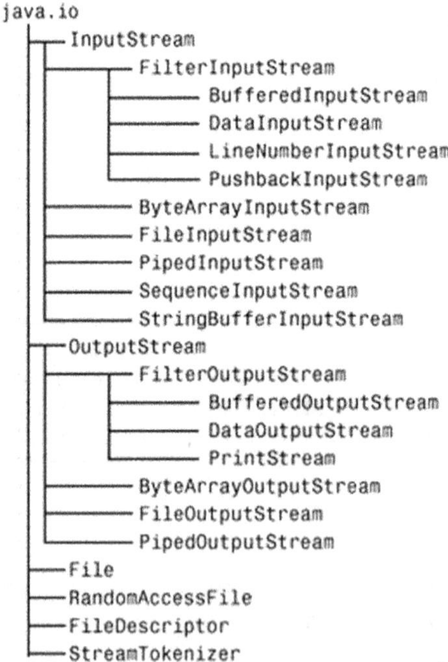

FIGURE 11.2 java.io package classes.

TABLE 11.4
Input and output streams

Stream Type	Stream Name	Description	Examples
Byte-Based Input Streams			
Input	FileInputStream	Reads bytes from a file	Reading binary data from a file
Input	BufferedInputStream	Buffers input bytes for more efficient reading	Reading large binary files
Input	DataInputStream	Reads primitive data types from an input stream	Reading data types like int, float
Input	ObjectInputStream	Deserializes primitive data and objects from an input stream	Reading serialized objects
Input	PipedInputStream	Reads bytes from a piped output stream	Inter-thread communication
Character-Based Input Streams			
Input	FileReader	Reads characters from a file	Reading text from a file
Input	BufferedReader	Buffers input characters for more efficient reading	Reading text files line-by-line
Input	InputStreamReader	Converts bytes to characters using a specified charset	Reading bytes as characters
Input	StringReader	Reads characters from a string	Reading characters from a string
Byte-Based Output Streams			
Output	FileOutputStream	Writes bytes to a file	Writing binary data to a file
Output	BufferedOutputStream	Buffers output bytes for more efficient writing	Writing large binary files
Output	DataOutputStream	Writes primitive data types to an output stream	Writing data types like int, float
Output	ObjectOutputStream	Serializes primitive data and objects to an output stream	Writing serialized objects
Output	PipedOutputStream	Writes bytes to a piped input stream	Inter-thread communication
Character-Based Output Streams			
Output	FileWriter	Writes characters to a file	Writing text to a file
Output	BufferedWriter	Buffers output characters for more efficient writing	Writing text files
Output	OutputStreamWriter	Converts characters to bytes using a specified charset	Writing characters as bytes
Output	StringWriter	Writes characters to a string buffer	Writing characters to a string
Mixed Streams			
Mixed	PrintStream	Provides convenient methods to write formatted data	System.out, System.err
Mixed	PrintWriter	Provides convenient methods to write formatted data	Writing formatted text output

The Java I/O package, java.io, encompasses a collection of classes designed for input and output operations. These classes facilitate reading and writing data to and from files, as well as handling other input and output sources. The classes in java.io are broadly categorized into three groups: input streams, output streams, and miscellaneous streams. Input streams are used for reading data, output streams for writing data, and miscellaneous streams serve other specialized purposes within the I/O framework.

11.2.1 Input Streams

Input streams in Java are responsible for reading data from a variety of input sources, such as files, strings, or memory. These input streams inherit from the `InputStream` class, which serves as a programming interface for reading bytes or arrays of bytes. The `InputStream` class provides methods for various operations, including reading bytes, marking locations in the stream, skipping bytes of input, determining the number of available bytes for reading, and resetting the current position within the stream. When you create an input stream, it is automatically opened, and you can explicitly close it using the `close()` method when no longer needed.

11.2.2 Output Streams

Output streams in Java are responsible for writing data to various output sources, such as files, strings, or memory. These output streams utilize the `OutputStream` class, which serves as a programming interface for writing bytes or arrays of bytes to the stream and flushing the stream. An output stream is automatically opened when created, and you can explicitly close it using the `close()` method when no longer needed.

11.2.3 Other Streams

The `java.io` package encompasses several other classes:

- `File`: Represents a file within the host system.
- `RandomAccessFile`: Enables access to a file for both reading and writing in a non-sequential manner.
- `StreamTokenizer`: Facilitates tokenization of the content within a stream, breaking it down into individual tokens.

11.3 FILE STREAM

Java Input/Output (I/O) is responsible for handling the input and output operations in Java programs. The Java I/O API, provided by the `java.io` package, offers classes for file handling and various input/output operations. Input streams are utilized to read data from a source, while output streams are employed to write data to a destination.

Streams in Java I/O are categorized into two main types:

- Byte Stream: These streams deal with individual bytes, typically 8 bits of data. Byte stream classes extend abstract classes such as `InputStream` and `OutputStream`.
- Character Stream: These streams handle single characters of data. Character stream classes extend abstract classes like `Reader` and `Writer`.

Each stream type offers functionalities for reading or writing data, with byte streams focusing on bytes and character streams operating on characters. These classes enable Java programs to interact with external data sources and destinations effectively. Table 11.5 tabulates the different byte stream classes.

11.3.1 Directories in Java

A directory serves as a container for files and other directories. In Java, the creation of directories is facilitated by two essential methods provided by the `File` class:

TABLE 11.5
Stream classes

Stream Class	Description
Buffered Input Stream	Used for buffered input stream.
Buffered Output Stream	Used for buffered output stream.
Data Input Stream	Contains method for reading Java standard datatype.
Data Output Stream	An output stream that contains method for writing Java standard data type.
File Input Stream	Input stream that reads from a file.
File Output Stream	Output stream that writes to a file.
Input Stream	Abstract class that describes stream input.
Output Stream	Abstract class that describes stream output.
Print Stream	Output Stream that contains print() and println() method.

- The `mkdir()` method creates a directory and returns `true` if the operation is successful, and `false` otherwise.
- The `mkdirs()` method creates a directory along with all its parent directories if they do not exist already.

These methods enable Java programs to organize and manage files and directories efficiently by providing functionality to create directories as needed.

Program

```
import java.io.File;
public class Test {
  void main(String[] args) {
    // Define the path for the new directory
    String directoryPath = "C:/jj/java";
    // Create a File object with the specified path
    File directory = new File(directoryPath);
    // Attempt to create the directory and any necessary parent directories
    if (directory.mkdirs()) {
      System.out.println("Directory created successfully.");
    } else {
      System.out.println("Directory creation failed or directory already
         exists.");
    }
  }
}
Output:
Directory created successfully.
```

In the above program, we performed an operation to create a directory named "java" within the "C:/jj/" drive using the `mkdirs()` method.

11.3.2 Listing Directories

The `list()` method provided by the File class in Java is used to obtain an array of strings naming the files and directories in the directory specified by the File object. When invoked, this method returns an array of strings containing the names of all files and directories present in the directory represented by the File object. Each string in the array corresponds to the name of a file or directory within the specified directory. If the directory is empty or does not exist, the method returns null.

Program

```
import java.io.File;
public class ListFilesExample {
  void main(String[] args) {
    // Define the path of the directory to be listed
    String directoryPath = "C:/jj";
    // Create a File object with the specified directory path
    File directory = new File(directoryPath);
    // Check if the File object is indeed a directory
    if (directory.isDirectory()) {
      // Get the list of files and directories
      String[] filesAndDirs = directory.list();
      // Check if the list is not null
      if (filesAndDirs != null) {
        System.out.println("Contents of directory " + directoryPath + ":");
        // Print the names of files and directories
        for (String name : filesAndDirs) {
          System.out.println(name);
        }
      } else {
        System.out.println("The directory is empty or an I/O error
           occurred.");
      }
    } else {
      System.out.println(directoryPath + " is not a directory.");
    }
  }
}
```

Output

```
Contents of directory C:/jj:
Demo.class
Demo.java
java
Test.class
Test.java
```

In the above example, the `list()` method is called on the File object `directory`, which represents the directory "C:/jj". The method returns an array of strings containing the names of files and directories within "C:/jj", which is then printed to the console.

Program

```
import java.io.File;
public class Test {
  void main(String[] args) {
    File f = null;
    try {
      // Initialize File object to represent the directory "C:/jj"
      f = new File("C:/jj");
      // Get the list of files and directories in the specified directory
      String[] filesAndDirs = f.list();
```

```
      // Check if the list is not null
      if (filesAndDirs != null) {
        System.out.println("Contents of directory C:/jj:");
        // Print each file and directory name
        for (String name : filesAndDirs) {
          System.out.println(name);
        }
      } else {
        System.out.println("The directory is empty or an I/O error
           occurred.");
      }
    } catch (Exception e) {
      // Print the stack trace of the exception to the standard error stream
      e.printStackTrace();
    }
  }
}
```

Output

```
Contents of directory C:/jj:
Demo.class
Demo.java
java
Test.class
Test.java
```

In the above program, we performed an operation to list the files and directories within the "C:/jj" directory. If successful, the names are printed, and any exceptions are handled with a stack trace output.

11.3.3 Standard Streams

In Java programming, there are three standard streams associated with the console:

1. System.out: This is the standard output stream, used for displaying regular output from the program. Data written to this stream is typically displayed on the console.
2. System.in: This is the standard input stream, used for reading input from the user via the console. Programs can read data from this stream to interact with the user.
3. System.err: This is the standard error stream, used for displaying error messages and diagnostic information. Unlike `System.out`, data written to this stream is typically displayed as error messages, making it useful for reporting errors and exceptions.

These standard streams provide a way for Java programs to interact with the console for input, output, and error handling.

11.4 JAVA BYTE STREAM CLASSES

In Java, byte streams are defined using two abstract classes: `InputStream` and `OutputStream`.

1. InputStream: This abstract class is the superclass of all classes representing an input stream of bytes. It defines the basic methods for reading bytes from a source. Subclasses of `InputStream` provide implementations for reading bytes from different sources such as files, network connections, or memory buffers.

2. OutputStream: Similarly, `OutputStream` is an abstract class that serves as the superclass of all classes representing an output stream of bytes. It defines the basic methods for writing bytes to a destination. Subclasses of `OutputStream` provide implementations for writing bytes to different destinations such as files, network connections, or memory buffers.

These abstract classes form the foundation for working with byte streams in Java, allowing developers to read from and write to various byte-based data sources and destinations. These stream classes define several key methods, among which two of the most important are:

a. read(): This method is used to read a byte of data from the input stream. It returns an integer value representing the byte read, or -1 if the end of the stream has been reached.
b. write(): The write() method is used to write a byte of data to the output stream. It takes an integer value representing the byte to be written as an argument.

These methods are fundamental for reading and writing bytes of data in input and output streams, respectively. They allow developers to interact with byte-based data sources and destinations in Java programs.

11.4.1 File Output Stream

The FileOutputStream class in Java is responsible for creating a file and writing data into it. If the specified file does not exist, the stream will create it before opening it for output.

There are two constructors available for creating FileOutputStream objects:

- Using a file name as a string: This constructor takes a file name as a string to create an output stream object for writing to the specified file. Here's an example:

```
OutputStream outputStream = new FileOutputStream("C:/io/test");
```

- Using a File object: This constructor takes a File object to create an output stream object for writing to the file represented by the File object. First, you need to create a File object using the File() method, and then pass it to the FileOutputStream constructor. Here's an example:

```
File file = new File("C:/io/test");
OutputStream outputStream = new FileOutputStream(file);
```

Both constructors create a FileOutputStream object that can be used to write data to the specified file.

Once the *OutputStream* object, then there is a list of predefined methods and they are tabulated in Table 11.6.

In Java, the FileOutputStream class is responsible for writing a stream of bytes to a file. It's a subclass of the OutputStream class in the java.io package. Using FileOutputStream, you can write bytes of data to a file in a sequential manner. It provides methods for writing bytes to the file, flushing the stream, and closing the stream after writing is complete. To use FileOutputStream, you typically create an instance of it by providing the path to the file you want to write to. Then, you can use methods like write() to write bytes to the file from a buffer or perform other operations as needed.

TABLE 11.6
OutputStream class methods

S.No	Method and Description
1	**public void close() throws IOException{}** Closes the file output stream.
2	**protected void finalize()throws IOException {}** This method cleans up the connection to the file.
3	**public void write(int w)throws IOException{}** writes the specified byte to the output stream.
4	**public void write(byte[] w)** Writes w.length bytes from the specified byte array to the OutputStream.

Program

```
import java.io.FileOutputStream;
import java.io.IOException;
public class FileOutputExample {
  void main(String[] args) {
    // The string to be written to the file
    String text = "Dr. Usharani Bhimavarapu!";
    // File path for the output file
    String filePath = "output.txt";
    // Create a FileOutputStream to write to the file
    try (FileOutputStream fos = new FileOutputStream(filePath)) {
      // Convert the string to bytes
      byte[] bytes = text.getBytes();
      // Write bytes to the file
      fos.write(bytes);
      System.out.println("Data has been written to " + filePath);
    } catch (IOException e) {
      // Handle potential IOExceptions
      e.printStackTrace();
    }
  }
}
```

Output

```
Data has been written to output.txt
Output.txt
Dr. Usharani Bhimavarapu!
```

In the above program, FileOutputStream is used to write the string “Dr. Usharani Bhimavarapu!” to the file “output.txt”. The string is first converted to bytes using the getBytes() method, and then the bytes are written to the file using the write() method. Finally, the output stream is closed to release any system resources associated with it.

11.4.1.1 Constructors

Table 11.7 tabulates the different constructors for FileOutputStream class.

11.4.1.2 Methods

Table 11.8 tabulates the predefined methods of the FileOutputStream class.

TABLE 11.7
FileOutputStream class constructors

Constructor	Description
FileOutputStream(File file)	Creates a file output stream to write to the file represented by the specified File object.
FileOutputStream(FileDescriptorfdObj)	Creates a file output stream to write to the specified file descriptor, which represents an existing connection to an actual file in the file system.
FileOutputStream(File file, boolean append)	Creates a file output stream to write to the file represented by the specified File object.
FileOutputStream(String name)	Creates a file output stream to write to the file with the specified name.
FileOutputStream(String name, boolean append)	Creates a file output stream to write to the file with the specified name.

TABLE 11.8
FileOutputStream class methods

Method	Description
protected void finalize()	Clean up the connection with the file output stream.
void write(byte[] arr)	Writes arr.length bytes from the byte array to the file output stream.
void write(byte[] arr, int off, int len)	Write len bytes from the byte array starting at an offset off to the file output stream.
void write(int b)	Writes the specified byte to the file output stream.
FileChannelgetChannel()	Return the file channel object associated with the file output stream.
FileDescriptorgetFD()	Return the file descriptor associated with the stream.
void close()	Closes the file output stream.

11.4.2 FileInputStream Class

In Java, FileInputStream is responsible for reading data and streams of bytes from a file. It's a built-in class defined in the java.io package. FileInputStream is a subclass of InputStream, which is a superclass for all input stream classes. Using FileInputStream, you can read bytes of data from a file in a sequential manner. It provides methods to read bytes from the file and perform various operations such as skipping bytes, marking positions in the stream, and resetting the stream to a previously marked position. To use FileInputStream, you typically create an instance of it by providing the path to the file you want to read from. Then, you can use methods like read() to read bytes from the file into a buffer or perform other operations as needed.

Program

```
import java.io.FileInputStream;
import java.io.IOException;
public class FileInputExample {
  void main(String[] args) {
    // Path of the input file
    String filePath = "example.txt";
    // Create a FileInputStream to read from the file
    try (FileInputStream fis = new FileInputStream(filePath)) {
      int byteRead;
      // Read bytes from the file until the end of the file is reached
      while ((byteRead = fis.read()) != -1) {
        // Convert byte to character and print it
        char character = (char) byteRead;
        System.out.print(character);
```

```
        }
        System.out.println(); // Print a newline for better output formatting
    } catch (IOException e) {
        // Handle potential IOExceptions
        e.printStackTrace();
    }
  }
}
example.txt consists of
This is to test
```
Output:
```
This is to test
```

In the above program, FileInputStream is used to read bytes from the file "example.txt", and each byte is converted to a character and printed to the console. Finally, the input stream is closed to release any system resources associated with it.

The FileInputStream class contains constructors and some functions as a FileInputStream class member function are tabulated in Table 11.9.

11.4.2.1 Methods

Table 11.10 tabulates the predefined methods of FileInputStream class.

Program

```
import java.io.FileInputStream;
import java.io.IOException;
public class FileInputExample {
  void main(String[] args) {
```

TABLE 11.9
Constructors of Java FileInputStream class

FileInputStream(File file)- creates an instance of FileInputStream by opening a connection to a specified file to read from this object.
FileInputStream(FileDescriptorfdobj)- creates an instance of FileInputStream by using the file descriptor.
FileInputStream(String fname)- creates an instance of FileInputStream by opening a connection to a specified file.

TABLE 11.10
FileInputStream class methods

Method	Description
int available()	Returns the estimated number of bytes that can be read from the input stream.
int read()	Read the byte of data from the input stream.
int read(byte[] b)	Read up to b.length bytes of data from the input stream.
int read(byte[] b, int off, int len)	Read up to len bytes of data from the input stream.
long skip(long x)	Discards x bytes of data from the input stream.
FileChannelgetChannel()	Return the unique FileChannel object associated with the file input stream.
FileDescriptorgetFD()	Return the FileDescriptor object.
protected void finalize()	Close method is called when there is no more reference to the file input stream.
void close()	Closes the stream.

```
    // Path of the input file
    String filePath = "input.txt";
    // Create a FileInputStream to read from the file
    try (FileInputStream fis = new FileInputStream(filePath)) {
      int byteRead;
      // Read bytes from the file until the end of the file is reached
      while ((byteRead = fis.read()) != -1) {
        // Convert byte to character and print it
        char character = (char) byteRead;
        System.out.print(character);
      }
      System.out.println(); // Print a newline for better output formatting
    } catch (IOException e) {
      // Handle potential IOExceptions
      e.printStackTrace();
    }
  }
}
input.txt
This is to test
```

Output

```
This is to test
```

In the above program we read data from a file named "input.txt" using the FileInputStream class. In the main method, a try-catch block is used to handle any exceptions that may occur during file handling. Within the try block, a FileInputStream object named "fis" is created to establish a connection to the "input.txt" file. Inside a while loop, the read() method of FileInputStream is called to read bytes from the file one by one. The read byte is then cast to a character and printed to the console using System.out.print(). This process continues until the read() method returns -1, indicating the end of the file. After reading is complete, the FileInputStream object is closed using the close() method to release any system resources associated with the file input stream. In case of any exceptions, the catch block catches the exception and calls the getStackTrace() method on the exception object to print the stack trace to the standard error stream.

Program

```
import java.io.FileInputStream;
import java.io.IOException;
public class FileInputAvailableExample {
  void main(String[] args) {
    String filePath = "input.txt";
    try (FileInputStream fis = new FileInputStream(filePath)) {
      // Print available bytes at the beginning
      System.out.println("beginning: " + fis.available());
      // Read three bytes from the file
      fis.read(new byte[3]);
      // Print available bytes after reading
      System.out.println("end: " + fis.available());
    } catch (IOException e) {
      e.printStackTrace();
    }
  }
}
```

```
input.txt
This is to test
Output
beginning: 15
end: 12
```

In the above program the FileInputStream class reads data from a file named "input.txt". Within the main method, a try-catch block is utilized to handle potential exceptions that may arise during file operations. Inside the try block, a FileInputStream object named "fis" is created to establish a connection to the "input.txt" file. Following that, the program prints the available number of bytes in the FileInputStream before and after reading some bytes from the file. This is accomplished by calling the available() method on the FileInputStream object. Initially, we printed the available bytes at the beginning of the file, and then read three bytes from the file using the read() method. Finally, the FileInputStream object is closed using the close() method to release any system resources associated with the file input stream. In case any exceptions occur during the file handling process, the catch block catches the exception and prints the stack trace to the standard error stream using the getStackTrace() method.

Program

```
import java.io.FileInputStream;
import java.io.IOException;
public class FileInputSkipExample {
  void main(String[] args) {
    String filePath = "input.txt";
    try (FileInputStream input = new FileInputStream(filePath)) {
      // Skip the first 3 bytes
      input.skip(3);
      int byteData;
      // Read and print bytes from the file
      while ((byteData = input.read()) != -1) {
        System.out.print((char) byteData);
      }
    } catch (IOException e) {
      e.printStackTrace();
    }
  }
}
input.txt
This is to test
Output
s to test
```

In the above program FileInputStream object reads data from a file named "input.txt". Inside the main method, a try-catch block is used to handle any exceptions that may occur during file operations. Within the try block, a FileInputStream object named "input" is created to establish a connection to the "input.txt" file. Then calls the skip(3) method on the FileInputStream object, which skips the first three bytes in the file. Inside the while loop, we read bytes from the file one by one until the end of the file is reached (i.e., until read() returns -1). Each byte is cast to a character and printed to the standard output stream. Once all bytes have been read from the file, the FileInputStream object is closed using the close() method to release any system resources associated with the file input stream. In case of any exceptions during the file handling process, the catch block catches the exception and prints the stack trace to the standard error stream using the getStackTrace() method.

11.4.3 BufferedInputStream Class

The BufferedInputStream class in Java is used to read data from an input stream efficiently by using buffering. It is typically used in conjunction with other input stream classes like FileInputStream. BufferedInputStream creates an internal buffer, or a temporary storage area, where it stores a group of bytes read from the underlying input stream.

When the read() method is called, BufferedInputStream reads bytes from the internal buffer rather than directly from the input source, such as a file. If the data requested is not available in the buffer, BufferedInputStream will read a larger chunk of data from the underlying input stream into the buffer. This reduces the number of disk or network reads, which can significantly improve performance, especially when working with large files or streams.

Program

```
import java.io.BufferedInputStream;
import java.io.FileInputStream;
import java.io.IOException;
public class BufferedInputStreamExample {
  void main(String[] args) {
    String filePath = "input.txt";
    try (BufferedInputStream bis = new BufferedInputStream(new FileInputStream(filePath))) {
      int byteData;
      // Read bytes from the file until the end is reached
      while ((byteData = bis.read()) != -1) {
        System.out.print((char) byteData);
      }
    } catch (IOException e) {
      e.printStackTrace();
    }
  }
}
input.txt
This is to test
Output
This is to test
```

We wrap the FileInputStream with a BufferedInputStream to improve reading performance. Inside the while loop, we use the read() method of BufferedInputStream to read bytes from the file until the end of the file is reached. Finally, we close the BufferedInputStream, which also closes the underlying FileInputStream.

Note: A Buffered Input Stream reads data from other Input Stream, but a FileInputStream reads from a file

Note: Buffered Input Stream is buffered, but File Input Stream is not.

Table 11.11 tabulated the constructors of the BufferedInputStream class in Java:

Table 11.12 tabulated the predefined methods of the BufferedInputStream class in Java:

Program

```
import java.io.BufferedInputStream;
import java.io.FileInputStream;
import java.io.IOException;
public class BufferedInputStreamExample {
```

TABLE 11.11
BufferedInputStream class constructors

Constructor	Description
BufferedInputStream(InputStream is)	Creates a BufferedInputStream and saves the 'is' stream for later use.
BufferedInputStream(InputStreamis, int size)	Creates a BufferedInputStream with a specified size and stores the 'is' parameter stream for later use.

TABLE 11.12
BufferedInputStream methods

Method	Description
int available()	Returns the estimate number of bytes available to read.
void close()	Closes the BufferedInputStream.
void mark(int readLimit)	Marks the current position to read from the input stream.
booleanmarkSupported()	Checks whether the stream supports the mark() and reset() methods.
int read()	Reads a byte of data from the input stream.
int read(byte[] b)	Reads the specified byte from the input array.
int read(byte[] b, int off, int len)	Reads the len bytes of data from the array starting from specified off position.
byte[] readAllBytes()	Reads all the remaining bytes from the input stream.
byte[] readNBytes(int len)	Reads upto the specified number of bytes.
int readNBytes(bytes[]b, int off, int len)	Reads upto the specified length of bytes from the byte array starting from the offset position.
long skip(long n)	Slips or discards the specified number of bytes during the read operation.
void skipNBytes(long n)	Skips or discards up to the specified number of bytes during the read operation.
long transferTo(OutputStream out)	Reads all the bytes from the input stream and writes it to the specified output stream in the same order.

```
  void main(String[] args) {
    String filePath = "output.txt";
    try (BufferedInputStream bis = new BufferedInputStream(new
    FileInputStream(filePath))) {
      int byteData;
      // Read bytes from the file until the end is reached
      while ((byteData = bis.read()) != -1) {
        System.out.print((char) byteData);
      }
    } catch (IOException e) {
      e.printStackTrace();
    }
  }
}
output.txt
This is to test
```

Output

```
This is to test
```

In the above program, we performed an operation to efficiently read data from a file using `BufferedInputStream`. We created a `FileInputStream` for "output.txt," wrapped it in a `BufferedInputStream` for improved performance, and then read and printed the data byte by byte.

Finally, we handled any exceptions that occurred during the process to ensure proper resource management.

Program

```
import java.io.BufferedInputStream;
import java.io.FileInputStream;
import java.io.IOException;
public class BufferedInputStreamExample {
  void main(String[] args) {
    String filePath = "test.txt";
    try (BufferedInputStream bis = new BufferedInputStream(new
FileInputStream(filePath))) {
      // Print the number of bytes available for reading
      System.out.println("Bytes available at the beginning: " + bis.
         available());
      // Read three bytes from the file
      bis.read();
      bis.read();
      bis.read();
      // Print the number of bytes available for reading after reading
      three bytes
      System.out.println("Bytes available after reading three bytes: " +
         bis.available());
    } catch (IOException e) {
      e.printStackTrace();
    }
  }
}
```

test.txt

```
This is to test
```

Output

```
Bytes available at the beginning: 15
Bytes available after reading three bytes: 12
```

In the above program, we performed an operation to read data from a file using `BufferedInputStream`. We read and displayed the number of bytes available before and after reading three bytes from the file, using the `available()` and `read()` methods.

11.4.4 Buffered Output Stream Class

The BufferedOutputStream class in Java provides buffering for output streams. It increases the efficiency of writing data to an output stream by reducing the number of write operations performed directly on the underlying output destination, such as a file or network socket.

BufferedOutputStream maintains an internal buffer of a fixed size, typically 8192 bytes (or 8 KB). When data is written to the BufferedOutputStream, it is first stored in the internal buffer rather than being immediately written to the output destination. This buffering reduces the number of write operations performed on the output destination, which can significantly improve performance, especially when writing large amounts of data.

Once the internal buffer is full, or when the flush() method is called, the entire buffer is written to the underlying output destination. This operation is typically more efficient than writing individual bytes directly to the output destination because it reduces the overhead associated with each write operation.

Program

```
import java.io.BufferedOutputStream;
import java.io.FileOutputStream;
import java.io.IOException;
public class BufferedOutputStreamExample {
  void main(String[] args) {
    String filePath = "output.txt";
    String data = "This is a test string to write to the file.";
    // Convert the string data to a byte array
    byte[] byteArray = data.getBytes();
    try   (BufferedOutputStream   bos   =   new   BufferedOutputStream(new
FileOutputStream(filePath))) {
      // Write the byte array to the buffered output stream
      bos.write(byteArray);
      // Flush the buffered data to ensure all data is written to the file
      bos.flush();
    } catch (IOException e) {
      e.printStackTrace();
    }
  }
}
After executing the program output.txt file contains the text
This is a test string to write to the file.
```

In the above program, we created a FileOutputStream object to write data to a file named "output. txt". We then wrap the FileOutputStream with a BufferedOutputStream to improve writing performance. We use the write(byte[] b) method of BufferedOutputStream to write the data to the internal buffer. Finally, we call the flush() method to ensure that all buffered data is written to the file and close the BufferedOutputStream, which also closes the underlying FileOutputStream.

Table 11.13 tabulates the constructors of the Buffered Output Stream class.

Table 11.14 tabulates the predefined methods of the Buffered Output Stream class.

TABLE 11.13
Java buffered output stream class constructors

Constructor	Description
BufferedOutputStream(OutputStreamos)	Creates the new buffered output stream which is used for writing the data to the specified output stream.
BufferedOutputStream(OutputStreamos, int size)	Creates the new buffered output stream which is used for writing the data to the specified output stream with a specified buffer size.

TABLE 11.14
Java BufferedOutputStream class methods

Method	Description
void write(int b)	Writes the specified byte to the buffered output stream.
void write(byte[] b, int off, int len)	Writes the bytes from the specified byte-input stream into a specified byte array, starting with the given offset.
void flush()	Flushes the buffered output stream.

Program

```
import java.io.BufferedOutputStream;
import java.io.FileOutputStream;
import java.io.IOException;
public class BufferedOutputStreamExample {
  void main(String[] args) {
    // Path to the file
    String filePath = "out.txt";
    // Data to be written to the file
    String data = "testing";
    // Convert the string to a byte array
    byte[] byteArray = data.getBytes();
    // Using try-with-resources to ensure streams are closed properly
    try (FileOutputStream fout = new FileOutputStream(filePath);
        BufferedOutputStream bout = new BufferedOutputStream(fout)) {
      // Write the byte array to the buffered output stream
      bout.write(byteArray);
      // Flush the buffered data to ensure it's written to the file
      bout.flush();
    } catch (IOException e) {
      // Print stack trace if an exception occurs
      e.printStackTrace();
    }
  }
}
After executing the program out.txt file contains the text
testing
```

In the above program, we wrote data to a file using `BufferedOutputStream`. The string "testing" was converted into a byte array and written to the file "out.txt" through a buffered output stream. After execution, the "out.txt" file contained the text "testing."

11.5 JAVA CHARACTER STREAM CLASSES

Character streams are defined using two abstract classes: `Reader` and `Writer`. These classes provide a higher level of abstraction compared to byte streams, allowing developers to work with character-based data instead of bytes. Character streams are designed to handle Unicode characters properly, ensuring correct handling of character encoding and decoding.

These classes define various methods for reading and writing character-based data. By using character streams, developers can read and write characters from and to character-based sources and destinations, such as text files, network connections, and memory buffers. Character streams provide a more convenient and efficient way to handle text data in Java programs compared to byte streams. Table 11.15 tabulates the character stream classes and Table 11.16 tabulates the predefined methods in character stream classes.

11.5.1 Buffered Reader

`BufferedReader` is used to read text from an input stream efficiently. It buffers characters to provide efficient reading of characters, arrays, and lines. It's often used to read data from files or other character input streams where performance is critical.

TABLE 11.15
Character stream classes

Stream class	Description
BufferedReader	Handles buffered input stream.
BufferedWriter	Handles buffered output stream.
FileReader	Input stream that reads from file.
FileWriter	Output stream that writes to file.
InputStreamReader	Input stream that translates byte to character.
OutputStreamReader	Output stream that translates character to byte.
PrintWriter	Output Stream that contains print() and println() method.
Reader	Abstract class that defines character stream input.
Writer	Abstract class that defines character stream output.

TABLE 11.16
Input and output stream class methods

S.No	Method and Description
1	**public void close() throws IOException{}** This method closes the file output stream.
2	**protected void finalize()throws IOException {}** This method cleans up the connection to the file.
3	**public int read(int r)throws IOException{}** This method reads the specified byte of data from the InputStream.
4	**public int read(byte[] r) throws IOException{}** This method reads r.length bytes from the input stream into an array.
5	**public int available() throws IOException{}** Gives the number of bytes that can be read from this file input stream.

Program

```
import java.io.BufferedReader;
import java.io.FileReader;
import java.io.IOException;
public class BufferedReaderExample {
  void main(String[] args) {
    // Path to the file
    String filePath = "sr.txt";
    // Using try-with-resources to ensure BufferedReader is closed properly
    try (BufferedReader br = new BufferedReader(new FileReader(filePath))) {
      String line;
      // Read and print each line from the file
      while ((line = br.readLine()) != null) {
        System.out.println(line);
      }
    } catch (IOException e) {
      // Print stack trace if an exception occurs
      e.printStackTrace();
    }
  }
}
```

```
sr.txt
testing
Output:
testing
```

In the above program we read the contents of a file named `sr.txt` and prints each line to the console. The `FileReader` is used to open the file, and `readLine()` method reads each line one by one. The `while` loop continues until there are no more lines to read, and the `BufferedReader` is closed at the end to release resources.

11.5.2 Buffered Writer

`BufferedWriter` is used to write text to an output stream efficiently. It buffers characters to provide efficient writing of characters, arrays, and strings. This stream is useful when writing large amounts of text data to improve performance.

Program

```
import java.io.BufferedWriter;
import java.io.FileWriter;
import java.io.IOException;
public class BufferedWriterExample {
  void main(String[] args) {
    // Path to the file
    String filePath = "cr.txt";
    // Registration details
    String studentName = "Usharani";
    String courseDetails = "Java Programming";
    // Using try-with-resources to ensure BufferedWriter is closed properly
    try (BufferedWriter bw = new BufferedWriter(new FileWriter(filePath))) {
      // Write student name followed by a newline
      bw.write("Student Name: " + studentName);
      bw.newLine();
      // Write course details followed by a newline
      bw.write("Course Details: " + courseDetails);
      bw.newLine();
      // Flush the BufferedWriter to ensure all data is written to the file
      bw.flush();
    } catch (IOException e) {
      // Print stack trace if an exception occurs
      e.printStackTrace();
    }
  }
}
After executing the program the cr.txt file contains
Student Name: Usharani
Course Details: Java Programming
```

In the above program, a `BufferedWriter` is used to write registration details into a file named "cr.txt." The `BufferedWriter` is initialized using `FileWriter`, and inside the try block, the student's name and course details are written, each followed by a new line. The `flush()` method ensures the data is written properly to the file. If any exceptions occur, they are caught and the stack trace is printed.

11.5.3 FileReader

`FileReader` is a convenience class for reading character files. It uses the default character encoding and provides simple methods to read characters, arrays, and lines from a file.

Program

```
import java.io.FileReader;
import java.io.IOException;
public class FileReaderExample {
  void main(String[] args) {
    // Path to the file
    String filePath = "sr.txt";
    // Using try-with-resources to ensure FileReader is closed properly
    try (FileReader fr = new FileReader(filePath)) {
      int character;
      // Read characters one by one until end of file
      while ((character = fr.read()) != -1) {
        // Cast the integer to char and print it
        System.out.print((char) character);
      }
    } catch (IOException e) {
      // Print stack trace if an exception occurs
      e.printStackTrace();
    }
  }
}
sr.txt
testing
Output:
testing
```

In this program, we performed the task of reading the contents of the "sr.txt" file character by character using a `FileReader` and printed each character to the console. If an `IOException` occurs, we handle it by printing the stack trace.

11.5.4 FileWriter

`FileWriter` is a convenience class for writing character files. It uses the default character encoding and provides simple methods to write characters, arrays, and strings to a file.

Program

```
import java.io.FileWriter;
import java.io.IOException;
public class FileWriterExample {
  void main(String[] args) {
    // Path to the file
    String filePath = "cr.txt";
    // Using try-with-resources to ensure FileWriter is closed properly
    try (FileWriter fw = new FileWriter(filePath)) {
      // Student's name and course details
      String studentName = "Usharani";
```

```
      String courseDetails = "Course: Introduction to Java";
      // Write the student's name to the file
      fw.write("Student Name: " + studentName + "\n");
      // Write the course details to the file
      fw.write(courseDetails + "\n");
      // Optionally, you could use flush() here to ensure all data is written
      // fw.flush();
    } catch (IOException e) {
      // Print stack trace if an exception occurs
      e.printStackTrace();
    }
  }
}
After executing the program the cr.txt file contains
Student Name: Usharani
Course: Introduction to Java
```

In the above program, we performed the task of writing a student's name and course details to the "cr.txt" file using a `FileWriter`. The file will contain the student's name followed by the course details, and if an `IOException` occurs, it will be handled by printing the stack trace.

11.5.5 InputStreamReader

`InputStreamReader` bridges byte streams to character streams. It reads bytes and decodes them into characters using a specified charset, making it useful for reading text from byte-oriented streams.

Program

```
import java.io.BufferedReader;
import java.io.FileInputStream;
import java.io.InputStreamReader;
import java.io.IOException;
public class FileReaderExample {
  void main(String[] args) {
    // Path to the file
    String filePath = "sr.txt";
    // Using try-with-resources to ensure BufferedReader is closed properly
    try (FileInputStream fis = new FileInputStream(filePath);
        InputStreamReader isr = new InputStreamReader(fis, "UTF-8");
        BufferedReader br = new BufferedReader(isr)) {
      String line;
      // Read each line from the file and print it to the console
      while ((line = br.readLine()) != null) {
        System.out.println(line);
      }
    } catch (IOException e) {
      // Print stack trace if an exception occurs
      e.printStackTrace();
    }
  }
}
sr.txt
testing
```

Output:
```
testing
```

In this program, we read the contents of the "sr.txt" file line-by-line using a `BufferedReader`. We created a `FileInputStream` and wrapped it in an `InputStreamReader` to handle character encoding, and then read each line from the file, printing it to the console. If an `IOException` occurs, it is handled by printing the stack trace.

11.5.6 OutputStreamWriter

`OutputStreamWriter` bridges character streams to byte streams. It encodes characters into bytes using a specified charset, making it useful for writing text to byte-oriented streams.

Program

```
import java.io.BufferedWriter;
import java.io.FileOutputStream;
import java.io.IOException;
import java.io.OutputStreamWriter;
public class FileWriterExample {
  void main(String[] args) {
    // Path to the file
    String filePath = "cr.txt";
    // Registration details
    String studentName = "Usharani";
    String course = "Java Programming";
    // Using try-with-resources to ensure BufferedWriter is closed properly
    try (FileOutputStream fos = new FileOutputStream(filePath);
        OutputStreamWriter osw = new OutputStreamWriter(fos, "UTF-8");
        BufferedWriter bw = new BufferedWriter(osw)) {
      // Write the student's name and course information to the file
      bw.write("Student Name: " + studentName);
      bw.newLine();
      bw.write("Course: " + course);
      bw.newLine();
      // Flush the BufferedWriter to ensure all data is written to the file
      bw.flush();
    } catch (IOException e) {
      // Print stack trace if an exception occurs
      e.printStackTrace();
    }
  }
}
After executing the program the cr.txt file contains
Student Name: Usharani
Course: Java Programming
```

In this program, we performed the task of writing student registration details to the "cr.txt" file using a `BufferedWriter`. We created a `FileOutputStream` and wrapped it in an `OutputStreamWriter` to specify the character encoding, then used the `BufferedWriter` to write the student's name and course information. Finally, we ensured that all data was properly flushed to the file and handled any potential `IOException` by printing the stack trace.

11.5.7 PrintWriter

`PrintWriter` provides convenient methods to print formatted representations of objects to a text-output stream. It can be used for console output as well as writing to files.

Program

```
import java.io.FileWriter;
import java.io.IOException;
import java.io.PrintWriter;
public class PrintWriterExample {
  void main(String[] args) {
    // Path to the file
    String filePath = "rs.txt";
    // Registration details
    String studentName = "Usharani";
    String course = "Advanced Java";
    // Using try-with-resources to ensure PrintWriter is closed properly
    try (FileWriter fw = new FileWriter(filePath);
        PrintWriter pw = new PrintWriter(fw)) {
      // Write the student's name and course information to the file
      pw.println("Student Name: " + studentName);
      pw.println("Course: " + course);
      // No need to flush or close explicitly, as try-with-resources takes
      care of it
    } catch (IOException e) {
      // Print stack trace if an exception occurs
      e.printStackTrace();
    }
  }
}
After executing the program the rs.txt file contains
Student Name: Usharani
Course: Advanced Java
```

In the above program, we performed the task of writing student registration details to the "rs.txt" file using a `PrintWriter`. We created a `FileWriter` to specify the file path and then wrapped it in a `PrintWriter` to facilitate easy writing of formatted text. The student's name and course information were written to the file, and we utilized a try-with-resources statement to ensure proper resource management, including automatic closing of the writer to prevent resource leaks.

11.5.8 Reader

`Reader` is an abstract class for reading character streams. It provides basic methods to read characters, arrays, and lines. Subclasses include `BufferedReader`, `FileReader`, etc.

Program

```
import java.io.FileReader;
import java.io.IOException;
import java.io.Reader;
public class ReaderExample {
```

```
  void main(String[] args) {
    // Path to the file
    String filePath = "sr.txt";
    // Create a Reader object for reading the file
    try (Reader reader = new FileReader(filePath)) {
      int character;
      // Read characters one by one until the end of the file
      while ((character = reader.read()) != -1) {
        // Convert the int to a char and print it
        System.out.print((char) character);
      }
    } catch (IOException e) {
      // Print stack trace if an exception occurs
      e.printStackTrace();
    }
  }
}
sr.txt
testing
```
Output:
```
testing
```

In this program, we read characters from the "sr.txt" file using a `Reader` object. We created a `FileReader` to access the file and then read its content character by character in a loop until the end of the file was reached. Each character was converted from an integer to a character and printed to the console.

11.5.9 Writer

`Writer` is an abstract class for writing to character streams. It provides basic methods to write characters, arrays, and strings. Subclasses include `BufferedWriter`, `FileWriter`, etc.

Program

```
import java.io.FileWriter;
import java.io.IOException;
import java.io.Writer;
public class WriterExample {
  void main(String[] args) {
    // Path to the file
    String filePath = "cr.txt";
    // Create a Writer object for writing to the file
    try (Writer writer = new FileWriter(filePath)) {
      // Write data to the file
      writer.write("Student Name: Usharani\n");
      writer.write("Course: Cyber Security\n");
    } catch (IOException e) {
      // Print stack trace if an exception occurs
      e.printStackTrace();
    }
  }
}
After executing the program the cr.txt file contains
Student Name: Usharani
```

```
Course: Cyber Security
```

In this program, we are writing data to the "cr.txt" file using a `Writer` object. A `FileWriter` was created to facilitate writing text to the file, and we used the `write` method to add the student's name and course information. We employed a try-with-resources statement to ensure that the writer is properly closed after use, preventing resource leaks.

11.6 RANDOM-ACCESS FILE CLASS

The RandomAccessFile class in Java provides a convenient way to read from and write to a file at any specific location, hence allowing random access to the data stored in the file. Unlike other input and output streams, which provide sequential access to data, RandomAccessFile allows you to directly seek to a particular position within the file and perform read and write operations from that point.

Random access means that you can access the contents of the file in any order, rather than being limited to reading or writing sequentially from the beginning to the end of the file. This is particularly useful when working with large files or when you need to modify specific parts of a file without affecting the rest of its contents.

The RandomAccessFile class provides methods for both reading and writing data at a specified file pointer position. Some of the key methods provided by the RandomAccessFile class include:

- seek(long pos): Moves the file pointer to the specified position within the file.
- read(): Reads a byte of data from the current file pointer position.
- read(byte[] b): Reads an array of bytes from the current file pointer position into the specified byte array.
- write(int b): Writes a byte of data to the current file pointer position.
- write(byte[] b): Writes an array of bytes to the current file pointer position.

Program

```
import java.io.RandomAccessFile;
import java.io.IOException;
public class Main {
  void main(String[] args) {
    // Path to the file
    String filePath = "data.txt";
    // Create a RandomAccessFile object for reading and writing
    try (RandomAccessFile raf = new RandomAccessFile(filePath, "rw")) {
      // Move the file pointer to position 10 and write data
      raf.seek(10);
      raf.writeUTF("Dr.Usharani Bhimavarapu");
      // Move the file pointer back to position 10 to read data
      raf.seek(10);
      String data = raf.readUTF();  // Read data from the same position
      System.out.println("Data read from position 10: " + data);
    } catch (IOException e) {
      // Print stack trace if an exception occurs
      e.printStackTrace();
    }
  }
}
```

Output

```
Data read from position 10: Dr.Usharani Bhimavarapu
```

In the above example, we created a RandomAccessFile named "data.txt" in read-write mode. We then use the seek() method to move the file pointer to specific positions within the file (e.g., position 10 and position 20), where we write and read data respectively. Finally, we close the RandomAccessFile when done.

Syntax

```
RandomAccessFile objectname = new RandomAccessFile("file path", "mode");
```

11.6.1 Access Modes

Access modes in file handling refer to the permissions that dictate how a file can be accessed or manipulated, such as reading, writing, or appending. Common access modes include read-only, write-only, and read-write, which determine the type of operations allowed on the file. Table 11.7 tabulates the modes of the RandomAccessFile.

The RandomAccessFile class in Java provides functionality for working with files in a random-access manner, allowing both reading and writing operations. Unlike other file handling classes, RandomAccessFile extends the Object class and implements the DataInput and DataOutput interfaces, providing methods to support random-access operations.

A random-access file consists of a sequence of bytes, and it supports a special pointer known as the file pointer. This pointer indicates the current position or location within the file. The file pointer can be moved to any arbitrary position in the file before performing read or write operations. Initially, when a file is created, the file pointer is set to position zero, representing the beginning of the file.

As data is read from or written to the file using the read or write methods, the file pointer automatically advances to the next data item, typically the next byte in the file. This allows for efficient sequential reading and writing of data, as well as direct access to specific locations within the file for random-access operations.

RandomAccessFile provides methods for positioning the file pointer, reading and writing bytes, as well as reading and writing primitive data types. Some of the key methods provided by RandomAccessFile include:

- seek(long pos): Moves the file pointer to the specified position within the file.
- read(): Reads a byte of data from the current file pointer position.
- write(int b): Writes a byte of data to the current file pointer position.
- readInt(): Reads an integer value from the current file pointer position.
- writeInt(int v): Writes an integer value to the current file pointer position.

TABLE 11.17
Access modes of the RandomAccessFile

Mode	Description
R	Read mode.
rw	Read and write mode.
rwd	Read and write mode – synchronously. All updates to file should write to the disk synchronously.
rws	Read and write mode – synchronously. All updates to file or meta data should writeto the disk synchronously.

By leveraging the capabilities of RandomAccessFile, developers can efficiently work with files in a random-access manner, accessing data at specific locations within the file as needed for various file processing tasks.

Syntax

```
RandomAccessFile(File file, String mode)
```

Creates a random-access file stream specified by the File argument.

Table 11.18 tabulates the predefined methods for the random-access file.

Program

```
import java.io.RandomAccessFile;
import java.io.IOException;
public class Main {
  // Method to read bytes from a file starting at a specified position
  public static void readFromFile(String filePath, long position, int
  numBytes) {
    try (RandomAccessFile raf = new RandomAccessFile(filePath, "r")) {
      // Check if file size is enough for reading
      long fileLength = raf.length();
      if (position + numBytes > fileLength) {
        System.out.println("Error: Attempt to read beyond the file length.");
        return;
      }
      // Move the file pointer to the specified position
      raf.seek(position);
      byte[] b = new byte[numBytes];
      // Read bytes into the byte array
      raf.readFully(b);
      // Convert byte array to string and print
      String data = new String(b);
      System.out.println("Read data: " + data);
    } catch (IOException e) {
      // Print stack trace if an exception occurs
      e.printStackTrace();
    }
  }
  // Method to write data to a file starting at a specified position
  public static void writeToFile(String filePath, String data, long pos-
  ition) {
```

TABLE 11.18
Random-access file methods

Modifier	Method	Description
void	close()	Closes the specified random access file.
int	readInt()	Reads integer from specified file.
void	seek(long pos)	Sets the file-pointer offset, from the beginning of specified file.
int	read()	Reads a byte of data from specified file.

```
    try (RandomAccessFile raf = new RandomAccessFile(filePath, "rw")) {
      // Move the file pointer to the specified position
      raf.seek(position);
      // Write the string data to the file
      raf.write(data.getBytes());
    } catch (IOException e) {
      // Print stack trace if an exception occurs
      e.printStackTrace();
    }
  }
  void main(String[] args) {
    // File path
    final String filePath = "rs.txt";
    // Write data first to ensure the file has enough content
    writeToFile(filePath, "This is a sample content to avoid EOFException.", 0);
    // Read 18 bytes from position 0
    readFromFile(filePath, 0, 18);
    // Write data to position 31
    writeToFile(filePath, "This is to test the java files", 31);
  }
}
```

Output:

```
Read data: This is a sample c
```

In the above program we create a `RandomAccessFile` and performed read from and write to a file at a specific position. In the main method, we define a constant string representing the file path "test.txt" and calls the `readFromFile` method to read 18 bytes from the file starting at position 0. The `readFromFile` method opens the file in read mode, seeks to the specified position, reads the bytes into a byte array, and converts the data to a string for display. Next, `writeToFile` method is called to write the string "This is to test the java files" to the file starting at position 31. The `writeToFile` method opens the file in read-write mode, seeks to the specified position, and writes the string data as bytes to the file.

11.6.2 Seeking in a RandomAccessFile

In Java's RandomAccessFile class, the `seek()` method is used to move the file pointer to a specific position within the file. This allows for random-access operations, enabling reading or writing data at a particular location in the file.

The `seek()` method takes a `long` parameter representing the desired position within the file. After invoking `seek()`, subsequent read or write operations will occur at the specified position.

For example, to move the file pointer to the beginning of the file, you can use `seek(0)`. If you want to position the file pointer at a specific byte offset, you pass that offset as an argument to the `seek()` method.

Here's a syntax of using `seek()` to move the file pointer to a specific position:

```
try {
  RandomAccessFile file = new RandomAccessFile("example.txt", "rw");
  // Move file pointer to position 100
  file.seek(100);
  // Read 10 bytes from the file
  byte[] buffer = new byte[10];
  file.read(buffer);
  // Print the read data
```

```
  System.out.println(new String(buffer));
  // Move file pointer to position 200
  file.seek(200);
  // Write data at position 200
  file.write("Usharani".getBytes());
  file.close();
} catch (IOException e) {
  e.printStackTrace();
}
```

In the above code, the file pointer is moved to position 100 using `seek(100)`, and then 10 bytes are read from that position. Later, the file pointer is moved to position 200 using `seek(200)`, and the string " Usharani " is written at that position in the file.

Here is an example of seeking to a specific position in a Java RandomAccessFile:

```
RandomAccessFile file = new RandomAccessFile("c:\\io\\file.txt", "rw");
file.seek(200);
```

The above syntax creates a `RandomAccessFile` object named `file` that opens the file located at "c:\io\file.txt" in read-write mode. The `seek(200)` method moves the file pointer to the 200th byte of the file, allowing subsequent read or write operations to start from that position.

11.6.3 Get File Position

In Java's `RandomAccessFile` class, you can use the `getFilePointer()` method to retrieve the current position of the file pointer. This method returns a `long` value representing the index of the byte where the file pointer is currently positioned.

Here's the syntax demonstrating the usage of `getFilePointer()`:

```
try {
  RandomAccessFile file = new RandomAccessFile("example.txt", "r");
  // Read the current position of the file pointer
  long position = file.getFilePointer();
  // Print the current position
  System.out.println("Current position: " + position);
  file.close();
} catch (IOException e) {
  e.printStackTrace();
}
```

In the above code, `getFilePointer()` is called to retrieve the current position of the file pointer, and the result is stored in the variable `position`. This value represents the byte index where the file pointer is currently located within the file. Finally, the current position is printed to the console.

Program: reading the random access file content

```
import java.io.RandomAccessFile;
import java.io.IOException;
public class Main {
  void main(String[] args) {
    try {
      // Create a RandomAccessFile object in read-write mode
      RandomAccessFile raf = new RandomAccessFile("file.txt", "rw");
```

```
      // Move the file pointer to position 5
      raf.seek(5);
      // Write the string "this is to test" to the file at the current
      position
      String dataToWrite = "this is to test";
      raf.write(dataToWrite.getBytes());
      // Close the RandomAccessFile
      raf.close();
      // Create another RandomAccessFile object in read-only mode
      RandomAccessFile raf1 = new RandomAccessFile("file.txt", "r");
      // Move the file pointer to position 1
      raf1.seek(1);
      // Create a byte array to store the read data
      byte[] b = new byte[5];
      // Read 5 bytes from the file into the byte array
      raf1.read(b);
      // Close the RandomAccessFile
      raf1.close();
      // Print the string representation of the byte array
      String readData = new String(b);
      System.out.println("Read data: " + readData);
    } catch (IOException e) {
      // Handle IOExceptions
      e.printStackTrace();
    }
  }
}
```

Output:

```
Read data: his t
```

First we open "file.txt" in read-write mode, seeks to position 5, and writes the string "this is to test." Then, we reopens the file in read-only mode, seeks to position 1, reads 5 bytes into a byte array, and prints the resulting string.

Program

```
import java.io.RandomAccessFile;
import java.io.IOException;
public class RandomAccessFileExample {
  void main(String[] args) {
    try {
      // Create a RandomAccessFile object in read-write mode
      RandomAccessFile raf = new RandomAccessFile("file.txt", "rw");
      // Write the string "this is to test" to the file using writeUTF
      raf.writeUTF("this is to test");
      // Move the file pointer back to position 0
      raf.seek(0);
      // Read a line of text from the file starting at position 0
      String readData = raf.readUTF();
      // Print the read data
      System.out.println("Read data: " + readData);
      // Move the file pointer back to position 0
      raf.seek(0);
      // Overwrite the file content with the string "Java"
```

```
      raf.writeUTF("Java");
      // Move the file pointer back to position 0
      raf.seek(0);
      // Read the updated content from the file
      String updatedData = raf.readUTF();
      // Print the updated data
      System.out.println("Updated data: " + updatedData);
      // Close the RandomAccessFile
      raf.close();
    } catch (IOException e) {
      // Handle IOExceptions
      e.printStackTrace();
    }
  }
}
```

Output:

```
Read data: this is to test
Updated data: Java
```

In the above we demonstrated the use of `RandomAccessFile` to write, read, and overwrite data in a file. First we created a file named "file.txt" in read-write mode and writes the string "this is to test" using `writeUTF`. After reading the content back, we overwrite the file with the string "Java," read the updated content, and print both the original and updated data to the console.

Program

```
import java.io.RandomAccessFile;
import java.io.IOException;
public class RandomAccessFileExample {
  void main(String[] args) {
    try {
      // Create RandomAccessFile objects in read-write mode
      RandomAccessFile raf = new RandomAccessFile("file.txt", "rw");
      RandomAccessFile raf1 = new RandomAccessFile("file.txt", "rw");
      // Use raf to write data at a specific position
      raf.seek(5);  // Move file pointer to position 5
      raf.write("vijayawada".getBytes());  // Write "vijayawada" at pos-
                                              ition 5
      raf.close();  // Close the file
      // Use raf1 to write data at the end of the file
      raf1.seek(raf1.length());  // Move file pointer to the end of the file
      raf1.write("students".getBytes());  // Write "students" at the end of
                                            the file
      raf1.close(); // Close the file
    } catch (IOException e) {
      // Handle IOExceptions
      e.printStackTrace();
    }
  }
}
```

Output:

```
File.txt:
..... vijayawadastudents
```

In the above program we demonstrated the use of `RandomAccessFile` to write data to a specific position in a file. First was created two `RandomAccessFile` objects in read-write mode, using the first to write the string "vijayawada" starting at position 5 in "file.txt" and then closing it. The second `RandomAccessFile` writes the string "students" at the end of the file, effectively appending it, before closing as well.

Program

```
import java.io.FileWriter;
import java.io.FileReader;
import java.io.IOException;
public class FileReadWriteExample {
  void main(String[] args) {
    // Write data to the file
    try {
      FileWriter fw = new FileWriter("test.txt");
      fw.write("this is to test");
      fw.close(); // Close the FileWriter to release system resources
      // Read data from the file
      FileReader fr = new FileReader("test.txt");
      int ch;
      while ((ch = fr.read()) != -1) {
        System.out.print((char) ch); // Print each character read from
           the file
      }
      fr.close(); // Close the FileReader to release system resources
    } catch (IOException e) {
      e.printStackTrace(); // Handle IOExceptions
    }
  }
}
Output:
this is to test
```

In the above program we demonstrated basic file operations using `FileWriter` and `FileReader` in Java. First, wrote the string "this is to test" to a file named "test.txt" and then reads the content back character by character, printing it to the console. Both the `FileWriter` and `FileReader` are closed after their respective operations to ensure proper resource management.

Program

```
import java.io.CharArrayWriter;
import java.io.FileWriter;
import java.io.IOException;
public class MultiFileWriterExample {
  void main(String[] args) {
    // Create a CharArrayWriter to buffer characters in memory
    CharArrayWriter out = new CharArrayWriter();
    try {
      // Write data to the CharArrayWriter
      out.write("this is to test");
      // Create FileWriter objects for multiple files
      FileWriter f1 = new FileWriter("f1.txt");
      FileWriter f2 = new FileWriter("f2.txt");
```

```
        FileWriter f3 = new FileWriter("f3.txt");
        FileWriter f4 = new FileWriter("f4.txt");
        // Write the content of CharArrayWriter to each FileWriter
        out.writeTo(f1);
        out.writeTo(f2);
        out.writeTo(f3);
        out.writeTo(f4);
        // Close each FileWriter to release system resources
        f1.close();
        f2.close();
        f3.close();
        f4.close();
      } catch (IOException e) {
        e.printStackTrace(); // Handle IOExceptions
      } finally {
          out.close();
      }
    }
}
```

In the above program we demonstrated the use of `CharArrayWriter` to write the same string to multiple files in Java. We first wrote the string "this is to test" to a `CharArrayWriter` and then created several `FileWriter` objects for different files. The content of the `CharArrayWriter` is then written to each file, and all resources are properly closed to prevent memory leaks.

11.7 STREAM GATHERERES

The "Stream Gatherers" feature introduced in Java 22, outlined in JEP 461, addresses several important needs related to flexibility, efficiency, and maintainability when working with streams in Java. Here are the key needs fulfilled by the Stream Gatherers feature:

Needs for Stream Gatherers in Java 22

- Custom Intermediate Operations: Traditional Java streams provide a set of predefined intermediate operations (such as `filter`, `map`, `flatMap`, etc.) that allow developers to transform and manipulate data flowing through the stream pipeline. However, in certain cases, developers may need to apply custom logic or operations that aren't provided by the standard API. The Stream Gatherers feature fills this gap by enabling developers to define and integrate custom intermediate operations seamlessly into their stream pipelines.
- Enhanced Stream Composition: Java streams support a fluent and declarative style of programming, where operations can be chained together to form complex data processing pipelines. Before Java 22, customizing stream behavior beyond the standard operations required creating additional utility methods or resorting to less expressive approaches. Stream Gatherers enhance stream composition by allowing developers to encapsulate and reuse complex stream logic as gatherers, improving code readability and maintainability.
- Code Reusability and Encapsulation: Modern software development emphasizes code reusability and encapsulation to improve modularity and reduce redundancy. With Stream Gatherers, developers can encapsulate complex stream processing logic into reusable gatherer functions, promoting a more modular design approach. This enables clearer separation of concerns and facilitates easier unit testing and debugging of stream operations.
- Performance Optimization: Efficient stream processing is critical for applications dealing with large datasets or requiring real-time data processing. Stream Gatherers enhance performance

optimization by allowing developers to optimize custom operations directly within the stream pipeline. This can lead to improved throughput and reduced latency in data-intensive applications.
- Support for Functional Programming Paradigms: Java promotes functional programming paradigms through features like lambdas and streams, which simplify concurrent and parallel programming tasks. Stream Gatherers further support these paradigms by providing a mechanism to encapsulate functional behavior within reusable components. This encourages a more functional style of programming, where operations are expressed as transformations on data streams.

Program

```
import java.util.List;
import java.util.stream.Collectors;
import java.util.stream.Stream;
public class Demo {
  void main(String[] args) {
    // Create a stream of strings
    Stream<String> stream = Stream.of("DR.", "Usha", "Rani", "Bhimavarapu");
    // Collect elements into an unmodifiable list
    List<String>      collectedList      =      stream.collect(Collectors.
    toUnmodifiableList());
    System.out.println("Collected List: " + collectedList);
    // Create another stream
    Stream<Integer> numberStream = Stream.of(1, 2, 3, 4, 5);
    // Collect elements into an unmodifiable set
    var collectedSet = numberStream.collect(Collectors.toUnmodifiableSet());
    System.out.println("Collected Set: " + collectedSet);
  }
}
Output:
Collected List: [DR., Usha, Rani, Bhimavarapu]
Collected Set: [2, 3, 4, 5, 1]
```

The above program demonstrates the use of Java streams and `Collectors` to create unmodifiable collections. First, we created a stream of strings and collected them into an unmodifiable list. Then, we created a stream of integers and collected them into an unmodifiable set. The output displays both the list and the set.

Program

```
import java.util.*;
import java.util.stream.*;
class Demo {
  void main(String a[]) {
    List<Integer> numbers = List.of(1, 2, 3, 4, 5);
    List<Integer> doubled = numbers.stream()
        .collect(Collectors.collectingAndThen(
            Collectors.toList(),
            list  ->  list.stream().map(n  ->  n  *  2).collect(Collectors.
toList())
        ));
    System.out.println(doubled);
  }
}
```

```
Output
[2, 4, 6, 8, 10]
```

We first collect a list of integers using `Collectors.toList()`, and then transform this list by doubling each number. Later we use `collectingAndThen` to apply this transformation and then print the resulting list, which contains each original integer multiplied by 2.

Program

```
import java.util.*;
import java.util.stream.*;
class Demo {
  void main(String a[]) {
        List<String> strings = List.of("a", "bb", "ccc", "dddd");
    List<String> result = strings.stream()
        .collect(Collectors.collectingAndThen(
            Collectors.toList(),
            list->list.stream().filter(s->s.length()>2).collect(Collectors.
toList())
        ));
    System.out.println(result);
  }
}
Output
[ccc, dddd]
```

We applied filters to list of strings with a length of 2 or less. First we collect all strings into a list and then process this list to retain only strings longer than two characters.

Program

```
import java.util.*;
import java.util.stream.*;
class Demo {
  void main(String a[]) {
        List<String> strings = List.of("Ammulu", "Bhimavarapu", "Chinni",
"Daddy");
    Map<Character, List<String>> grouped = strings.stream()
        .collect(Collectors.collectingAndThen(
            Collectors.groupingBy(s -> s.charAt(0)),
            map -> map
        ));
    System.out.println(grouped);
  }
}
Output:
{A=[Ammulu], B=[Bhimavarapu], C=[Chinni], D=[ Daddy]}
```

We group a list of strings based on their starting character using `Collectors.groupingBy` and later creates a map where each key is the first character of the strings, and each value is a list of strings starting with that character.

Program

```
import java.util.*;
import java.util.stream.*;
class Demo {
  void main(String a[]) {
        List<Integer> numbers = List.of(1, 2, 3, 4, 5, 6);
    Map<Boolean, List<Integer>> partitioned = numbers.stream()
        .collect(Collectors.collectingAndThen(
            Collectors.partitioningBy(n -> n % 2 == 0),
            map -> map
        ));
    System.out.println(partitioned);
  }
}
Output
{false=[1, 3, 5], true=[2, 4, 6]}
```

In the above program we partitioned a list of integers into two groups based on whether the numbers are even or odd. We used `Collectors.partitioningBy` to create a map with boolean keys indicating even (`true`) or odd (`false`) numbers.

Program

```
import java.util.*;
import java.util.stream.*;
class Demo {
  void main(String a[]) {
        List<String> strings = List.of("one", "two", "three");
    String result = strings.stream()
        .collect(Collectors.collectingAndThen(
            Collectors.joining(", "),
            s -> "[" + s + "]"
        ));
    System.out.println(result);
  }
}
Output:
[one, two, three]
```

In the above program we created a list of strings and used Java streams to concatenate them into a single string with comma separators. The `collectingAndThen` method formats the concatenated string by enclosing it in square brackets.

11.8 MEDICAL APPLICATIONS

11.8.1 Case Study 1

COVID-19 Data collection and store the data in .csv file

```
import java.io.FileWriter;
import java.io.IOException;
import java.util.Random;
public class Covid19DatasetGenerator {
```

```
  void main(String[] args) {
    try (FileWriter writer = new FileWriter("covid19_dataset.csv"))
{     writer.write("Age,Gender,Fever,Cough,DifficultyBreathing,Fatigue,Bod
         yAches,LossOfTasteOrSmell,SoreThroat,TestResult\n");
      Random random = new Random();
      for (int i = 0; i < 1000; i++) {
        int age = random.nextInt(80) + 18;
        String gender = random.nextBoolean()? "Male" : "Female";
        boolean fever = random.nextBoolean();
        boolean cough = random.nextBoolean();
        boolean difficultyBreathing = random.nextBoolean();
        boolean fatigue = random.nextBoolean();
        boolean bodyAches = random.nextBoolean();
        boolean lossOfTasteOrSmell = random.nextBoolean();
        boolean soreThroat = random.nextBoolean();
        String testResult = random.nextBoolean()? "Positive" : "Negative";
        writer.write(String.format("%d,%s,%s,%s,%s,%s,%s,%s,%s,%s\n",
            age, gender, fever? "Yes" : "No", cough? "Yes" : "No",
            difficultyBreathing? "Yes" : "No", fatigue? "Yes" : "No",
            bodyAches? "Yes" : "No", lossOfTasteOrSmell? "Yes" : "No",
            soreThroat? "Yes" : "No", testResult));
      }
    } catch (IOException e) {
      e.printStackTrace();
    }
  }
}
```

Covid19DatasetGenerator generates a synthetic dataset of COVID-19 cases and writes it to a CSV file named "covid19_dataset.csv". It uses a `FileWriter` to create the file and writes headers for the dataset, which include attributes such as age, gender, and various symptoms. A `Random` object is used to generate random data for 1000 entries, including random ages between 18 and 97, random gender, and random boolean values for symptoms like fever, cough, difficulty breathing, fatigue, body aches, loss of taste or smell, and sore throat. Each entry also includes a random COVID-19 test result, either "Positive" or "Negative". The program handles any potential `IOException` that might occur during file operations.

11.8.2 Case Study 2

Data collection in Excel file

```
import org.apache.poi.ss.usermodel.*;
import org.apache.poi.xssf.usermodel.XSSFWorkbook;
import java.io.FileOutputStream;
import java.io.IOException;
import java.util.ArrayList;
import java.util.List;
class DepressionRecord {
  private int age;
  private String gender;
  private String maritalStatus;
  private String employmentStatus;
  private String educationLevel;
  private boolean familyHistoryOfDepression;
  private boolean sleepDisturbances;
```

```
  private boolean appetiteChanges;
  private boolean lossOfInterestOrPleasure;
  private boolean fatigueOrLossOfEnergy;
  private boolean feelingsOfWorthlessnessOrGuilt;
  private boolean difficultyConcentrating;
  private boolean suicidalThoughts;
  private boolean depressionDiagnosis;
  public DepressionRecord(int age, String gender, String maritalStatus,
     String employmentStatus, String educationLevel,
     boolean familyHistoryOfDepression, boolean sleepDisturbances, boolean
appetiteChanges,
     boolean lossOfInterestOrPleasure, boolean fatigueOrLossOfEnergy,
     boolean feelingsOfWorthlessnessOrGuilt, boolean difficultyConcentrating,
     boolean suicidalThoughts, boolean depressionDiagnosis) {
    this.age = age;
    this.gender = gender;
    this.maritalStatus = maritalStatus;
    this.employmentStatus = employmentStatus;
    this.educationLevel = educationLevel;
    this.familyHistoryOfDepression = familyHistoryOfDepression;
    this.sleepDisturbances = sleepDisturbances;
    this.appetiteChanges = appetiteChanges;
    this.lossOfInterestOrPleasure = lossOfInterestOrPleasure;
    this.fatigueOrLossOfEnergy = fatigueOrLossOfEnergy;
    this.feelingsOfWorthlessnessOrGuilt = feelingsOfWorthlessnessOrGuilt;
    this.difficultyConcentrating = difficultyConcentrating;
    this.suicidalThoughts = suicidalThoughts;
    this.depressionDiagnosis = depressionDiagnosis;
  }
  public int getAge() { return age; }
  public String getGender() { return gender; }
  public String getMaritalStatus() { return maritalStatus; }
  public String getEmploymentStatus() { return employmentStatus; }
  public String getEducationLevel() { return educationLevel; }
  public boolean isFamilyHistoryOfDepression() { return
     familyHistoryOfDepression; }
  public boolean isSleepDisturbances() { return sleepDisturbances; }
  public boolean isAppetiteChanges() { return appetiteChanges; }
  public boolean isLossOfInterestOrPleasure() { return
     lossOfInterestOrPleasure; }
  public boolean isFatigueOrLossOfEnergy() { return fatigueOrLossOfEnergy; }
  public boolean isFeelingsOfWorthlessnessOrGuilt() { return
     feelingsOfWorthlessnessOrGuilt; }
  public boolean isDifficultyConcentrating() { return difficultyConcentrating; }
  public boolean isSuicidalThoughts() { return suicidalThoughts; }
  public boolean isDepressionDiagnosis() { return depressionDiagnosis; }
}
public class DepressionDataset {
  void main(String[] args) {
    List<DepressionRecord> records = new ArrayList<>();
    // Add records to the list (In a real application, this data might come
    from user input or a database)
    records.add(new DepressionRecord(25, "Female", "Single", "Employed",
"Bachelor's", true, true, true, true, true, true, true, true, true));
```

```
    records.add(new DepressionRecord(30, "Male", "Married", "Unemployed",
    "Master's", false, true, false, true, true, false, true, false, false));
    try (Workbook workbook = new XSSFWorkbook()) {
      Sheet sheet = workbook.createSheet("DepressionData");
      String[] headers = {"Age", "Gender", "Marital Status", "Employment
         Status", "Education Level", "Family History of Depression", "Sleep
         Disturbances", "Appetite Changes", "Loss of Interest or Pleasure",
         "Fatigue or Loss of Energy", "Feelings of Worthlessness or Guilt",
         "Difficulty  Concentrating",  "Suicidal  Thoughts",  "Depression
         Diagnosis"};
      Row headerRow = sheet.createRow(0);
      for (int i = 0; i < headers.length; i++) {
        Cell cell = headerRow.createCell(i);
        cell.setCellValue(headers[i]);
      }
      int rowNum = 1;
      for (DepressionRecord record : records) {
        Row row = sheet.createRow(rowNum++);
        row.createCell(0).setCellValue(record.getAge());
        row.createCell(1).setCellValue(record.getGender());
        row.createCell(2).setCellValue(record.getMaritalStatus());
        row.createCell(3).setCellValue(record.getEmploymentStatus());
        row.createCell(4).setCellValue(record.getEducationLevel());
        row.createCell(5).setCellValue(record.isFamilyHistoryOfDepress
        ion());
        row.createCell(6).setCellValue(record.isSleepDisturbances());
        row.createCell(7).setCellValue(record.isAppetiteChanges());
        row.createCell(8).setCellValue(record.
          isLossOfInterestOrPleasure());
        row.createCell(9).setCellValue(record.isFatigueOrLossOfEnergy());
        row.createCell(10).setCellValue(record.isFeelingsOfWorthlessnessOr
          Guilt());
        row.createCell(11).setCellValue(record.isDifficultyConcentrating());
        row.createCell(12).setCellValue(record.isSuicidalThoughts());
        row.createCell(13).setCellValue(record.isDepressionDiagnosis());
      }
      try (FileOutputStream fileOut = new FileOutputStream("DepressionData.
        xlsx")) {
        workbook.write(fileOut);
      }
      System.out.println("DepressionData.xlsx written successfully.");
    } catch (IOException e) {
      e.printStackTrace();
    }
  }
}
```

DepressionDataset application generates an Excel spreadsheet named "DepressionData.xlsx" containing data on depression symptoms. It defines a `DepressionRecord` class to represent individual records with various attributes such as age, gender, and specific symptoms related to depression. The main method initializes a list of `DepressionRecord` instances and populates it with sample data. Using Apache POI, it creates an Excel workbook and sheet, writes the header row with column names, and iterates through the records to populate each row with data. Finally, the program writes the workbook to a file and handles any potential `IOException`.

11.8.3 Case Study 3

Data collection in .txt file

```
import java.io.File;
import java.io.FileWriter;
import java.io.IOException;
import java.util.Random;
public class VitaminDeficiencyData {
  void main(String[] args) {
    int ageRangeStart = 20;
    int ageRangeEnd = 80;
    double sunExposureRangeStart = 0.0;
    double sunExposureRangeEnd = 5.0; // Hours per day
    int dietaryVitaminDIntakeRangeStart = 0;
    int dietaryVitaminDIntakeRangeEnd = 400; // IU per day
    double serumVitaminDLevelRangeStart = 12.0;
    double serumVitaminDLevelRangeEnd = 80.0; // ng/mL
    String[] symptoms = {"Bone Pain", "Muscle Weakness", "Fatigue",
       "Depression", "Hair Loss"};
    int numSamples = 100;
    String data = "";
    for (int i = 0; i < numSamples; i++) {
      data += generateSampleData(ageRangeStart, ageRangeEnd,
          sunExposureRangeStart, sunExposureRangeEnd,
          dietaryVitaminDIntakeRangeStart, dietaryVitaminDIntakeRangeEnd,
          serumVitaminDLevelRangeStart, serumVitaminDLevelRangeEnd,
          symptoms) + "\n";
    }
    try {
      File file = new File("vitamin_deficiency_data.txt");
      FileWriter writer = new FileWriter(file);
      writer.write(data);
      writer.close();
      System.out.println("Sample vitamin deficiency data generated and stored
         in vitamin_deficiency_data.txt");
    } catch (IOException e) {
      e.printStackTrace();
    }
  }
  private static String generateSampleData(int ageRangeStart, int
ageRangeEnd, double sunExposureRangeStart, double sunExposureRangeEnd, int
dietaryVitaminDIntakeRangeStart, int dietaryVitaminDIntakeRangeEnd, double
serumVitaminDLevelRangeStart, double serumVitaminDLevelRangeEnd,
          String[] symptoms) {
    Random random = new Random();
    int age = random.nextInt(ageRangeEnd - ageRangeStart + 1) + ageRangeStart;
    String gender = random.nextBoolean() ? "Male" : "Female";
    double sunExposure = random.nextDouble() * (sunExposureRangeEnd -
       sunExposureRangeStart) + sunExposureRangeStart;
    int dietaryVitaminDIntake = random.nextInt(dietaryVitaminDIntakeRan
       geEnd - dietaryVitaminDIntakeRangeStart + 1) + dietaryVitaminDIn
       takeRangeStart; double serumVitaminDLevel = random.nextDouble()
       * (serumVitaminDLevelRangeEnd - serumVitaminDLevelRangeStart) +
       serumVitaminDLevelRangeStart;
    StringBuilder symptomString = new StringBuilder();
```

```
    for (String symptom : symptoms) {
      symptomString.append(random.nextBoolean() ? "Yes," : "No,");
    }
    return age + "," + gender + "," + sunExposure + "," + dietaryVitaminDIntake
       + "," +
       serumVitaminDLevel + "," + symptomString.toString();
  }
}
```

The application "VitaminDeficiencyData" generates a dataset of simulated vitamin D deficiency data and stores it in a text file named "vitamin_deficiency_data.txt". It defines ranges for age, sun exposure, dietary vitamin D intake, and serum vitamin D levels, and specifies a set of possible symptoms. The main method generates 100 samples of data within these ranges using a helper method `generateSampleData`, which produces random values for each attribute and concatenates them into a comma-separated string. This data is then written to a file using a `FileWriter`, and any potential `IOException` is handled.

12 Abstract Window Toolkit

12.1 INTRODUCTION

Java AWT (Abstract Window Toolkit) is a set of APIs used by Java programmers to create graphical user interfaces (GUIs) and rich user interface (UI) components. It is part of Java's standard library and provides a platform-independent way to create and manage windows, buttons, text fields, and other UI components. AWT is one of the earliest Java libraries for building GUIs, predating the more modern Swing library.

AWT's platform independence, simplicity, and robust event-handling capabilities make it a valuable tool for developing basic graphical user interfaces in Java. Its ability to integrate with native code and manage layout efficiently further enhances its utility, especially for simpler applications and legacy systems.

Java's Abstract Window Toolkit (AWT) is widely used for creating graphical user interfaces (GUIs) and handling user interaction in Java applications. Below are some key applications of AWT:

12.1.1 Components of AWT

1. Containers: These are components that can hold other components, such as windows and panels. Examples include `Frame`, `Panel`, and `Applet`.
2. Components: These are the individual elements of the GUI, such as buttons, labels, text fields, and lists. Examples include `Button`, `Label`, `TextField`, and `List`.
3. Layout Managers: These control the positioning and sizing of components within containers. Examples include `FlowLayout`, `BorderLayout`, `GridLayout`, and `CardLayout`.
4. Event Handling: AWT provides a robust event-handling mechanism to respond to user inputs like mouse clicks, keyboard inputs, and window actions. This includes listeners such as `ActionListener`, `MouseListener`, and `KeyListener`.

12.1.2 The Need for Using AWT

1. Platform Independence: AWT allows developers to create applications that can run on any operating system with a Java Virtual Machine (JVM), providing a consistent look and feel across platforms.
2. Basic GUI Development: For simple applications or those requiring lightweight GUIs, AWT provides the essential tools needed without the overhead of more complex libraries like Swing or JavaFX.

DOI: 10.1201/9781003544319-12

3. Event Handling: AWT provides a robust and easy-to-use event-handling mechanism that allows applications to respond to user actions, such as button clicks and key presses.
4. Integration with Native Code:AWT components are heavyweight, meaning they are tied to the native windowing system. This can be advantageous when integrating Java applications with native applications or libraries.
5. Legacy Support: Many older Java applications were built using AWT. Understanding AWT is essential for maintaining and updating these legacy systems.

12.2 ADVANTAGES OF AWT

Java's Abstract Window Toolkit (AWT) offers several advantages for developing graphical user interfaces (GUIs) and handling user interactions. Here are some key benefits:

1. Platform Independence:
   AWT allows developers to create applications that can run on any operating system with a Java Virtual Machine (JVM). This ensures that the GUI looks and behaves consistently across different platforms.
2. Lightweight and Simple:
   For applications with basic GUI requirements, AWT provides a straightforward and lightweight framework. This can be advantageous when developing simple applications or prototyping user interfaces.
3. Integration with Native Code:
   AWT components are heavyweight, meaning they are directly mapped to native operating system components. This can facilitate better integration with native applications and libraries, leveraging the strengths of the underlying platform.
4. Event Handling Mechanism:
   AWT provides a robust and easy-to-use event-handling mechanism, allowing developers to efficiently handle user inputs like mouse clicks, keyboard strokes, and window actions. This makes it easier to build interactive applications.
5. Basic Layout Management:
   AWT offers several layout managers (e.g., `FlowLayout`, `BorderLayout`, `GridLayout`) that help in arranging GUI components within containers. These layout managers simplify the process of designing user interfaces that adapt to different screen sizes and resolutions.
6. Legacy Support:
   AWT is one of the oldest GUI toolkits in Java, meaning many legacy systems and applications are built using it. Knowledge of AWT is essential for maintaining and updating these older applications.
7. Simplified API for Basic Applications:
   AWT's API is relatively straightforward for basic applications, making it easier for beginners to learn and start creating GUIs quickly. The simplicity of AWT components makes it suitable for small projects and educational purposes.

12.3 APPLICATIONS OF AWT

1. Desktop Applications:
   - Simple GUI Applications: AWT is suitable for creating simple desktop applications with basic graphical user interfaces. These applications often involve basic components like buttons, text fields, labels, and simple event handling.

- Prototyping: AWT can be used to quickly prototype the user interface of desktop applications before moving to more complex GUI frameworks like Swing or JavaFX.

2. Educational Tools:
   - Teaching and Learning: AWT provides an easy entry point for beginners learning about GUI development in Java. It is often used in educational environments to teach the basics of event-driven programming and GUI design.
   - Interactive Tutorials: Simple educational applications and interactive tutorials can be developed using AWT to provide a hands-on learning experience.
3. Utilities and Tools:
   - Custom Tools: Developers can use AWT to create small utility programs and tools that require a graphical user interface, such as calculators, text editors, and file explorers.
   - System Monitoring: Applications for monitoring system resources, such as CPU usage or memory consumption, can be developed using AWT.
4. Data Visualization:
   - Graphing and Charting: AWT can be used to develop applications that visualize data through simple graphs and charts. These applications are useful in fields like finance, engineering, and scientific research.
   - Statistical Tools: Basic statistical analysis tools with graphical outputs can be created using AWT.
5. Custom Components and Widgets:
   - Custom GUI Components: Developers can create custom GUI components and widgets using AWT, providing more control over the appearance and behavior of the application's user interface.
   - Reusable Libraries: AWT can be used to develop reusable libraries of custom components that can be integrated into other Java applications.
6. Games and Simulations:
   - Simple Games: Basic games and simulations can be developed using AWT. These applications often involve handling user input, rendering graphics, and managing game states.
   - Educational Simulations: AWT can be used to create educational simulations and interactive learning tools that help visualize complex concepts and processes.

12.4 FEATURES OF JAVA AWT

1. Platform Independence:
   AWT is platform-independent, meaning that AWT applications can run on any operating system that supports Java without requiring any modifications.
2. Lightweight Components:
   AWT includes a set of lightweight components (like buttons, text fields, and labels) that are rendered using the native GUI components of the operating system, ensuring a native look and feel.
3. Event Handling:
   AWT provides a robust event-handling mechanism to manage user interactions such as mouse clicks, key presses, and other actions. It uses the delegation event model, where event handling is delegated to listener objects.
4. Layouts:
   AWT provides several layout managers (like FlowLayout, BorderLayout, GridLayout, etc.) that help in arranging GUI components within a container. Layout managers make it easy to design flexible and adaptable user interfaces.

5. Graphics and Drawing:
   AWT includes classes for drawing and rendering graphics, such as lines, rectangles, ovals, and other shapes. It also supports custom rendering and image processing.
6. Containers and Components:
   AWT consists of containers (such as Frame, Panel, and Applet) and components (such as Button, TextField, Label, etc.) that form the building blocks of an AWT application.
7. Accessibility:
   AWT components are designed to be accessible, supporting assistive technologies such as screen readers, making applications more usable for people with disabilities.
8. Integration with Native Code:
   AWT can integrate with native code through the Java Native Interface (JNI), allowing developers to access and use platform-specific features not available in the standard Java API.
9. Basic GUI Components:
   AWT provides a rich set of basic GUI components, including buttons, checkboxes, choice lists, text areas, scrollbars, and more, enabling developers to build interactive user interfaces.

12.5 AWT PACKAGES

1. `java.awt`
   Core package for the Abstract Window Toolkit (AWT) containing classes for basic GUI components, layout managers, and painting.
2. `java.awt.event`
   Provides classes and interfaces for event handling, including various event types (e.g., mouse, key, action events) and their listeners.
3. `java.awt.geom`
   Contains classes for defining and performing operations on geometric objects, useful for custom graphics and shapes.
4. `java.awt.image`
   Offers classes for creating, manipulating, and observing images, facilitating image processing and display.
5. `java.awt.datatransfer`
   Provides classes and interfaces for transferring data between and within applications, supporting clipboard operations and data flavors.
6. `java.awt.dnd`
   Supports drag-and-drop operations, including drag sources and drop targets, enabling intuitive data transfer within GUIs.

These packages collectively enable the creation and management of graphical user interfaces and handle user interactions in Java applications.

12.6 CONTAINER CLASSES IN AWT

In Java AWT (Abstract Window Toolkit), a container is a component that can contain other components such as buttons, text fields, labels, and other containers. Containers provide a way to organize and arrange the components in a graphical user interface (GUI).

The importance of containers in Java AWT lies in their ability to manage the layout and organization of components within a GUI. They allow developers to create structured and visually appealing user interfaces by arranging components in specific layouts such as BorderLayout, FlowLayout, GridLayout, etc.

Containers play a crucial role in developing applications as they provide the structure and organization needed to create intuitive and user-friendly interfaces. They allow developers to control the placement and arrangement of components, manage user interactions, and ensure proper resizing and scaling of the GUI elements across different screen sizes and resolutions. In Java AWT, there are several types of containers available for organizing and managing components in a graphical user interface (GUI). Here are the main container classes in Java AWT:

12.6.1 Frame

A `Frame` is a top-level window with a title and a border that can act as the main window for the GUI application.In AWT (Abstract Window Toolkit), The key features of a `Frame` are:

1. Top-Level Window: A `Frame` in AWT represents the main window of an application, providing a window with a title bar, borders, and standard window controls (minimize, maximize, close).
2. Resizable and Closable: It allows the user to resize the window, close it, and perform windowing operations like minimizing and maximizing, controlled by the window manager.
3. Contains Components: A `Frame` can hold various AWT components like buttons, text fields, panels, etc., allowing developers to build the user interface within the `Frame`.

Program

```
import java.awt.*;
import java.awt.event.*;
public class FrameExample {
  void main(String[] args) {
  // Create a new Frame
  Frame frame = new Frame("Frame Example");

  // Set the size of the frame
  frame.setSize(300, 200);

  // Set the background color of the frame
  frame.setBackground(Color.LIGHT_GRAY);

  // Set the layout to FlowLayout
  frame.setLayout(new FlowLayout());

  // Create a Button and add it to the frame
  Button button = new Button("Usha");
  frame.add(button);

  // Add a WindowListener to handle window closing
  frame.addWindowListener(new WindowAdapter() {
    @Override
    public void windowClosing(WindowEvent e) {
    System.exit(0);
    }
  });

  // Make the frame visible
  frame.setVisible(true);
  }
}
```

Output

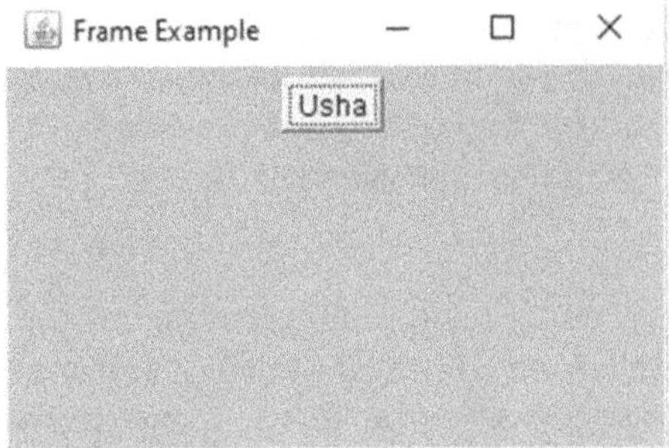

In the above program we created a frame window titled "Frame Example" with a size of 300 by 200 pixels and a light gray background. The layout is set to `FlowLayout`, which arranges components in a left-to-right flow, similar to lines of text in a paragraph. A button labeled "Click Me" is added to the frame. Finally, the frame is made visible to the user.

12.6.2 Panel

A `Panel` is a simple container class that can hold other AWT components. The key features of a `Panel` in AWT (Abstract Window Toolkit):

1. Lightweight Container: `Panel` is a lightweight container that is used to organize and hold AWT components (like buttons, labels, etc.) within a section of a window or applet.
2. Layout Management: It uses layout managers (such as `FlowLayout`, `GridLayout`, etc.) to control the positioning and sizing of components within the panel.
3. Nested Containers: `Panel` can be used as a nested container inside other containers (like `Frame` or another `Panel`), allowing for flexible and complex UI layouts.

Program

```
import java.awt.*;
public class PanelExample {
  void main(String[] args) {
  // Create a new Frame with the title "Panel Example"
  Frame frame = new Frame("Panel Example");

  // Set the size of the frame
  frame.setSize(300, 200);

  // Create a new Panel
  Panel panel = new Panel();

  // Set the background color of the panel to cyan
  panel.setBackground(Color.CYAN);

  // Create two Buttons and add them to the panel
  Button button1 = new Button("Button 1");
  Button button2 = new Button("Button 2");
  panel.add(button1);
  panel.add(button2);
```

```
  // Add the panel to the frame
  frame.add(panel);

  // Make the frame visible
  frame.setVisible(true);
  }
}
```

Output

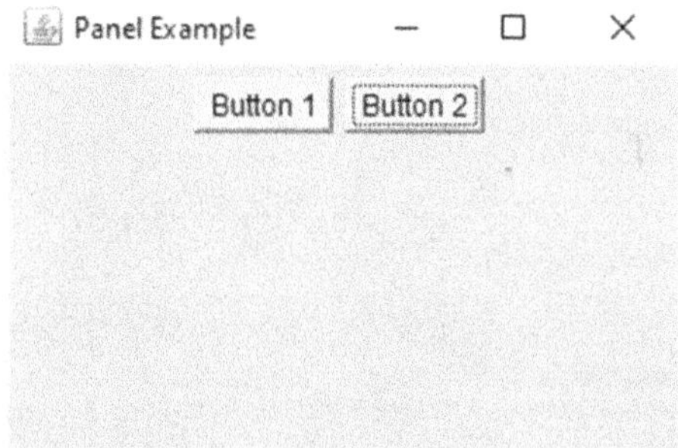

In the above program we created a `Frame` titled "Panel Example" with a size of 300 by 200 pixels. Within the frame, a `Panel` is created and set to have a cyan background. The panel includes two buttons labeled "Button 1" and "Button 2." The panel is then added to the frame, and finally, the frame is made visible to the user.

12.6.3 Dialog

A `Dialog` is a pop-up window that can be modal (blocking user input to other windows) or modeless (allowing user input to other windows). The key features of a `Dialog` in AWT (Abstract Window Toolkit):

1. Pop-Up Window: `Dialog` represents a pop-up window that can be used to display messages, prompts, or request user input. It typically appears over its parent `Frame` or `Applet`.
2. Modal and Non-Modal: `Dialog` can be modal (blocking interaction with other windows until it is closed) or non-modal (allowing interaction with other windows while it is open), controlled by setting its modality.
3. Customizable: It provides the ability to add components and customize their appearance and behavior, such as adding buttons for user actions (e.g., OK, Cancel) and setting its layout and size.

Program

```
import java.awt.*;
import java.awt.event.WindowAdapter;
import java.awt.event.WindowEvent;
public class DialogExample {
  void main(String[] args) {
  // Create the main frame with the title "Dialog Example"
  Frame frame = new Frame("Dialog Example");
  frame.setSize(300, 200);
  frame.setLayout(new FlowLayout());
  // Create a modal dialog with the title "My Dialog"
  final Dialog dialog = new Dialog(frame, "My Dialog", true);
  dialog.setSize(200, 100);
  dialog.setLayout(new FlowLayout());
  dialog.setBackground(Color.PINK);
```

```
  // Add a label to the dialog
  Label label = new Label("This is a dialog");
  dialog.add(label);
  // Display the dialog
  dialog.setVisible(true);
  // Display the main frame
  frame.setVisible(true);
  }
}
```

Output

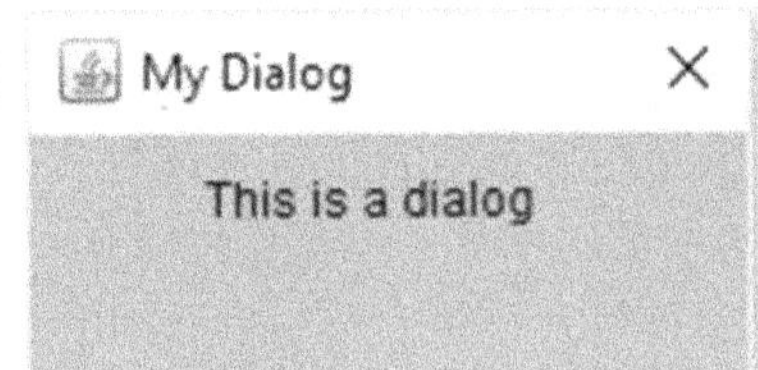

In the above program we created a `Frame` titled "Dialog Example" and within it, a modal `Dialog` titled "My Dialog" with a size of 200 by 100 pixels. The dialog has a pink background and a `FlowLayout`. A `Label` with the text "This is a dialog" is added to the dialog. Finally, the dialog is made visible to the user.

12.6.4 Window

In Java AWT, a `Window` is a top-level container that represents a graphical window with no title or border. It's often used for creating custom pop-up windows or dialog boxes. The key features of a `Window` in AWT (Abstract Window Toolkit):

1. Top-Level Container: `Window` serves as a basic top-level container that can hold other AWT components. It is used as the basis for creating more specific window types like `Frame` and `Dialog`.
2. No Decorations: Unlike `Frame`, `Window` does not include built-in window decorations such as title bars, borders, or control buttons. It provides a plain, undecorated window, which can be useful for custom window designs.
3. Customizable Size and Position: `Window` allows for manual control of its size and position on the screen. Developers can programmatically set its size, position, and visibility as needed for their application.

Program

```
import java.awt.*;
import java.awt.event.*;
public class ColorChangeExample {
  void main(String[] args) {
  // Create a new Frame
  Frame frame = new Frame("Color Change Example");

  // Set the layout to FlowLayout
  frame.setLayout(new FlowLayout());
  // Create a Button to change the background color
  Button changeColorButton = new Button("Change Color");

  // Add an ActionListener to the button to handle click events
```

```
  changeColorButton.addActionListener(new ActionListener() {
    private boolean isDefaultColor = true;

    @Override
    public void actionPerformed(ActionEvent e) {
    // Change the background color of the frame
    if (isDefaultColor) {
      frame.setBackground(Color.CYAN); // Change to cyan
    } else {
      frame.setBackground(Color.LIGHT_GRAY); // Change to light gray
    }
    // Toggle the color state
    isDefaultColor = !isDefaultColor;
    }
  });
  // Add the button to the frame
  frame.add(changeColorButton);
  // Set the frame size and make it visible
  frame.setSize(300, 200);
  frame.setVisible(true);
  // Handle the window closing event
  frame.addWindowListener(new WindowAdapter() {
    @Override
    public void windowClosing(WindowEvent e) {
    System.exit(0);
    }
  });
  }
}
```

Output

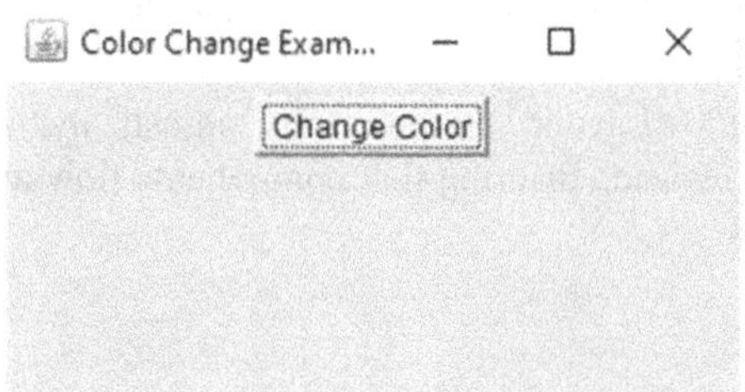

In the above program, we created a simple GUI application using AWT that allows users to change the background color of a frame by clicking a button. The `ColorChangeExample` class sets up a frame with a "Change Color" button, and an `ActionListener` toggles the frame's background color between cyan and light gray each time the button is clicked.

12.7 LAYOUT OF AWT

In Java AWT and Swing, layout managers are used to define the positions and sizes of components within a container. They determine how components are arranged relative to each other and the container itself. The layout managers are important and necessary in developing applications:

1. Platform Independence: Layout managers ensure that the GUI components are positioned correctly regardless of the platform or screen resolution. They handle the differences in window sizes and fonts across different operating systems, ensuring a consistent user experience.

2. Adaptability: Layout managers automatically adjust the layout of components when the window is resized. This makes the GUIs more responsive and adaptable to changes in the window size, ensuring that components remain visible and usable even when the window size changes.
3. Ease of Maintenance: Using layout managers simplifies the process of modifying and maintaining GUIs. Since layout managers handle the positioning of components, you can focus on designing the interface without worrying about the exact pixel coordinates of each component.
4. Scalability: Layout managers support the addition and removal of components dynamically at runtime. This allows you to add or remove components as needed without affecting the overall layout of the interface.
5. Cross-Platform Compatibility: Java's layout managers are designed to work consistently across different platforms, ensuring that the GUIs look and behave the same way on all supported systems.

Layout managers play a crucial role in creating flexible, responsive, and platform-independent GUIs in Java applications. They simplify the development process and help ensure that the applications provide a consistent and user-friendly interface across different environments. The most commonly used layout managers are described below.

12.7.1 FlowLayout

`FlowLayout` arranges components in a left-to-right flow, like lines of text in a paragraph.

The key features of `FlowLayout` in AWT (Abstract Window Toolkit):

1. Simple Layout: `FlowLayout` arranges components in a left-to-right flow, wrapping them to the next line when the current line is filled. It's a straightforward layout manager that arranges components in rows.
2. Alignment Options: It provides options for aligning components horizontally within the container: `LEFT`, `CENTER`, and `RIGHT`. This allows control over the alignment of components within each row.
3. Dynamic Resizing: `FlowLayout` automatically adjusts the arrangement of components when the container is resized, ensuring that components flow and wrap appropriately as the window's size changes.

Program

```
import java.awt.*;
import java.awt.event.*;
public class FlowLayoutExample {
  void main(String[] args) {
  // Create a new Frame
  Frame frame = new Frame("FlowLayout Example");

  // Set the layout to FlowLayout
  frame.setLayout(new FlowLayout());
  // Create two buttons with different background colors
  Button javaButton = new Button("Java");
  javaButton.setBackground(Color.CYAN); // Set background color to cyan

  Button pythonButton = new Button("Python");
  pythonButton.setBackground(Color.MAGENTA); // Set background color to
                                                magenta
```

```
  // Add the buttons to the frame
  frame.add(javaButton);
  frame.add(pythonButton);
  // Set the frame size and make it visible
  frame.setSize(300, 100);
  frame.setVisible(true);
  // Handle the window closing event
  frame.addWindowListener(new WindowAdapter() {
    @Override
    public void windowClosing(WindowEvent e) {
    System.exit(0);
    }
  });
  }
}
```

Output

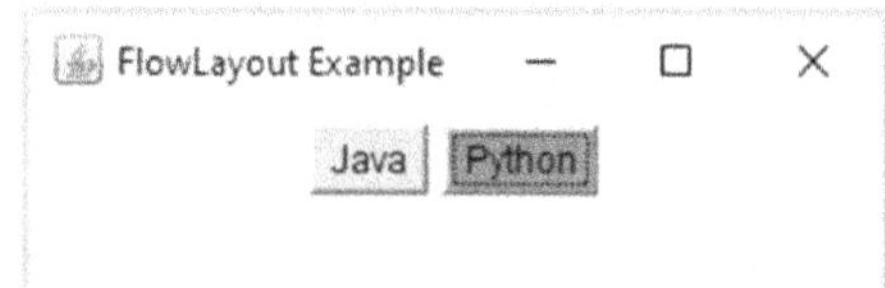

In the above program a `Frame` titled "FlowLayout Example" is created and its layout is set to `FlowLayout`. Two `Button` components labeled "Java" and "Python" are created with cyan and magenta backgrounds, respectively. These buttons are added to the frame. The frame is then sized to 300 by 100 pixels and made visible to the user.

12.7.2 BorderLayout

`BorderLayout` arranges components in five regions: north, south, east, west, and center.

The key features of `BorderLayout` in AWT (Abstract Window Toolkit):

1. Five Regions: `BorderLayout` divides the container into five distinct regions: `NORTH`, `SOUTH`, `EAST`, `WEST`, and `CENTER`. Each region can hold one component, with the `CENTER` region expanding to fill any remaining space.
2. Component Resizing: Components added to the `NORTH` and `SOUTH` regions are sized to fit the full width of the container, while those in the `EAST` and `WEST` regions are sized to fit the full height. The component in the `CENTER` region expands to fill any remaining space.
3. Simple Layout Management: `BorderLayout` provides a straightforward way to manage the placement and resizing of components, making it easy to create layouts where components are positioned around a central area.

Program

```
import java.awt.*;
import java.awt.event.*;
public class BorderLayoutExample {
  void main(String[] args) {
  // Create a new Frame
  Frame frame = new Frame("BorderLayout Example");

  // Set the layout to BorderLayout
```

```
    frame.setLayout(new BorderLayout());
    // Create buttons with different background colors and labels
    Button northButton = new Button("North");
    northButton.setBackground(Color.RED); // Set background color to red
    Button southButton = new Button("South");
    southButton.setBackground(Color.BLUE); // Set background color to blue
    Button eastButton = new Button("East");
    eastButton.setBackground(Color.GREEN); // Set background color to green
    Button westButton = new Button("West");
    westButton.setBackground(Color.ORANGE); // Set background color to orange
    Button centerButton = new Button("Center");
    centerButton.setBackground(Color.PINK); // Set background color to pink
    // Add buttons to the corresponding regions of the frame
    frame.add(northButton, BorderLayout.NORTH);
    frame.add(southButton, BorderLayout.SOUTH);
    frame.add(eastButton, BorderLayout.EAST);
    frame.add(westButton, BorderLayout.WEST);
    frame.add(centerButton, BorderLayout.CENTER);
    // Set the frame size and make it visible
    frame.setSize(400, 300);
    frame.setVisible(true);
    // Handle the window closing event
    frame.addWindowListener(new WindowAdapter() {
      @Override
      public void windowClosing(WindowEvent e) {
      System.exit(0);
      }
    });
    }
}
```

Output

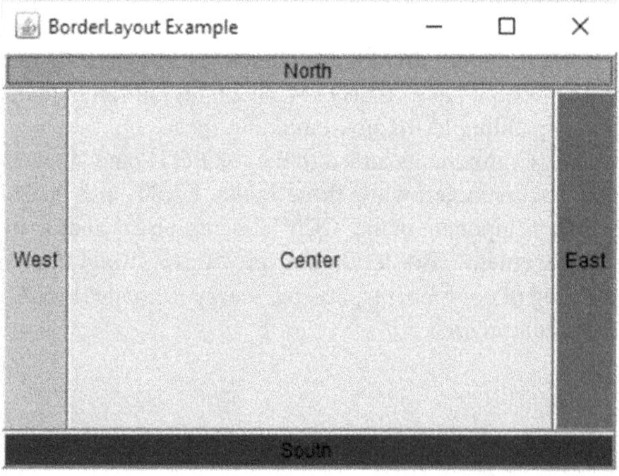

In the above program a `Frame` titled "BorderLayout Example" is created and its layout is set to `BorderLayout`. Five `Button` components are created with different background colors and labels indicating their position: "North" (red), "South" (blue), "East" (green), "West" (orange), and "Center" (pink). These buttons are added to the corresponding regions of the frame. The frame is then sized to 400 by 300 pixels and made visible to the user.

12.7.3 GridLayout

GridLayout` arranges components in a grid of cells, each of equal size. The key features of `GridLayout` in AWT (Abstract Window Toolkit):

1. Uniform Grid: `GridLayout` arranges components in a grid with equal-sized cells. Components are placed in rows and columns, and each cell has the same size.
2. Flexible Row and Column Configuration: You can specify the number of rows and columns when creating a `GridLayout`. If the number of components exceeds the specified rows and columns, it automatically adjusts to fit the components within the grid.
3. Equal Component Sizing: All components within a `GridLayout` are resized to fit into their respective cells, ensuring uniformity and alignment. This makes it ideal for creating consistent and organized layouts.

Program

```
import java.awt.*;
import java.awt.event.*;
public class GridLayoutExample {
  void main(String[] args) {
  // Create a new Frame
  Frame frame = new Frame("GridLayout Example");
  // Set the layout to GridLayout with 2 rows and 2 columns
  frame.setLayout(new GridLayout(2, 2));
  // Create buttons with different background colors and labels
  Button javaButton = new Button("Java");
  javaButton.setBackground(Color.CYAN); // Set background color to cyan
  Button pythonButton = new Button("Python");
  pythonButton.setBackground(Color.MAGENTA); // Set background color to
                                              magenta
  Button cppButton = new Button("C++");
  cppButton.setBackground(Color.YELLOW); // Set background color to yellow
  Button dataStructuresButton = new Button("Data Structures");
  dataStructuresButton.setBackground(Color.ORANGE); // Set background
                                                     color to orange
  // Add buttons to the frame
  frame.add(javaButton);
  frame.add(pythonButton);
  frame.add(cppButton);
  frame.add(dataStructuresButton);
  // Set the frame size and make it visible
  frame.setSize(300, 200);
  frame.setVisible(true);
  // Handle the window closing event
  frame.addWindowListener(new WindowAdapter() {
    @Override
    public void windowClosing(WindowEvent e) {
    System.exit(0);
    }
  });
  }
}
```

Output

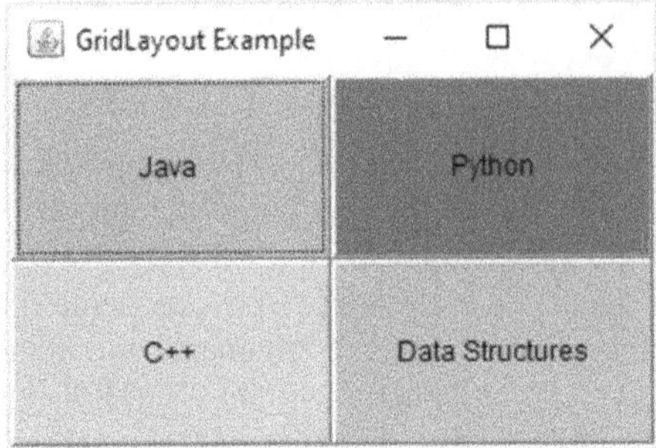

In the above program we created a `Frame` titled "GridLayout Example" and its layout is set to a 2x2 grid. Four `Button` components are created with different background colors and labels indicating programming courses: "Java" (cyan), "Python" (magenta), "C++" (yellow), and "Data Structures" (orange). These buttons are added to the frame in a grid layout. The frame is then sized to 300 by 200 pixels and made visible to the user.

12.7.4 CardLayout

`CardLayout` manages multiple components (cards) that share the same display space. The key features of `CardLayout` in AWT:

1. Card-Based Navigation: `CardLayout` allows you to stack multiple components (cards) on top of each other and switch between them. Each component can be thought of as a "card" in a deck, with only one card visible at a time.
2. Simple Navigation Methods: It provides methods like `next()`, `previous()`, `first()`, and `last()` to navigate through the cards. You can also switch directly to a specific card using a name or index.
3. Dynamic Layout Management: `CardLayout` manages the visibility and layout of the cards dynamically. When a new card is shown, the previously visible card is hidden, making it suitable for creating tabbed or wizard-style interfaces where different content is presented in a single container.

Program

```
import java.awt.*;
import java.awt.event.*;
public class CardLayoutExample {
  void main(String[] args) {
  // Create a new Frame
  Frame frame = new Frame("CardLayout Example");

  // Set the layout to CardLayout
  frame.setLayout(new CardLayout());
  // Create two Panels with light gray background
  Panel panel1 = new Panel();
  panel1.setBackground(Color.LIGHT_GRAY);
  panel1.add(new Label("Register"));
  Panel panel2 = new Panel();
  panel2.setBackground(Color.LIGHT_GRAY);
  panel2.add(new Label("Courses"));
```

```
    // Add panels to the frame with identifiers
    frame.add(panel1, "Register");
    frame.add(panel2, "Courses");
    // Set the layout to display the "Courses" panel
    CardLayout cardLayout = (CardLayout) frame.getLayout();
    cardLayout.show(frame, "Courses");
    // Set the frame size and make it visible
    frame.setSize(300, 200);
    frame.setVisible(true);
    // Handle the window closing event
    frame.addWindowListener(new WindowAdapter() {
      @Override
      public void windowClosing(WindowEvent e) {
      System.exit(0);
      }
    });
    }
}
```

Output

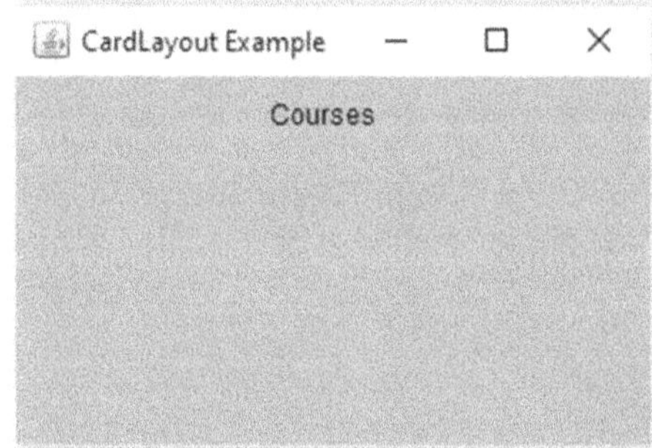

In the above program we created a `Frame` titled "CardLayout Example", and its layout is set to `CardLayout`. Two `Panel` components, each with a light gray background, are created: `panel1` contains a "Register" label, and `panel2` contains a "Courses" label. These panels are added to the frame with identifiers "Register" and "Courses". The `CardLayout` is then set to display the "Courses" panel. Finally, the frame is sized to 300 by 200 pixels and made visible to the user.

12.7.5 GridBagLayout

`GridBagLayout` is a flexible layout manager that aligns components vertically and horizontally, without requiring that the components be of the same size. The key features of `GridBagLayout` in AWT:

1. Flexible Grid System: `GridBagLayout` arranges components in a flexible grid of rows and columns. Unlike `GridLayout`, it allows components to span multiple rows or columns and can adjust their sizes based on their grid constraints.
2. Fine-Grained Control: It provides detailed control over component placement and resizing through `GridBagConstraints`, which specify how a component should be positioned and how it should resize relative to other components in the grid.
3. Complex Layouts: `GridBagLayout` is suitable for creating complex and non-uniform layouts where components of varying sizes and proportions need to be arranged in a grid-like fashion. It can handle intricate UI designs with diverse component arrangements.

Program

```
import java.awt.*;
import java.awt.event.*;
public class GridBagLayoutExample {
  void main(String[] args) {
  // Create a new Frame
  Frame frame = new Frame("GridBagLayout Example");
  // Set the layout to GridBagLayout
  frame.setLayout(new GridBagLayout());
  // Create GridBagConstraints
  GridBagConstraints gbc = new GridBagConstraints();
  gbc.fill = GridBagConstraints.BOTH;
  gbc.insets = new Insets(5, 5, 5, 5); // Padding around components
  // Create buttons with different background colors
  Button button1 = new Button("Java");
  button1.setBackground(Color.CYAN);

  Button button2 = new Button("Python");
  button2.setBackground(Color.MAGENTA);

  Button button3 = new Button("C++");
  button3.setBackground(Color.YELLOW);

  Button button4 = new Button("Data Structures");
  button4.setBackground(Color.ORANGE);
  // Add buttons to the frame with GridBagConstraints
  gbc.gridx = 0; // Column
  gbc.gridy = 0; // Row
  frame.add(button1, gbc);
  gbc.gridx = 1;
  gbc.gridy = 0;
  frame.add(button2, gbc);
  gbc.gridx = 0;
  gbc.gridy = 1;
  frame.add(button3, gbc);
  gbc.gridx = 1;
  gbc.gridy = 1;
  frame.add(button4, gbc);
  // Set the frame size and make it visible
  frame.setSize(300, 200);
  frame.setVisible(true);
  // Handle the window closing event
  frame.addWindowListener(new WindowAdapter() {
    @Override
    public void windowClosing(WindowEvent e) {
    System.exit(0);
    }
  });
  }
}
```

Output

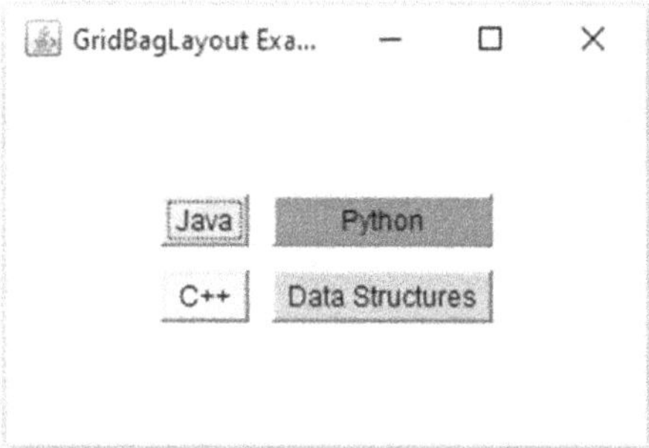

In the above program a `Frame` titled "GridBagLayout Example" is created, and its layout is set to `GridBagLayout`. Four buttons are created with different background colors: "Java" (cyan), "Python" (magenta), "C++" (yellow), and "Data Structures" (orange). Each button is added to the frame at specified grid positions using `GridBagConstraints`. The frame is then set to a size of 300 by 200 pixels and made visible.

12.7.6 BoxLayout

`BoxLayout` arranges components either vertically or horizontally. The key features of `BoxLayout` in AWT:

1. Linear Arrangement: `BoxLayout` arranges components either vertically or horizontally in a single row or column, providing a simple way to align components in a straight line.
2. Component Alignment: It allows components to be aligned along the baseline, center, or other specified positions within the container, facilitating flexible and consistent spacing and alignment.
3. Resizable Components: Components within a `BoxLayout` can grow or shrink according to their preferred sizes and the available space, making it easy to manage layouts with varying component sizes while maintaining a linear arrangement.

Program

```
import java.awt.*;
import java.awt.event.*;
public class BoxLayoutExample {
  void main(String[] args) {
  // Create a new Frame
  Frame frame = new Frame("BoxLayout Example");
  // Create a Panel with BoxLayout set to Y_AXIS (vertical)
  Panel panel = new Panel();
  panel.setLayout(new BoxLayout(panel, BoxLayout.Y_AXIS));
  // Create buttons with different background colors
  Button button1 = new Button("Java");
  button1.setBackground(Color.CYAN);

  Button button2 = new Button("Python");
  button2.setBackground(Color.MAGENTA);
  // Add buttons to the panel
  panel.add(button1);
  panel.add(button2);
```

```
  // Add the panel to the frame
  frame.add(panel);
  // Set the frame size and make it visible
  frame.setSize(300, 200);
  frame.setVisible(true);
  // Handle the window closing event
  frame.addWindowListener(new WindowAdapter() {
    @Override
    public void windowClosing(WindowEvent e) {
    System.exit(0);
    }
  });
  }
}
```

Output

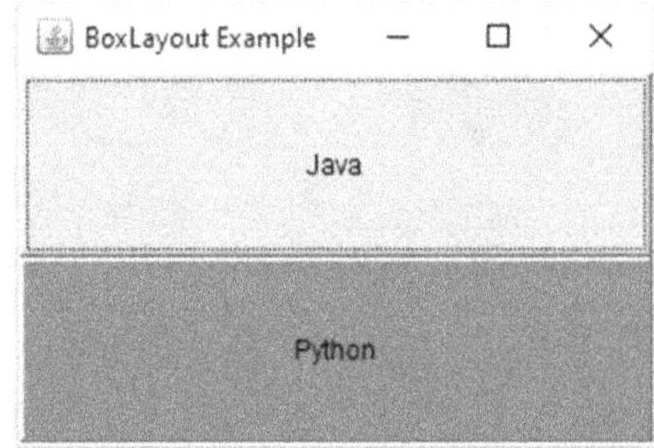

In the above program a `Frame` titled "BoxLayout Example" is created, and a `Panel` with a vertical `BoxLayout` is added to it. Two buttons are created: "Java" (cyan background) and "Python" (magenta background). These buttons are added to the panel. Finally, the panel is added to the frame, the frame's size is set to 300 by 200 pixels, and the frame is made visible.

12.7.7 GroupLayout

`GroupLayout` is a layout manager that arranges the components in a hierarchical manner. The key features of `GroupLayout` are:

1. Flexible Layout Management: `GroupLayout` allows for precise control over component positioning by organizing components into horizontal and vertical groups. This enables complex and flexible arrangements where components can be aligned and spaced according to specific constraints.
2. Automatic Sizing and Alignment: It automatically adjusts component sizes and alignments based on their preferred sizes and constraints, ensuring that components are properly aligned and spaced without requiring manual adjustments.
3. Integrated with GUI Builders: `GroupLayout` is particularly useful in GUI builders (like NetBeans) where it simplifies the design process by visually arranging components and managing their layout, making it easier to create sophisticated and responsive user interfaces.

Program

```
import javax.swing.*;
import javax.swing.GroupLayout.Alignment;
import java.awt.*;
```

```
public class GroupLayoutExample {
  void main(String[] args) {
  // Create a JFrame with the title "GroupLayout Example"
  JFrame frame = new JFrame("GroupLayout Example");
  frame.setDefaultCloseOperation(JFrame.EXIT_ON_CLOSE);
  // Create a JPanel and set its layout to GroupLayout
  JPanel panel = new JPanel();
  GroupLayout layout = new GroupLayout(panel);
  panel.setLayout(layout);
  // Create buttons with different background colors
  JButton button1 = new JButton("Java");
  button1.setBackground(Color.CYAN);
  JButton button2 = new JButton("Python");
  button2.setBackground(Color.MAGENTA);
  // Define the horizontal group
  layout.setHorizontalGroup(
    layout.createSequentialGroup()
    .addContainerGap()
    .addGroup(layout.createParallelGroup(Alignment.LEADING)
      .addComponent(button1)
      .addComponent(button2))
    .addContainerGap()
  );
  // Define the vertical group
  layout.setVerticalGroup(
    layout.createSequentialGroup()
    .addContainerGap()
    .addComponent(button1)
    .addPreferredGap(LayoutStyle.ComponentPlacement.RELATED)
    .addComponent(button2)
    .addContainerGap()
  );
  // Add the panel to the frame
  frame.add(panel);
  // Set the frame size and make it visible
  frame.setSize(300, 100);
  frame.setVisible(true);
  }
}
```

Output

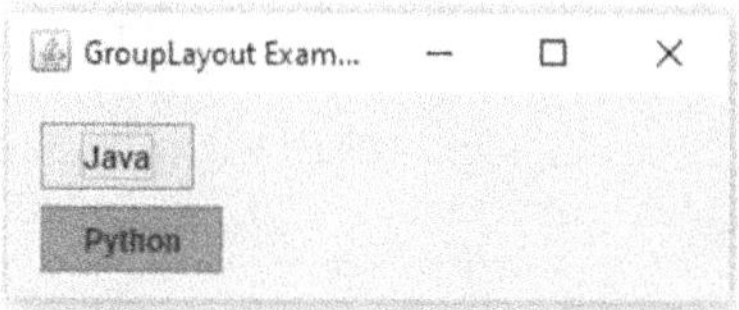

In the above program a `Frame` titled "GroupLayout Example" is created, containing a `JPanel` with a `GroupLayout`. Two buttons, "Java" (cyan background) and "Python" (magenta background), are added to the panel. The layout is set to create gaps automatically between components and container edges. The horizontal group is set to display the buttons sequentially, and the vertical group is set to align the buttons in parallel. The panel is added to the frame, which is sized to 300 by 100 pixels and made visible.

12.7.8 SpringLayout

`SpringLayout` is a flexible layout manager designed for use by GUI builders. The key features of `SpringLayout`are:

1. Flexible Layout Constraints: `SpringLayout` allows for precise control over component positioning using a set of flexible constraints, or "springs," which define the relative positions of components based on their distances from each other and from the container's edges.
2. Dynamic Layout Adjustment: The layout manager adjusts components dynamically as the container is resized or as components are added or removed, maintaining the specified constraints and ensuring a responsive layout.
3. Complex Layouts: It enables the creation of complex and adaptive layouts by specifying constraints for each component, allowing for more sophisticated designs where components' positions and sizes are governed by relative relationships rather than fixed coordinates.

Program

```
import javax.swing.*;
import java.awt.*;
import java.awt.event.*;
public class SpringLayoutExample {
  void main(String[] args) {
  // Create a JFrame with the title "SpringLayout Example"
  JFrame frame = new JFrame("SpringLayout Example");
  frame.setDefaultCloseOperation(JFrame.EXIT_ON_CLOSE);
  // Create a JPanel and set its layout to SpringLayout
  JPanel panel = new JPanel();
  SpringLayout layout = new SpringLayout();
  panel.setLayout(layout);
  // Create buttons with different background colors
  JButton button1 = new JButton("Java");
  button1.setBackground(Color.CYAN);
  JButton button2 = new JButton("Python");
  button2.setBackground(Color.MAGENTA);
  // Add buttons to the panel
  panel.add(button1);
  panel.add(button2);
  // Define SpringLayout constraints for button1
  layout.putConstraint(SpringLayout.NORTH, button1, 10, SpringLayout.
     NORTH, panel);
  layout.putConstraint(SpringLayout.WEST, button1, 10, SpringLayout.WEST,
     panel);
  // Define SpringLayout constraints for button2
  layout.putConstraint(SpringLayout.NORTH, button2, 0, SpringLayout.NORTH,
     button1);
  layout.putConstraint(SpringLayout.WEST, button2, 20, SpringLayout.EAST,
     button1);
  // Add the panel to the frame
  frame.add(panel);
  // Set the frame size and make it visible
  frame.setSize(300, 100);
  frame.setVisible(true);
  }
}
```

Output

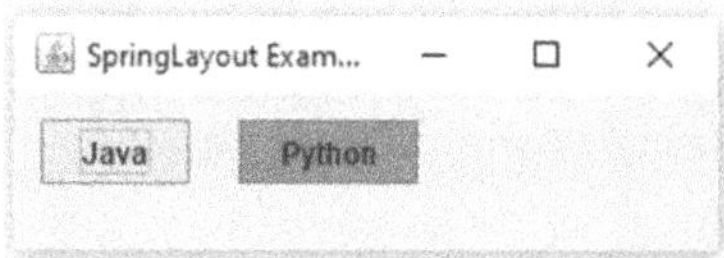

In the above program a `JFrame` titled "SpringLayout Example" contains a `JPanel` with a `SpringLayout`. Two buttons, "Java" (cyan background) and "Python" (magenta background), are added to the panel. The layout constraints position the "Java" button 10 pixels from the top-left corner of the panel, and the "Python" button 20 pixels to the right of the "Java" button, aligned vertically. The panel is added to the frame, which is sized to 300 by 100 pixels and made visible.

12.7.9 Absolute Layout

Absolute Layout allows precise placement of components by specifying exact coordinates. The key features of `Absolute Layout` are:

1. Fixed Positioning: In Absolute Layout, components are positioned at specific coordinates (x, y) within the container. This allows for precise control over the placement and size of each component, but it requires manual specification of coordinates and dimensions.
2. No Automatic Layout Management: Unlike other layout managers, Absolute Layout does not automatically adjust or manage the sizes or positions of components when the container is resized. Components remain fixed in their specified positions and sizes, which can lead to layout issues if the container's dimensions change.
3. Simple and Direct: While offering precise control, Absolute Layout is straightforward and easy to implement for simple interfaces where components do not need to adjust dynamically. However, it is generally less flexible and scalable for complex or responsive UI designs compared to other layout managers.

Program

```
import java.awt.*;
import java.awt.event.*;
public class AbsoluteLayoutExample {
  void main(String[] args) {
  // Create a Frame with the title "AbsoluteLayout Example"
  Frame frame = new Frame("AbsoluteLayout Example");
  frame.setLayout(null);  // Set layout to null for absolute positioning
  // Create buttons with different background colors
  Button button1 = new Button("Java");
  button1.setBackground(Color.CYAN);
  Button button2 = new Button("Python");
  button2.setBackground(Color.MAGENTA);
  // Set size and position for button1
  button1.setBounds(50, 50, 80, 30);  // x, y, width, height
  // Set size and position for button2
  button2.setBounds(150, 50, 80, 30);  // x, y, width, height
  // Add buttons to the frame
  frame.add(button1);
  frame.add(button2);
  // Set the frame size and make it visible
```

```
  frame.setSize(300, 150);
  frame.setVisible(true);
  // Add a window listener to handle the closing event
  frame.addWindowListener(new WindowAdapter() {
    public void windowClosing(WindowEvent e) {
    System.exit(0);
    }
  });
  }
}
```

Output

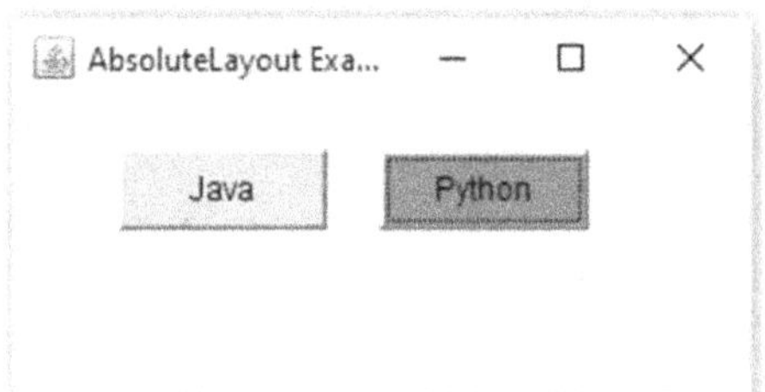

In the above program a `Frame` titled "AbsoluteLayout Example" has its layout set to `null`, enabling absolute positioning. Two buttons, "Java" (cyan background) and "Python" (magenta background), are added to the frame. The "Java" button is positioned at (50, 50) with dimensions 80x30 pixels, while the "Python" button is positioned at (150, 50) with the same dimensions. The frame is set to a size of 300x150 pixels and made visible.

12.8 COMPONENTS OF AWT

In Java AWT, components are the building blocks used to create graphical user interfaces (GUIs). Components represent various visual elements such as buttons, labels, text fields, checkboxes, menus, and more. They are the user interface elements with which users interact to perform actions or provide input.

The importance of components in Java AWT lies in their role in creating interactive and visually appealing user interfaces for Java applications.

1. User Interaction: Components enable users to interact with the application by clicking buttons, entering text, selecting options, and performing other actions.
2. Visual Representation: Components provide a visual representation of various GUI elements, making it easy for users to understand and navigate through the application.
3. Event Handling: Components generate events in response to user actions, such as button clicks or text input. These events can be handled by event listeners to execute specific actions or trigger application logic.
4. Customization: Components can be customized in terms of appearance, size, color, font, and layout to match the design requirements and aesthetics of the application.
5. Modularity: Components can be reused across different parts of the application or in multiple applications, promoting modularity and code reusability.
6. Hierarchy: Components can be organized hierarchically, allowing for the creation of complex user interfaces with nested containers and subcomponents.

12.8.1 Label

A `Label` is a non-editable text component. The key features of `Label` in AWT (Abstract Window Toolkit):

1. Text Display: `Label` is used to display a single line of text or an image. It is typically used to provide information or labels next to other components, such as text fields or buttons.
2. Non-Editable: Unlike other components like `TextField` or `TextArea`, `Label` is non-editable. It simply shows text or images without user interaction, making it ideal for static display purposes.
3. Alignment and Styling: `Label` allows text alignment options such as left, center, or right alignment. You can also customize its font, color, and other properties to match the design of your user interface.

Program

```
import java.awt.*;
import java.awt.event.*;
public class LabelExample {
  void main(String[] args) {
  // Create a Frame with the title "Label Example"
  Frame frame = new Frame("Label Example");
  frame.setLayout(new FlowLayout()); // Set layout to FlowLayout
  // Create a Label with the text "Course Registration Form"
  Label label = new Label("Course Registration Form");
  label.setBackground(Color.CYAN); // Set background color to cyan
  // Add the label to the frame
  frame.add(label);
  // Set the frame size and make it visible
  frame.setSize(300, 100);
  frame.setVisible(true);
  // Add a window listener to handle the closing event
  frame.addWindowListener(new WindowAdapter() {
    public void windowClosing(WindowEvent e) {
    System.exit(0);
    }
  });
  }
}
```

Output

Label Example

Course Registration Form

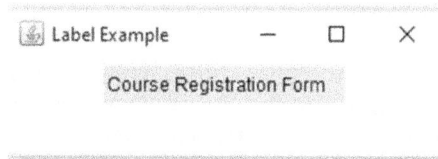

In the above program we created a `Frame` titled "Label Example" with a `Label` that reads "Course Registration Form" and has a cyan background. The label is added to the frame, which uses a `FlowLayout` for arranging components. The frame is set to a size of 300x100 pixels and made visible.

12.8.2 Button

A `Button` is a push-button control that triggers an action event when clicked. The key features of `Button` in AWT (Abstract Window Toolkit):

1. Interactive Element: `Button` is an interactive component that allows users to trigger actions when clicked. It can execute specific code or perform operations when the user interacts with it.
2. Customizable Text and Appearance: You can set the text or label displayed on the button, and customize its appearance, including its size, font, and color. This allows you to tailor the button's look to fit the design of your application.
3. Event Handling: `Button` supports event handling, where you can attach `ActionListener` objects to handle button click events. This enables you to define custom behavior in response to user actions, such as submitting a form or initiating a process.

Program

```
import java.awt.*;
import java.awt.event.*;
public class ButtonExample {
  void main(String[] args) {
  // Create a Frame with the title "Button Example"
  Frame frame = new Frame("Button Example");
  frame.setLayout(new FlowLayout());  // Set layout to FlowLayout
  // Create a Button with the label "Submit"
  Button button = new Button("Submit");
  button.setBackground(Color.GREEN);  // Set background color to green
  // Add the button to the frame
  frame.add(button);
  // Set the frame size and make it visible
  frame.setSize(200, 100);
  frame.setVisible(true);
  // Add a window listener to handle the closing event
  frame.addWindowListener(new WindowAdapter() {
    public void windowClosing(WindowEvent e) {
    System.exit(0);
    }
  });
  }
}
```

Output

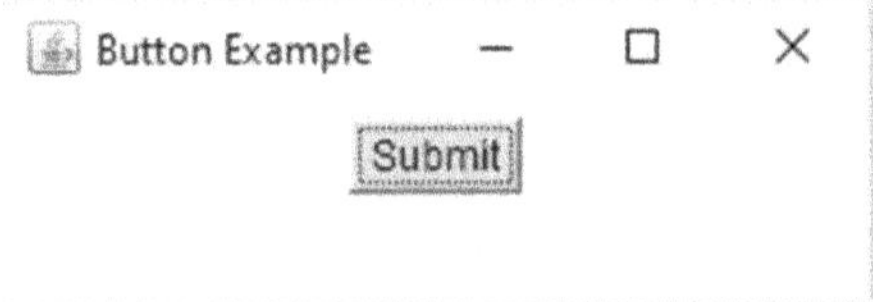

In the above program we created a `Frame` titled "Button Example", and a `Button` labeled "Submit" with a green background is added to it. The frame uses a `FlowLayout` to arrange its components. The frame is set to a size of 200x100 pixels and is made visible.

12.8.3 TextField

A `TextField` allows the user to enter a single line of text. The key features of `TextField` in AWT (Abstract Window Toolkit):

1. Single-Line Input: `TextField` provides a single-line area where users can enter and edit text. It is commonly used for user input such as entering names, search queries, or short pieces of information.
2. Customizable Size and Columns: You can specify the number of columns for the `TextField`, which determines its width. This allows you to adjust the size of the text field according to your design needs and the expected length of input.
3. Event Handling and Validation: `TextField` supports event handling through `ActionListener` and other listeners, enabling you to respond to user interactions and validate input. This makes it easy to implement functionality such as data submission or real-time input validation.

Program

```
import java.awt.*;
import java.awt.event.*;
public class TextFieldExample {
  void main(String[] args) {
  // Create a Frame with the title “TextField Example”
  Frame frame = new Frame(“TextField Example”);
  frame.setLayout(new FlowLayout());  // Set layout to FlowLayout
  // Create a TextField with placeholder text
  TextField textField = new TextField(“Enter your name”);
  textField.setBackground(Color.YELLOW);  // Set background color to yellow
  // Add the TextField to the frame
  frame.add(textField);
  // Set the frame size and make it visible
  frame.setSize(300, 100);
  frame.setVisible(true);
  // Add a window listener to handle the closing event
  frame.addWindowListener(new WindowAdapter() {
    public void windowClosing(WindowEvent e) {
    System.exit(0);
    }
  });
  }
}
```

Output

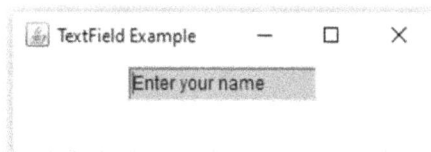

In the above program we created a `Frame` titled “TextField Example” and added a `TextField` with the placeholder text “Enter your name” and a yellow background. The frame uses a `FlowLayout` to manage its components. The frame is sized to 300x100 pixels and made visible.

12.8.4 TextArea

A `TextArea` allows the user to enter multiple lines of text. The key features of `TextArea`are:

1. Multi-Line Input: `TextArea` allows users to enter and edit multiple lines of text, making it suitable for longer input such as comments, descriptions, or large blocks of data.

2. Scroll Capability: It supports scrolling when the text exceeds the visible area of the text area. This ensures users can view and edit all text content without requiring a fixed-size input field.
3. Customizable Line and Column Size: You can set the number of rows and columns for the `TextArea`, which controls its size and how much text can be displayed at once. This flexibility allows you to tailor the component to fit various design requirements and text entry needs.

Program

```
import java.awt.*;
import java.awt.event.*;
public class TextAreaExample {
  void main(String[] args) {
  // Create a Frame with the title "TextArea Example"
  Frame frame = new Frame("TextArea Example");
  frame.setLayout(new FlowLayout()); // Set layout to FlowLayout
  // Create a TextArea with placeholder text, 5 rows, and 30 columns
  TextArea textArea = new TextArea("Enter your experience", 5, 30);
  textArea.setBackground(Color.PINK); // Set background color to pink
  // Add the TextArea to the frame
  frame.add(textArea);
  // Set the frame size and make it visible
  frame.setSize(400, 200);
  frame.setVisible(true);
  // Add a window listener to handle the closing event
  frame.addWindowListener(new WindowAdapter() {
    public void windowClosing(WindowEvent e) {
    System.exit(0);
    }
  });
  }
}
```

Output

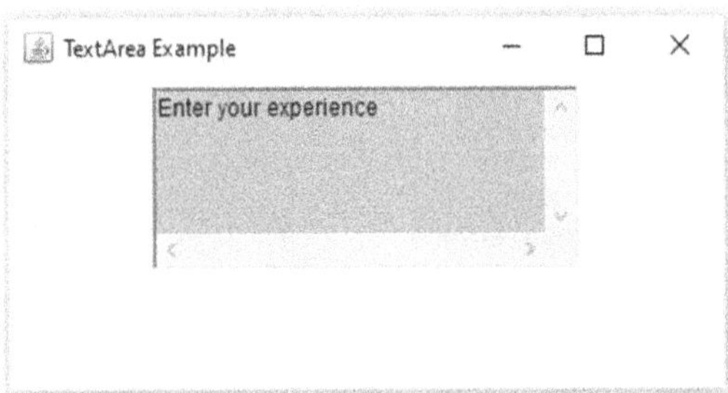

In the above program we created a `Frame` titled "TextArea Example" and added a `TextArea` with the placeholder text "Enter your experience", sized 5 rows by 30 columns, and a pink background. The frame uses a `FlowLayout` to manage its components. The frame is sized to 400x200 pixels and made visible.

12.8.5 Checkbox

A `Checkbox` allows the user to make a binary choice, i.e., a choice between one of two possible options. The key features of `Checkbox` are:

1. Binary Choice: `Checkbox` allows users to make a binary choice, either selecting (checked) or deselecting (unchecked) an option. It is commonly used for options that are not mutually exclusive, where multiple checkboxes can be selected at once.
2. Labeling: Each `Checkbox` can be associated with a text label, which describes the option or choice it represents. This helps users understand the purpose of the checkbox and what action they are selecting.
3. State Handling: `Checkbox` supports event handling through `ItemListener`, allowing you to respond to changes in its state (checked or unchecked). This enables you to execute specific actions based on the user's selections, such as updating other components or triggering events.

Program

```
import java.awt.*;
import java.awt.event.*;
public class CourseSelectionAWT {
  void main(String[] args) {
  // Create a new Frame
  Frame frame = new Frame("Checkbox Example");
  // Set the layout of the frame to FlowLayout
  frame.setLayout(new FlowLayout());
  // Create a label for "Courses"
  Label courseLabel = new Label("Courses:");
  // Create checkboxes for Java and Python courses
  Checkbox javaCheckbox = new Checkbox("Java");
  Checkbox pythonCheckbox = new Checkbox("Python");
  // Add components to the frame
  frame.add(courseLabel);
  frame.add(javaCheckbox);
  frame.add(pythonCheckbox);
  // Set frame size and make it visible
  frame.setSize(300, 200);
  frame.setVisible(true);
  // Add window listener to close the frame
  frame.addWindowListener(new WindowAdapter() {
    public void windowClosing(WindowEvent windowEvent) {
    System.exit(0);
    }
  });
  }
}
```

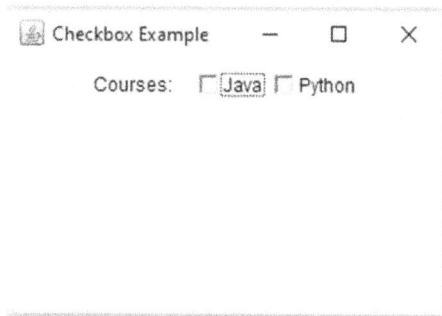

Output

Checkbox Example

Courses: Java Python

In the above program we created a simple AWT Frame with a FlowLayout that arranges components from left to right. Later we added a Label ("Courses") and two checkboxes for Java and Python course selection. The frame also includes a WindowListener to allow closing the window when the user clicks the close button.

12.8.6 CheckboxGroup

A `CheckboxGroup` allows the user to select only one checkbox from a group of checkboxes. The key features of `CheckboxGroup` are:

1. Mutual Exclusivity: `CheckboxGroup` allows for the grouping of multiple `Checkbox` components so that only one checkbox in the group can be selected at a time. This creates a mutually exclusive set of choices, similar to radio buttons.
2. Shared State: Within a `CheckboxGroup`, all checkboxes share a common state. Selecting one checkbox automatically deselects any previously selected checkbox in the same group, ensuring that only one option is active at a time.
3. State Management: `CheckboxGroup` provides methods to manage the selection state, such as `getSelectedCheckbox()` to retrieve the currently selected checkbox and `setSelectedCheckbox(Checkbox checkbox)` to programmatically select a specific checkbox within the group. This allows for control and manipulation of the selection state programmatically.

Program

```
import java.awt.*;
import java.awt.event.*;
public class CheckboxGroupExample {
  void main(String[] args) {
  // Create a Frame with the title "CheckboxGroup Example"
  Frame frame = new Frame("CheckboxGroup Example");
  frame.setLayout(new FlowLayout());  // Set layout to FlowLayout
  // Create a CheckboxGroup
  CheckboxGroup group = new CheckboxGroup();
  // Create two Checkboxes with the same CheckboxGroup
  Checkbox checkbox1 = new Checkbox("Java", group, false);
  checkbox1.setBackground(Color.ORANGE);  // Set background color to orange
  Checkbox checkbox2 = new Checkbox("Python", group, false);
  checkbox2.setBackground(Color.ORANGE);  // Set background color to orange
  // Add the Checkboxes to the frame
  frame.add(checkbox1);
  frame.add(checkbox2);
  // Set the frame size and make it visible
  frame.setSize(300, 100);
  frame.setVisible(true);
  // Add a window listener to handle the closing event
  frame.addWindowListener(new WindowAdapter() {
    public void windowClosing(WindowEvent e) {
    System.exit(0);
    }
  });
  }
}
```

Output

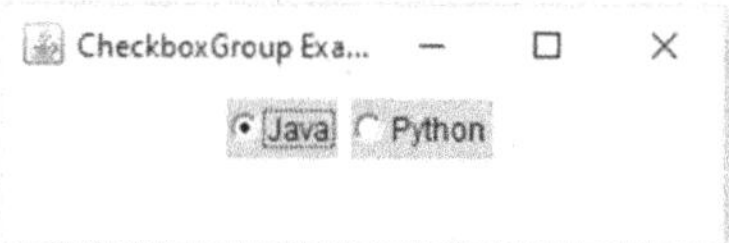

In the above program we created a `Frame` titled "CheckboxGroup Example" and added two checkboxes labeled "Java" and "Python", grouped together in a `CheckboxGroup` so only one can be selected at a time. Both checkboxes have an orange background. The frame uses a `FlowLayout` for its components, is sized to 300x100 pixels, and is made visible.

12.8.7 Choice

A `Choice` is a pop-up menu that lets the user choose one option from a list of options. The key features of `Choice` in AWT:

1. Drop-Down List: `Choice` provides a drop-down list of items from which users can select a single option. It displays a compact list of choices that expands when clicked, making it ideal for saving space in a user interface.
2. Item Management: You can dynamically add, remove, and modify items in the `Choice` list using methods such as `addItem()`, `removeItem()`, and `insertItem()`. This allows for flexible management of the options available to users.
3. Event Handling: `Choice` supports event handling through `ItemListener`, enabling you to respond to user selections. This allows you to execute specific actions or update other components based on the user's choice from the drop-down list.

Program

```
import java.awt.*;
import java.awt.event.*;
public class ChoiceExample {
  void main(String[] args) {
  // Create a Frame with the title "Choice Example"
  Frame frame = new Frame("Choice Example");
  frame.setLayout(new FlowLayout()); // Set layout to FlowLayout
  // Create a Choice dropdown menu
  Choice choice = new Choice();
  choice.add("Java");
  choice.add("Python");
  choice.add("C++");
  // Set background color of the Choice dropdown menu
  choice.setBackground(Color.MAGENTA);
  // Add the Choice dropdown menu to the frame
  frame.add(choice);
  // Set the frame size and make it visible
  frame.setSize(300, 100);
  frame.setVisible(true);
  // Add a window listener to handle the closing event
  frame.addWindowListener(new WindowAdapter() {
    public void windowClosing(WindowEvent e) {
    System.exit(0);
    }
```

```
  });
  }
}
```

Output

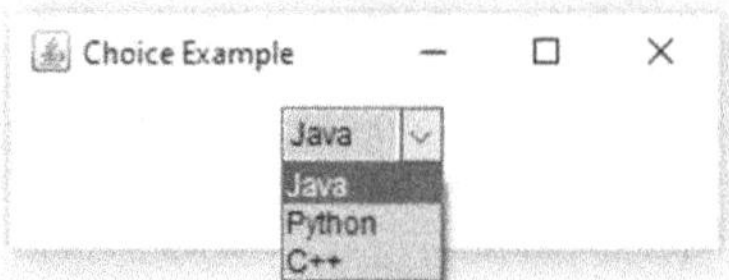

In the above program we created a `Frame` titled "Choice Example" and added a `Choice` drop-down menu with options "Java," "Python," and "C++," setting the drop-down's background color to magenta. The frame uses a `FlowLayout` for its components, is sized to 300x100 pixels, and is made visible.

12.8.8 List

A `List` allows the user to select one or more items from a list. The key features of `List` in AWT (Abstract Window Toolkit):

1. Multiple Selection Modes: `List` can be configured to allow single or multiple selections. Users can choose one or more items from the list based on the selection mode set (`MULTIPLE_INTERVAL_SELECTION`, `SINGLE_SELECTION`, etc.).
2. Scrollable List: `List` provides scrollbars automatically when the number of items exceeds the visible area. This ensures that users can scroll through and view all available items in the list.
3. Dynamic Item Management: You can add, remove, and modify items in a `List` using methods such as `add()`, `remove()`, and `insert()`. This flexibility allows you to update the list of options programmatically based on user interactions or other application events.

Program

```
import java.awt.*;
public class ListExample {
  void main(String[] args) {
  // Create a Frame with the title "List Example"
  Frame frame = new Frame("List Example");
  frame.setLayout(new FlowLayout()); // Set layout to FlowLayout
  // Create a List component
  List list = new List();
  list.add("Java");
  list.add("Python");
  list.add("C++");
  list.add("Data Structures");
  // Set background color of the List
  list.setBackground(Color.CYAN);
  // Add the List component to the frame
  frame.add(list);
  // Set the frame size and make it visible
  frame.setSize(300, 200);
  frame.setVisible(true);
  // Add a window listener to handle the closing event
  frame.addWindowListener(new WindowAdapter() {
```

```
    public void windowClosing(WindowEvent e) {
    System.exit(0);
    }
  });
  }
}
```

Output

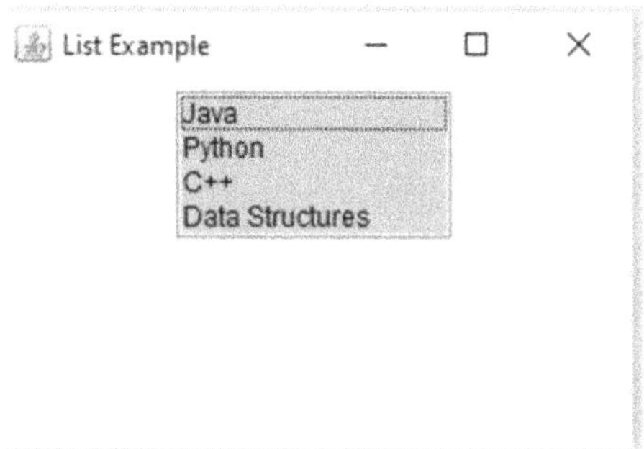

In the above program we created a `Frame` titled “List Example” and added a `List` component with items “Java,” “Python,” “C++,” and “Data Structures,” setting the list’s background color to cyan. The frame uses a `FlowLayout` for its components, is sized to 300x200 pixels, and is made visible.

12.8.9 Canvas

A `Canvas` is a blank rectangular area where users can draw or trap input events. The key features of `Canvas` in AWT:

1. Custom Drawing: `Canvas` provides a blank area where you can perform custom drawing and graphics operations using Java’s Graphics class. It is commonly used for creating custom graphical interfaces or visual elements.
2. Flexible Size: You can set the size of a `Canvas` to fit the specific needs of your application. This allows for precise control over the drawing area and ensures that it can be resized or adjusted as required.
3. Event Handling: `Canvas` supports event handling for user interactions, such as mouse and keyboard events. This makes it possible to create interactive graphics and respond to user input within the canvas area.

Program

```
import java.awt.*;
import java.awt.event.*;
public class CanvasExample {
  void main(String[] args) {
  // Create a Frame with the title "Canvas Example"
  Frame frame = new Frame("Canvas Example");
  frame.setLayout(new FlowLayout());  // Set layout to FlowLayout
  // Create a custom Canvas component
  Canvas canvas = new Canvas() {
    @Override
    public void paint(Graphics g) {
    super.paint(g);
    // Set the color to red
```

```
    g.setColor(Color.RED);
    // Draw a rectangle at coordinates (50, 50) with width 100 and height 100
    g.fillRect(50, 50, 100, 100);
    }
  };

  // Set the background color of the Canvas to light gray
  canvas.setBackground(Color.LIGHT_GRAY);
  // Set the size of the Canvas
  canvas.setSize(300, 200);
  // Add the Canvas to the Frame
  frame.add(canvas);
  // Set the Frame size and make it visible
  frame.setSize(300, 200);
  frame.setVisible(true);
  // Add a window listener to handle the closing event
  frame.addWindowListener(new WindowAdapter() {
    public void windowClosing(WindowEvent e) {
    System.exit(0);
    }
  });
  }
}
```

Output

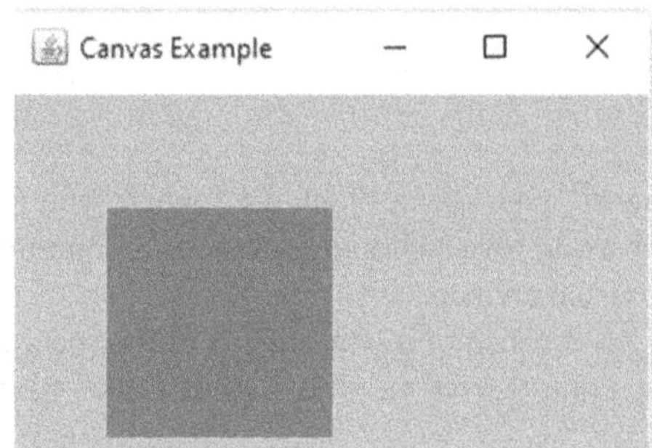

In the above program we created a `Frame` titled "Canvas Example" and added a custom `Canvas` component. The `Canvas` is overridden to draw a red rectangle at coordinates (50, 50) with a width of 100 pixels and a height of 100 pixels. The canvas's background color is set to light gray. The frame uses a `FlowLayout` for its components, is sized to 300x200 pixels, and is made visible.

12.8.10 Scrollbar

A `Scrollbar` provides a way to adjust the visible portion of a component or content area. The key features of `Scrollbar` in AWT:

1. Scrolling Functionality: `Scrollbar` provides a mechanism for scrolling through content that exceeds the visible area of a container. It allows users to navigate through a range of values or a long list of items by moving the scrollbar thumb.
2. Adjustable Orientation: `Scrollbar` can be oriented horizontally or vertically, depending on the direction in which scrolling is required. This flexibility allows for integration into both vertical and horizontal scrolling interfaces.

3. Customizable Parameters: You can customize the `Scrollbar` with parameters such as the minimum and maximum values, the visible amount, and the unit and block increments. This allows you to fine-tune its behavior and appearance to fit specific application needs.

Program

```
import java.awt.*;
import java.awt.event.*;
public class ScrollbarExample {
  void main(String[] args) {
  // Create a Frame with the title "Scrollbar Example"
  Frame frame = new Frame("Scrollbar Example");
  frame.setLayout(new FlowLayout()); // Set layout to FlowLayout
  // Create a Scrollbar component
  Scrollbar scrollbar = new Scrollbar();

  // Set the background color of the Scrollbar to pink
  scrollbar.setBackground(Color.PINK);
  // Add the Scrollbar to the Frame
  frame.add(scrollbar);
  // Set the size of the Frame and make it visible
  frame.setSize(300, 200);
  frame.setVisible(true);
  // Add a window listener to handle the closing event
  frame.addWindowListener(new WindowAdapter() {
    public void windowClosing(WindowEvent e) {
    System.exit(0);
    }
  });
  }
}
```

Output

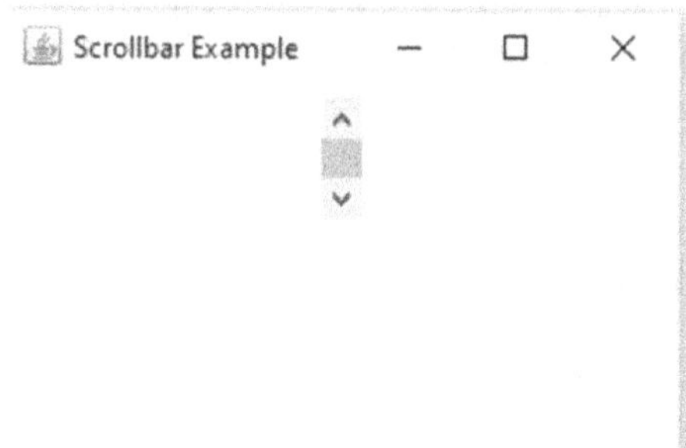

In the above program we created a `Frame` titled "Scrollbar Example" and added a `Scrollbar` component. The background color of the scrollbar is set to pink. The frame uses a `FlowLayout` for its components, is sized to 300x200 pixels, and is made visible.

12.8.11 Menu

A `Menu` is a drop-down menu in a menu bar. The key features of `Menu` in AWT:

1. Hierarchical Structure: `Menu` provides a way to organize related actions or commands in a hierarchical structure, typically accessed through a drop-down list from a menu bar. This

allows for the grouping of related functionalities into categories, enhancing usability and organization.

2. Menu Items: Within a `Menu`, you can add `MenuItem` components (or other nested menus), which represent individual actions or commands. This allows users to interact with various options and perform specific tasks based on their selection.
3. Event Handling: `Menu` supports event handling through `ActionListener` and other event listeners, enabling you to define custom behaviors for each menu item. This allows you to respond to user selections and execute corresponding actions within your application.

Program

```
import java.awt.*;
import java.awt.event.ActionEvent;
import java.awt.event.ActionListener;
import java.awt.event.*;
public class MenuExample {
  void main(String[] args) {
  // Create a Frame with the title "Menu Example"
  Frame frame = new Frame("Menu Example");
  // Create a MenuBar
  MenuBar menuBar = new MenuBar();
  // Create a Menu titled "Courses"
  Menu coursesMenu = new Menu("Courses");
  // Create MenuItems for the Menu
  MenuItem javaMenuItem = new MenuItem("Java");
  MenuItem pythonMenuItem = new MenuItem("Python");
  // Add ActionListener to MenuItems
  javaMenuItem.addActionListener(new ActionListener() {
    public void actionPerformed(ActionEvent e) {
    System.out.println("Java selected");
    }
  });
  pythonMenuItem.addActionListener(new ActionListener() {
    public void actionPerformed(ActionEvent e) {
    System.out.println("Python selected");
    }
  });
  // Add MenuItems to the Menu
  coursesMenu.add(javaMenuItem);
  coursesMenu.add(pythonMenuItem);
  // Add the Menu to the MenuBar
  menuBar.add(coursesMenu);
  // Set the MenuBar for the Frame
  frame.setMenuBar(menuBar);
  // Set the size of the Frame and make it visible
  frame.setSize(300, 100);
  frame.setVisible(true);
  // Add a window listener to handle the closing event
  frame.addWindowListener(new WindowAdapter() {
    public void windowClosing(WindowEvent e) {
    System.exit(0);
    }
  });
  }
}
```

Output

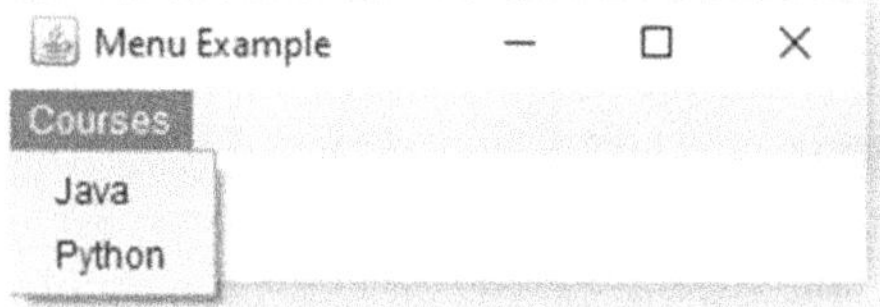

In the above program we created a `Frame` titled "Menu Example" and added a `MenuBar` component. Inside the menu bar, a menu titled "Courses" is created and populated with two menu items: "Java" and "Python". The frame is sized to 300x100 pixels and made visible.

12.8.12 MenuItem

A `MenuItem` is an item in a menu. The key features of `MenuItem` in AWT:

1. Command Execution: `MenuItem` represents an individual option within a `Menu` that triggers a specific action or command when selected by the user. This allows for executing tasks or initiating processes within the application.
2. Customizable Label and Icon: You can set a label text and optionally an icon for a `MenuItem`, allowing you to customize its appearance and provide clear, descriptive options for users. This enhances usability and helps in organizing commands effectively.
3. Event Handling: `MenuItem` supports event handling through `ActionListener`, enabling you to define custom behavior when a menu item is selected. This allows you to execute specific code in response to user interactions with the menu item.

Program

```
import java.awt.*;
import java.awt.event.*;
public class MenuItemExample {
  void main(String[] args) {
  // Create a Frame with the title "MenuItem Example"
  Frame frame = new Frame("MenuItem Example");
  // Create a MenuBar
  MenuBar menuBar = new MenuBar();
  // Create a Menu titled "Courses"
  Menu coursesMenu = new Menu("Courses");
  // Create MenuItems for the Menu
  MenuItem javaMenuItem = new MenuItem("Java");
  MenuItem pythonMenuItem = new MenuItem("Python");
  // Remove the unsupported setBackground calls
  // javaMenuItem.setBackground(Color.YELLOW); // Not supported
  // pythonMenuItem.setBackground(Color.YELLOW); // Not supported
  // Add ActionListener to MenuItems
  javaMenuItem.addActionListener(new ActionListener() {
    public void actionPerformed(ActionEvent e) {
    System.out.println("Java selected");
    }
  });
  pythonMenuItem.addActionListener(new ActionListener() {
    public void actionPerformed(ActionEvent e) {
    System.out.println("Python selected");
```

```
    }
  });
  // Add MenuItems to the Menu
  coursesMenu.add(javaMenuItem);
  coursesMenu.add(pythonMenuItem);
  // Add the Menu to the MenuBar
  menuBar.add(coursesMenu);
  // Set the MenuBar for the Frame
  frame.setMenuBar(menuBar);
  // Set the size of the Frame and make it visible
  frame.setSize(300, 100);
  frame.setVisible(true);
  // Add a window listener to handle the closing event
  frame.addWindowListener(new WindowAdapter() {
    public void windowClosing(WindowEvent e) {
    System.exit(0);
    }
  });
  }
}
```

Output

MenuItem Example
Courses
Java
Python

In the above program we created a `Frame` titled "MenuItem Example" and added a `MenuBar` component. Inside the menu bar, a menu titled "Courses" is created and populated with two menu items: "Java" and "Python". Both menu items have a background color of yellow. The frame is sized to 300x100 pixels and made visible.

12.8.13 FileDialog

A `FileDialog` is a dialog window from which the user can select a file. The key features of `FileDialog` in AWT:

1. File Selection: `FileDialog` provides a standard dialog window for users to select files or directories. It allows users to browse the file system and choose files or directories, making it easier to open or save files in an application.
2. Customizable Dialog Type: You can configure `FileDialog` to function as either an "open" or "save" dialog. This allows you to present different options to the user depending on whether they are opening an existing file or saving a new file.
3. Directory and File Filtering: `FileDialog` allows you to filter files based on their types or extensions. This enables users to view and select only certain types of files, streamlining the file selection process and improving user experience.

Program

```
import java.awt.*;
import java.awt.event.*;
public class FileDialogExample {
```

```
void main(String[] args) {
// Create the main frame
Frame frame = new Frame("FileDialog Example");

// Set the size of the frame
frame.setSize(300, 100);

// Set the layout of the frame
frame.setLayout(new FlowLayout());

// Create a FileDialog with the frame as the parent
FileDialog fileDialog = new FileDialog(frame, "Select a File", FileDialog.
   LOAD);

// Set the background color of the file dialog (this will affect the
component's display in some systems)
fileDialog.setBackground(Color.LIGHT_GRAY);

// Show the file dialog
fileDialog.setVisible(true);

// Add a WindowListener to handle closing the frame
frame.addWindowListener(new WindowAdapter() {
  public void windowClosing(WindowEvent we) {
  frame.dispose();
  }
});

// Make the frame visible
frame.setVisible(true);
}
}
```

Output

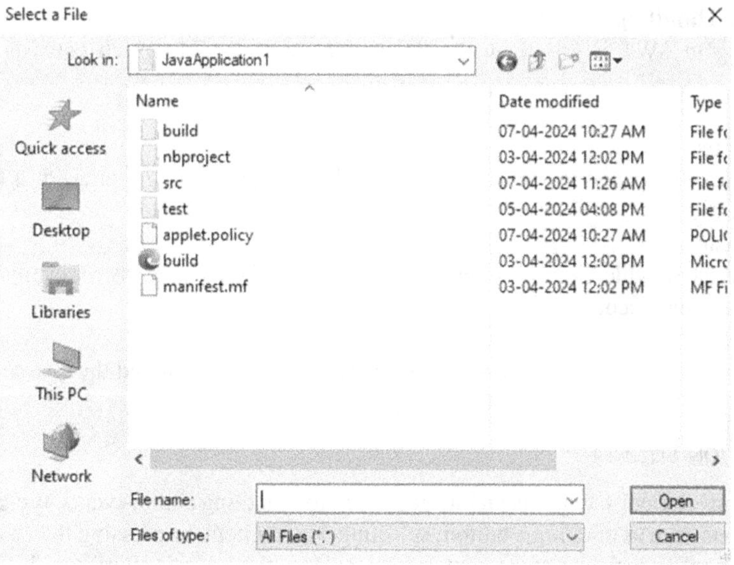

In the above program a `FileDialog` is instantiated with the parent frame, a title “Select a File”, and the mode set to `LOAD`. The background color of the file dialog is set to light gray. The frame is sized to 300x100 pixels and made visible along with the file dialog.

12.9 EVENT HANDLING

Event handling in Java AWT is crucial because it allows applications to respond to user interactions and other events, making the application interactive and dynamic. Without event handling, an application would not be able to respond to user actions such as clicks, key presses, mouse movements, and other interactions.

The importance of event handling in AWT are:

1. Interactivity:
   Event handling makes applications interactive. It allows the application to respond to user actions like clicking a button, entering text, selecting items, etc.
2. User Experience:
   Proper event handling enhances the user experience by providing immediate feedback and appropriate responses to user actions.
3. Control Flow Management:
   It helps manage the flow of the application by performing specific actions in response to user events, such as opening a new window, updating a display, or saving data.
4. Customization:
   Developers can customize how their application behaves in response to different events, allowing for flexible and feature-rich applications.
5. Separation of Logic:
   Event handling separates user interface code from application logic, making the code cleaner, more organized, and easier to maintain.
6. Asynchronous Processing:
   Events are processed asynchronously, meaning the application can handle multiple events occurring at the same time, improving performance and responsiveness.

How Event Handling Works in AWT

Event handling in AWT is based on the delegation event model, which consists of three main components:

1. Event Source:
   The object that generates an event. This could be a button being clicked, a text field being edited, etc.
2. Event Listener:
   An interface in which the event handler method is defined. It listens for events and is notified when the event occurs.
3. Event Object:
   Contains information about the event, such as the type of event and the source of the event.

12.9.1 Action Listener

In Java AWT, an `ActionListener` is an interface used for handling action events, typically associated with user actions such as clicking a button, selecting a menu item, or pressing the Enter key in a text field. The `ActionListener` interface contains a single method, `actionPerformed(ActionEvent e)`, which must be implemented by any class that wishes to handle action events. When an action event occurs, the `actionPerformed` method is invoked, passing an `ActionEvent` object that contains information about the event, including the source of the event and a command string that provides additional context.

The primary role of an `ActionListener` is to define the behavior that should occur when an action is performed. This allows developers to separate the logic of what should happen from the components that trigger the actions, promoting modularity and reusability in the code. Action listeners are registered with components using the `addActionListener` method, establishing a connection between the user action and the handling logic.

Program

```
import java.awt.*;
import java.awt.event.*;
public class ButtonClickEventExample {
  void main(String[] args) {
  // Create the main frame
  Frame frame = new Frame("Button Click Event Example");

  // Set the size of the frame
  frame.setSize(300, 200);

  // Set the layout of the frame
  frame.setLayout(new FlowLayout());

  // Create a button with the label "Click Me"
  Button button = new Button("Click Me");

  // Add an ActionListener to the button
  button.addActionListener(new ActionListener() {
    @Override
    public void actionPerformed(ActionEvent e) {
    // Change the background color of the button to red
    button.setBackground(Color.RED);
    }
  });

  // Add the button to the frame
  frame.add(button);

  // Add a WindowListener to handle closing the frame
  frame.addWindowListener(new WindowAdapter() {
    public void windowClosing(WindowEvent we) {
    frame.dispose();
    }
  });

  // Make the frame visible
  frame.setVisible(true);
  }
}
```

Output

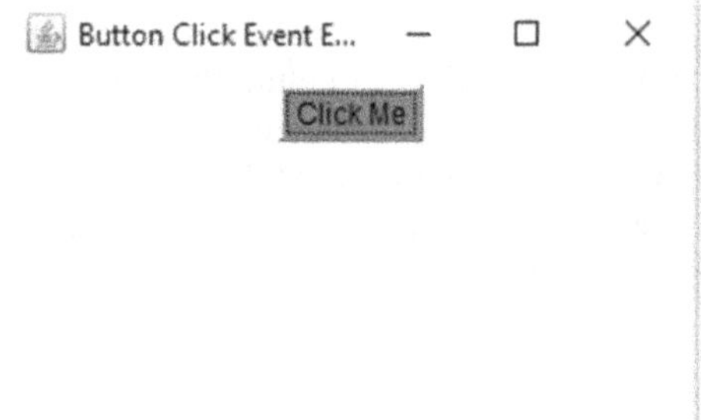

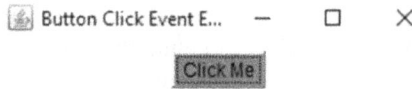

In the above program we created a `Frame` titled "Button Click Event Example" and added a button labeled "Click Me" to it. Upon clicking the button, its background color changes to red. This behavior is achieved by adding an `ActionListener` to the button that sets its background color when triggered. Finally, the frame is sized to 300x200 pixels and made visible.

Program

```
import java.awt.*;
import java.awt.event.*;
public class MenuSelectionEventExample {
  void main(String[] args) {
  // Create the main frame
  Frame frame = new Frame("Menu Selection Event Example");

  // Set the size of the frame
  frame.setSize(300, 200);

  // Create a menu bar
  MenuBar menuBar = new MenuBar();

  // Create a menu and add it to the menu bar
  Menu fileMenu = new Menu("File");
  menuBar.add(fileMenu);

  // Create a menu item and add it to the menu
  MenuItem openMenuItem = new MenuItem("Open");
  fileMenu.add(openMenuItem);

  // Add an ActionListener to the menu item
  openMenuItem.addActionListener(new ActionListener() {
    @Override
    public void actionPerformed(ActionEvent e) {
    // Print message to the console when menu item is selected
    System.out.println("File -> Open selected");
    }
  });

  // Set the menu bar for the frame
  frame.setMenuBar(menuBar);

  // Add a WindowListener to handle closing the frame
```

```
    frame.addWindowListener(new WindowAdapter() {
      public void windowClosing(WindowEvent we) {
      frame.dispose();
      }
    });

    // Make the frame visible
    frame.setVisible(true);
  }
}
```

Output

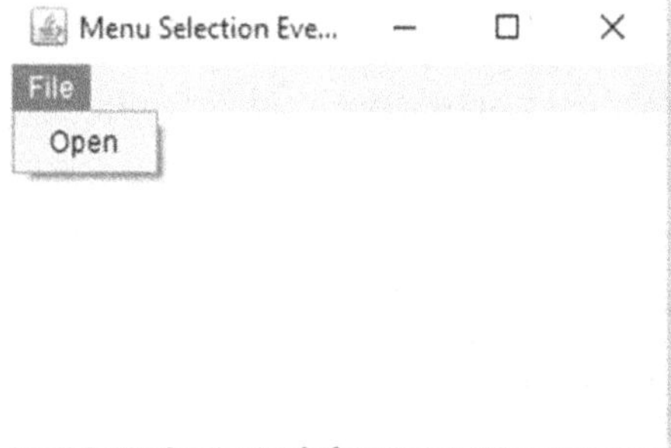


```
File -> Open selected
```

In the above program we created a `Frame` titled "Menu Selection Event Example" with a `MenuBar`. The menu bar contains a `Menu` titled "File", which in turn includes a `MenuItem` labeled "Open". An `ActionListener` is added to the "Open" menu item to listen for selection events. When the "Open" menu item is selected, it prints "File -> Open selected" to the console. Finally, the frame is set to a specific size and made visible.

12.9.2 Focus Listener

A `FocusListener` in Java AWT is an interface that receives focus events, which occur when a component gains or loses keyboard focus. The `FocusListener` interface includes two methods: `focusGained(FocusEvent e)` and `focusLost(FocusEvent e)`. These methods must be implemented by any class that wants to handle focus events. The `focusGained` method is called when a component gains focus, allowing developers to define specific behavior when the component becomes the target for keyboard input. Conversely, the `focusLost` method is called when a component loses focus, enabling the implementation of actions to be taken when the component is no longer in focus. This can be particularly useful for validating input when the user moves away from a text field, updating the user interface to reflect the change in focus, or ensuring that certain actions are only available when a component is active. By implementing the `FocusListener` interface, developers can create more interactive and user-friendly applications, where the user interface responds appropriately to the user's focus changes.

Program

```
import java.awt.*;
import java.awt.event.*;
public class FocusEventExample {
  void main(String[] args) {
```

```
  // Create a Frame
  Frame frame = new Frame("FocusListener Example");
  // Create a TextField
  TextField textField = new TextField("Enter Name", 20);
  // Create a Label to display focus information
  Label focusLabel = new Label();
  // Add FocusListener to the TextField
  textField.addFocusListener(new FocusListener() {
    // This method is called when the TextField gains focus
    public void focusGained(FocusEvent e) {
    focusLabel.setText("TextField gained focus!");
    }
    // This method is called when the TextField loses focus
    public void focusLost(FocusEvent e) {
    focusLabel.setText("TextField lost focus!");
    }
  });
  // Add components to the Frame
  frame.add(textField, BorderLayout.NORTH);
  frame.add(focusLabel, BorderLayout.SOUTH);
  // Set the size of the Frame and make it visible
  frame.setSize(300, 100);
  frame.setVisible(true);
  // Add a window listener to handle the closing event
  frame.addWindowListener(new WindowAdapter() {
    public void windowClosing(WindowEvent e) {
    System.exit(0);
    }
  });
  }
}
```

Output

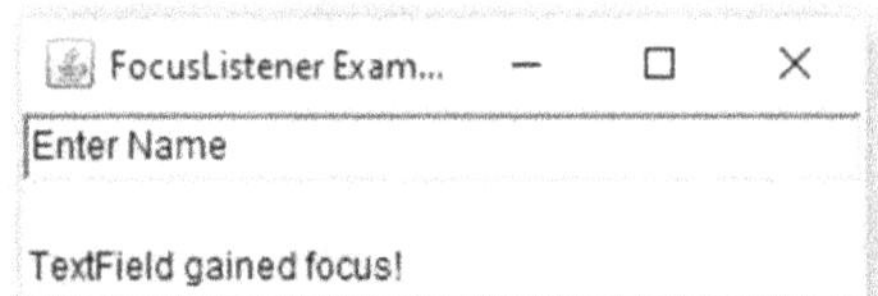

This program demonstrates how to use a FocusListener in AWT to detect focus events on a TextField. When the TextField gains or loses focus, the respective methods `focusGained` and `focusLost` update a Label to reflect the focus state. We included a WindowListener to close the application properly when the window is closed.

12.9.3 Item Listener

An `ItemListener` in Java AWT is an interface designed to handle item events, which are triggered when the state of an item changes. Item events typically occur with components such as checkboxes, radio buttons, choice lists, and other selection items. The `ItemListener` interface has a single method, `itemStateChanged(ItemEvent e)`, which must be implemented by any class that wants to respond to item state changes. When an item is selected or deselected, the `itemStateChanged` method is invoked, allowing the program to react to these changes. This can involve updating the user interface, performing calculations, or any other logic that needs to respond to the selection state of the item. By implementing the `ItemListener` interface, developers can create dynamic and responsive user interfaces where actions are contingent upon the user's selection or deselection of items within the component. This interaction enhances the interactivity and usability of the application, providing immediate feedback and functionality based on user input.

Program

```
import java.awt.*;
import java.awt.event.*;
public class CheckboxItemEventExample {
  void main(String[] args) {
  // Create the frame with the title "Checkbox Item Event Example"
  Frame frame = new Frame("Checkbox Item Event Example");

  // Set the size of the frame
  frame.setSize(300, 200);

  // Create a checkbox labeled "Agree"
  Checkbox checkbox = new Checkbox("Agree");

  // Add an ItemListener to the checkbox
  checkbox.addItemListener(new ItemListener() {
    @Override
    public void itemStateChanged(ItemEvent e) {
    // Check the state of the checkbox and print a message accordingly
    if (checkbox.getState()) {
      System.out.println("Checkbox is selected.");
    } else {
      System.out.println("Checkbox is deselected.");
    }
    }
  });

  // Add the checkbox to the frame
  frame.add(checkbox, BorderLayout.CENTER);

  // Add a WindowListener to handle closing the frame
  frame.addWindowListener(new WindowAdapter() {
    public void windowClosing(WindowEvent we) {
    frame.dispose();
    }
  });

  // Make the frame visible
  frame.setVisible(true);
  }
}
```

Output

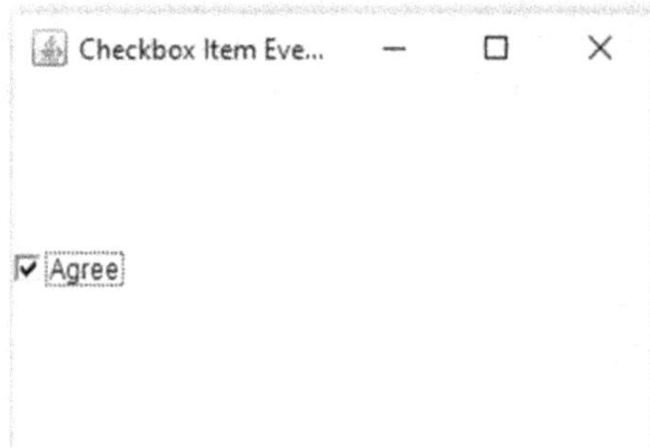

In the above program we created a `Frame` titled "Checkbox Item Event Example" and added a checkbox labeled "Agree." When the checkbox state changes (either selected or deselected), it prints a message indicating the new state. This behavior is defined using an `ItemListener` added to the checkbox. Finally, the frame is sized to 300x200 pixels and made visible.

Program

```
import java.awt.*;
import java.awt.event.*;
public class ChoiceItemEventExample {
  void main(String[] args) {
  // Create the frame with the title "Choice Item Event Example"
  Frame frame = new Frame("Choice Item Event Example");

  // Set the size of the frame
  frame.setSize(300, 200);

  // Create a Choice component with options "Red", "Green", and "Blue"
  Choice colorChoice = new Choice();
  colorChoice.add("Red");
  colorChoice.add("Green");
  colorChoice.add("Blue");

  // Create a Label to display the chosen color
  Label colorLabel = new Label("Choose a color");

  // Add an ItemListener to the Choice component
  colorChoice.addItemListener(new ItemListener() {
    @Override
    public void itemStateChanged(ItemEvent e) {
    // Get the selected item
    String selectedColor = colorChoice.getSelectedItem();

    // Change the label's text color based on the selected item
    switch (selectedColor) {
      case "Red":
      colorLabel.setForeground(Color.RED);
      break;
      case "Green":
      colorLabel.setForeground(Color.GREEN);
      break;
      case "Blue":
```

```
            colorLabel.setForeground(Color.BLUE);
            break;
          }
        }
      });

      // Set the layout manager for the frame
      frame.setLayout(new FlowLayout());

      // Add the Choice and Label to the frame
      frame.add(colorChoice);
      frame.add(colorLabel);

      // Add a WindowListener to handle closing the frame
      frame.addWindowListener(new WindowAdapter() {
        public void windowClosing(WindowEvent we) {
        frame.dispose();
        }
      });

      // Make the frame visible
      frame.setVisible(true);
      }
    }
```

Output

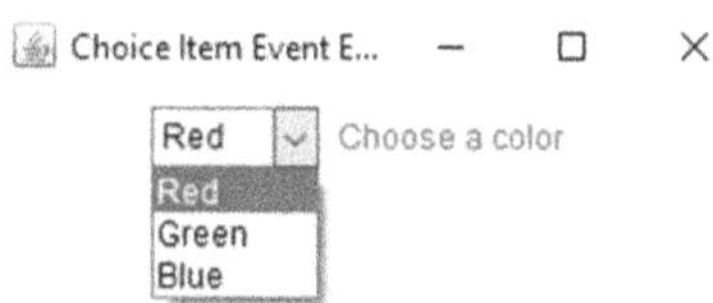

In the above program we created a `Frame` titled "Choice Item Event Example" and added a `Choice` component with options "Red", "Green", and "Blue". A `Label` titled "Choose a color" is also added. When an item in the choice is selected, it changes the color of the label text accordingly. This behavior is implemented using an `ItemListener` added to the choice. The frame is then sized to 300x200 pixels and displayed.

Program

```
import java.awt.*;
import java.awt.event.*;
public class ListSelectionEventExample {
  void main(String[] args) {
  // Create the frame with the title "List Selection Event Example"
  Frame frame = new Frame("List Selection Event Example");

  // Set the size of the frame
  frame.setSize(300, 200);

  // Create a List component with options "Java", "Python", and "C++"
  List languageList = new List();
```

```
  languageList.add("Java");
  languageList.add("Python");
  languageList.add("C++");

  // Add an ItemListener to the List component
  languageList.addItemListener(new ItemListener() {
    @Override
    public void itemStateChanged(ItemEvent e) {
    // Print the selected item to the console
    System.out.println("Selected item: " + languageList.getSelectedItem());
    }
  });

  // Set the layout manager for the frame
  frame.setLayout(new FlowLayout());

  // Add the List to the frame
  frame.add(languageList);

  // Add a WindowListener to handle closing the frame
  frame.addWindowListener(new WindowAdapter() {
    public void windowClosing(WindowEvent we) {
    frame.dispose();
    }
  });

  // Make the frame visible
  frame.setVisible(true);
  }
}
```

Output

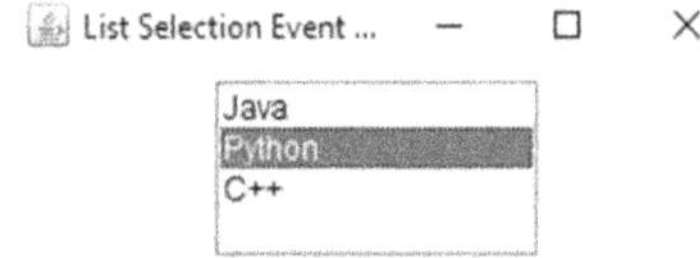

In the above program we created a `Frame` titled "List Selection Event Example" and added a `List` component containing options "Java", "Python", and "C++". An `ItemListener` is attached to the list, which listens for item state changes. When an item is selected, it prints the selected item to the console. Finally, the frame is sized to 300x200 pixels and displayed.

Program

```
import java.awt.*;
import java.awt.event.*;
public class ItemEventExample {
  void main(String[] args) {
  // Create the frame with the title "Item Event Example"
  Frame frame = new Frame("Item Event Example");
```

```
// Set the size of the frame
frame.setSize(300, 200);

// Create a Choice component with color options
Choice colorChoice = new Choice();
colorChoice.add("Red");
colorChoice.add("Green");
colorChoice.add("Blue");

// Add an ItemListener to the Choice component
colorChoice.addItemListener(new ItemListener() {
  @Override
  public void itemStateChanged(ItemEvent e) {
  // Get the selected color
  String selectedColor = colorChoice.getSelectedItem();

  // Change the background color of the frame based on the selected color
  switch (selectedColor) {
    case "Red":
    frame.setBackground(Color.RED);
    break;
    case "Green":
    frame.setBackground(Color.GREEN);
    break;
    case "Blue":
    frame.setBackground(Color.BLUE);
    break;
  }
  }
});

// Set the layout manager for the frame
frame.setLayout(new FlowLayout());

// Add the Choice component to the frame
frame.add(colorChoice);

// Add a WindowListener to handle closing the frame
frame.addWindowListener(new WindowAdapter() {
  public void windowClosing(WindowEvent we) {
  frame.dispose();
  }
});

// Make the frame visible
frame.setVisible(true);
}
}
```

Output

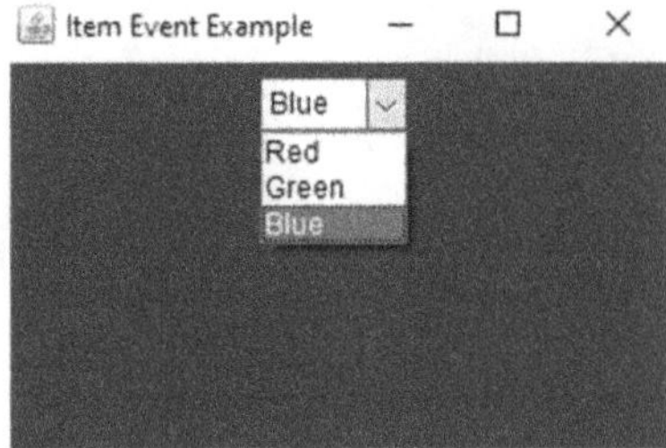

In the above program we created a `Frame` titled "Item Event Example" and a `Choice` component with options for selecting colors: "Red", "Green", and "Blue". An `ItemListener` is added to the choice component to detect item state changes. Depending on the selected color, the background color of the frame changes accordingly. The frame is then sized and displayed.

12.9.4 Windows Listener

A `WindowListener` in Java AWT (Abstract Window Toolkit) is an interface used to receive and handle various types of window events. These events are related to the changes in the state of a window, such as opening, closing, iconifying, deiconifying, activating, and deactivating the window.

The `WindowListener` interface defines seven methods:

```
`windowOpened(WindowEvent e)`,
`windowClosing(WindowEvent e)`,
`windowClosed(WindowEvent e)`,
`windowIconified(WindowEvent e)`,
`windowDeiconified(WindowEvent e)`,
`windowActivated(WindowEvent e)`,
and `windowDeactivated(WindowEvent e)`.
```

Each of these methods corresponds to a specific type of window event, allowing developers to implement custom behavior when these events occur. For example, `windowClosing` is often used to prompt the user to save changes before closing the application, while `windowIconified` and `windowDeiconified` might be used to manage resources when a window is minimized or restored. By implementing a `WindowListener`, developers can ensure that their applications respond appropriately to changes in the window state, enhancing user experience and ensuring proper resource management.

Program

```
import java.awt.*;
import java.awt.event.*;
public class WindowStateChangeEventExample {
  void main(String[] args) {
  // Create a Frame with the title "Window State Change Event Example"
  Frame frame = new Frame("Window State Change Event Example");
  // Set the size of the frame
  frame.setSize(400, 300);
  // Add a WindowStateListener to handle window state changes
  frame.addWindowStateListener(new WindowStateListener() {
    @Override
    public void windowStateChanged(WindowEvent e) {
    int newState = e.getNewState();
```

```
    // Check if the window is iconified
    if ((newState & Frame.ICONIFIED) == Frame.ICONIFIED) {
      System.out.println("Window iconified");
    }

    // Check if the window is deiconified
    if ((newState & Frame.NORMAL) == Frame.NORMAL) {
      System.out.println("Window deiconified");
    }
    }
  });
  // Add a WindowListener to handle closing the frame
  frame.addWindowListener(new WindowAdapter() {
    public void windowClosing(WindowEvent we) {
    frame.dispose();
    }
  });
  // Make the frame visible
  frame.setVisible(true);
  }
}
```

Output:

Window State Change Event Example

```
Window iconified
Window deiconified
Window deiconified
Window deiconified
Window deiconified
```

In the above program we created a `Frame` titled "Window State Change Event Example" and added a `WindowStateListener` to it. The listener checks if the window is iconified or deiconified using bitwise operations on the window state. If the window is iconified, it prints "Window iconified" to the console, and if it's deiconified, it prints "Window deiconified". Finally, the frame is set to a specific size and made visible.

12.9.5 Adjustment Listener

An `AdjustmentListener` in Java AWT is an interface used to handle adjustment events generated by adjustable components like scrollbars and sliders. The interface contains a single method, `adjustmentValueChanged(AdjustmentEvent e)`, which is invoked whenever the value of an adjustable component changes. This listener is essential for providing dynamic and responsive user interfaces, allowing developers to execute specific actions in response to user interactions with adjustable components. For instance, when a user moves a scrollbar, the `adjustmentValueChanged` method can be implemented to update the displayed content accordingly. This real-time feedback is crucial for applications that require precise control over component values, such as custom controls, interactive data visualizations, and user interface adjustments. By implementing an `AdjustmentListener`, developers can enhance the interactivity and usability of their applications, ensuring that adjustments to component values are immediately reflected in the application's behavior and appearance.

Program

```
import java.awt.*;
import java.awt.event.*;
public class AdjustmentEventExample {
  void main(String[] args) {
  // Create a Frame with the title "Adjustment Event Example"
  Frame frame = new Frame("Adjustment Event Example");
  // Set the layout of the frame to BorderLayout
  frame.setLayout(new BorderLayout());
  // Create a vertical Scrollbar
  Scrollbar scrollbar = new Scrollbar(Scrollbar.VERTICAL);
  scrollbar.setMaximum(255); // Set the maximum value for the scrollbar
  // Add an AdjustmentListener to the scrollbar
  scrollbar.addAdjustmentListener(new AdjustmentListener() {
    @Override
    public void adjustmentValueChanged(AdjustmentEvent e) {
    // Get the scrollbar value
    int value = scrollbar.getValue();

    // Change the background color of the frame based on the scrollbar value
    // The color is determined by the value from the scrollbar (0 to 255)
    Color color = new Color(value, value, value); // Grayscale color
    frame.setBackground(color);
    }
  });
  // Add the scrollbar to the east side of the frame
  frame.add(scrollbar, BorderLayout.EAST);
  // Set the size of the frame
  frame.setSize(400, 300);
  // Add a WindowListener to handle closing the frame
  frame.addWindowListener(new WindowAdapter() {
    public void windowClosing(WindowEvent we) {
    frame.dispose();
    }
  });
  // Make the frame visible
  frame.setVisible(true);
  }
}
```

Output

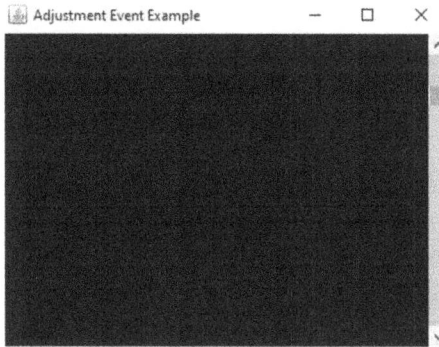

In the above program we created a `Frame` titled "Adjustment Event Example" and a vertical `Scrollbar`. An `AdjustmentListener` is added to the scrollbar to change the background color of the frame dynamically based on the scrollbar value. The frame's layout is set to BorderLayout, and the scrollbar is added to the east side of the frame. Finally, the frame is sized and displayed.

12.10 ADAPTER CLASSES IN JAVA AWT

Adapter classes in Java are abstract classes provided by the AWT framework that implement listener interfaces with empty method bodies. These classes include `MouseAdapter`, `KeyAdapter`, `FocusAdapter`, `WindowAdapter`, and others. The primary purpose of adapter classes is to simplify the creation of event listeners. When using listener interfaces, developers must implement all methods defined in the interface, even if they only need one or a few methods. This can lead to verbose and cluttered code. Adapter classes address this issue by providing default, empty implementations of all the interface methods, allowing developers to override only the methods they need.

The importance of adapter classes lies in their ability to streamline code and improve readability and maintainability. They reduce code, enabling developers to focus on the specific event-handling logic relevant to their application. For example, if a developer only needs to handle a mouse click event, they can extend `MouseAdapter` and override the `mouseClicked` method, leaving other methods like `mousePressed`, `mouseReleased`, etc., with their default empty implementations. This approach not only makes the code cleaner but also reduces the likelihood of errors that might arise from implementing unnecessary methods.

12.10.1 WindowAdapter

The `WindowAdapter` class in Java is a part of the AWT framework and serves as an abstract adapter class for receiving window events. This class provides default implementations for all methods defined in the `WindowListener` interface, which allows developers to handle window-related events such as opening, closing, activating, deactivating, iconifying, deiconifying, and gaining or losing focus. By extending `WindowAdapter`, developers can override only the methods they are interested in, without being forced to provide implementations for all the methods in the `WindowListener` interface. This leads to cleaner and more maintainable code, as it reduces code and focuses only on the relevant event-handling logic. The `WindowAdapter` class is particularly useful in simplifying the development process when dealing with window events in GUI applications, as it streamlines the creation of event listeners and enhances code readability.

Program

```
import java.awt.*;
import java.awt.event.*;
public class WindowAdapterExample extends Frame {
  public WindowAdapterExample() {
  // Set the title of the frame
  setTitle("Window Adapter Example");
  // Set the size of the frame
  setSize(300, 200);
  // Set the background color of the frame
  setBackground(Color.YELLOW);
  // Add a WindowListener using WindowAdapter to handle window closing event
  addWindowListener(new WindowAdapter() {
    @Override
    public void windowClosing(WindowEvent e) {
    // Exit the application when the window is closed
    System.exit(0);
    }
  });
  // Set the layout of the frame
  setLayout(new FlowLayout());
  // Make the frame visible
  setVisible(true);
  }
  void main(String[] args) {
  // Create an instance of WindowAdapterExample to show the frame
  new WindowAdapterExample();
  }
}
```

Output

In the above program we created a subclass of `Frame` titled "Window Adapter Example". The frame is set to a size of 300x200 pixels and given a yellow background color. An instance of `WindowAdapter` is added to handle the window closing event, which exits the application when triggered.

12.10.2 MouseAdapter

The `MouseAdapter` class in Java, part of the AWT (Abstract Window Toolkit) framework, is an abstract adapter class designed to handle mouse events. This class provides default (empty) implementations for all methods defined in the `MouseListener` and `MouseMotionListener` interfaces, which include methods for handling mouse clicks, presses, releases, entries, exits, and mouse movement and dragging events. By extending `MouseAdapter`, developers can override only the methods relevant to their application, without needing to implement every method from the interfaces. This approach simplifies the code, making it more concise and easier to manage, as it eliminates unnecessary method definitions and focuses solely on the event-handling logic that is needed. The `MouseAdapter` class is essential for developing responsive and interactive graphical user interfaces, as it provides a streamlined way to manage mouse interactions with components, enhancing the usability and functionality of Java-based applications.

Program

```
import java.awt.*;
import java.awt.event.*;
public class MouseAdapterExample extends Frame {
  public MouseAdapterExample() {
  // Set the title of the frame
  setTitle("Mouse Adapter Example");
  // Set the size of the frame
  setSize(300, 200);
  // Set the background color of the frame
  setBackground(Color.LIGHT_GRAY);
  // Add a MouseListener using MouseAdapter to handle mouse events
  addMouseListener(new MouseAdapter() {
    @Override
    public void mouseClicked(MouseEvent e) {
    // Change the background color to blue when the mouse is clicked
    setBackground(Color.BLUE);
    }
  });
  // Set the layout of the frame
  setLayout(new FlowLayout());
  // Make the frame visible
  setVisible(true);
  // Add a WindowListener to handle window closing event
  addWindowListener(new WindowAdapter() {
    @Override
    public void windowClosing(WindowEvent e) {
    // Exit the application when the window is closed
    System.exit(0);
    }
  });
  }
  void main(String[] args) {
  // Create an instance of MouseAdapterExample to show the frame
  new MouseAdapterExample();
  }
}
```

Output

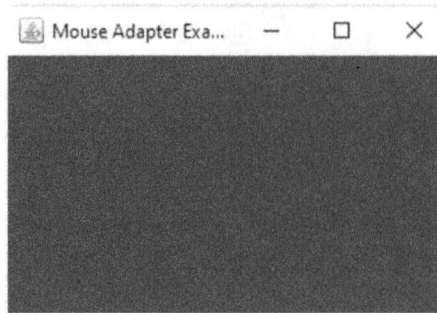

In the above program we extended the `Frame` class, creating a window titled "Mouse Adapter Example" with dimensions 300x200 pixels. Then we added a `MouseListener` through `MouseAdapter`, specifically handling the `mouseClicked` event, which sets the background color to blue when triggered.

12.10.3 KeyAdapter

The `KeyAdapter` class in Java, part of the AWT (Abstract Window Toolkit) framework, is an abstract adapter class designed to handle keyboard events. This class provides default (empty) implementations for all methods defined in the `KeyListener` interface, which include methods for handling key presses, key releases, and key typing events. By extending `KeyAdapter`, developers can override only the methods relevant to their specific application needs, without having to implement every method from the `KeyListener` interface. This approach simplifies the code by eliminating unnecessary method definitions, making it more concise and easier to manage. The `KeyAdapter` class is particularly useful in scenarios where only a subset of keyboard events need to be handled, allowing developers to focus on the specific logic required for those events. It enhances the efficiency of handling keyboard interactions within Java-based applications, contributing to the creation of responsive and user-friendly interfaces.

Program

```
import java.awt.*;
import java.awt.event.*;
public class KeyAdapterExample extends Frame {
  public KeyAdapterExample() {
  // Set the title of the frame
  setTitle("Key Adapter Example");
  // Set the size of the frame
  setSize(300, 200);
  // Set the background color of the frame
  setBackground(Color.LIGHT_GRAY);
  // Add a KeyListener using KeyAdapter to handle key events
  addKeyListener(new KeyAdapter() {
    @Override
    public void keyPressed(KeyEvent e) {
    // Check if the space key is pressed
    if (e.getKeyCode() == KeyEvent.VK_SPACE) {
      // Change the background color to green
      setBackground(Color.GREEN);
    }
```

```
    }
  });
  // Set the layout of the frame
  setLayout(new FlowLayout());
  // Make the frame visible
  setVisible(true);
  // Add a WindowListener to handle window closing event
  addWindowListener(new WindowAdapter() {
    @Override
    public void windowClosing(WindowEvent e) {
    // Exit the application when the window is closed
    System.exit(0);
    }
  });
  }
  void main(String[] args) {
  // Create an instance of KeyAdapterExample to show the frame
  new KeyAdapterExample();
  }
}
```

Output

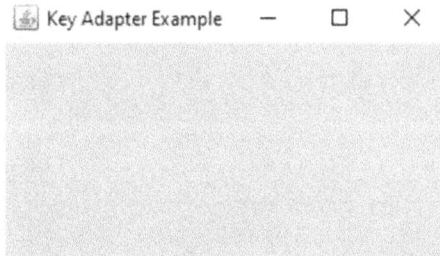

Key Adapter Example

In the above program we extended the `Frame` class, creating a window titled "Key Adapter Example" with dimensions 300x200 pixels. The program adds a `KeyListener` through `KeyAdapter`, specifically handling the `keyPressed` event. When the space key is pressed (`KeyEvent.VK_SPACE`), the background color changes to green.

12.10.4 MouseMotionAdapter

The `MouseMotionAdapter` class in Java, part of the AWT framework, is an abstract adapter class designed to handle mouse motion events. This class provides default (empty) implementations for all methods defined in the `MouseMotionListener` interface, which include methods for handling mouse movements (`mouseMoved`) and mouse drag events (`mouseDragged`). By extending `MouseMotionAdapter`, developers can override only the methods they need, without the necessity to implement both methods from the `MouseMotionListener` interface. This approach streamlines the development process by reducing code and focusing on the specific logic required for handling mouse motion. The `MouseMotionAdapter` is particularly useful in graphical applications where precise tracking of the mouse's position or drag actions is essential, such as in drawing applications, games, or custom UI components. It simplifies the creation of responsive and interactive user interfaces by allowing developers to easily manage and respond to mouse motion events.

Program

```
import java.awt.*;
import java.awt.event.*;
public class MouseMotionAdapterExample extends Frame {
  public MouseMotionAdapterExample() {
  // Set the title of the frame
  setTitle("Mouse Motion Adapter Example");
  // Set the size of the frame
  setSize(300, 200);
  // Set the initial background color of the frame
  setBackground(Color.WHITE);
  // Add a MouseMotionListener using MouseMotionAdapter to handle mouse
  motion events
  addMouseMotionListener(new MouseMotionAdapter() {
    @Override
    public void mouseMoved(MouseEvent e) {
    // Get the mouse coordinates
    int x = e.getX();
    int y = e.getY();
    // Change the background color based on mouse coordinates
    if (x > 150 && y > 100) {
      setBackground(Color.RED);
    } else {
      setBackground(Color.WHITE);
    }
    }
  });
  // Set the layout of the frame (optional in this case as no additional
  components are added)
  setLayout(new FlowLayout());
  // Make the frame visible
  setVisible(true);
  // Add a WindowListener to handle window closing event
  addWindowListener(new WindowAdapter() {
    @Override
    public void windowClosing(WindowEvent e) {
    // Exit the application when the window is closed
    System.exit(0);
    }
  });
  }
  void main(String[] args) {
  // Create an instance of MouseMotionAdapterExample to show the frame
  new MouseMotionAdapterExample();
  }
}
```

Output

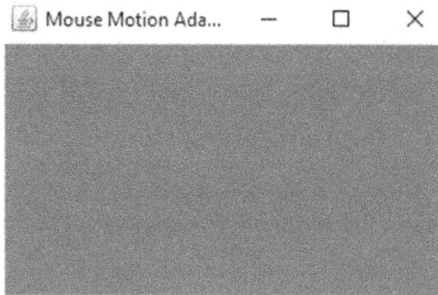

In the above program we are extending the `Frame` class, and creates a window titled "Mouse Motion Adapter Example" with dimensions 300x200 pixels. Then adds a `MouseMotionListener` via `MouseMotionAdapter`, specifically handling the `mouseMoved` event. If the mouse coordinates are greater than (150, 100), the background color changes to red; otherwise, it changes to white.

12.10.5 FocusAdapter

The `FocusAdapter` class in Java's AWT framework is an abstract adapter class designed to simplify the handling of focus events. This class provides default, empty implementations of the methods in the `FocusListener` interface, which includes `focusGained` and `focusLost` methods. When a developer extends `FocusAdapter`, they can override only the methods they are interested in, rather than implementing all methods of the `FocusListener` interface. This approach reduces code and enhances code readability, making it easier to manage focus-related events such as when a component gains or loses focus. The `FocusAdapter` is particularly useful in large applications where only specific focus events need to be handled, streamlining the development process and improving maintainability.

Program

```
import java.awt.*;
import java.awt.event.*;
public class FocusAdapterExample extends Frame {
  public FocusAdapterExample() {
  // Set the title of the frame
  setTitle("Focus Adapter Example");
  // Set the size of the frame
  setSize(300, 200);
  // Set the initial background color of the frame
  setBackground(Color.WHITE);
  // Add a FocusListener using FocusAdapter to handle focus events
  addFocusListener(new FocusAdapter() {
    @Override
    public void focusGained(FocusEvent e) {
    // Change the background color to yellow when the frame gains focus
    setBackground(Color.YELLOW);
    }
    @Override
    public void focusLost(FocusEvent e) {
    // Change the background color to white when the frame loses focus
    setBackground(Color.WHITE);
    }
  });
```

```
  // Set the layout of the frame (optional in this case as no additional
components are added)
  setLayout(new FlowLayout());
  // Make the frame visible
  setVisible(true);
  // Add a WindowListener to handle window closing event
  addWindowListener(new WindowAdapter() {
    @Override
    public void windowClosing(WindowEvent e) {
    // Exit the application when the window is closed
    System.exit(0);
    }
  });
  }
  void main(String[] args) {
  // Create an instance of FocusAdapterExample to show the frame
  new FocusAdapterExample();
  }
}
```

Output

In the above program we extended the `Frame` class to create a window titled “Focus Adapter Example” with dimensions 300x200 pixels. Then added a `FocusListener` using `FocusAdapter`, which changes the background color to yellow when the frame gains focus and to white when it loses focus.

12.10.6 ContainerAdapter

The `ContainerAdapter` class in Java’s AWT library serves as an abstract adapter class for receiving container events. It implements the `ContainerListener` interface and provides default, empty implementations for all methods within the interface. This includes methods such as `componentAdded` and `componentRemoved`, which are invoked when components are added to or removed from a container.

By extending `ContainerAdapter`, developers can create custom container event listeners more efficiently. They only need to override the specific methods they are interested in handling, rather than implementing the entire `ContainerListener` interface. This approach reduces code verbosity and enhances code readability, as developers can focus solely on the logic related to the events they wish to handle.

The `ContainerAdapter` is particularly beneficial in scenarios where only certain container events need to be handled, allowing for cleaner and more concise event handling code. It is commonly used in applications with complex user interfaces to manage dynamic changes in container contents.

Program

```
import java.awt.*;
import java.awt.event.*;
public class ContainerAdapterExample extends Frame {
  public ContainerAdapterExample() {
  // Set the title of the frame
  setTitle("Container Adapter Example");
  // Set the size of the frame
  setSize(300, 200);
  // Set the layout manager (FlowLayout is used for this example)
  setLayout(new FlowLayout());
  // Create an instance of MyPanel and add it to the frame
  MyPanel panel = new MyPanel();
  add(panel);
  // Make the frame visible
  setVisible(true);
  // Add a WindowListener to handle window closing event
  addWindowListener(new WindowAdapter() {
    @Override
    public void windowClosing(WindowEvent e) {
    // Exit the application when the window is closed
    System.exit(0);
    }
  });
  }
  // Custom Panel class that changes its color on mouse click
  class MyPanel extends Panel {
  public MyPanel() {
    // Set the initial background color of the panel
    setBackground(Color.BLUE);
    // Add a MouseListener to change the color on mouse click
    addMouseListener(new MouseAdapter() {
    @Override
    public void mouseClicked(MouseEvent e) {
      // Change the panel's background color to red on mouse click
      setBackground(Color.RED);
    }
    });
  }
  }
  void main(String[] args) {
  // Create an instance of ContainerAdapterExample to show the frame
  new ContainerAdapterExample();
  }
}
```

Output

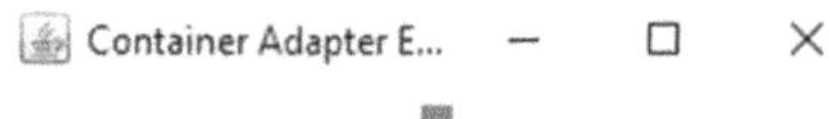

In the above program we extended the `Frame` class, generating a window titled "Container Adapter Example" with dimensions of 300x200 pixels. The frame incorporates a custom `MyPanel` class, extending `Panel`, which sets its background color to blue and registers a `MouseListener` to change its color to red upon mouse click. Finally, the frame is set to be visible.

12.10.7 Component Adapter

The `ComponentAdapter` class in Java's AWT library provides an abstract adapter class for receiving component events. It implements the `ComponentListener` interface and offers default, empty implementations for all its methods. These methods include `componentResized`, `componentMoved`, `componentShown`, and `componentHidden`, each corresponding to different component-related events.

By extending `ComponentAdapter`, developers can create custom component event listeners more efficiently. They only need to override the specific methods they are interested in handling, rather than implementing the entire `ComponentListener` interface. This approach reduces code verbosity and enhances code readability, as developers can focus solely on the logic related to the events they wish to handle.

The `ComponentAdapter` class is particularly useful in scenarios where only certain component events need to be handled. It allows developers to streamline event handling code, making it easier to manage changes and interactions with individual components within a graphical user interface.

Program

```
import java.awt.*;
import java.awt.event.*;
public class ComponentResizingEventExample extends Frame {
  private Label label;
  public ComponentResizingEventExample() {
  // Set the title of the frame
  setTitle("Component Resizing Event Example");
  // Set the layout manager for the frame
  setLayout(new FlowLayout());
  // Create a label with initial text
  label = new Label("Resize Me");
  // Add the label to the frame
  add(label);
  // Add a ComponentListener to the label using ComponentAdapter
  label.addComponentListener(new ComponentAdapter() {
    @Override
    public void componentResized(ComponentEvent e) {
```

```
    // Update the label's text to show its current width and height
    label.setText("Width: " + label.getWidth() + ", Height: " + label.
    getHeight());
    }
  });
  // Set the size of the frame
  setSize(300, 200);
  // Make the frame visible
  setVisible(true);
  // Add a WindowListener to handle window closing
  addWindowListener(new WindowAdapter() {
    @Override
    public void windowClosing(WindowEvent e) {
    // Exit the application when the window is closed
    System.exit(0);
    }
  });
  }
  void main(String[] args) {
  // Create an instance of ComponentResizingEventExample to show the frame
  new ComponentResizingEventExample();
  }
}
```

Output

```
Component Resizin...   —   ☐   ✕
        Width: 127, Height: 23
```

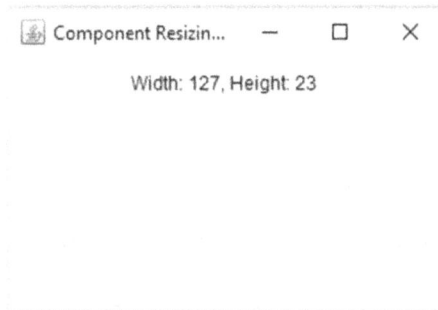

In the above program we created a `Frame` titled "Component Resizing Event Example" containing a `Label` with the text "Resize Me". The label's `ComponentListener` listens for resizing events using a `ComponentAdapter`. When the label is resized, we display the text showing its current width and height. Finally, the frame is set to a specific size and made visible.

12.11 MEDICAL APPLICATIONS

12.11.1 Case Study 1

The risk of diabetes includes severe complications such as cardiovascular disease, nerve damage, kidney failure, and vision loss. Early intervention through lifestyle changes and medical management is essential to mitigate these health threats. The parameters analyzed to identify the risk are:

1. **BMI**: The user's Body Mass Index.
2. **Blood Pressure**: The user's blood pressure, provided as systolic/diastolic values.
3. **Fasting Blood Sugar**: The user's fasting blood sugar level.
4. **Post-Prandial Blood Sugar**: The user's blood sugar level after eating.
5. **Family History**: Check whether the user has a family history of diabetes.

6. **Physical Activity**: Check whether the user engages in regular physical activity.
7. **Smoker**: Check whether the user is a smoker.
8. **Diabetic**: Check whether the user has been diagnosed with diabetes.

Program

```
import java.awt.*;
import java.awt.event.*;
import java.io.FileNotFoundException;
import java.io.FileOutputStream;
import java.io.PrintStream;
import java.util.ArrayList;
public class HealthDataCollector extends Frame implements ActionListener {
  Label titleLabel, ageLabel, genderLabel, bmiLabel, bloodPressureLabel,
    fastingBloodSugarLabel, postPrandialBloodSugarLabel,
    familyHistoryLabel, physicalActivityLabel, smokerLabel, diabeticLabel;
  TextField ageField, bmiField, bloodPressureField, fastingBloodSugarField,
    postPrandialBloodSugarField;
  Choice genderChoice, familyHistoryChoice, physicalActivityChoice,
     smokerChoice, diabeticChoice;
  Button submitButton;
  // Data storage
  ArrayList<HealthData> dataList = new ArrayList<>();
  public HealthDataCollector() {
  super("Health Data Collection");
  // Create UI components
  titleLabel = new Label("Health Data Collection");
  ageLabel = new Label("Age:");
  genderLabel = new Label("Gender:");
  bmiLabel = new Label("BMI:");
  bloodPressureLabel = new Label("Blood Pressure:");
  fastingBloodSugarLabel = new Label("Fasting Blood Sugar:");
  postPrandialBloodSugarLabel = new Label("Post-Prandial Blood Sugar:");
  familyHistoryLabel = new Label("Family History:");
  physicalActivityLabel = new Label("Physical Activity:");
  smokerLabel = new Label("Smoker:");
  diabeticLabel = new Label("Diabetic:");
  ageField = new TextField(10);
  bmiField = new TextField(10);
  bloodPressureField = new TextField(10);
  fastingBloodSugarField = new TextField(10);
  postPrandialBloodSugarField = new TextField(10);
  genderChoice = new Choice();
  genderChoice.add("Male");
  genderChoice.add("Female");
  familyHistoryChoice = new Choice();
  familyHistoryChoice.add("Yes");
  familyHistoryChoice.add("No");
  physicalActivityChoice = new Choice();
  physicalActivityChoice.add("Yes");
  physicalActivityChoice.add("No");
  smokerChoice = new Choice();
  smokerChoice.add("Yes");
  smokerChoice.add("No");
```

```
  diabeticChoice = new Choice();
  diabeticChoice.add("Yes");
  diabeticChoice.add("No");
  submitButton = new Button("Submit");
  // Layout components
  setLayout(new GridLayout(11, 2));
  add(titleLabel);
  add(new Label(""));
  add(ageLabel);
  add(ageField);
  add(genderLabel);
  add(genderChoice);
  add(bmiLabel);
  add(bmiField);
  add(bloodPressureLabel);
  add(bloodPressureField);
  add(fastingBloodSugarLabel);
  add(fastingBloodSugarField);
  add(postPrandialBloodSugarLabel);
  add(postPrandialBloodSugarField);
  add(familyHistoryLabel);
  add(familyHistoryChoice);
  add(physicalActivityLabel);
  add(physicalActivityChoice);
  add(smokerLabel);
  add(smokerChoice);
  add(diabeticLabel);
  add(diabeticChoice);
  add(submitButton);
  submitButton.addActionListener(this);
  }
public void actionPerformed(ActionEvent e) {
  if (e.getSource() == submitButton) {
  // Extract data from UI components with improved error handling
  try {
    String ageStr = ageField.getText();
    int age = Integer.parseInt(ageStr);
    if (age < 18 || age > 100) {
  throw new NumberFormatException("Invalid age (must be between 18 and
     100)");
    }
    String gender = genderChoice.getSelectedItem();
    String bmiStr = bmiField.getText();
    double bmi = Double.parseDouble(bmiStr);
    String bloodPressureStr = bloodPressureField.getText();
    String[] bloodPressureValues = bloodPressureStr.split("/");
    if (bloodPressureValues.length != 2) {
  throw new NumberFormatException("Invalid blood pressure format (sys-
tolic/diastolic)");
    }
    int systolicBP = Integer.parseInt(bloodPressureValues[0]);
    int diastolicBP = Integer.parseInt(bloodPressureValues[1]);
    String fastingBloodSugarStr = fastingBloodSugarField.getText();
    double fastingBloodSugar = Double.parseDouble(fastingBloodSugarStr);
```

```
      String    postPrandialBloodSugarStr    =    postPrandialBloodSugarField.
getText();
      double postPrandialBloodSugar = Double.parseDouble(postPrandialBloodS
ugarStr);
      String familyHistory = familyHistoryChoice.getSelectedItem();
      String physicalActivity = physicalActivityChoice.getSelectedItem();
      String smoker = smokerChoice.getSelectedItem();
      String diabetic = diabeticChoice.getSelectedItem(); // This should be
         pre-populated as "No"
      // Diabetes risk calculation (replace with a more comprehensive model)
      double riskScore = calculateDiabetesRisk(age, gender, bmi, systolicBP,
         diastolicBP,       fastingBloodSugar,       postPrandialBloodSugar,
         familyHistory, physicalActivity, smoker);
      // Interpret risk score and display results
      String riskMessage;
      if (riskScore < 0.2) {
    riskMessage = "You have a low risk of developing diabetes.";
      } else if (riskScore < 0.5) {
    riskMessage = "You have a moderate risk of developing diabetes. Consider
        consulting a healthcare professional for further evaluation.";
      } else {
    riskMessage = "You have a high risk of developing diabetes. We strongly
        recommend consulting a healthcare professional for a proper diagnosis
        and discussing risk management strategies.";
      }
      showInfoDialog(riskMessage);
      clearFields();
    } catch (NumberFormatException ex) {
      showErrorDialog("Invalid data format! Please check your entries.");
    } catch (Exception ex) { // Catch other potential exceptions
      showErrorDialog("An error occurred. Please try again.");
      ex.printStackTrace(); // Log the exception for debugging
    }
    } else if (e.getSource() == resetButton) {
    clearFields();
    }
}
      // Create a HealthData object and store the data
      HealthData data = new HealthData(age, gender, bmi, bloodPressureStr,
        fastingBloodSugarStr,    postPrandialBloodSugarStr,    familyHistory,
        physicalActivity, smoker, diabetic);
      dataList.add(data);
      // Optional: Write data to CSV file
      writeDataToCSV(dataList);
      // Clear the form for next entry
      ageField.setText("");
      bmiField.setText("");
      bloodPressureField.setText("");
      fastingBloodSugarField.setText("");
      postPrandialBloodSugarField.setText("");
      showInfoDialog("Data submitted successfully!");
    }
```

The `HealthDataCollector` program is a Java-based GUI application designed to collect and analyze various health-related data. It gathers user information such as age, gender, BMI, blood pressure, fasting and post-prandial blood sugar levels, family history of diseases, physical activity, smoking status, and diabetic status. This information is validated and then used to calculate a diabetes risk score, which is interpreted and presented to the user.

12.11.2 Case Study 2

Low bone mineral density (BMD) significantly raises the risk of fractures and osteoporosis, compromising bone strength and overall skeletal health. Early detection and preventive measures, such as proper nutrition and weight-bearing exercises, are crucial for mitigating these risks. The parameters used to store and possibly analyze the user's BMD data to understand bone health and density are:

1. **Weight**: The user's weight in kilograms.
2. **Height**: The user's height in centimeters.
3. **Hip BMD**: The user's Bone Mass Density at the hip, measured in grams per square centimeter (g/cm²).
4. **Spine BMD**: The user's Bone Mass Density at the spine, measured in grams per square centimeter (g/cm²).

Program

```
import java.awt.*;
import java.awt.event.*;
import java.util.ArrayList;
public class BMDCalculator extends Frame implements ActionListener {
  // UI components
  Label titleLabel, nameLabel, ageLabel, genderLabel, weightLabel,
heightLabel, hipBMDLabel, spineBMDLabel;
  TextField nameField, ageField, weightField, heightField, hipBMDField,
spineBMDField;
  Choice genderChoice;
  Button calculateButton, resetButton;
  // Data storage (replace with actual BMD data class if needed)
  ArrayList<BMDRecord> bmdRecords = new ArrayList<>();
  public BMDCalculator() {
  super("Bone Mass Density Calculator");
  // Create UI components
  titleLabel = new Label("Bone Mass Density Calculator", Label.CENTER);
  nameLabel = new Label("Name:");
  ageLabel = new Label("Age (years):");
  genderLabel = new Label("Gender:");
  weightLabel = new Label("Weight (kg):");
  heightLabel = new Label("Height (cm):");
  hipBMDLabel = new Label("Hip BMD (g/cm²):");
  spineBMDLabel = new Label("Spine BMD (g/cm²):");
  nameField = new TextField(20);
  ageField = new TextField(3);
  weightField = new TextField(5);
  heightField = new TextField(5);
  hipBMDField = new TextField(5);
  spineBMDField = new TextField(5);
  genderChoice = new Choice();
  genderChoice.add("Male");
  genderChoice.add("Female");
```

```
  calculateButton = new Button("Calculate");
  resetButton = new Button("Reset");
  // Layout components (modify as needed)
  setLayout(new GridLayout(10, 2, 5, 5));
  add(titleLabel);
  add(new Label(""));
  add(nameLabel);
  add(nameField);
  add(ageLabel);
  add(ageField);
  add(genderLabel);
  add(genderChoice);
  add(weightLabel);
  add(weightField);
  add(heightLabel);
  add(heightField);
  add(hipBMDLabel);
  add(hipBMDField);
  add(spineBMDLabel);
  add(spineBMDField);
  add(calculateButton);
  add(resetButton);
  calculateButton.addActionListener(this);
  resetButton.addActionListener(this);
  }
  public void actionPerformed(ActionEvent e) {
  if (e.getSource() == calculateButton) {
    // Extract data from UI components
    String name = nameField.getText();
    String ageStr = ageField.getText();
    String gender = genderChoice.getSelectedItem();
    String weightStr = weightField.getText();
    String heightStr = heightField.getText();
    String hipBMDStr = hipBMDField.getText();
    String spineBMDStr = spineBMDField.getText();
    // Basic validation (replace with appropriate BMD data processing)
    if  (name.isEmpty()  ||  ageStr.isEmpty()  ||  weightStr.isEmpty()  ||
      heightStr.isEmpty() || hipBMDStr.isEmpty() || spineBMDStr.isEmpty()) {
  showErrorDialog("Please fill in all fields.");
  return;
    }
    try {
  int age = Integer.parseInt(ageStr);
  double weight = Double.parseDouble(weightStr);
  double height = Double.parseDouble(heightStr);
  double hipBMD = Double.parseDouble(hipBMDStr);
  double spineBMD = Double.parseDouble(spineBMDStr);
  // (Optional) Perform BMD calculations based on gender, age, etc.
  // Create a BMD record (replace with actual data structure if needed)
  BMDRecord record = new BMDRecord(name, age, gender, weight, height,
hipBMD, spineBMD);
  bmdRecords.add(record);
  // Display results (replace with meaningful interpretation)
  showInfoDialog("BMD data for " + name + " has been recorded.");
  clearFields();
```

```
    } catch (NumberFormatException ex) {
  showErrorDialog("Invalid data format. Please enter numbers only.");
    }
  } else if (e.getSource() == resetButton) {
    clearFields();
  }
  }
  private void showErrorDialog(String message) {
  Dialog errorDialog = new Dialog(this, "Error");
  errorDialog.setLayout(new FlowLayout());
  errorDialog.add(new Label(message));
  errorDialog.setSize(300, 100);
  errorDialog.setLocationRelativeTo(this);
  errorDialog.setVisible(true);
  }
  private void showInfoDialog(String message) {
  Dialog infoDialog = new Dialog(this, "Information");
  infoDialog.setLayout(new FlowLayout());
  infoDialog.add(new Label(message));
  infoDialog.setSize(300, 100);
  infoDialog.setLocationRelativeTo(this);
  infoDialog.setVisible(true);
  }
private void clearFields() {
  nameField.setText("");
  ageField.setText("");
  weightField.setText("");
  heightField.setText("");
  hipBMDField.setText("");
  spineBMDField.setText("");
}
void main(String[] args) {
  BMDCalculator calculator = new BMDCalculator();
  calculator.setSize(400, 300);
  calculator.setVisible(true);
}
}
```

The `BMDCalculator` application is a Java-based graphical user interface application designed to calculate and record Bone Mass Density (BMD) data. It extends the `Frame` class and implements the `ActionListener` interface to handle user interactions. The user interface includes fields for entering personal information such as name, age, gender, weight, height, and BMD values for the hip and spine, as well as buttons for calculation and resetting the fields. When the calculate button is pressed, the program validates the input, performs basic calculations, and stores the data in an `ArrayList` of `BMDRecord` objects, providing feedback via dialog boxes. The reset button clears all input fields.

12.11.3 Case Study 3

Smoking significantly increases the risk of lung cancer, heart disease, and chronic respiratory conditions, reducing overall life expectancy. Understanding these risks is crucial for making informed decisions about smoking cessation and health improvement. Theparameters are used to calculate the disease risk.

1. **Smoker Status**: Check whether the user is a smoker.
2. **Years Smoked**: The number of years the user has been smoking.
3. **Daily Cigarettes**: The number of cigarettes the user smokes per day.

Program

```
import java.awt.*;
import java.awt.event.*;
import java.util.ArrayList;
public class SmokingDiseaseDetector extends Frame implements ActionListener {
  // UI components
  Label titleLabel, ageLabel, genderLabel, smokerLabel, yearsSmokedLabel,
dailyCigarettesLabel;
  TextField ageField, yearsSmokedField, dailyCigarettesField;
  Choice genderChoice, smokerChoice;
  Button calculateButton, resetButton;
  // Data storage
  ArrayList<SmokingData> smokingDataList = new ArrayList<>();
  public SmokingDiseaseDetector() {
  super("Smoking Disease Detector");
  // Create UI components
  titleLabel = new Label("Smoking Disease Detector", Label.CENTER);
  ageLabel = new Label("Age:");
  genderLabel = new Label("Gender:");
  smokerLabel = new Label("Smoker:");
  yearsSmokedLabel = new Label("Years Smoked:");
  dailyCigarettesLabel = new Label("Daily Cigarettes:");
  ageField = new TextField(3);
  yearsSmokedField = new TextField(3);
  dailyCigarettesField = new TextField(3);
  genderChoice = new Choice();
  genderChoice.add("Male");
  genderChoice.add("Female");
  smokerChoice = new Choice();
  smokerChoice.add("Yes");
  smokerChoice.add("No");
  calculateButton = new Button("Calculate");
  resetButton = new Button("Reset");
  // Layout components
  setLayout(new GridLayout(8, 2, 5, 5));
  add(titleLabel);
  add(new Label(""));
  add(ageLabel);
  add(ageField);
  add(genderLabel);
  add(genderChoice);
  add(smokerLabel);
  add(smokerChoice);
  add(yearsSmokedLabel);
  add(yearsSmokedField);
  add(dailyCigarettesLabel);
  add(dailyCigarettesField);
  add(calculateButton);
  add(resetButton);
```

```
  calculateButton.addActionListener(this);
  resetButton.addActionListener(this);
  }
  public void actionPerformed(ActionEvent e) {
  if (e.getSource() == calculateButton) {
    // Extract data from UI components
    String ageStr = ageField.getText();
    String gender = genderChoice.getSelectedItem();
    String smoker = smokerChoice.getSelectedItem();
    String yearsSmokedStr = yearsSmokedField.getText();
    String dailyCigarettesStr = dailyCigarettesField.getText();
    // Basic validation
    if (ageStr.isEmpty() || yearsSmokedStr.isEmpty() || dailyCigarettesStr.
       isEmpty()) {
  showErrorDialog("Please fill in all fields.");
  return;
    }
    try {
  int age = Integer.parseInt(ageStr);
  int yearsSmoked = Integer.parseInt(yearsSmokedStr);
  int dailyCigarettes = Integer.parseInt(dailyCigarettesStr);
  // Calculate disease risk based on smoking data
  double    diseaseRisk    =    calculateDiseaseRisk(age,    yearsSmoked,
     dailyCigarettes);
  // Create a SmokingData object and store the data
  SmokingData data = new SmokingData(age, gender, smoker, yearsSmoked,
     dailyCigarettes, diseaseRisk);
  smokingDataList.add(data);
  // Display results
  showInfoDialog("Disease risk calculated: " + diseaseRisk);
  clearFields();
    } catch (NumberFormatException ex) {
  showErrorDialog("Invalid data format. Please enter numbers only.");
    }
  } else if (e.getSource() == resetButton) {
    clearFields();
  }
  }
double baseRisk = 0.1;  // Base risk of developing smoking-related diseases
  double ageFactor = (double) age / 100;  // Ageing increases risk
  double packYears = yearsSmoked * (dailyCigarettes / 20.0);  // Calculate
                                                               pack-years
  double smokingFactor = packYears * 0.05;  // Pack-years contribute to risk
  return baseRisk + ageFactor + smokingFactor;  // Combine factors for a
                                                   basic risk estimate
  }
  private void showErrorDialog(String message) {
  Dialog errorDialog = new Dialog(this, "Error");
  errorDialog.setLayout(new FlowLayout());
  errorDialog.add(new Label(message));
  errorDialog.setSize(300, 100);
  errorDialog.setLocationRelativeTo(this);
  errorDialog.setVisible(true);
  }
  private void showInfoDialog(String message) {
  Dialog infoDialog = new Dialog(this, "Information");
```

```
  infoDialog.setLayout(new FlowLayout());
  infoDialog.add(new Label(message));
  infoDialog.setSize(300, 100);
  infoDialog.setLocationRelativeTo(this);
  infoDialog.setVisible(true);
  }
  private void clearFields() {
  ageField.setText("");
  yearsSmokedField.setText("");
  dailyCigarettesField.setText("");
  }
  void main(String[] args) {
  SmokingDiseaseDetector detector = new SmokingDiseaseDetector();
  detector.setSize(400, 300);
  detector.setVisible(true);
  }
}
public class SmokingData {
  private int age;
  private String gender;
  private String smoker;
  private int yearsSmoked;
  private int dailyCigarettes;
  private double diseaseRisk;
  public SmokingData(int age, String gender, String smoker, int yearsSmoked,
int dailyCigarettes, double diseaseRisk) {
  this.age = age;
  this.gender = gender;
  this.smoker = smoker;
  this.yearsSmoked = yearsSmoked;
  this.dailyCigarettes = dailyCigarettes;
  this.diseaseRisk = diseaseRisk;
  }
  public int getAge() {
  return age;
  }
  public String getGender() {
  return gender;
  }
  public String getSmoker() {
  return smoker;
  }
  public int getYearsSmoked() {
  return yearsSmoked;
  }
  public int getDailyCigarettes() {
  return dailyCigarettes;
  }
  public double getDiseaseRisk() {
  return diseaseRisk;
  }
  @Override
  public String toString() {
  return "SmokingData{" +
  "age=" + age +
```

```
    ", gender='" + gender + '\'' +
    ", smoker='" + smoker + '\'' +
    ", yearsSmoked=" + yearsSmoked +
    ", dailyCigarettes=" + dailyCigarettes +
    ", diseaseRisk=" + diseaseRisk +
    '}';
  }
}
```

The `SmokingDiseaseDetector` application is a Java-based GUI application that evaluates the risk of developing smoking-related diseases. It extends the `Frame` class and implements the `ActionListener` interface for user interaction handling. The interface includes fields for age, gender, smoking status, years smoked, and daily cigarettes, along with buttons for calculating risk and resetting inputs. Upon calculating, it validates inputs, computes disease risk based on smoking data, and stores this information in an `ArrayList` of `SmokingData` objects. Results are displayed to the user through dialog boxes, while the reset button clears all fields for new entries.

13 Swings

13.1 INTRODUCTION

Java Swing stands as a robust and highly favored graphical user interface (GUI) toolkit, renowned for its prowess in developing desktop applications. As an integral part of the Java Foundation Classes (JFC), it furnishes developers with an extensive array of components and layout managers, facilitating the creation of diverse GUIs. One of its hallmark attributes is its platform independence, making it compatible with any operating system that supports Java.

A notable feature of Java Swing is its provision of a pluggable look and feel, affording developers the flexibility to tailor the GUI to suit user preferences. Furthermore, it offers a robust event-handling mechanism, empowering developers to effectively manage events triggered by graphical components.

Notably, Swing is labeled as "lightweight" due to its self-contained implementation in Java, rendering it independent of underlying operating systems for rendering GUI components.

As a prominent member of the Java Foundation Classes, Swing empowers developers to create versatile and dynamic desktop applications across various platforms. Its pluggable look and feel feature allows for extensive customization of the GUI to align with user preferences, while robust event-handling mechanisms ensure seamless interaction with graphical elements.

Furthermore, Swing offers a selection of layout managers such as BorderLayout, FlowLayout, GridLayout, CardLayout, and BoxLayout, enabling developers to design sophisticated and user-friendly GUI layouts that adapt to diverse screen resolutions and user preferences.

Swing has gained immense popularity among developers tasked with creating visually appealing graphical user interfaces (GUIs) for commercial software applications.

- Swing is a comprehensive set of API, encompassing a wide array of classes and interfaces tailored for GUI development.
- It serves as a powerful tool for designing interactive and user-friendly graphical interfaces.
- Swing extends the functionality of the Abstract Window Toolkit (AWT), introducing new and enhanced components to elevate the aesthetics and functionality of GUIs.
- The library empowers developers to build standalone Swing GUI applications, as well as servlets and applets.
- Swing adopts a model/view design architecture, facilitating the separation of data presentation and user interaction.
- It offers greater portability and flexibility compared to AWT, leveraging the underlying AWT framework.
- Entirely implemented in Java, Swing ensures platform independence, and its lightweight components contribute to efficient resource utilization.

DOI: 10.1201/9781003544319-13

- Swing boasts support for a pluggable look and feel, allowing developers to customize the appearance of GUI components to suit various design preferences.
- It provides a rich assortment of components, including tables, lists, scroll panes, color choosers, tabbed panes, and more.
- Following the Model-View-Controller (MVC) architectural pattern, Swing promotes a modular and scalable approach to GUI development.

13.1.1 Advantages of Java Swing

Java Swing offers numerous benefits for developing graphical user interfaces (GUIs) in Java. Some of its key advantages include:

1. Cross-Platform Compatibility: Since Swing is written purely in Java, it enjoys platform independence. This means Swing-based applications can seamlessly run on any platform supporting Java without requiring any platform-specific modifications.
2. Flexible Appearance: One of Swing's standout features is its pluggable look and feel functionality. This allows developers to tailor the appearance of their GUI components to match specific design preferences or branding requirements, ensuring a consistent and professional look across different platforms.
3. Extensive Component Library: Swing boasts a rich collection of components, ranging from basic ones like buttons and text fields to more advanced elements such as trees, tables, and spinners. Additionally, it supports multimedia components, offering versatility in GUI design.
4. Layout Management: With Swing, developers have access to various layout managers that facilitate the organization and arrangement of GUI components. These layout managers simplify the process of creating visually appealing and user-friendly interfaces by automatically handling component positioning and resizing.
5. Robust Event Handling: Swing provides a robust event-handling mechanism, empowering developers to respond effectively to user interactions like mouse clicks and keystrokes. This event-driven model enhances the interactivity and responsiveness of Swing-based applications.
6. Customizability: Swing components are highly customizable, enabling developers to fine-tune their appearance and behavior to suit specific application requirements. This flexibility allows for the creation of tailored GUIs that align perfectly with the application's design objectives.

13.1.2 Disadvantages of Java Swing

Java Swing, despite its many advantages, also comes with some notable drawbacks:

1. Performance Overhead: Due to the need to run on the Java Virtual Machine (JVM), Swing applications may suffer from performance issues, especially in resource-intensive scenarios or when dealing with large datasets. This overhead can lead to slower response times compared to native applications.
2. Non-Native Look and Feel: While Swing's pluggable look and feel feature offers customization options, achieving a truly native appearance can be challenging. Swing applications may look and behave differently from native applications on the same platform, potentially causing inconsistency and user confusion.
3. Steep Learning Curve: Although Swing is relatively easy for Java developers to grasp, beginners may find its complex component hierarchy and layout managers daunting. Creating sophisticated GUIs with Swing requires a deep understanding of its various components and their interactions.

4. Resource Consumption: Swing applications often demand substantial system resources, including memory and processing power. This resource-intensive nature can be problematic for devices with limited capabilities or in scenarios where scalability is a concern, such as enterprise-grade applications.
5. Limited Mobile Support: As a desktop-oriented GUI toolkit, Swing lacks robust support for mobile devices. Developers aiming to create cross-platform applications spanning both desktop and mobile environments may encounter challenges in adapting Swing-based interfaces for mobile platforms, potentially necessitating alternative solutions.

13.1.3 MVC Model

Swing components adhere to the Model-View-Controller (MVC) architecture, which separates the visual component into three distinct aspects:

1. View: This aspect determines the appearance of the component when rendered on the screen. It encompasses the visual representation of the component.
2. Controller: The controller aspect dictates how the component reacts to user interactions. It handles user inputs and triggers appropriate actions or responses.
3. Model: This aspect encapsulates the state information associated with the component. It represents the underlying data or properties of the component.

In the context of user interfaces, these three main aspects are considered:

- UI Elements: These are the fundamental visual elements that users interact with. Swing provides a comprehensive range of UI elements, from basic to complex, catering to various application requirements.
- Layouts: Layouts define the arrangement of UI elements on the screen, ensuring a cohesive and organized appearance. They play a crucial role in determining the final look and feel of the graphical user interface (GUI).
- Behavior: Behavior refers to the events that occur when users interact with UI elements. It encompasses event-handling mechanisms, allowing developers to define responses to user actions effectively.

Throughout the development process, understanding and addressing these aspects are essential for creating intuitive, user-friendly, and visually appealing Swing-based applications.

13.2 APPLICATIONS OF JAVA SWING

Java Swing is a versatile toolkit for building graphical user interfaces (GUIs) in Java. It is part of the Java Foundation Classes (JFC) and provides a rich set of components for creating desktop applications. Here are some key applications of Java Swing:

1. Desktop Applications: Swing is widely used to develop standalone desktop applications such as text editors, media players, and office productivity tools. Examples include NetBeans IDE and JDownloader.
2. Graphical User Interfaces (GUIs): Swing allows developers to create sophisticated, visually appealing user interfaces with components like buttons, tables, trees, and text fields. It supports various layout managers in arranging components in complex layouts.

3. Data Visualization: Swing can be used to build applications that require data visualization, such as charts, graphs, and dashboards. Libraries like JFreeChart can be integrated with Swing to enhance data representation.
4. Simulation and Modeling: Swing is useful in scientific and engineering applications for creating simulation tools and modeling environments. These applications often require intricate interfaces to manage complex data and operations.
5. Educational Software: Swing is utilized in creating educational tools and software for learning and teaching purposes. Examples include interactive tutorials, quizzes, and e-learning platforms.
6. Game Development: While not as common as other frameworks, Swing can be used for developing simple 2D games and educational games due to its rich set of GUI components and event-handling capabilities.

Swing's cross-platform nature, ease of use, and an extensive component library make it a popular choice for developing a wide range of desktop applications. Java Swing finds extensive application in the development of desktop applications, catering to diverse domains such as billing systems, inventory management, and real-time control of mechanical devices. Moreover, Swing is a preferred choice for crafting mobile applications, ranging from interactive games to utility tools like calculators, owing to its versatility and rich feature set.

Furthermore, Swing facilitates the creation of network-based applications aimed at managing clients within a network environment. From client-server architectures to distributed systems, Swing empowers developers to architect robust and scalable solutions tailored to their specific networking requirements.

By leveraging Swing's capabilities, developers can build applications that seamlessly operate across different platforms, ensuring widespread accessibility and ease of deployment.

13.3 FEATURES OF JAVA SWING

Some notable features of Java Swing include:

1. Platform Independence: Java Swing is renowned for its platform independence, allowing applications developed with Swing to run seamlessly on any platform that supports Java. Whether it's Windows, macOS, Linux, or any other Java-compatible operating system, Swing-based applications can operate effortlessly.
2. . Lightweight Components: Swing offers a collection of lightweight components designed for ease of use and customization. These components are engineered to be memory-efficient and consume minimal processing power, ensuring optimal performance for Swing-based applications.
3. Pluggable Look and Feel: With Java Swing, developers have the flexibility to customize the appearance of their GUIs to align with user preferences. The framework provides a pluggable look and feel feature, enabling developers to choose from various pre-built themes.
4. Layout Managers: Java Swing equips developers with a suite of layout managers, facilitating the organization of graphical components within a GUI. These layout managers empower developers to create adaptable and responsive user interfaces capable of adjusting to diverse screen sizes and resolutions.
5. Robust Event-Handling Mechanism: Swing boasts a robust event-handling mechanism that empowers developers to manage events generated by graphical components effectively. By registering event listeners, developers can detect and respond to user interactions with the GUI, enhancing the overall interactivity and responsiveness of Swing-based applications.

13.4 JAVA SWING PACKAGES

Some commonly used packages in Java Swing include:

1. javax.swing: This package encompasses the core components of Swing, featuring essential elements like JButton, JLabel, JTable, JList, along with classes for constructing top-level containers such as JFrame and JDialog.
2. javax.swing.event: Responsible for handling events generated by Swing components, this package houses event listener interfaces, event adapter classes, and event objects essential for event management within Swing-based applications.
3. javax.swing.border: Offering classes for border creation around Swing components, this package provides options for crafting various border types including line borders, enhancing the visual presentation of Swing elements.
4. javax.swing.layout: Focused on layout management within Swing, this package provides classes for creating and managing layout managers essential for organizing graphical components effectively. It includes popular layout managers like BorderLayout, FlowLayout, GridLayout, BoxLayout, and CardLayout.
5. javax.swing.plaf: Dedicated to the pluggable look and feel feature of Swing, this package classes for managing look and feel themes, offering customization options, and providing default look and feel themes tailored to different platforms.
6. javax.swing.text: Designed for creating and managing text components within Swing, this package contains classes for text-related functionalities such as text fields, text areas, and other text-based components, facilitating text manipulation and display in Swing applications.
7. javax.swing.table: Specifically tailored for managing tables in Swing applications, this package offers classes for creating and managing JTable instances, along with components like TableModel, TableColumn, and TableCellRenderer, ensuring efficient handling and presentation of tabular data within Swing interfaces.

13.5 CONTAINER CLASS

A container class in Java is any class that can hold or contain other components within it. When building GUI applications, at least one container class is required to organize and manage the components effectively.

13.5.1 JPanel

Panels are used to organize and group components within a window. They provide a way to structure the layout of components and manage their placement.

Program

```
import javax.swing.JButton;
import javax.swing.JFrame;
import javax.swing.JLabel;
import javax.swing.JPanel;
public class PanelExample {
  void main(String[] args) {
  // Create a JFrame with a title
  JFrame frame = new JFrame("Panel Example");
  // Set default close operation and size of the frame
```

```
  frame.setDefaultCloseOperation(JFrame.EXIT_ON_CLOSE);
  frame.setSize(300, 200);
  // Create a JPanel to hold components
  JPanel panel = new JPanel();
  // Create and add buttons to the panel
  JButton button1 = new JButton("Button 1");
  JButton button2 = new JButton("Button 2");
  panel.add(button1);
  panel.add(button2);
  // Create and add a label to the panel
  JLabel label = new JLabel("Label 1");
  panel.add(label);
  // Add the panel to the frame
  frame.add(panel);
  // Make the frame visible
  frame.setVisible(true);
  }
}
```

Output:

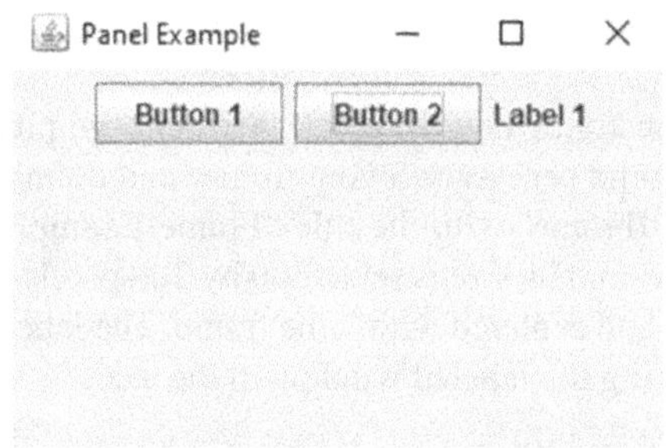

The above program creates a simple graphical user interface using Java Swing. It starts by importing the necessary Swing library and defining the `PanelExample` class. Inside the `main` method, it creates a `JFrame` with the title "Panel Example" and sets its default close operation and size. A `JPanel` is instantiated to group components together. Three components are added to the panel: two buttons labeled "Button 1" and "Button 2", and a label labeled "Label 1". The panel is then added to the frame, and the frame is made visible, displaying the window with the grouped components.

13.5.2 JFrame

Frames are fully functioning windows that typically include features such as icons, titles, and menu bars. They serve as the main window for an application and provide the user interface for interacting with the program.

Program

```
import javax.swing.JFrame;
import javax.swing.JLabel;
import javax.swing.SwingConstants;
public class FrameExample {
  void main(String[] args) {
  // Create a JFrame with a title
  JFrame frame = new JFrame("Frame Example");
  // Set default close operation and size of the frame
```

```
    frame.setDefaultCloseOperation(JFrame.EXIT_ON_CLOSE);
    frame.setSize(400, 200);
    // Create a JLabel with text and center it
    JLabel label = new JLabel("This is a frame window", SwingConstants.
       CENTER);
    // Add the label to the frame
    frame.add(label);
    // Make the frame visible
    frame.setVisible(true);
    }
}
```

Output

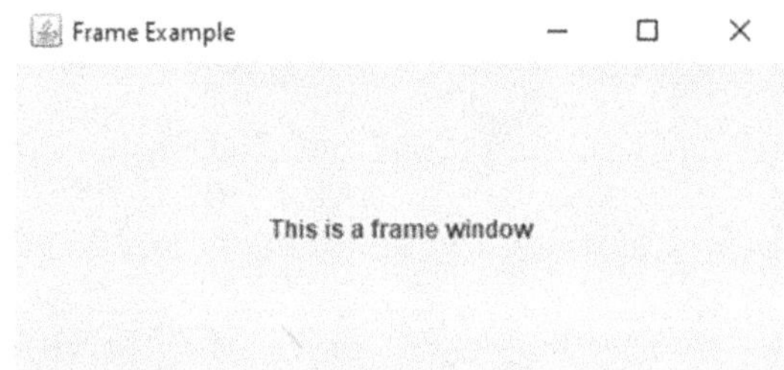

The above program demonstrates how to create a simple graphical user interface using Java Swing. It begins by importing the necessary Swing library and defining the `FrameExample` class. Inside the `main` method, a `JFrame` with the title "Frame Example" is created, its default close operation is set to exit on close, and its size is set to 400 by 200 pixels. A `JLabel` with the text "This is a frame window" is created and centered within the frame. The label is added to the frame, and the frame is made visible, displaying the labeled window to the user.

13.5.3 JDialog

JDialog is a top-level window with a title and a border that typically takes some form of input from the user.

Program

```
import javax.swing.*;
import java.awt.*;
public class DialogExample {
  void main(String[] args) {
  JFrame frame = new JFrame("Dialog Example");
  JButton button = new JButton("Open Dialog");
  button.setBackground(Color.MAGENTA);
  JDialog dialog = new JDialog(frame, "Course Registration", true);
  JLabel label = new JLabel("Select your course:");
  JComboBox<String> comboBox = new JComboBox<>(new String[]{"Java",
     "Python", "C++"});
  JButton okButton = new JButton("OK");
  okButton.addActionListener(e -> dialog.dispose());
  dialog.setLayout(new FlowLayout());
  dialog.add(label);
  dialog.add(comboBox);
  dialog.add(okButton);
```

```
  frame.add(button);
  frame.setSize(300, 100);
  frame.setDefaultCloseOperation(JFrame.EXIT_ON_CLOSE);
  frame.setVisible(true);
  }
}
```

Output

Dialog Example

Open Dialog

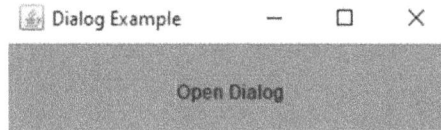

The `DialogExample` program demonstrates the use of a JDialog in a Java Swing application. A JFrame titled "Dialog Example" contains a JButton labeled "Open Dialog" with a magenta background. When the button is clicked, a modal JDialog titled "Course Registration" opens. This dialog includes a JLabel prompting the user to select a course, a JComboBox with options ("Java", "Python", "C++"), and an OK button that closes the dialog when clicked. The main frame is set to a size of 300x100 pixels, configured to close the application upon exit, and made visible. This program shows how to create and display a modal dialog for course selection.

13.6 COMPONENTS OF JAVA SWING

Java Swing components are essential for creating graphical user interfaces (GUIs) in Java. They provide a rich set of pre-built UI elements, such as buttons, text fields, labels, and menus, that can be easily customized and arranged to create complex GUIs. These components are responsible for handling user input, displaying data, and responding to events. They are also highly customizable, allowing developers to change their appearance, behavior, and layout to suit their needs. Additionally, Swing components are platform-independent, meaning they can run on any operating system that supports Java. They also provide a robust event-handling mechanism, allowing developers to respond to user interactions and other events. Furthermore, Swing components are highly reusable, making it easy to build and maintain large GUI applications. They also provide a wide range of layout managers, making it easy to arrange components in a variety of layouts.

13.6.1 JButton

JButton is a push button used to perform an action when clicked. The main features are:

1. Event-Driven: `JButton` triggers actions when clicked, commonly used with `ActionListener` for handling events.
2. Customizable Appearance: Supports text, icons, and allows customization of colors, fonts, and borders.
3. Interactive Component: Provides focus and accessibility features, including tooltips and keyboard mnemonics for user interaction.

Program

```
import javax.swing.JButton;
import javax.swing.JFrame;
import java.awt.Color;
public class ButtonExample {
```

```
  void main(String[] args) {
  // Create a new JFrame
  JFrame frame = new JFrame("Button Example");
  // Create a new JButton with text
  JButton button = new JButton("Enroll in Java Course");
  // Set the background color of the button
  button.setBackground(Color.CYAN);
  // Add the button to the JFrame
  frame.add(button);
  // Set the default close operation and size of the JFrame
  frame.setDefaultCloseOperation(JFrame.EXIT_ON_CLOSE);
  frame.setSize(300, 200);
  // Make the JFrame visible
  frame.setVisible(true);
  }
}
```

Output

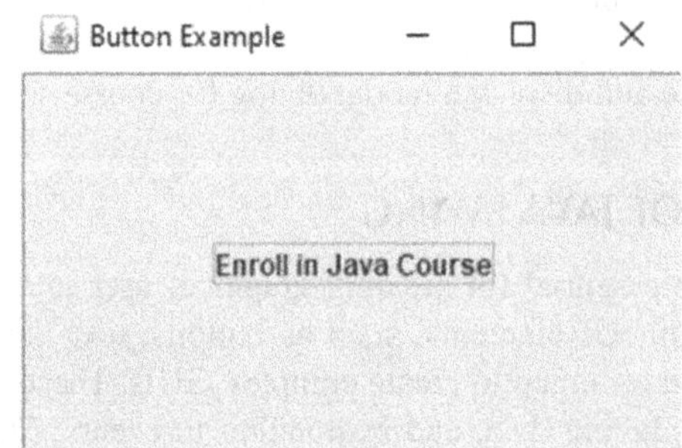

This Java program creates a graphical user interface (GUI) using the Swing library. The program starts by creating a new JFrame, which is a window that can contain other GUI components. The JFrame is given the title "Button Example". A new JButton is then created with the text "Enroll in Java Course". The button's background color is set to cyan. Finally, the button is added to the JFrame, which is then set to a fixed size and made visible, allowing the user to interact with it.

13.6.2 JLabel

JLabel is a display area for a short text string or an image, or both. The main features are:

1. Display Text and Images: `JLabel` is used to display static text, icons, or both without user interaction.
2. Customizable Appearance: Allows customization of font, text color, alignment, and borders for a tailored look.
3. No Event Handling: Unlike buttons, `JLabel` does not trigger events, making it ideal for displaying information without interaction.

Program

```
import javax.swing.JFrame;
import javax.swing.JLabel;
import java.awt.Color;
import java.awt.Font;
public class LabelExample {
```

```
  void main(String[] args) {
  // Create a new JFrame
  JFrame frame = new JFrame("Label Example");
  // Create a new JLabel with the desired text
  JLabel label = new JLabel("Welcome to the Computer Science Department");
  // Set the label's font color to blue
  label.setForeground(Color.BLUE);
  // Set the font of the label (optional, for better visual)
  label.setFont(new Font("Arial", Font.BOLD, 16));
  // Add the label to the JFrame
  frame.add(label);
  // Set the default close operation and size of the JFrame
  frame.setDefaultCloseOperation(JFrame.EXIT_ON_CLOSE);
  frame.setSize(400, 100);
  // Make the JFrame visible
  frame.setVisible(true);
  }
}
```

Output

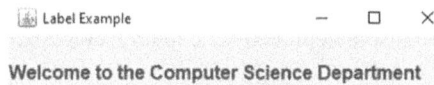

Label Example

Welcome to the Computer Science Department

This Java program displays a window with a label that shows the text "Welcome to the Computer Science Department" in blue color. The window is set to a fixed size and when the user closes the window, the program terminates.

13.6.3 JTextField

JTextField is a component that allows the editing of a single line of text. The main features are:

1. User Input: `JTextField` allows users to enter and edit a single line of text in a GUI application.
2. Customizable Appearance: Supports customization of text, font, color, and size, with options to set placeholder text or limit the number of characters.
3. Event Handling: Can handle events like text input or pressing "Enter" through listeners such as `ActionListener` or `DocumentListener` for real-time input processing.

Program

```
import javax.swing.JFrame;
import javax.swing.JTextField;
import java.awt.Color;
public class TextFieldExample {
  void main(String[] args) {
  // Create a new JFrame
  JFrame frame = new JFrame("Text Field Example");
  // Create a new JTextField with the initial text
  JTextField textField = new JTextField("Enter course name");
  // Set the background color of the text field to light gray
  textField.setBackground(Color.LIGHT_GRAY);
  // Add the text field to the JFrame
  frame.add(textField);
```

```
  // Set the default close operation and size of the JFrame
  frame.setDefaultCloseOperation(JFrame.EXIT_ON_CLOSE);
  frame.setSize(300, 100);
  // Make the JFrame visible
  frame.setVisible(true);
  }
}
```

Output

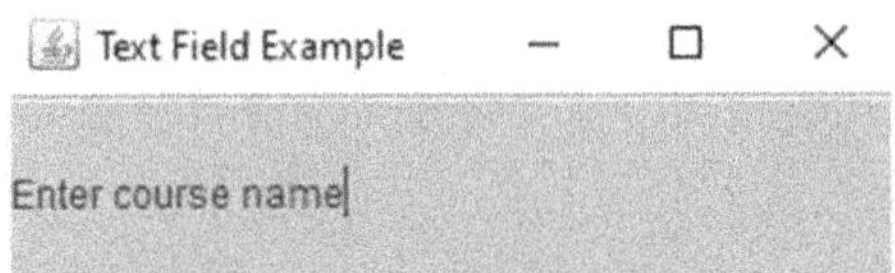

This Java program displays a window with a text field that is initially filled with the text "Enter course name". The text field has a light gray background and the window is set to a fixed size. When the user closes the window, the program terminates.

13.6.4 JTextArea

JTextArea is a multiline area to display/edit text. The main features are:

1. Multiline Text Input: `JTextArea` allows users to enter and edit multiple lines of text, unlike `JTextField`, which is limited to one line.
2. Customizable Layout: Supports line wrapping, customizable rows and columns, font, and background color for flexible text formatting.
3. Event Handling: Provides support for handling events like text changes through `DocumentListener` and supports copy-paste operations for user input.

Program

```
import javax.swing.JFrame;
import javax.swing.JTextArea;
import javax.swing.JScrollPane;
import java.awt.Color;
public class TextAreaExample {
  void main(String[] args) {
  // Create a new JFrame with the title "TextArea Example"
  JFrame frame = new JFrame("TextArea Example");
  // Create a new JTextArea with placeholder text
  JTextArea textArea = new JTextArea("Describe your programming experience");
  // Set the background color of the JTextArea to pink
  textArea.setBackground(Color.PINK);
  // Wrap the JTextArea in a JScrollPane to enable scrolling
  JScrollPane scrollPane = new JScrollPane(textArea);
  // Add the JScrollPane (which contains the JTextArea) to the JFrame
  frame.add(scrollPane);
  // Set the default close operation, size of the JFrame, and make it visible
  frame.setDefaultCloseOperation(JFrame.EXIT_ON_CLOSE);
  frame.setSize(400, 200);
  frame.setVisible(true);
  }
}
```

Output

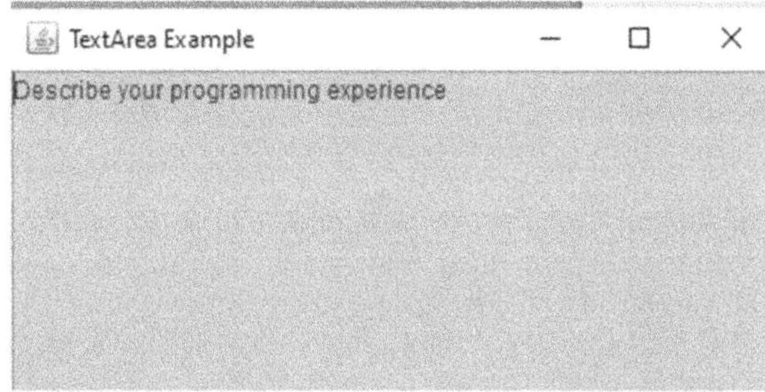

The `TextAreaExample` program demonstrates the use of a JTextArea in a Java Swing application. It creates a JFrame titled "TextArea Example" and adds a pink-background JTextArea with the placeholder text "Describe your programming experience," wrapped in a JScrollPane. The frame is set to a size of 400x200 pixels, configured to close the application on exit, and made visible.

13.6.5 JPasswordField

JPasswordField is a text field that echoes each character with an echo character, typically used for password input. The main features are:

1. Secure Text Input: `JPasswordField` is designed for entering sensitive information like passwords, where the characters are hidden or masked (usually displayed as dots or asterisks).
2. Customizable Masking: You can customize the masking character (e.g., `setEchoChar(char c)`), allowing different symbols to be displayed instead of the actual password characters.
3. Event Handling: It supports event handling through `ActionListener` or `DocumentListener`, allowing validation or processing when the user inputs or submits the password.

Program

```
import javax.swing.JFrame;
import javax.swing.JPasswordField;
import java.awt.Color;
public class PasswordFieldExample {
  void main(String[] args) {
  // Create a new JFrame with the title "PasswordField Example"
  JFrame frame = new JFrame("PasswordField Example");
  // Create a new JPasswordField with placeholder text
  JPasswordField passwordField = new JPasswordField("Enter your password");
  // Set the background color of the JPasswordField to yellow
  passwordField.setBackground(Color.YELLOW);
  // Add the JPasswordField to the JFrame
  frame.add(passwordField);
  // Set the default close operation, size of the JFrame, and make it visible
  frame.setDefaultCloseOperation(JFrame.EXIT_ON_CLOSE);
  frame.setSize(300, 100);
  frame.setVisible(true);
  }
}
```

Output

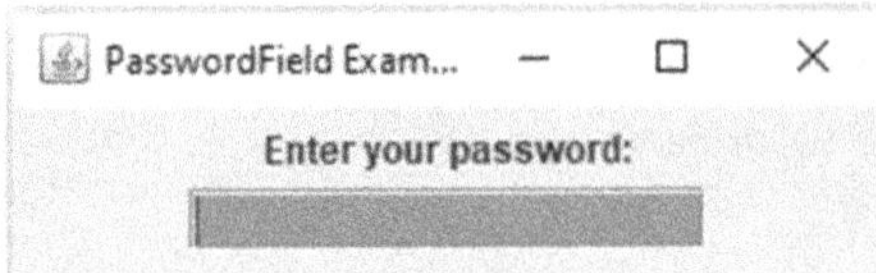

The `PasswordFieldExample` program demonstrates the use of a JPasswordField in a Java Swing application. It creates a JFrame titled "PasswordField Example" and adds a yellow background JPasswordField with the placeholder text "Enter your password." The frame is set to a size of 300x100 pixels, configured to close the application on exit, and made visible.

13.6.6 JCheckBox

JCheckBox is a component that can be selected or deselected. The main features are:

1. Selectable Option: `JCheckBox` allows users to select or deselect an option, providing a boolean choice (checked or unchecked).
2. Multiple Selection: Supports independent multiple selections, where users can check or uncheck multiple checkboxes in a group.
3. Event Handling: Captures state changes (checked/unchecked) through `ItemListener` or `ActionListener` for event-driven behavior.

Program

```
import javax.swing.JFrame;
import javax.swing.JCheckBox;
import java.awt.Color;
public class CheckBoxExample {
  void main(String[] args) {
  // Create a new JFrame with the title "CheckBox Example"
  JFrame frame = new JFrame("CheckBox Example");
  // Create a new JCheckBox with the label "computer courses"
  JCheckBox checkBox = new JCheckBox("computer courses");
  // Set the background color of the JCheckBox to green
  checkBox.setBackground(Color.GREEN);
  // Add the JCheckBox to the JFrame
  frame.add(checkBox);
  // Set the default close operation, size of the JFrame, and make it visible
  frame.setDefaultCloseOperation(JFrame.EXIT_ON_CLOSE);
  frame.setSize(300, 100);
  frame.setVisible(true);
  }
}
```

Output

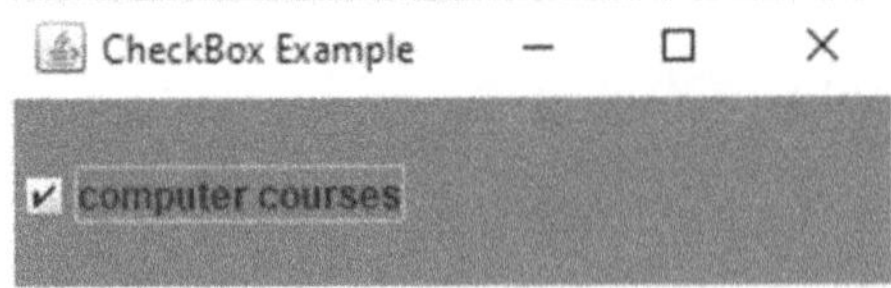

The above Java program creates a basic graphical user interface with a single checkbox. Inside this class, we created a checkbox with the label "computer courses" and set its background color to green. Finally, a window (JFrame) is created, the checkbox is added to it, and the window is sized, configured to close when you press the 'X' button, and displayed on the screen.

13.6.7 JRadioButton

JRadioButton is a button that can be selected or deselected, and is used in groups. The main features are:

1. Single Selection: `JRadioButton` allows users to select only one option from a group, ensuring mutually exclusive choices when grouped with other radio buttons.
2. Grouped Behavior: Typically used with `ButtonGroup` to ensure only one button can be selected at a time within the group.
3. Event Handling: Captures selection changes through `ActionListener` or `ItemListener` to handle actions when a radio button is selected or deselected.

Program

```
import javax.swing.JFrame;
import javax.swing.JRadioButton;
import javax.swing.ButtonGroup;
import java.awt.FlowLayout;
import java.awt.Color;
public class RadioButtonExample {
  void main(String[] args) {
  // Create a new JFrame with the title "RadioButton Example"
  JFrame frame = new JFrame("RadioButton Example");
  // Set the layout manager to FlowLayout
  frame.setLayout(new FlowLayout());
  // Create two JRadioButton instances with labels "Java" and "JSP"
  JRadioButton radioButton1 = new JRadioButton("Java");
  JRadioButton radioButton2 = new JRadioButton("JSP");
  // Set the background color of the radio buttons to orange
  radioButton1.setBackground(Color.ORANGE);
  radioButton2.setBackground(Color.ORANGE);
  // Create a ButtonGroup to group the radio buttons together
  ButtonGroup group = new ButtonGroup();
  group.add(radioButton1);
  group.add(radioButton2);
  // Add the radio buttons to the JFrame
  frame.add(radioButton1);
  frame.add(radioButton2);
  // Set the default close operation, size of the JFrame, and make it visible
  frame.setDefaultCloseOperation(JFrame.EXIT_ON_CLOSE);
  frame.setSize(300, 100);
  frame.setVisible(true);
  }
}
```

Output

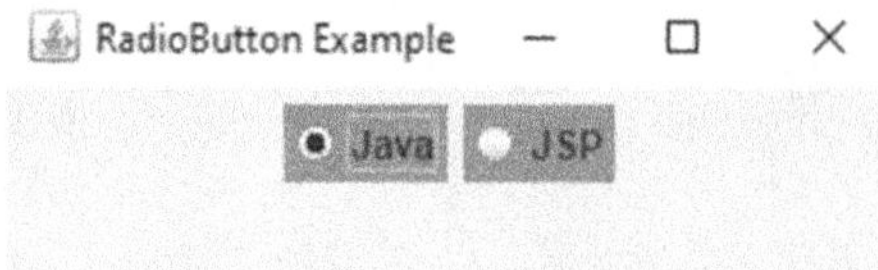

In the above program we created a JFrame titled "RadioButton Example" and initialized two radio buttons labeled "Java" and "JSP," both with an orange background. These radio buttons are grouped together using a ButtonGroup to ensure mutual exclusivity. The frame's layout is set to FlowLayout, and the radio buttons are added to the frame. The frame is sized to 300x100 pixels, configured to close the application upon exit, and made visible.

13.6.8 JList

JList is a component that displays a list of items and allows the user to select one or more items. The main features are:

1. List Display: `JList` allows the display of a scrollable list of items, where users can select one or multiple options from the list.
2. Single or Multiple Selections: Supports both single-selection and multiple-selection modes, allowing flexibility in user interaction.
3. Customizable Rendering: The appearance of list items can be customized using a custom `ListCellRenderer`, allowing you to modify how each item is displayed.

Program

```
import javax.swing.JFrame;
import javax.swing.JList;
import javax.swing.JScrollPane;
import java.awt.Color;
public class ListExample {
  void main(String[] args) {
  // Create a new JFrame with the title "List Example"
  JFrame frame = new JFrame("List Example");
  // Create an array of course names for the JList
  String[] courses = {"Java", "C++", "Python", "JavaScript", "Ruby"};
  // Initialize the JList with the array of course names
  JList<String> list = new JList<>(courses);
  // Set the background color of the JList to cyan
  list.setBackground(Color.CYAN);
  // Wrap the JList in a JScrollPane to allow for scrolling if needed
  JScrollPane scrollPane = new JScrollPane(list);
  // Add the JScrollPane to the JFrame
  frame.add(scrollPane);
  // Set the default close operation, size of the JFrame, and make it visible
  frame.setDefaultCloseOperation(JFrame.EXIT_ON_CLOSE);
  frame.setSize(300, 200);
  frame.setVisible(true);
  }
}
```

Output

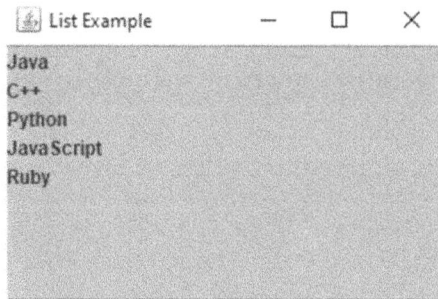

In the above program we created a JFrame titled "List Example" and initialized a JList with an array of course names. The list's background color is set to cyan. The list is displayed within a JScrollPane to enable scrolling if needed. The frame is sized to 300x200 pixels, configured to close the application upon exit, and made visible.

13.6.9 JTable

JTable is a component that displays data in a two-dimensional table format. The main features are:

1. Tabular Data Display: `JTable` allows the presentation of data in a tabular format with rows and columns, supporting both editable and non-editable cells.
2. Customizable Structure: The table's structure, including columns and cell content, can be customized using `TableModel` and `TableCellRenderer`, allowing flexible data representation.
3. Built-in Features: Provides built-in support for features such as sorting, filtering, and cell editing, enhancing data interaction and management.

Program

```
import javax.swing.JFrame;
import javax.swing.JTable;
import javax.swing.JScrollPane;
import javax.swing.table.DefaultTableModel;
import java.awt.Color;
public class TableExample {
  void main(String[] args) {
  // Create a new JFrame with the title "Table Example"
  JFrame frame = new JFrame("Table Example");
  // Define column names for the JTable
  String[] columnNames = {"Course Name", "Duration(months)", "Instructor"};
  // Define data for the JTable
  Object[][] data = {
    {"Java", "3", "A"},
    {"C++", "2", "B"},
    {"Python", "4", "C"},
    {"JavaScript", "3 ", "D"},
    {"Ruby", "1 ", "E"}
  };
  // Create a DefaultTableModel with the data and column names
  DefaultTableModel model = new DefaultTableModel(data, columnNames);
  // Initialize the JTable with the model
```

```
  JTable table = new JTable(model);
  // Set the background color of the JTable to light gray
  table.setBackground(Color.LIGHT_GRAY);
  // Wrap the JTable in a JScrollPane to allow for scrolling if needed
  JScrollPane scrollPane = new JScrollPane(table);
  // Add the JScrollPane to the JFrame
  frame.add(scrollPane);
  // Set the default close operation, size of the JFrame, and make it visible
  frame.setDefaultCloseOperation(JFrame.EXIT_ON_CLOSE);
  frame.setSize(400, 200);
  frame.setVisible(true);
  }
}
```

Output

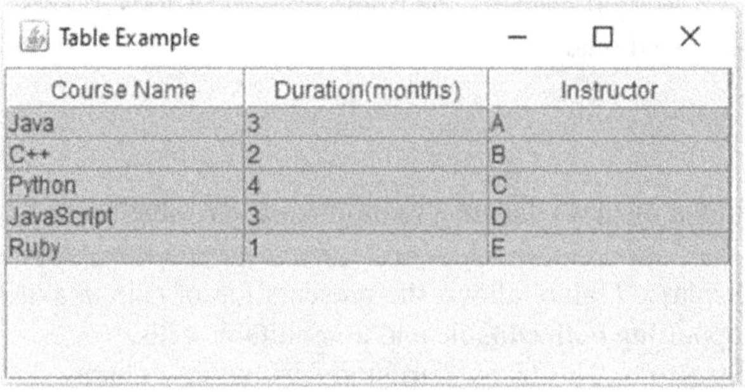

Table Example

Course Name	Duration(months)	Instructor
Java	3	A
C++	2	B
Python	4	C
JavaScript	3	D
Ruby	1	E

In the above program we created a JFrame titled "Table Example" and initialized a JTable with data and column names. The table's background color is set to light gray. The table is displayed within a JScrollPane to enable scrolling if needed. The frame is sized to 400x200 pixels, configured to close the application upon exit, and made visible.

13.6.10 JSlider

JSlider is a component that lets the user graphically select a value by sliding a knob within a bounded interval. The main features are:

1. Value Selection: `JSlider` allows users to select a value from a range by sliding a knob along a track, providing a visual way to choose numeric values.
2. Customizable Range and Tick Marks: You can set the minimum, maximum, and increment values, as well as customize tick marks and labels for precise value selection.
3. Event Handling: Supports event handling through `ChangeListener` to respond to changes in the slider's value, enabling real-time updates or actions based on user input.

Program

```
import javax.swing.JFrame;
import javax.swing.JSlider;
import javax.swing.JPanel;
import java.awt.Color;
public class SliderExample {
  void main(String[] args) {
  // Create a new JFrame with the title "Slider Example"
```

```
  JFrame frame = new JFrame("Slider Example");

  // Create a JSlider with a range from 0 to 100 and an initial value of 50
  JSlider slider = new JSlider(0, 100, 50);

  // Set the background color of the JSlider to pink
  slider.setBackground(Color.PINK);

  // Create a JPanel to hold the JSlider
  JPanel panel = new JPanel();
  panel.add(slider);

  // Add the JPanel to the JFrame
  frame.add(panel);

  // Set the default close operation, size of the JFrame, and make it visible
  frame.setDefaultCloseOperation(JFrame.EXIT_ON_CLOSE);
  frame.setSize(400, 100);
  frame.setVisible(true);
  }
}
```

Output

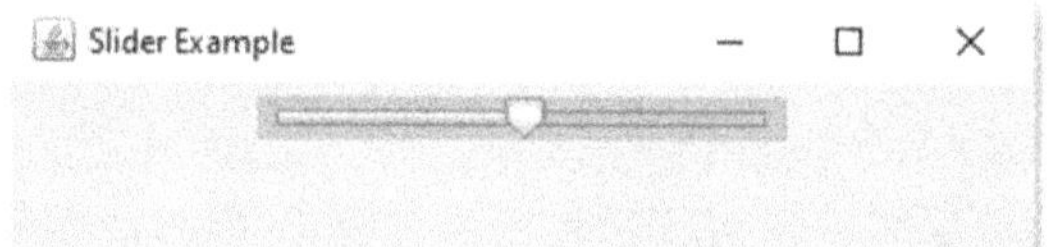

In the above program we created a JFrame titled "Slider Example" and initialized a JSlider with a range from 0 to 100, setting its initial value to 50. The slider's background color is set to pink. The slider is added to the frame, which is sized to 400x100 pixels, configured to close the application upon exit, and made visible.

13.6.11 JProgressBar

JProgressBar is a component that visually displays the progress of some task. The main features are:

1. Progress Indication: `JProgressBar` visually represents the progress of a task or operation, showing how much of a process is complete as a percentage.
2. Customizable Range: Allows you to set the minimum and maximum values, as well as the current progress, enabling dynamic updates to reflect the progress of ongoing tasks.
3. Various Styles: Supports different styles such as determinate (for known progress) and indeterminate (for unknown progress), providing flexibility in how progress is displayed.

Program

```
import javax.swing.JFrame;
import javax.swing.JProgressBar;
import javax.swing.JPanel;
import java.awt.Color;
```

```
public class ProgressBarExample {
  void main(String[] args) {
  // Create a new JFrame with the title "ProgressBar Example"
  JFrame frame = new JFrame("ProgressBar Example");

  // Create a JProgressBar with a range from 0 to 100 and an initial value of 75
  JProgressBar progressBar = new JProgressBar(0, 100);
  progressBar.setValue(75);
  progressBar.setStringPainted(true); // Display the progress bar's value
                                         as a string
  progressBar.setBackground(Color.GREEN); // Set the background color of
                                             the progress bar

  // Create a JPanel to hold the JProgressBar
  JPanel panel = new JPanel();
  panel.add(progressBar);

  // Add the JPanel to the JFrame
  frame.add(panel);

  // Set the default close operation, size of the JFrame, and make it visible
  frame.setDefaultCloseOperation(JFrame.EXIT_ON_CLOSE);
  frame.setSize(300, 100);
  frame.setVisible(true);
  }
}
```

Output

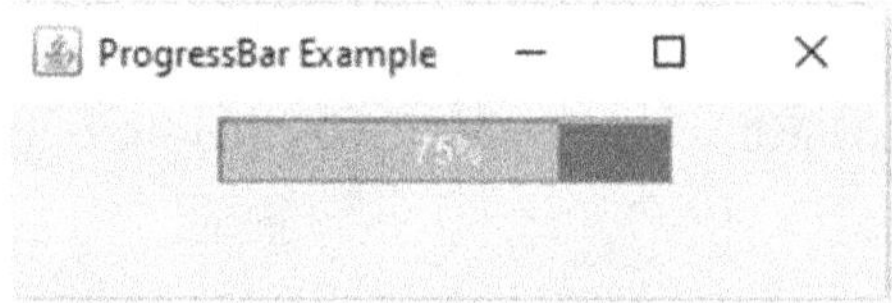

In the above program we created a JFrame titled "ProgressBar Example" and initialized a JProgressBar with a range from 0 to 100, setting its value to 75. The progress bar is configured to display a string representing its value and has a green background color. The progress bar is added to the frame, which is sized to 300x100 pixels, set to close the application upon exit, and made visible.

13.6.12 JTree

JTree is a component that presents a hierarchical view of data. The main features are:

1. Hierarchical Data Display: `JTree` displays data in a tree-like structure with nodes that can have child nodes, allowing the representation of hierarchical relationships.
2. Expandable Nodes: Supports expandable and collapsible nodes, enabling users to navigate through different levels of the hierarchy dynamically.
3. Customizable Rendering: The appearance and behavior of tree nodes can be customized using `TreeCellRenderer` and `TreeModel`, allowing tailored visual representation and interaction.

Program

```
import javax.swing.JFrame;
import javax.swing.JScrollPane;
import javax.swing.JTree;
import javax.swing.tree.DefaultMutableTreeNode;
import javax.swing.tree.DefaultTreeModel;
import java.awt.Color;
public class TreeExample {
  void main(String[] args) {
  // Create the root node
  DefaultMutableTreeNode rootNode = new DefaultMutableTreeNode("Courses");

  // Create child nodes
  DefaultMutableTreeNode javaNode = new DefaultMutableTreeNode("Java");
  DefaultMutableTreeNode pythonNode = new DefaultMutableTreeNode("Python");

  // Add child nodes to the root node
  rootNode.add(javaNode);
  rootNode.add(pythonNode);

  // Create a JTree with the root node
  JTree tree = new JTree(rootNode);
  tree.setBackground(Color.ORANGE); // Set the background color of the tree

  // Create a JScrollPane to enable scrolling if needed
  JScrollPane scrollPane = new JScrollPane(tree);

  // Create a JFrame
  JFrame frame = new JFrame("Tree Example");
  frame.setDefaultCloseOperation(JFrame.EXIT_ON_CLOSE);
  frame.setSize(300, 200);

  // Add the JScrollPane (containing the JTree) to the JFrame
  frame.add(scrollPane);

  // Make the frame visible
  frame.setVisible(true);
  }
}
```

Output

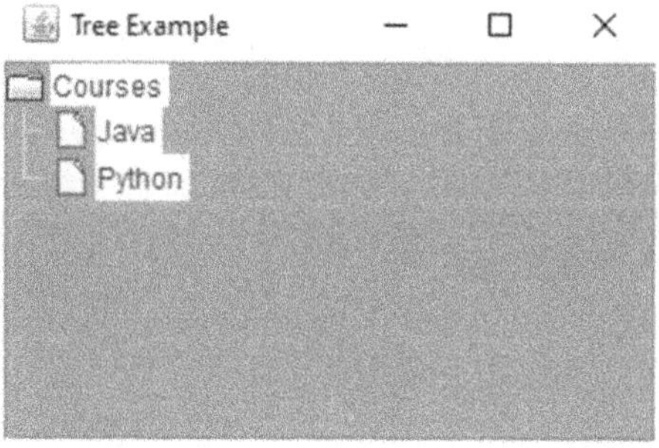

Tree Example

Courses
Java
Python

In the above program we created a JFrame titled "Tree Example" and initialized a root node labeled "Courses". Two child nodes, "Java" and "Python", are added to the root node. A JTree is instantiated with the root node and displayed within a JScrollPane. The background color of the tree is set to orange. The frame is sized to 300x200 pixels, configured to close the application upon exit, and made visible.

13.6.13 JMenuBar

JMenuBar is a menu bar to which menus are added. The main features are:

1. Menu Container: `JMenuBar` serves as a container for `JMenu` components, which represent the main menu items of an application's menu bar, typically placed at the top of a window.
2. Menu Organization: Allows the organization of menus into a hierarchical structure, where each `JMenu` can contain multiple `JMenuItem` components and submenus.
3. Customizable: Supports customization of menu items, including adding icons, accelerators (keyboard shortcuts), and event listeners to handle user interactions with menu items.

Program

```
import javax.swing.JFrame;
import javax.swing.JMenu;
import javax.swing.JMenuBar;
import javax.swing.JMenuItem;
import java.awt.Color;
public class MenuBarExample {
  void main(String[] args) {
  // Create a JFrame
  JFrame frame = new JFrame("MenuBar Example");
  frame.setDefaultCloseOperation(JFrame.EXIT_ON_CLOSE);
  frame.setSize(300, 200);
  // Create a JMenuBar
  JMenuBar menuBar = new JMenuBar();
  menuBar.setBackground(Color.YELLOW); // Set background color to yellow

  // Create a JMenu
  JMenu menu = new JMenu("Courses");

  // Create JMenuItems
  JMenuItem javaItem = new JMenuItem("Java");
  JMenuItem pythonItem = new JMenuItem("Python");

  // Add JMenuItems to JMenu
  menu.add(javaItem);
  menu.add(pythonItem);

  // Add JMenu to JMenuBar
  menuBar.add(menu);

  // Set the JMenuBar for the JFrame
  frame.setJMenuBar(menuBar);

  // Make the frame visible
```

```
  frame.setVisible(true);
  }
}
```

Output

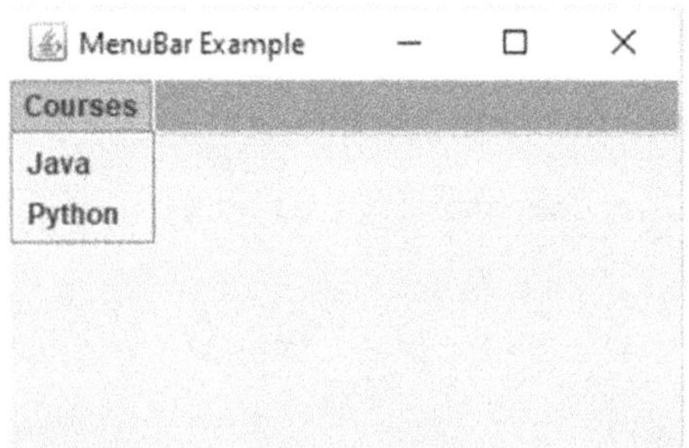

In the above program we created a JFrame titled "MenuBar Example" and added a JMenuBar to it. Within the menu bar, a JMenu labeled "Courses" is added, containing two JMenuItems: "Java" and "Python". The menu bar's background color is set to yellow. The frame's menu bar is set using the `setJMenuBar` method. The frame is then sized to 300x200 pixels, set to close the application upon exit, and made visible.

13.6.14 JPopupMenu

JPopupMenu is a pop-up menu that is activated when the user right-clicks on a component. The main features are:

1. Contextual Menus: `JPopupMenu` displays a context-sensitive menu that appears upon user interaction, such as a right-click or a specific event, providing additional options relevant to the current context.
2. Dynamic Content: Can dynamically populate and display menu items (`JMenuItem`, `JCheckBoxMenuItem`, `JRadioButtonMenuItem`) based on the context or user actions, allowing flexible and interactive menu options.
3. Customizable Behavior: Supports customization of appearance and behavior, including adding event listeners to handle menu item selections and managing menu visibility and positioning.

Program

```
import javax.swing.JFrame;
import javax.swing.JMenuItem;
import javax.swing.JPopupMenu;
import java.awt.event.MouseAdapter;
import java.awt.event.MouseEvent;
public class PopupMenuExample {
  void main(String[] args) {
  // Create a JFrame
  JFrame frame = new JFrame("PopupMenu Example");
  frame.setDefaultCloseOperation(JFrame.EXIT_ON_CLOSE);
  frame.setSize(300, 200);
  // Create a JPopupMenu
  JPopupMenu popupMenu = new JPopupMenu();
  // Create JMenuItems
  JMenuItem javaItem = new JMenuItem("Java");
```

```
  JMenuItem pythonItem = new JMenuItem("Python");
  // Add JMenuItems to JPopupMenu
  popupMenu.add(javaItem);
  popupMenu.add(pythonItem);
  // Add MouseListener to JFrame to show popup menu on right-click
  frame.addMouseListener(new MouseAdapter() {
    @Override
    public void mouseReleased(MouseEvent e) {
    if (e.isPopupTrigger()) {
      popupMenu.show(e.getComponent(), e.getX(), e.getY());
    }
    }
  });
  // Make the frame visible
  frame.setVisible(true);
  }
}
```

Output

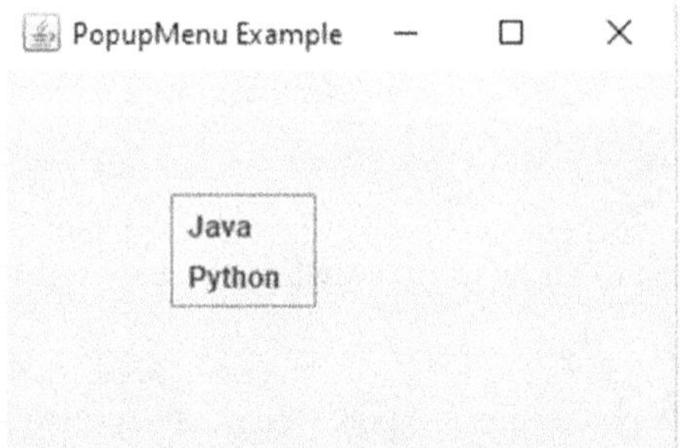

In the above program we created a JFrame titled "PopupMenu Example" and a JPopupMenu with two JMenuItems: "Java" and "Python". Includes a MouseAdapter to detect mouse events; when the right mouse button is released, it triggers the pop-up menu to appear at the mouse location. The main frame is set to a size of 300x200 pixels, configured to close the application upon exit, and made visible.

13.6.15 JScrollPane

JScrollPane provides a scrollable view of a component. The main features are:

1. Scrollable View: `JScrollPane` provides a scrollable view of its contained component, allowing users to navigate through content that exceeds the visible area by using scroll bars.
2. Automatic Scroll Bars: Automatically displays horizontal and/or vertical scroll bars as needed based on the size of the contained component and the viewport dimensions.
3. Flexible Content: Can be used to wrap various components such as `JTextArea`, `JTable`, or custom components, enabling scroll functionality for any content that requires it.

Program

```
import javax.swing.JFrame;
import javax.swing.JScrollPane;
import javax.swing.JTextArea;
import javax.swing.ScrollPaneConstants;
import java.awt.Dimension;
public class ScrollPaneExample {
```

```
  void main(String[] args) {
  // Create the main JFrame
  JFrame frame = new JFrame("ScrollPane Example");
  frame.setSize(300, 200);
  frame.setDefaultCloseOperation(JFrame.EXIT_ON_CLOSE);
  // Create a JTextArea
  JTextArea textArea = new JTextArea(10, 20);
  textArea.setText("This is a JTextArea inside a JScrollPane.\nYou can type
     or add more text to see the scrollbar in action.");

  // Create a JScrollPane and add the JTextArea to it
  JScrollPane scrollPane = new JScrollPane(textArea);

  // Set the vertical scrollbar policy to always show
  scrollPane.setVerticalScrollBarPolicy(ScrollPaneConstants.VERTICAL_
     SCROLLBAR_ALWAYS);

  // Add the JScrollPane to the frame
  frame.add(scrollPane);
  // Make the frame visible
  frame.setVisible(true);
  }
}
```

Output

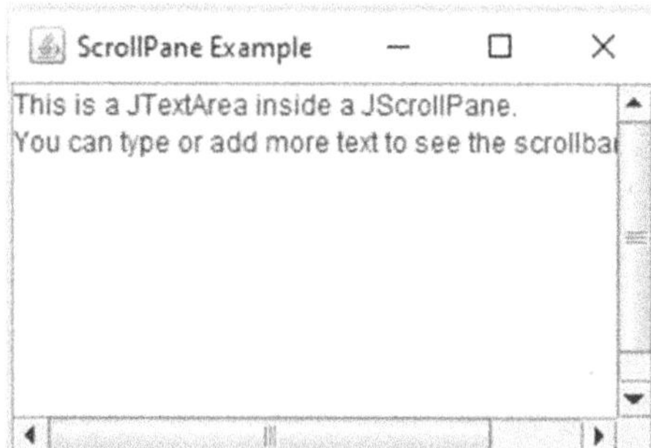

In the above program, inside the frame, a JTextArea with 10 rows and 20 columns is added to a JScrollPane. The vertical scrollbar is always visible due to the `setVerticalScrollBarPolicy` method. The JScrollPane is then added to the frame. The frame is set to a size of 300x200 pixels, configured to close the application upon exit, and made visible.

13.6.16 JSeparator

JSeparator is a horizontal or vertical line used to separate groups of components in a container. The main features are:

1. Visual Divider: `JSeparator` is used to visually divide or group components within a container, providing a clear separation between different sections or items in a user interface.
2. Orientation Options: Can be oriented either horizontally or vertically, allowing it to fit into different layouts and design needs depending on the visual separation required.
3. Customizable Appearance: Supports customization of its appearance, including color and thickness, to match the design and style of the surrounding components and overall UI.

Program

```
import javax.swing.JFrame;
import javax.swing.JPanel;
import javax.swing.JButton;
import javax.swing.JSeparator;
import javax.swing.BoxLayout;
import java.awt.Dimension;
public class SeparatorExample {
  void main(String[] args) {
  // Create the main JFrame
  JFrame frame = new JFrame("Separator Example");
  frame.setSize(300, 200);
  frame.setDefaultCloseOperation(JFrame.EXIT_ON_CLOSE);

  // Create a JPanel with a vertical BoxLayout
  JPanel panel = new JPanel();
  panel.setLayout(new BoxLayout(panel, BoxLayout.Y_AXIS));

  // Create two buttons
  JButton button1 = new JButton("Button 1");
  JButton button2 = new JButton("Button 2");

  // Create a JSeparator
  JSeparator separator = new JSeparator(JSeparator.VERTICAL);

  // Add the buttons and separator to the panel
  panel.add(button1);
  panel.add(separator);
  panel.add(button2);

  // Add the panel to the frame
  frame.add(panel);

  // Make the frame visible
  frame.setVisible(true);
  }
}
```

Output

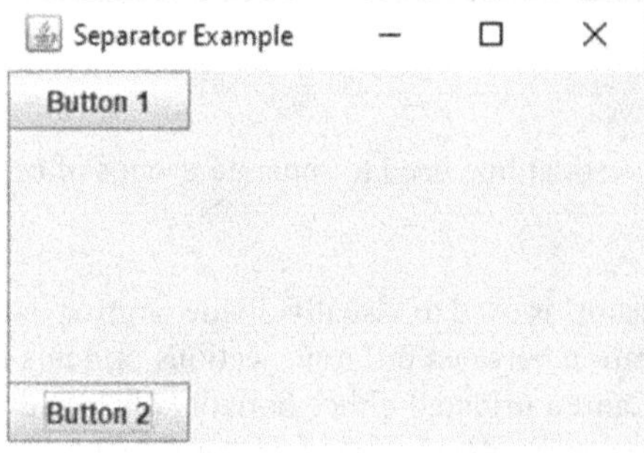

In the above program, inside the frame, a JPanel with a vertical BoxLayout is added. The panel contains two buttons ("Button 1" and "Button 2") with a JSeparator between them. This separator visually separates the two buttons. The panel is then added to the frame. The frame is set to a size of 300x200 pixels, configured to close the application upon exit, and made visible.

13.6.17 JToolBar

JToolBar is a component that contains buttons and other controls that perform common tasks. The main features are:

1. Quick Access: `JToolBar` provides a set of commonly used tools or actions in a compact, easily accessible area, typically positioned at the top or side of an application window.
2. Customizable Components: Can contain various components such as `JButton`, `JLabel`, and `JComboBox`, allowing for flexible arrangement of tools and actions with custom icons, text, and separators.
3. Docking and Floating: Supports docking and floating functionality, enabling users to move the toolbar to different locations within the window or detach it as a separate floating window for improved accessibility and usability.

Program

```
import javax.swing.JFrame;
import javax.swing.JToolBar;
import javax.swing.JButton;
import javax.swing.BorderFactory;
import java.awt.BorderLayout;
public class ToolBarExample {
  void main(String[] args) {
  // Create the main JFrame
  JFrame frame = new JFrame("ToolBar Example");
  frame.setSize(300, 100);
  frame.setDefaultCloseOperation(JFrame.EXIT_ON_CLOSE);
  frame.setLayout(new BorderLayout());

  // Create a JToolBar
  JToolBar toolBar = new JToolBar();

  // Create two buttons
  JButton button1 = new JButton("Java");
  JButton button2 = new JButton("Python");

  // Add buttons to the toolBar
  toolBar.add(button1);
  toolBar.addSeparator();  // Add a separator between buttons
  toolBar.add(button2);

  // Add the toolBar to the frame at the top (north)
  frame.add(toolBar, BorderLayout.NORTH);

  // Make the frame visible
  frame.setVisible(true);
  }
}
```

Output

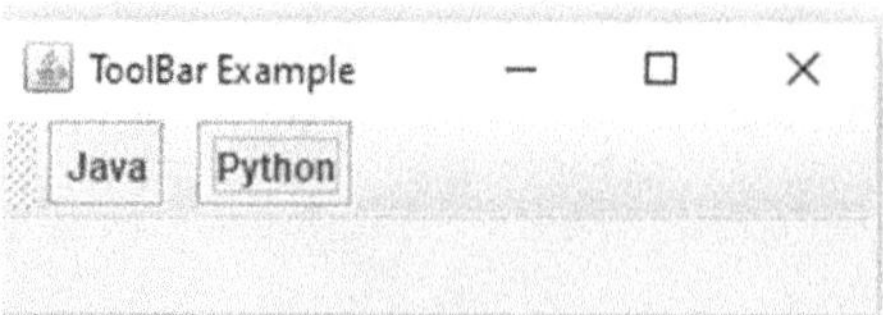

In the above program, a JToolBar is added to the frame, containing two buttons labeled "Java" and "Python", with a separator between them. The toolbar is positioned at the top (north) of the frame. The frame is set to a size of 300x100 pixels, configured to close the application upon exit, and made visible.

13.6.18 JEditorPane

JEditorPane is a text component that allows the editing of styled text. The main features are:

1. Versatile Text Editing: `JEditorPane` provides a component for displaying and editing rich text content, including HTML, plain text, and styled documents, supporting various content types and formatting.
2. Content Loading: Capable of loading content from a URL or file, making it suitable for displaying web pages or external resources directly within a Swing application.
3. Customizable and Extendable: Allows customization through `HTMLEditorKit` and `StyledEditorKit`, and supports extending its functionality with custom document models and content renderers for specialized needs.

Program

```
import javax.swing.JFrame;
import javax.swing.JEditorPane;
import javax.swing.JScrollPane;
import java.io.IOException;
public class EditorPaneExample {
  void main(String[] args) {
  // Create the main JFrame
  JFrame frame = new JFrame("EditorPane Example");
  frame.setSize(400, 300);
  frame.setDefaultCloseOperation(JFrame.EXIT_ON_CLOSE);
  // Create a JEditorPane to display HTML content
  JEditorPane editorPane = new JEditorPane();
  editorPane.setContentType("text/html");

  // Set the HTML content
  String htmlContent = "<html><body>"
    + "<h1>Course Syllabus</h1>"
    + "<p>Welcome to the programming courses!</p>"
    + "<h2>Java Programming</h2>"
    + "<ul>"
    + "<li>Introduction to Java</li>"
    + "<li>Object-Oriented Programming</li>"
    + "<li>Java GUI Programming</li>"
    + "</ul>"
    + "<h2>Python Programming</h2>"
```

```
        + "<ul>"
        + "<li>Introduction to Python</li>"
        + "<li>Data Structures and Algorithms</li>"
        + "<li>Web Development with Python</li>"
        + "</ul>"
        + "</body></html>";
      editorPane.setText(htmlContent);
      // Wrap the JEditorPane in a JScrollPane
      JScrollPane scrollPane = new JScrollPane(editorPane);

      // Add the JScrollPane to the frame
      frame.add(scrollPane);

      // Make the frame visible
      frame.setVisible(true);
      }
}
```

Output

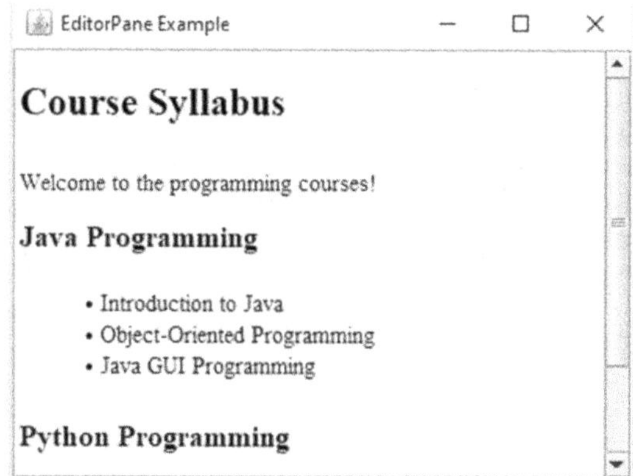

In the above program, inside the frame, a JEditorPane is initialized to display HTML content, specifically a sample course syllabus with Java and Python programming courses. This JEditorPane is wrapped in a JScrollPane to add scroll functionality. The JScrollPane is added to the frame. The frame is set to a size of 400x300 pixels, configured to close the application upon exit, and made visible.

13.6.19 JTabbedPane

JTabbedPane` is a Swing component in Java used to create tabbed panels, allowing multiple components to be organized in a tabular format within a single container. The main features are:

1. Tabbed Interface: `JTabbedPane` allows for organizing and displaying multiple components in a tabbed layout, where each tab represents a different panel or view, making it easy to switch between different sections or functionalities.
2. Dynamic Tab Management: Supports adding, removing, and reordering tabs dynamically, enabling flexible user interface design and interaction based on user needs or application state.
3. Customizable Appearance: Provides options for customizing tab placement (top, bottom, left, right), tab content, and tab titles, including icons and text, to fit the overall design and usability requirements of the application.

Program

```
import javax.swing.JFrame;
import javax.swing.JPanel;
import javax.swing.JTabbedPane;
import java.awt.BorderLayout;
import java.awt.Color;
public class TabbedPaneExample {
  void main(String[] args) {
  // Create the main JFrame
  JFrame frame = new JFrame("JTabbedPane Example");
  frame.setSize(300, 200);
  frame.setDefaultCloseOperation(JFrame.EXIT_ON_CLOSE);
  frame.setLayout(new BorderLayout());
  // Create JTabbedPane
  JTabbedPane tabbedPane = new JTabbedPane();
  // Create panels
  JPanel panel1 = new JPanel();
  panel1.setBackground(Color.LIGHT_GRAY);
  tabbedPane.addTab("Register", panel1);
  JPanel panel2 = new JPanel();
  panel2.setBackground(Color.LIGHT_GRAY);
  tabbedPane.addTab("Courses", panel2);
  // Add the JTabbedPane to the frame
  frame.add(tabbedPane, BorderLayout.CENTER);
  // Make the frame visible
  frame.setVisible(true);
  }
}
```

Output

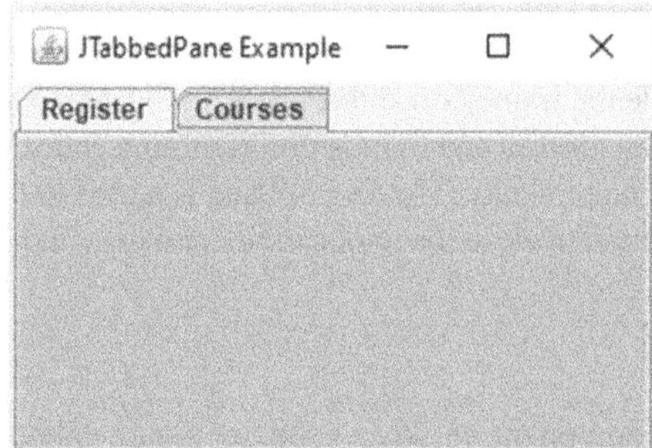

A JFrame titled "JTabbedPane Example" is set up with a BorderLayout. A JTabbedPane is created and two JPanel instances, `panel1` and `panel2`, are added to it, each with a light gray background. The panels are labeled "Register" and "Courses". The JTabbedPane is added to the center of the frame. The frame is configured to be 300x200 pixels in size, set to close the application when exited, and made visible.

13.6.20 JComboBox

JComboBox is a component that combines a button or editable field and a drop-down list. The main features are:

1. Drop-Down List: `JComboBox` provides a drop-down list of options from which users can select a single item, combining the functionality of a text field and a list.

2. Editable Option: Can be configured as editable, allowing users to type their own values in addition to selecting from the predefined list, or non-editable, restricting users to the given options.
3. Customizable Items: Supports customization of the list items with text and icons, and allows for dynamic updates to the item list, making it flexible for various user interface requirements.

Program

```
import javax.swing.JFrame;
import javax.swing.JComboBox;
import java.awt.Color;
public class ComboBoxExample {
  void main(String[] args) {
  // Create a new JFrame with the title "ComboBox Example"
  JFrame frame = new JFrame("ComboBox Example");
  // Create an array of course names for the JComboBox
  String[] courses = {"Java", "C++", "Python", "JavaScript", "Ruby"};
  // Initialize the JComboBox with the array of course names
  JComboBox<String> comboBox = new JComboBox<>(courses);
  // Set the background color of the JComboBox to magenta
  comboBox.setBackground(Color.MAGENTA);
  // Add the JComboBox to the JFrame
  frame.add(comboBox);
  // Set the default close operation, size of the JFrame, and make it visible
  frame.setDefaultCloseOperation(JFrame.EXIT_ON_CLOSE);
  frame.setSize(300, 100);
  frame.setVisible(true);
  }
}
```

Output

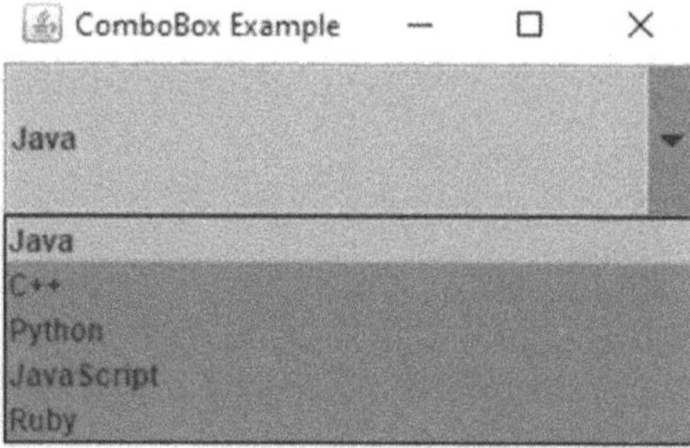

In the above program, we created a JFrame titled "ComboBox Example" and initialized a JComboBox with an array of course names. The combo box's background color is set to magenta. The combo box is added to the frame. The frame is sized to 300x100 pixels, configured to close the application upon exit, and made visible.

13.7 EVENTHANDLING FOR JAVA SWINGS

Event handling is essential for creating dynamic and interactive user interfaces in Java Swings. By implementing event listeners, developers can create applications that respond to user input, making them more user-friendly and engaging. Event handling is crucial in Java Swings as it allows for the creation of interactive and responsive user interfaces. By handling events, Swing components can detect user actions, such as button clicks or key presses, and react accordingly. This is achieved through the use of event listeners, which are interfaces that define methods to be executed when a specific event occurs. Some of the event handlers are discussed below.

13.7.1 Action Listener

In Java GUI development, an ActionListener is a key concept for handling user interactions with specific components. It's like a listener waiting for an action to happen. Imagine a button—the ActionListener acts as a responder waiting for the user to click it.

When you implement the ActionListener interface in your class, the user should define a method called actionPerformed. This method is what gets called whenever the user performs an action on the registered component, like clicking a button or selecting a menu item.

To use an ActionListener, you typically follow these steps:

1. Create a class that implements the ActionListener interface.
2. Register this class as a listener with the GUI component (e.g., using button.addActionListener (yourListenerObject)).
3. Override the actionPerformed method in your class to define the specific actions you want to happen when the user interacts with the component.

13.7.1.1 JButton with ActionListener

A `JButton` needs an `ActionListener` to know what to do when it's clicked. The `ActionListener` listens for the click and runs the code you've set for the button's action, making it respond to user interaction.

Program

```
import javax.swing.JButton;
import javax.swing.JFrame;
import javax.swing.JOptionPane;
import javax.swing.JPanel;
import java.awt.event.ActionEvent;
import java.awt.event.ActionListener;
public class RegisterButtonExample {
  void main(String[] args) {
  // Create the main JFrame
  JFrame frame = new JFrame("Register Button Example");
  frame.setSize(300, 100);
  frame.setDefaultCloseOperation(JFrame.EXIT_ON_CLOSE);
  // Create a JPanel to hold the button
  JPanel panel = new JPanel();
  // Create the JButton with label "Register"
  JButton registerButton = new JButton("Register");
  // Add ActionListener to handle button click
  registerButton.addActionListener(new ActionListener() {
    @Override
    public void actionPerformed(ActionEvent e) {
    // Display a pop-up message when the button is clicked
    JOptionPane.showMessageDialog(frame, "Congratulations on successfully
       registering for a computer course!");
    }
  });
```

```
    // Add the button to the panel
    panel.add(registerButton);
    // Add the panel to the frame
    frame.add(panel);
    // Make the frame visible
    frame.setVisible(true);
    }
}
```

Output

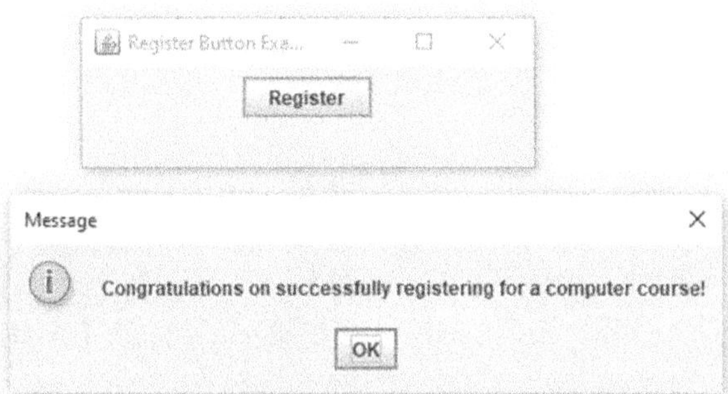

In the above program we displayed a window with a single button labeled "Register". When the button is clicked, a pop-up message appears congratulating the user on successfully registering for a computer course. The program uses a JFrame to create the window, a JButton to create the button, and an ActionListener to handle the button click event. The window is set to a fixed size and will close when the user clicks the close button.

13.7.1.2 JRadioButton with ActionListener

A `JRadioButton` requires an `ActionListener` to respond to user selections. This listener helps the program react whenever a radio button is chosen, updating the application's state accordingly and ensuring the right action is taken based on the selected option.

Program

```
import javax.swing.JButton;
import javax.swing.JFrame;
import javax.swing.JOptionPane;
import javax.swing.JPanel;
import javax.swing.JRadioButton;
import javax.swing.ButtonGroup;
import java.awt.event.ActionEvent;
import java.awt.event.ActionListener;
public class RadioButtonExample {
  void main(String[] args) {
  // Create the main JFrame
  JFrame frame = new JFrame("RadioButton Example");
  frame.setSize(300, 150);
  frame.setDefaultCloseOperation(JFrame.EXIT_ON_CLOSE);
  // Create a JPanel to hold the radio buttons
  JPanel panel = new JPanel();
  // Create two JRadioButtons
  JRadioButton pythonButton = new JRadioButton("Python");
  JRadioButton javaButton = new JRadioButton("Java");
```

```
    // Group the radio buttons
    ButtonGroup group = new ButtonGroup();
    group.add(pythonButton);
    group.add(javaButton);
    // Add ActionListener to handle button clicks
    ActionListener radioButtonListener = new ActionListener() {
      @Override
      public void actionPerformed(ActionEvent e) {
      // Display a pop-up message showing the selected course
      JRadioButton selectedButton = (JRadioButton) e.getSource();
      JOptionPane.showMessageDialog(frame, "Selected course: " +
         selectedButton.getText());
      }
    };
    // Attach the ActionListener to both radio buttons
    pythonButton.addActionListener(radioButtonListener);
    javaButton.addActionListener(radioButtonListener);
    // Add the radio buttons to the panel
    panel.add(pythonButton);
    panel.add(javaButton);
    // Add the panel to the frame
    frame.add(panel);
    // Make the frame visible
    frame.setVisible(true);
    }
}
```

Output

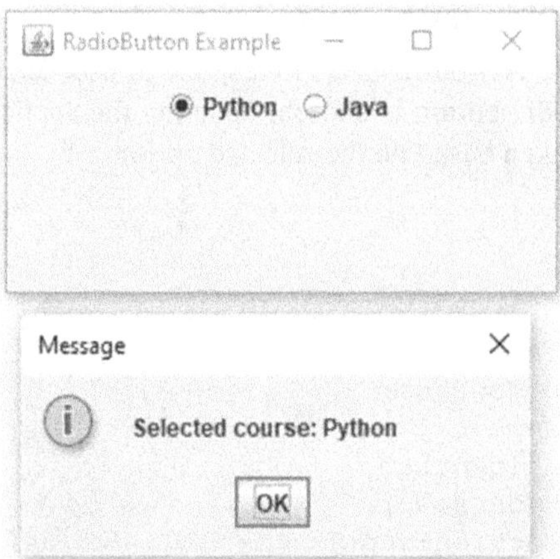

The radio buttons are grouped together, allowing only one to be selected at a time. When a radio button is clicked, a pop-up message appears displaying the selected course. In this program we use a JFrame to create the window, JRadioButtons to create the radio buttons, and an ActionListener to handle the button click event. The window is set to a fixed size and will close when the user clicks the close button.

13.7.1.3 JToggleButton with ActionListener

A `JToggleButton` needs an `ActionListener` to respond to changes in its toggle state, whether it's selected or deselected. This listener enables the application to take specific actions based on whether the button is in the on or off position.

Program

```
import javax.swing.JButton;
import javax.swing.JFrame;
import javax.swing.JOptionPane;
import javax.swing.JPanel;
import javax.swing.JToggleButton;
import java.awt.event.ActionEvent;
import java.awt.event.ActionListener;
public class ToggleButtonExample {
  void main(String[] args) {
  // Create the main JFrame
  JFrame frame = new JFrame("ToggleButton Example");
  frame.setSize(300, 150);
  frame.setDefaultCloseOperation(JFrame.EXIT_ON_CLOSE);
  // Create a JPanel to hold the toggle button
  JPanel panel = new JPanel();
  // Create a JToggleButton with the label "Enroll"
  JToggleButton toggleButton = new JToggleButton("Enroll");
  // Add ActionListener to handle button clicks
  ActionListener toggleButtonListener = new ActionListener() {
    @Override
    public void actionPerformed(ActionEvent e) {
    if (toggleButton.isSelected()) {
      // Display a pop-up message indicating enrollment
      JOptionPane.showMessageDialog(frame, "You are enrolled in the course.");
    } else {
      // Display a pop-up message indicating unenrollment
      JOptionPane.showMessageDialog(frame, "You are no longer enrolled in
         the course.");
    }
    }
  };
  // Attach the ActionListener to the toggle button
  toggleButton.addActionListener(toggleButtonListener);
  // Add the toggle button to the panel
  panel.add(toggleButton);
  // Add the panel to the frame
  frame.add(panel);
  // Make the frame visible
  frame.setVisible(true);
  }
}
```

Output

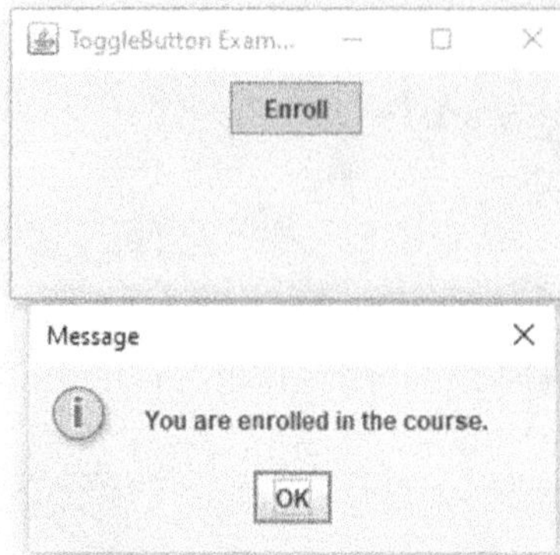

In this Java program we display a window with a toggle button labeled "Enroll". When the button is clicked, it toggles between selected and deselected states. If the button is selected, a pop-up message appears indicating that the user is enrolled in the course. If the button is deselected, a message appears indicating that the user is no longer enrolled.

13.7.1.4 JEditorPane with ActionListener

A `JEditorPane` typically uses a `DocumentListener` to respond to changes in the text content or formatting. Additionally, an `ActionListener` can handle actions like button clicks that interact with the editor, allowing the application to react to user inputs effectively.

Program

```
import javax.swing.*;
import java.awt.*;
import java.awt.event.ActionEvent;
import java.awt.event.ActionListener;
import java.awt.event.MouseAdapter;
import java.awt.event.MouseEvent;
public class EditorPaneExample {
  void main(String[] args) {
  // Create the main JFrame
  JFrame frame = new JFrame("EditorPane Example");
  frame.setSize(400, 300);
  frame.setDefaultCloseOperation(JFrame.EXIT_ON_CLOSE);
  // Create a JEditorPane to display HTML content
  JEditorPane editorPane = new JEditorPane();
  editorPane.setContentType("text/html");
  editorPane.setText("<html><body><h1>Course Syllabus</h1><p>Java and
     Python Programming Courses</p></body></html>");
  editorPane.setEditable(false); // Make the editor pane non-editable
  // Create a JPopupMenu with "Copy" and "Paste" options
  JPopupMenu popupMenu = new JPopupMenu();
  JMenuItem copyItem = new JMenuItem("Copy");
  JMenuItem pasteItem = new JMenuItem("Paste");

  // Add action listener to "Copy" menu item
  copyItem.addActionListener(new ActionListener() {
    @Override
    public void actionPerformed(ActionEvent e) {
```

```
    editorPane.copy(); // Perform copy operation
    }
  });
  // Add action listener to "Paste" menu item
  pasteItem.addActionListener(new ActionListener() {
    @Override
    public void actionPerformed(ActionEvent e) {
    editorPane.paste(); // Perform paste operation
    }
  });
  // Add menu items to popup menu
  popupMenu.add(copyItem);
  popupMenu.add(pasteItem);
  // Add mouse listener to show popup menu on right-click
  editorPane.addMouseListener(new MouseAdapter() {
    @Override
    public void mousePressed(MouseEvent e) {
    showPopup(e);
    }
    @Override
    public void mouseReleased(MouseEvent e) {
    showPopup(e);
    }
    private void showPopup(MouseEvent e) {
    if (SwingUtilities.isRightMouseButton(e)) {
      popupMenu.show(editorPane, e.getX(), e.getY());
      // Show popup menu at mouse location
    }
    }
  });
  // Add the JEditorPane to a JScrollPane for scrolling
  JScrollPane scrollPane = new JScrollPane(editorPane);
  // Add the JScrollPane to the frame
  frame.add(scrollPane, BorderLayout.CENTER);
  // Make the frame visible
  frame.setVisible(true);
  }
}
```

Output

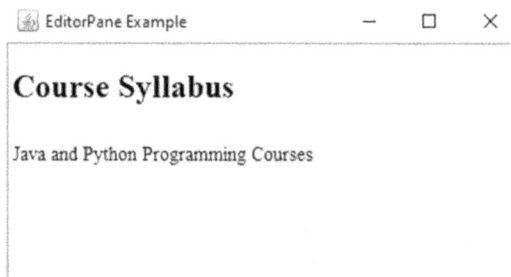

In the above Java program we created a GUI with a JFrame and a JEditorPane that displays HTML content. The JEditorPane is set to be non-editable and has a mouse listener that detects right-clicks. When a right-click is detected, a context menu (JPopupMenu) is shown with "Copy" and

"Paste" options. The "Copy" and "Paste" options are functional and can be used to copy and paste text from the JEditorPane.

13.7.1.5 JComboBox with ActionListener

A `JComboBox` requires an `ActionListener` to respond when a user selects an item from the drop-down list. This listener enables the application to take specific actions based on the chosen option, ensuring the program reacts appropriately to user selections.

Program

```
import javax.swing.*;
import java.awt.*;
import java.awt.event.ActionEvent;
import java.awt.event.ActionListener;
public class ComboBoxExample {
  void main(String[] args) {
  // Create the main JFrame
  JFrame frame = new JFrame("ComboBox Example");
  frame.setSize(300, 150);
  frame.setDefaultCloseOperation(JFrame.EXIT_ON_CLOSE);
  frame.setLayout(new FlowLayout());
  // Create a JComboBox with a list of programming courses
  String[] courses = {"Java", "Python", "C++", "JavaScript"};
  JComboBox<String> comboBox = new JComboBox<>(courses);
  comboBox.setBackground(Color.WHITE); // Set background color to white
  // Add an ActionListener to the JComboBox
  comboBox.addActionListener(new ActionListener() {
    @Override
    public void actionPerformed(ActionEvent e) {
    // Get the selected item and display it in a message dialog
    String selectedCourse = (String) comboBox.getSelectedItem();
    JOptionPane.showMessageDialog(frame, "Selected Course: " +
       selectedCourse);
    }
  });
  // Add the JComboBox to the JFrame
  frame.add(comboBox);
  // Make the frame visible
  frame.setVisible(true);
  }
}
```

Output

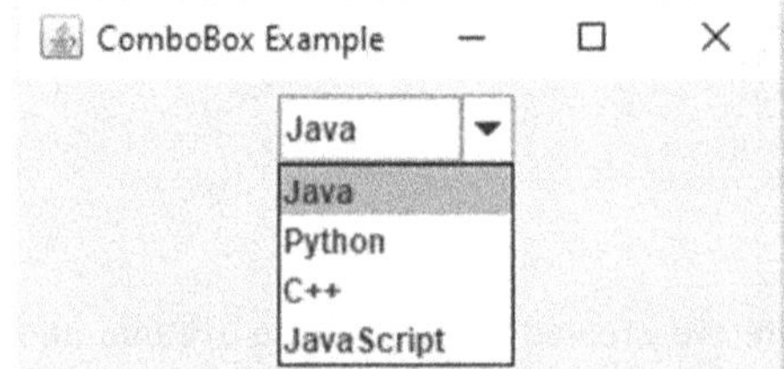

In the above Java program we created a JFrame with a FlowLayout and added a JComboBox to it, which is populated with a list of programming courses. The JComboBox is set to have a white background and an ActionListener is added to it, which will trigger when an item is selected from the drop-down list. When an item is selected, a message dialog will pop up displaying the selected course. The JFrame is then set to a fixed size and made visible, allowing the user to interact with the JComboBox.

13.7.1.6 JPopupMenu with ActionListener

A `JPopupMenu` needs an `ActionListener` to handle user interactions with its menu items. This listener triggers specific actions when a menu item is selected, ensuring the application responds appropriately to context-sensitive choices made by the user.

Program

```
import javax.swing.*;
import java.awt.*;
import java.awt.event.ActionEvent;
import java.awt.event.ActionListener;
import java.awt.event.MouseAdapter;
import java.awt.event.MouseEvent;
public class PopupMenuExample {
  void main(String[] args) {
  // Create the main JFrame
  JFrame frame = new JFrame("PopupMenu Example");
  frame.setSize(400, 300);
  frame.setDefaultCloseOperation(JFrame.EXIT_ON_CLOSE);
  frame.setLayout(new BorderLayout());
  // Create a JTextArea and wrap it in a JScrollPane
  JTextArea textArea = new JTextArea();
  textArea.setBackground(Color.WHITE); // Set background color to white
  JScrollPane scrollPane = new JScrollPane(textArea);
  // Create a JPopupMenu with a single JMenuItem
  JPopupMenu popupMenu = new JPopupMenu();
  JMenuItem registerItem = new JMenuItem("Register");
  popupMenu.add(registerItem);
  // Add an ActionListener to the JMenuItem
  registerItem.addActionListener(new ActionListener() {
    @Override
    public void actionPerformed(ActionEvent e) {
    JOptionPane.showMessageDialog(frame, "Registration Successful!");
    }
  });
  // Add a MouseAdapter to the JTextArea to show the JPopupMenu on right-click
  textArea.addMouseListener(new MouseAdapter() {
    @Override
    public void mouseReleased(MouseEvent e) {
    if (SwingUtilities.isRightMouseButton(e)) {
      popupMenu.show(textArea, e.getX(), e.getY());
    }
    }
  });
  // Add the JScrollPane to the JFrame
  frame.add(scrollPane, BorderLayout.CENTER);
  // Make the frame visible
```

```
  frame.setVisible(true);
  }
}
```

Output

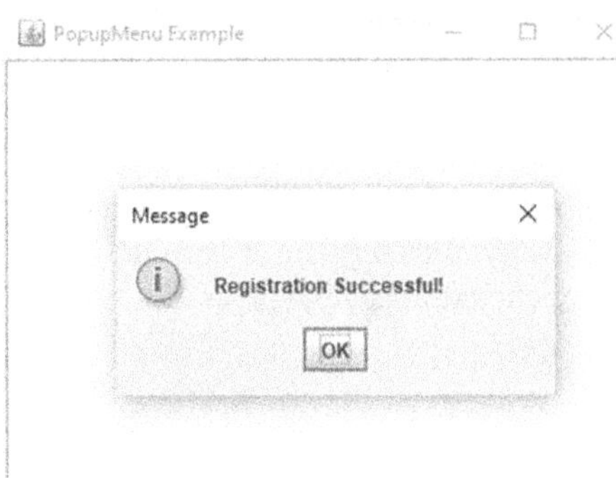

In the above Java program we created a JFrame with a BorderLayout and added a JTextArea to it, which is wrapped in a JScrollPane. The JTextArea is set to have a white background. A JPopupMenu is created and a JMenuItem "Register" is added to it. When the "Register" item is clicked, a message dialog will pop up displaying a success message. The JPopupMenu is then set as the pop-up menu for the JTextArea, which means it will appear when the user right-clicks on the JTextArea. Finally, the JFrame is set to a fixed size and made visible, allowing the user to interact with the JTextArea and the pop-up menu.

13.7.1.7 JToolBar with ActionListener

A `JToolBar` requires an `ActionListener` to manage user interactions with its buttons. This listener executes specific actions when a button is clicked, enabling functionalities like tool execution or command triggering directly from the toolbar.

Program

```
import javax.swing.*;
import java.awt.event.ActionEvent;
import java.awt.event.ActionListener;
public class ToolBarToggleButtonExample {
  void main(String[] args) {
  // Create the main JFrame
  JFrame frame = new JFrame("ToolBar ToggleButton Example");
  frame.setSize(400, 200);
  frame.setDefaultCloseOperation(JFrame.EXIT_ON_CLOSE);
  frame.setLayout(new BorderLayout());
  // Create a JToolBar
  JToolBar toolBar = new JToolBar();
  // Create a JToggleButton
  JToggleButton toggleButton = new JToggleButton("Register");
  toolBar.add(toggleButton);
  // Add ActionListener to the JToggleButton
  toggleButton.addActionListener(new ActionListener() {
    @Override
    public void actionPerformed(ActionEvent e) {
    if (toggleButton.isSelected()) {
      JOptionPane.showMessageDialog(frame, "Registration Successful!");
    }
```

```
    }
  });
  // Add the JToolBar to the top of the JFrame
  frame.add(toolBar, BorderLayout.PAGE_START);
  // Make the frame visible
  frame.setVisible(true);
  }
}
```

Output

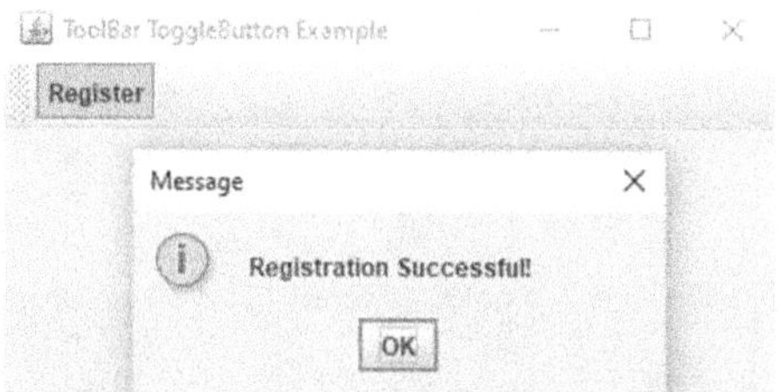

In the above program a JToggleButton "Register" is added to the JToolBar. When the JToggleButton is selected, a message dialog will pop up displaying a success message. The JToolBar is added to the top of the JFrame using the BorderLayout.PAGE_START constant. The JFrame is then set to a fixed size and made visible, allowing the user to interact with the JToggleButton.

13.7.1.8 JDesktopPane with ActionListener

A `JDesktopPane` typically does not use an `ActionListener` directly since it serves as a container for internal frames rather than interactive components. However, individual components within the `JDesktopPane`, such as buttons or menus, can use `ActionListener` to handle user actions within those internal frames.

Program

```
import javax.swing.*;
import java.awt.event.ActionEvent;
import java.awt.event.ActionListener;
public class DesktopPaneExample {
  void main(String[] args) {
  // Create the main JFrame
  JFrame frame = new JFrame("DesktopPane Example");
  frame.setSize(600, 400);
  frame.setDefaultCloseOperation(JFrame.EXIT_ON_CLOSE);
  frame.setLayout(null);
  // Create a JDesktopPane
  JDesktopPane desktopPane = new JDesktopPane();
  // Create a JInternalFrame
  JInternalFrame internalFrame = new JInternalFrame("Registration", true,
    true, true, true);
  internalFrame.setSize(300, 150);
  internalFrame.setLayout(null);
  // Create a JButton
  JButton registerButton = new JButton("Register");
  registerButton.setBounds(100, 50, 100, 30);
  // Add ActionListener to the JButton
  registerButton.addActionListener(new ActionListener() {
```

```
    @Override
    public void actionPerformed(ActionEvent e) {
    JOptionPane.showMessageDialog(internalFrame, "Registration Successful!");
    }
  });
  // Add the JButton to the JInternalFrame
  internalFrame.add(registerButton);
  // Add the JInternalFrame to the JDesktopPane
  desktopPane.add(internalFrame);
  // Make the JInternalFrame visible
  internalFrame.setVisible(true);
  // Add the JDesktopPane to the JFrame
  frame.add(desktopPane);
  // Make the JFrame visible
  frame.setVisible(true);
  }
}
```

Output

DesktopPane Example

In the above program the JDesktopPane is used to hold a JInternalFrame, which is a window that can be moved and resized within the JDesktopPane. The JInternalFrame has a title "Registration" and contains a JButton labeled "Register". When the button is clicked, a JOptionPane is displayed with a success message. The JDesktopPane is added to the JFrame, which is set to exit when closed and is made visible at the end of the program.

13.7.2 Focus Listener

A FocusListener is an interface in Java that is used to receive focus events, which occur when a component gains or loses focus. Focus refers to the state of a component where it is ready to receive input from the user. When a component gains focus, it is highlighted and ready to accept input, whereas when it loses focus, it is no longer highlighted and input is not accepted. The FocusListener interface has two methods: focusGained() and focusLost(). The focusGained() method is called when a component gains focus, and the focusLost() method is called when a component loses focus. These methods can be overridden to perform specific actions when a component gains or loses focus. For example, a text field may display a default value when it loses focus and clear the value when it gains focus. FocusListeners are commonly used in GUI applications to validate user input, update the display, or perform other actions based on the focus state of components.

13.7.2.1 JTextField with FocusListener

A `JTextField` requires a `FocusListener` to detect when it gains or loses focus. This allows for actions such as validation or user feedback based on focus changes, helping to manage input focus and improve user interaction.

Program

```
import javax.swing.*;
import java.awt.*;
import java.awt.event.FocusEvent;
import java.awt.event.FocusListener;
public class FocusListenerExample {
  void main(String[] args) {
  // Create the main JFrame
  JFrame frame = new JFrame("FocusListener Example");
  frame.setSize(300, 100);
  frame.setDefaultCloseOperation(JFrame.EXIT_ON_CLOSE);
  frame.setLayout(new FlowLayout());
  // Create a JTextField
  JTextField textField = new JTextField("Type here", 20);

  // Add a FocusListener to the JTextField
  textField.addFocusListener(new FocusListener() {
    @Override
    public void focusGained(FocusEvent e) {
    // Change background color to yellow when focus is gained
    textField.setBackground(Color.YELLOW);
    }
    @Override
    public void focusLost(FocusEvent e) {
    // Change background color to white when focus is lost
    textField.setBackground(Color.WHITE);
    }
  });
  // Add the JTextField to the JFrame
  frame.add(textField);
  // Make the JFrame visible
  frame.setVisible(true);
  }
}
```

Output

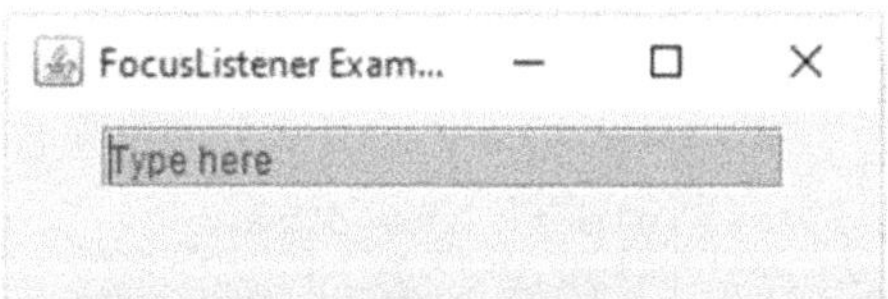

In the above program the JTextField is added to the JFrame with a FlowLayout. A FocusListener is added to the JTextField to change its background color when it gains or loses focus. When the JTextField gains focus, its background color changes to yellow, and when it loses focus, it changes back to white.

13.7.2.2 JFormattedTextField with FocusListener

A `JFormattedTextField` requires a `FocusListener` to handle events when it gains or loses focus. This allows for dynamic validation or formatting of input based on the focus state, ensuring accurate data entry and providing user feedback.

Program

```
import javax.swing.*;
import java.awt.*;
import java.awt.event.FocusEvent;
import java.awt.event.FocusListener;
import javax.swing.text.NumberFormatter;
import java.text.NumberFormat;
public class FormattedTextFieldExample {
  void main(String[] args) {
  // Create the main JFrame
  JFrame frame = new JFrame("FormattedTextField Example");
  frame.setSize(300, 100);
  frame.setDefaultCloseOperation(JFrame.EXIT_ON_CLOSE);
  frame.setLayout(new FlowLayout());
  // Create a NumberFormat for integer values
  NumberFormat numberFormat = NumberFormat.getIntegerInstance();

  // Create a NumberFormatter using the NumberFormat
  NumberFormatter numberFormatter = new NumberFormatter(numberFormat);
  numberFormatter.setAllowsInvalid(false); // Prevent invalid input

  // Create a JFormattedTextField with the NumberFormatter
  JFormattedTextField formattedTextField = new JFormattedTextField(number
     Formatter);
  formattedTextField.setColumns(10); // Set the number of columns

  // Add a FocusListener to the JFormattedTextField
  formattedTextField.addFocusListener(new FocusListener() {
    @Override
    public void focusGained(FocusEvent e) {
    // Change background color to yellow when focus is gained
    formattedTextField.setBackground(Color.YELLOW);
    }
    @Override
    public void focusLost(FocusEvent e) {
    // Change background color to white when focus is lost
    formattedTextField.setBackground(Color.WHITE);
    }
  });
  // Add the JFormattedTextField to the JFrame
  frame.add(formattedTextField);
  // Make the JFrame visible
  frame.setVisible(true);
  }
}
```

Output

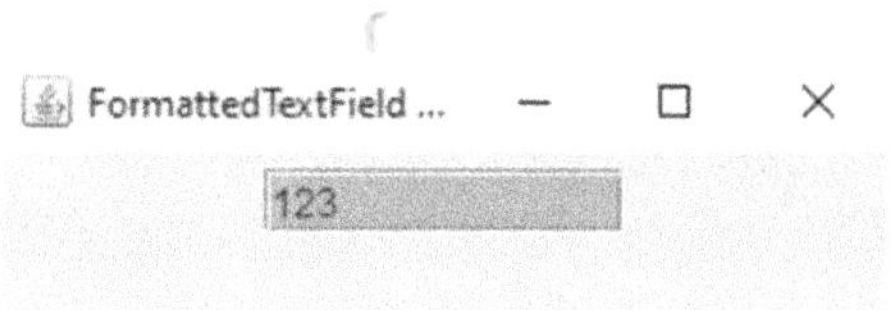

In the above program the JFormattedTextField is set to accept integer values and is added to the JFrame with a FlowLayout. A FocusListener is added to the JFormattedTextField to change its background color when it gains or loses focus. When the JFormattedTextField gains focus, its background color changes to yellow, and when it loses focus, it changes back to white.

13.7.3 Document Listener

A DocumentListener is an interface in Java that listens for changes to a document, typically a text component such as a JTextField or JTextArea. It is used to track changes to the document, such as insertions, removals, and changes to the document's content. The DocumentListener interface has three methods: insertUpdate, removeUpdate, and changedUpdate. These methods are called when the document is changed, inserted into, or removed from, respectively. DocumentListeners are often used to validate user input, update other components based on the document's content, or to perform other actions in response to changes to the document. They can be added to a document using the addDocumentListener method. DocumentListeners are typically used in conjunction with a document, which is an interface that represents a document, such as a text component. The document interface provides methods for inserting, removing, and retrieving content from the document. DocumentListeners are a powerful tool for tracking and responding to changes to a document in a Java application. They provide a way to react to changes to a document in real-time, allowing for more dynamic and interactive user interfaces.

13.7.3.1 JTextArea with DocumentListener

A `JTextArea` requires a `DocumentListener` to monitor changes in the text content. This enables real-time updates or validations as users modify the text, allowing for dynamic responses to text input.

Program

```
import javax.swing.*;
import javax.swing.event.DocumentEvent;
import javax.swing.event.DocumentListener;
import java.awt.*;
public class DocumentListenerExample {
  void main(String[] args) {
  // Create the main JFrame
  JFrame frame = new JFrame("DocumentListener Example");
  frame.setSize(400, 300);
  frame.setDefaultCloseOperation(JFrame.EXIT_ON_CLOSE);
  frame.setLayout(new BorderLayout());
  // Create a JTextArea and wrap it in a JScrollPane
  JTextArea textArea = new JTextArea(10, 30);
  JScrollPane scrollPane = new JScrollPane(textArea);
  // Add a DocumentListener to the JTextArea's Document
  textArea.getDocument().addDocumentListener(new DocumentListener() {
    @Override
    public void insertUpdate(DocumentEvent e) {
```

```
    updateText();
    }
    @Override
    public void removeUpdate(DocumentEvent e) {
    updateText();
    }
    @Override
    public void changedUpdate(DocumentEvent e) {
    updateText();
    }
    // Method to display a message dialog with the updated text
    private void updateText() {
    SwingUtilities.invokeLater(() -> {
      String text = textArea.getText();
      JOptionPane.showMessageDialog(frame, "Text updated:\n" + text);
    });
    }
  });
  // Add the JScrollPane to the JFrame
  frame.add(scrollPane, BorderLayout.CENTER);
  // Make the JFrame visible
  frame.setVisible(true);
  }
}
```

Output

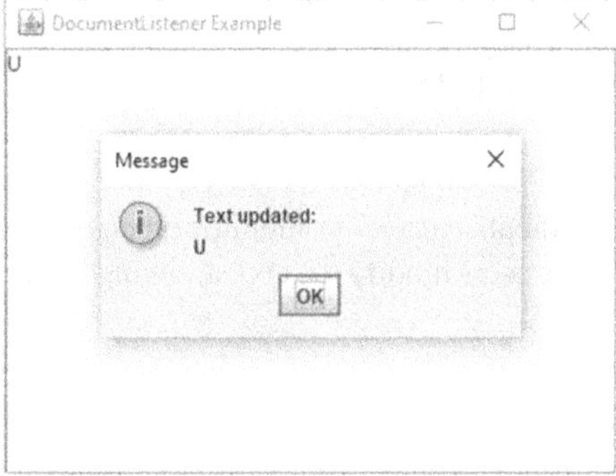

In the above program first JTextArea is added to the JFrame with a JScrollPane. A DocumentListener is added to the JTextArea's document to detect changes to the text. The updateText method is called whenever the text is changed, inserted into, or removed from. The updateText method displays a message dialog with the updated text.

13.7.4 Item Listener

An ItemListener is an interface in Java that listens for changes to a component, typically a checkbox, radio button, or combo box. It is used to track changes to the component's selection state, such as when an item is selected or deselected. The ItemListener interface has one method: itemStateChanged. This method is called when the component's selection state changes. ItemListeners are often used to perform an action when an item is selected or deselected, such as enabling or disabling other components. They can be added to a component using the addItemListener method. ItemListeners are typically used with components that have a selection state, such as JCheckBox, JRadioButton, and JComboBox. The itemStateChanged method receives an ItemEvent object, which provides information about the item that changed and its new state. ItemListeners are a powerful tool for tracking and responding to changes to a component's selection state in a Java application. They provide a way to react to changes to a component in real-time, allowing for more dynamic and interactive user interfaces.

13.7.4.1 JCheckBox with ItemListener

A `JCheckBox` requires an `ItemListener` to detect changes in its selection state. This listener enables you to execute specific actions when the check box is checked or unchecked, ensuring that your application responds appropriately to user choices.

Program

```
import javax.swing.*;
import java.awt.*;
import java.awt.event.ItemEvent;
import java.awt.event.ItemListener;
public class CheckBoxExample {
  void main(String[] args) {
  // Create the main JFrame
  JFrame frame = new JFrame("CheckBox Example");
  frame.setSize(300, 100);
  frame.setDefaultCloseOperation(JFrame.EXIT_ON_CLOSE);
  frame.setLayout(new FlowLayout());
  // Create a JCheckBox with a label "Enroll in Course"
  JCheckBox checkBox = new JCheckBox("Enroll in Course");
  checkBox.setBackground(Color.GREEN);
  // Add an ItemListener to the JCheckBox
  checkBox.addItemListener(new ItemListener() {
    @Override
    public void itemStateChanged(ItemEvent e) {
    if (e.getStateChange() == ItemEvent.SELECTED) {
      // Checkbox is selected
      JOptionPane.showMessageDialog(frame, "You are enrolled in the course.");
    } else {
      // Checkbox is deselected
      JOptionPane.showMessageDialog(frame, "You are no longer enrolled in
         the course.");
    }
    }
  });
  // Add the JCheckBox to the JFrame
  frame.add(checkBox);
  // Make the JFrame visible
  frame.setVisible(true);
  }
}
```

Output

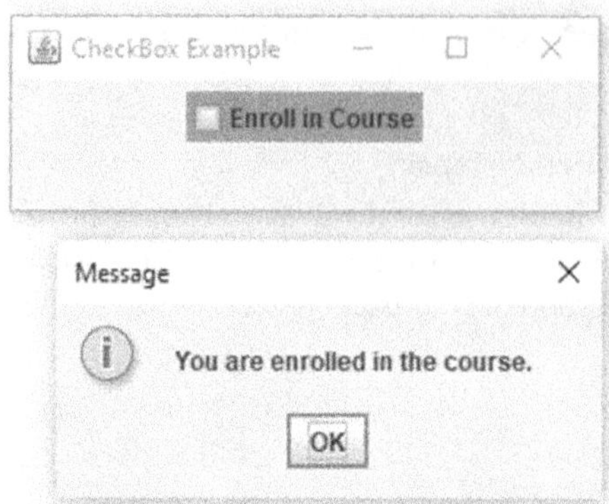

In the above program we created a JCheckBox and added to the JFrame with a FlowLayout and a green background. An ItemListener is added to the JCheckBox to detect changes to its selection state. When the JCheckBox is selected, a message dialog appears saying the user is enrolled in the course. When the JCheckBox is deselected, a message dialog appears saying the user is no longer enrolled.

13.7.5 Change Listener

A ChangeListener is an interface in Java that listens for changes to a component, typically a spinner, slider, or tabbed pane. It is used to track changes to the component's state, such as when the value of a spinner changes or the selected tab changes. The ChangeListener interface has one method: stateChanged. This method is called when the component's state changes. ChangeListeners are often used to perform an action when the component's state changes, such as updating a label or enabling/disabling other components. They can be added to a component using the addChangeListener method. ChangeListeners are typically used with components that have a changing state, such as JSpinner, JSlider, and JTabbedPane. The stateChanged method receives a ChangeEvent object, which provides information about the source of the change. ChangeListeners are a powerful tool for tracking and responding to changes to a component's state in a Java application.

13.7.5.1 JSlider with ChangeListener

A `JSlider` requires a `ChangeListener` to respond to changes in its value. This listener allows you to update the application state or perform actions based on the current slider position, ensuring real-time feedback and interaction.

Program

```
import javax.swing.*;
import javax.swing.event.ChangeEvent;
import javax.swing.event.ChangeListener;
import java.awt.*;
public class SliderExample {
  void main(String[] args) {
  // Create the main JFrame
  JFrame frame = new JFrame("Slider Example");
  frame.setSize(400, 200);
  frame.setDefaultCloseOperation(JFrame.EXIT_ON_CLOSE);
  frame.setLayout(new BorderLayout());
```

```
  // Create a JSlider with range 0 to 100 and initial value 50
  JSlider slider = new JSlider(JSlider.HORIZONTAL, 0, 100, 50);
  slider.setPaintTicks(true);
  slider.setPaintLabels(true);
  slider.setMajorTickSpacing(20);
  slider.setMinorTickSpacing(5);
  // Add a ChangeListener to the JSlider
  slider.addChangeListener(new ChangeListener() {
    @Override
    public void stateChanged(ChangeEvent e) {
    int value = slider.getValue();
    // Show the new value in a message dialog
    JOptionPane.showMessageDialog(frame, "Slider Value: " + value);
    }
  });
  // Add the JSlider to the frame
  frame.add(slider, BorderLayout.CENTER);
  // Make the JFrame visible
  frame.setVisible(true);
  }
}
```

Output

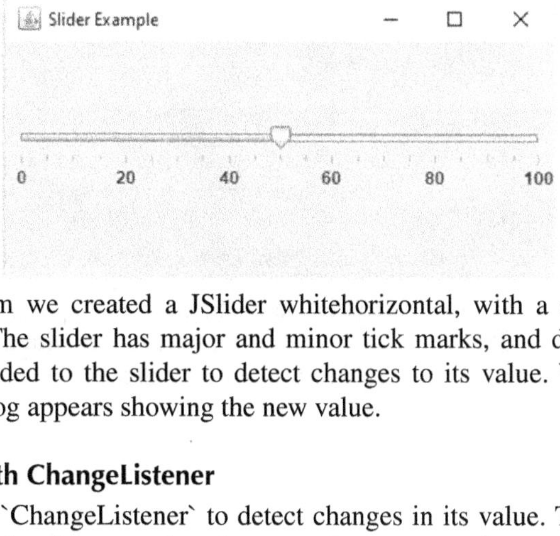

Slider Example

0 20 40 60 80 100

In the above program we created a JSlider whitehorizontal, with a range of 0 to 100, and an initial value of 50. The slider has major and minor tick marks, and displays its value labels. A ChangeListener is added to the slider to detect changes to its value. When the slider's value changes, a message dialog appears showing the new value.

13.7.5.2 JSpinner with ChangeListener

A `JSpinner` requires a `ChangeListener` to detect changes in its value. This listener enables the application to react or update its state when the user selects a new value, ensuring dynamic handling of user input.

Program

```
import javax.swing.*;
import javax.swing.event.ChangeEvent;
import javax.swing.event.ChangeListener;
import java.awt.*;
public class SpinnerExample {
  void main(String[] args) {
  // Create the main JFrame
  JFrame frame = new JFrame("Spinner Example");
  frame.setSize(300, 150);
```

```
  frame.setDefaultCloseOperation(JFrame.EXIT_ON_CLOSE);
  frame.setLayout(new FlowLayout());
  // Create a SpinnerNumberModel with a range of 0 to 100 and an initial
  value of 0
  SpinnerNumberModel model = new SpinnerNumberModel(0, 0, 100, 1);
  JSpinner spinner = new JSpinner(model);
  spinner.setBackground(Color.YELLOW);
  // Add a ChangeListener to the JSpinner
  spinner.addChangeListener(new ChangeListener() {
    @Override
    public void stateChanged(ChangeEvent e) {
    int value = (Integer) spinner.getValue();
    // Show the new value in a message dialog
    JOptionPane.showMessageDialog(frame, "Spinner Value: " + value);
    }
  });
  // Add the JSpinner to the frame
  frame.add(spinner);
  // Make the JFrame visible
  frame.setVisible(true);
  }
}
```

Output

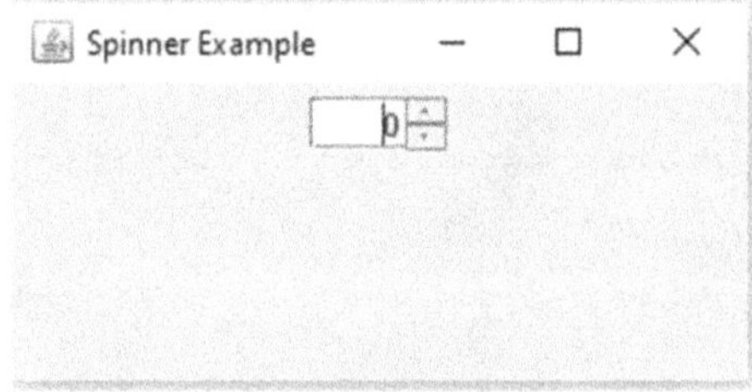

In the above program we demonstrated the use of JSpinner and ChangeListener to create a interactive GUI component. The JSpinner uses a SpinnerNumberModel with a range of 0 to 100, and an initial value of 0. The spinner has a yellow background. A ChangeListener is added to the spinner to detect changes to its value. When the spinner's value changes, a message dialog appears showing the new value.

13.7.5.3 JTabbedPane with ChangeListener

A `JTabbedPane` requires a `ChangeListener` to detect when the selected tab changes. This listener allows the application to update or respond based on the active tab, ensuring dynamic content adjustment and interaction according to the user's tab selection.

Program

```
import javax.swing.*;
import javax.swing.event.ChangeEvent;
import javax.swing.event.ChangeListener;
import java.awt.*;
public class TabbedPaneExample {
  void main(String[] args) {
  // Create the main JFrame
  JFrame frame = new JFrame("TabbedPane Example");
```

```
    frame.setSize(400, 300);
    frame.setDefaultCloseOperation(JFrame.EXIT_ON_CLOSE);
    frame.setLayout(new BorderLayout());
    // Create a JTabbedPane
    JTabbedPane tabbedPane = new JTabbedPane();
    // Create first JPanel and add it to the first tab
    JPanel panel1 = new JPanel();
    JLabel label1 = new JLabel("Content of Tab 1");
    panel1.add(label1);
    tabbedPane.addTab("Tab 1", panel1);
    // Create second JPanel and add it to the second tab
    JPanel panel2 = new JPanel();
    JLabel label2 = new JLabel("Content of Tab 2");
    panel2.add(label2);
    tabbedPane.addTab("Tab 2", panel2);
    // Add ChangeListener to JTabbedPane
    tabbedPane.addChangeListener(new ChangeListener() {
      @Override
      public void stateChanged(ChangeEvent e) {
      int selectedIndex = tabbedPane.getSelectedIndex();
      // Show the selected tab index in a message dialog
      JOptionPane.showMessageDialog(frame, "Selected Tab Index: " +
        selectedIndex);
      }
    });
    // Add the JTabbedPane to the JFrame
    frame.add(tabbedPane, BorderLayout.CENTER);
    // Make the JFrame visible
    frame.setVisible(true);
    }
}
```

Output

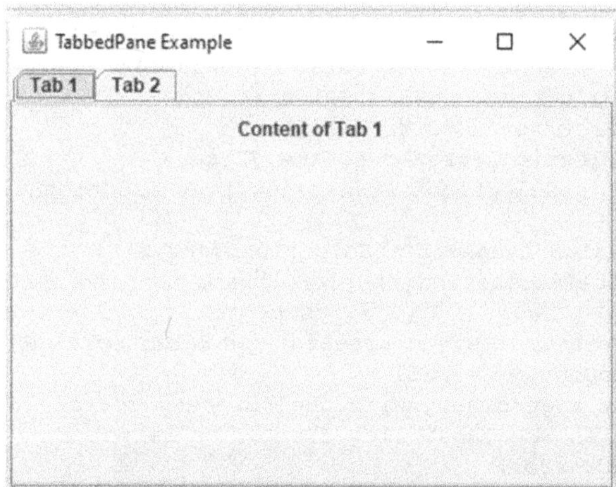

In the above program the JTabbedPane has two tabs, each containing a JPanel with a JLabel. A ChangeListener is added to the JTabbedPane to detect changes to the selected tab. When the selected tab changes, a message dialog appears showing the index of the new tab.

13.7.6 List Selection Listener

A ListSelectionListener is an interface in Java that defines a method to handle list selection events. It is used with JList components to detect changes in the selection of list items. The interface has one method, valueChanged(ListSelectionEvent e), which is called when the selection changes. This method is called whenever the user selects or deselects an item in the list. The ListSelectionEvent object passed to the method provides information about the change. The method can query the event to determine what items were selected or deselected. The listener can then perform actions based on the new selection, such as updating other components. ListSelectionListeners are typically added to JLists using the addListSelectionListener method. The listener is notified whenever the selection changes, allowing it to respond to user input. By using a ListSelectionListener, you can create interactive GUI components that respond to user selection.

13.7.6.1 JList with ListSelectionListener

A `JList` requires a `ListSelectionListener` to respond to changes in the selected items. This listener enables the application to perform actions or updates based on the user's selection, providing real-time interaction and feedback when the selection changes.

Program

```
import javax.swing.*;
import javax.swing.event.ListSelectionEvent;
import javax.swing.event.ListSelectionListener;
import java.awt.*;
public class ListSelectionExample {
  void main(String[] args) {
  // Create the main JFrame
  JFrame frame = new JFrame("List Selection Example");
  frame.setSize(300, 200);
  frame.setDefaultCloseOperation(JFrame.EXIT_ON_CLOSE);
  frame.setLayout(new BorderLayout());
  // Create a JList with a list of courses
  String[] courses = {"Java", "Python", "C++", "JavaScript", "Ruby"};
  JList<String> courseList = new JList<>(courses);
  courseList.setSelectionMode(ListSelectionModel.SINGLE_SELECTION);
  courseList.setBackground(Color.WHITE);
  // Add a ListSelectionListener to the JList
  courseList.addListSelectionListener(new ListSelectionListener() {
    @Override
    public void valueChanged(ListSelectionEvent e) {
    if (!e.getValueIsAdjusting()) { // Check if the selection event is
                                       complete
      String selectedCourse = courseList.getSelectedValue();
      if (selectedCourse != null) {
      // Show a message dialog with the selected course
      JOptionPane.showMessageDialog(frame, "Selected Course: " +
         selectedCourse);
      }
    }
    }
  });
```

```
  // Add the JList to a JScrollPane to handle scrolling
  JScrollPane scrollPane = new JScrollPane(courseList);
  // Add the JScrollPane to the JFrame
  frame.add(scrollPane, BorderLayout.CENTER);
  // Make the JFrame visible
  frame.setVisible(true);
  }
}
```

Output

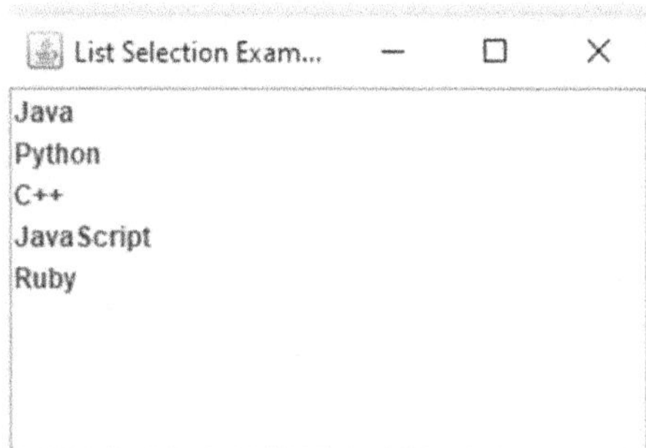

The JList displays a list of courses and allows the user to select one course at a time. When the user selects a course, a message dialog appears showing the selected course. We used a ListSelectionListener to detect changes in the list selection. The listener is added to the JList and responds to selection events by displaying a message dialog.

13.7.7 Mouse Listener

A MouseListener in Java is an interface that receives and handles mouse events such as clicks, presses, releases, entering, and exiting a component. It includes five methods: `mouseClicked(MouseEvent e)`, `mousePressed(MouseEvent e)`, `mouseReleased(MouseEvent e)`, `mouseEntered(MouseEvent e)`, and `mouseExited(MouseEvent e)`, which can be implemented to define specific behaviors when these mouse events occur.

13.7.7.1 JPopupMenu with Mouse Listener

A `JPopupMenu` with a `MouseListener` is needed to display the pop-up menu when the user right-clicks (`mousePressed` event) on a specific component. The `MouseListener` detects the mouse event and triggers the `JPopupMenu` to appear at the current cursor location.

Program

```
import javax.swing.*;
import java.awt.event.*;
public class PopupMenuExample {
  void main(String[] args) {
  // Create the main JFrame
  JFrame frame = new JFrame("PopupMenu Example");
  frame.setSize(400, 300);
  frame.setDefaultCloseOperation(JFrame.EXIT_ON_CLOSE);
  // Create a JTextArea
  JTextArea textArea = new JTextArea();
  textArea.setText("Right-click to see the popup menu with Cut, Copy, and
     Paste options.");
```

```
textArea.setLineWrap(true);
textArea.setWrapStyleWord(true);
// Create a JPopupMenu and add Cut, Copy, and Paste menu items
JPopupMenu popupMenu = new JPopupMenu();

JMenuItem cutItem = new JMenuItem("Cut");
cutItem.addActionListener(e -> textArea.cut());
popupMenu.add(cutItem);

JMenuItem copyItem = new JMenuItem("Copy");
copyItem.addActionListener(e -> textArea.copy());
popupMenu.add(copyItem);

JMenuItem pasteItem = new JMenuItem("Paste");
pasteItem.addActionListener(e -> textArea.paste());
popupMenu.add(pasteItem);
// Add a MouseListener to show the JPopupMenu on right-click
textArea.addMouseListener(new MouseAdapter() {
  @Override
  public void mousePressed(MouseEvent e) {
  if (e.isPopupTrigger()) {
    popupMenu.show(e.getComponent(), e.getX(), e.getY());
  }
  }
  @Override
  public void mouseReleased(MouseEvent e) {
  if (e.isPopupTrigger()) {
    popupMenu.show(e.getComponent(), e.getX(), e.getY());
  }
  }
});
// Add the JTextArea to the JFrame inside a JScrollPane
JScrollPane scrollPane = new JScrollPane(textArea);
frame.add(scrollPane);
// Make the JFrame visible
frame.setVisible(true);
}
}
```

Output

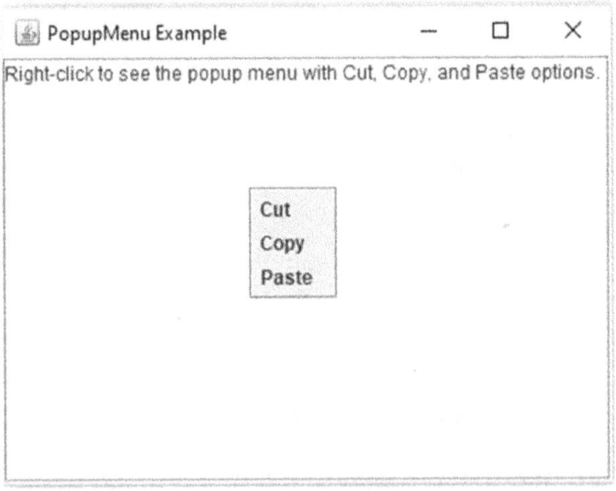

PopupMenu Example

Right-click to see the popup menu with Cut, Copy, and Paste options.

Cut
Copy
Paste

In the above program we used a mouse listener that detects right-clicks. When a right-click is detected, a context menu (JPopupMenu) is shown with "Cut", "Copy", and "Paste" options. The "Cut", "Copy", and "Paste" options are functional and can be used to manipulate text in the JTextArea.

13.8 MEDICAL CASE STUDY

13.8.1 Case Study 1

Collect the diabetes dataset using Swing application

Program

```
import javax.swing.*;
import java.awt.*;
import java.awt.event.*;
import java.io.*;
public class DiabetesDataCollector extends JFrame implements ActionListener {
  // Text fields for user input
  private JTextField tfAge, tfBMI, tfBloodPressure, tfFastingBloodSugar,
    tfPostPrandialBloodSugar, tfFamilyHistory, tfPhysicalActivity,
    tfSmoker, tfDiabetic;
  private JComboBox<String> cbGender;
  private JButton btnSave;
  public DiabetesDataCollector() {
  // Setting up the frame
  setTitle("Diabetes Data Collector");
  setLayout(new GridLayout(11, 2));
  setSize(400, 400);
  setDefaultCloseOperation(JFrame.EXIT_ON_CLOSE);
  // Adding labels and input fields to the frame
  add(new JLabel("Age:"));
  tfAge = new JTextField();
  add(tfAge);
  add(new JLabel("Gender:"));
  cbGender = new JComboBox<>(new String[] {"Male", "Female", "Other"});
  add(cbGender);
  add(new JLabel("BMI:"));
  tfBMI = new JTextField();
  add(tfBMI);
  add(new JLabel("Blood Pressure:"));
  tfBloodPressure = new JTextField();
  add(tfBloodPressure);
  add(new JLabel("Fasting Blood Sugar:"));
  tfFastingBloodSugar = new JTextField();
  add(tfFastingBloodSugar);
  add(new JLabel("Postprandial Blood Sugar:"));
  tfPostPrandialBloodSugar = new JTextField();
  add(tfPostPrandialBloodSugar);
  add(new JLabel("Family History (Yes/No):"));
  tfFamilyHistory = new JTextField();
  add(tfFamilyHistory);
  add(new JLabel("Physical Activity (Yes/No):"));
  tfPhysicalActivity = new JTextField();
  add(tfPhysicalActivity);
```

```
  add(new JLabel("Smoker (Yes/No):"));
  tfSmoker = new JTextField();
  add(tfSmoker);
  add(new JLabel("Diabetic (Yes/No):"));
  tfDiabetic = new JTextField();
  add(tfDiabetic);
  // Save button
  btnSave = new JButton("Save");
  btnSave.addActionListener(this);
  add(btnSave);
  setVisible(true);
  }
  @Override
  public void actionPerformed(ActionEvent e) {
  if (e.getSource() == btnSave) {
    try {
    // Write input data to a file
    BufferedWriter writer = new BufferedWriter(new FileWriter("diabetes_
       data.txt", true));
    writer.write(
      tfAge.getText() + "," +
      cbGender.getSelectedItem() + "," +
      tfBMI.getText() + "," +
      tfBloodPressure.getText() + "," +
      tfFastingBloodSugar.getText() + "," +
      tfPostPrandialBloodSugar.getText() + "," +
      tfFamilyHistory.getText() + "," +
      tfPhysicalActivity.getText() + "," +
      tfSmoker.getText() + "," +
      tfDiabetic.getText() + "\n"
    );
    writer.close();
    // Show a confirmation dialog
    JOptionPane.showMessageDialog(this, "Data saved successfully");
    // Clear input fields
    tfAge.setText("");
    cbGender.setSelectedIndex(0);
    tfBMI.setText("");
    tfBloodPressure.setText("");
    tfFastingBloodSugar.setText("");
    tfPostPrandialBloodSugar.setText("");
    tfFamilyHistory.setText("");
    tfPhysicalActivity.setText("");
    tfSmoker.setText("");
    tfDiabetic.setText("");
    } catch (IOException ex) {
    ex.printStackTrace();
    JOptionPane.showMessageDialog(this, "Error saving data");
    }
  }
  }
  void main(String[] args) {
  new DiabetesDataCollector();
  }
}
```

The `DiabetesDataCollector` program is a Java Swing application designed to collect and store diabetes-related health data from users. The program features a graphical user interface with input fields for age, gender, BMI, blood pressure, fasting blood sugar, postprandial blood sugar, family history, physical activity, smoking status, and diabetic status. Users can enter their information and save it by clicking the "Save" button, which writes the data to a text file. The program validates the input, provides a confirmation dialog upon successful data saving, and clears the input fields for the next entry. This application is useful for collecting and organizing health data for diabetes risk assessment or management.

13.8.2 Case Study 2

Neurological disorders encompass a broad range of conditions affecting the brain, spine, and nerves, with varying risk factors such as genetic predisposition, lifestyle factors (like diet and exercise), environmental influences (such as toxins), and age-related changes contributing to their development. Identifying specific risks often involves evaluating family medical history, lifestyle habits, and environmental exposures to understand susceptibility and potential preventive measures.

Program

```
import javax.swing.*;
import java.awt.*;
import java.awt.event.*;
public class Neuro Disorder Detector extends JFrame {
  private JTextField ageField;
  private JTextField symptomsField;
  private JButton detectButton;
  private JLabel resultLabel;
  public NeuroDisorderDetector() {
  super("Neuro Disorder Detector");
  setLayout(new FlowLayout());
  // Create UI components
  JLabel ageLabel = new JLabel("Age:");
  ageField = new JTextField(5);
  JLabel symptomsLabel = new JLabel("Symptoms:");
  symptomsField = new JTextField(20);
  detectButton = new JButton("Detect");
  detectButton.addActionListener(new DetectButtonListener());
  resultLabel = new JLabel("");
  // Add UI components to the frame
  add(ageLabel);
  add(ageField);
  add(symptomsLabel);
  add(symptomsField);
  add(detectButton);
  add(resultLabel);
  setSize(400, 200);
  setDefaultCloseOperation(EXIT_ON_CLOSE);
  setVisible(true);
  }
  private class DetectButtonListener implements ActionListener {
  public void actionPerformed(ActionEvent e) {
    // Get user input
    int age = Integer.parseInt(ageField.getText());
```

```
    String symptoms = symptomsField.getText();
    // Detect neuro disorder based on user input
    String disorder = detectNeuroDisorder(age, symptoms);
    // Display result
    resultLabel.setText("You may have " + disorder);
  }
  }
private String detectNeuroDisorder(int age, String symptoms) {
  // Define a list of possible neuro disorders
  String[] disorders = {"Alzheimer's disease", "Parkinson's disease",
     "Multiple Sclerosis", "Epilepsy", "Stroke"};
  // Define a list of symptoms for each disorder
  String[][] symptomsList = {
  {"memory loss", "confusion", "difficulty with communication"},
  // Alzheimer's disease
  {"tremors", "rigidity", "bradykinesia"}, // Parkinson's disease
  {"vision problems", "muscle weakness", "numbness or tingling"},
  // Multiple Sclerosis
  {"seizures", "loss of consciousness", "confusion"}, // Epilepsy
  {"sudden weakness", "numbness or paralysis", "difficulty with speech"}
// Stroke
  };
  // Initialize a variable to store the detected disorder
  String detectedDisorder = "Unknown";
  // Loop through each disorder and check if the symptoms match
  for (int i = 0; i < disorders.length; i++) {
  boolean match = true;
  for (String symptom : symptomsList[i]) {
    if (!symptoms.toLowerCase().contains(symptom.toLowerCase())) {
    match = false;
    break;
    }
  }
  if (match) {
    detectedDisorder = disorders[i];
    break;
  }
  }
  // Return the detected disorder
  return detectedDisorder;
}
  void main(String[] args) {
  NeuroDisorderDetector detector = new NeuroDisorderDetector();
  }
}
```

The `Neuro Disorder Detector` is a Java Swing application that helps in identifying potential neurological disorders based on user input. Users provide their ages and symptoms through text fields in a simple graphical user interface. Upon clicking the "Detect" button, it compares the entered symptoms against predefined symptom lists for various neurological disorders such as Alzheimer's disease, Parkinson's disease, Multiple Sclerosis, Epilepsy, and Stroke. If a match is found, the corresponding disorder is displayed on the interface.

13.8.3 Case Study 3

Thyroid disorders refer to conditions affecting the thyroid gland, leading to either overproduction (hyperthyroidism) or underproduction (hypothyroidism) of thyroid hormones. The program evaluates the symptoms against predefined lists of symptoms for the following thyroid disorders:

1. **Hypothyroidism**: Symptoms include fatigue, weight gain, dry skin, and hair loss.
2. **Hyperthyroidism**: Symptoms include weight loss, nervousness, irritability, and heat intolerance.
3. **Thyroid Nodules**: Symptoms include a lump in the neck, difficulty swallowing, and pain in the neck.
4. **Thyroid Cancer**: Symptoms include a lump in the neck, difficulty swallowing, pain in the neck, and hoarseness.

These symptom lists are used to detect potential thyroid disorders

Program

```
import javax.swing.*;
import java.awt.*;
import java.awt.event.*;
public class ThyroidDetector extends JFrame {
  private JTextField ageField;
  private JTextField symptomsField;
  private JButton detectButton;
  private JLabel resultLabel;
  public ThyroidDetector() {
  super("Thyroid Detector");
  setLayout(new FlowLayout());
  // Create UI components
  JLabel ageLabel = new JLabel("Age:");
  ageField = new JTextField(5);
  JLabel symptomsLabel = new JLabel("Symptoms:");
  symptomsField = new JTextField(20);
  detectButton = new JButton("Detect");
  detectButton.addActionListener(new DetectButtonListener());
  resultLabel = new JLabel("");
  // Add UI components to the frame
  add(ageLabel);
  add(ageField);
  add(symptomsLabel);
  add(symptomsField);
  add(detectButton);
  add(resultLabel);
  setSize(400, 200);
  setDefaultCloseOperation(EXIT_ON_CLOSE);
  setVisible(true);
  }
  private class DetectButtonListener implements ActionListener {
  public void actionPerformed(ActionEvent e) {
    // Get user input
    int age = Integer.parseInt(ageField.getText());
```

```
    String symptoms = symptomsField.getText();
    // Detect thyroid disorder based on user input
    String disorder = detectThyroidDisorder(age, symptoms);
    // Display result
    resultLabel.setText("You may have " + disorder);
  }
  }
  private String detectThyroidDisorder(int age, String symptoms) {
  // Define a list of possible thyroid disorders
  String[] disorders = {"Hypothyroidism", "Hyperthyroidism", "Thyroid
    Nodules", "Thyroid Cancer"};
  // Define a list of symptoms for each disorder
  String[][] symptomsList = {
    {"fatigue", "weight gain", "dry skin", "hair loss"}, // Hypothyroidism
    {"weight loss", "nervousness", "irritability", "heat intolerance"}, //
    Hyperthyroidism
    {"lump in the neck", "difficulty swallowing", "pain in the neck"}, //
    Thyroid Nodules
    {"lump in the neck", "difficulty swallowing", "pain in the neck",
        "hoarseness"} // Thyroid Cancer
  };
  // Initialize a variable to store the detected disorder
  String detectedDisorder = "Unknown";
  // Loop through each disorder and check if the symptoms match
  for (int i = 0; i < disorders.length; i++) {
    boolean match = true;
    for (String symptom : symptomsList[i]) {
    if (!symptoms.toLowerCase().contains(symptom.toLowerCase())) {
      match = false;
      break;
    }
    }
    if (match) {
    detectedDisorder = disorders[i];
    break;
    }
  }
  // Return the detected disorder
  return detectedDisorder;
  }
  void main(String[] args) {
  ThyroidDetector detector = new ThyroidDetector();
  }
}
```

The `ThyroidDetector` is a Java Swing application designed to identify potential thyroid disorders based on user input. The interface includes text fields for the user's age and symptoms, a "Detect" button, and a label to display the result. When the button is clicked, the program evaluates the entered symptoms against predefined symptom lists for various thyroid conditions such as hypothyroidism, hyperthyroidism, thyroid nodules, and thyroid cancer. If the symptoms match a known disorder, the program updates the result label to indicate the potential condition.

14 Java Generics

14.1 INTRODUCTION

Generics provide a way to create classes, interfaces, and methods that can operate on different types without sacrificing type safety. This is achieved by allowing you to specify the type as a parameter when creating instances of classes or invoking methods.

The primary advantage of using generics is code reusability. With a generic class or method, you can write code that works with various data types, promoting flexibility and reducing redundancy. This is particularly useful when you want to create components that can adapt to different data types without compromising type checking at compile-time.

It's important to note that generics do not work directly with primitive types. However, Java provides wrapper classes (e.g., Integer for int, Float for Float) that can be used with generics to achieve the same effect when working with primitive types. This ensures that the benefits of generics can be extended to a wide range of scenarios in Java programming.

The conventions contribute to the maintainability and clarity of the codebase.

- E - Element:
  Often used in the context of collections (e.g., ArrayList, Set) where the type parameter represents the type of elements contained in the collection.
- K - Key, V - Value:
  Frequently employed in the context of Map implementations (e.g., HashMap, TreeMap), where K represents the type of keys and V represents the type of values stored in the Map.
- N - Number:
  Commonly used when the generic type is expected to be a numeric data type.
- T - Type:
  Used as a generic type parameter when the actual type is unspecified or can vary.
- S, U, V, etc.:
  When dealing with multiple generic types, following letters from the alphabet (S, U, V, etc.) are often used to represent the second, third, and fourth types, providing a clear sequence in the order of declaration.

Following these conventions makes the code more understandable for developers and aligns with the conventions used in standard Java libraries. Consistency in naming conventions enhances collaboration and readability, especially when working with code that involves generic types across different projects or libraries.

DOI: 10.1201/9781003544319-14

14.2 BOUNDED TYPES

Bounded type parameters in Java Generics allow you to restrict the type of the generic parameter to be a subtype of a particular class or to implement a specific interface. This provides additional control and ensures that the type used with generics adheres to certain constraints.

When you declare a bounded type parameter in Java Generics, you use the extends keyword followed by the class or interface that you want to use as an upper bound for the type parameter. This restricts the type parameter to be a subtype of the specified class or to implement the specified interface.

Syntax

```
class Sample<T extends Number> {
  // class implementation
}
```

Where T extends Number means that T can be any type that is a subclass of Number or Number itself. This ensures that any type used for T must be compatible with the Number class. This restriction allows you to take advantage of the methods and properties of the upper-bounded class or interface within your generic class or method, while still providing the flexibility of using different subclasses of the specified type.

Program

```
// Generic class Test with a bounded type parameter T
class Test<T extends Number> {
  // Generic variable to store a numeric value
  private T value;
  // Constructor to initialize the generic variable
  public Test(T value) {
  this.value = value;
  }
  // Method to display the stored value
  public void display() {
  System.out.println("Value: " + value);
  }
}
// Main class to demonstrate the usage of the generic class
public class Main {
  void main(String[] args) {
  // Creating instances of the generic class with different numeric types
  Test<Integer> testInt = new Test<>(1);
  Test<Double> testDouble = new Test<>(1.1);
  Test<Float> testFloat = new Test<>(11.111f);
  // Displaying the values of each instance
  testInt.display();    // Output: Value: 1
  testDouble.display();  // Output: Value: 1.1
  testFloat.display();  // Output: Value: 11.111
  }
}
Output:
value: 1
value: 1.1
value: 11.111
```

This Java program showcases the implementation of a generic class named test with a bounded type parameter. The type parameter T is constrained to be a subtype of the Number class, ensuring that only numeric types can be used with instances of the test class. The generic class contains a constructor to initialize the generic variable and a display method to print the stored value. In the Main class, three instances of the generic class are created with different numeric types—Integer, Double, and Float. Each instance is initialized with a specific numeric value, and the display method is invoked to print the respective values.

Program

```
import java.util.ArrayList;
import java.util.Collection;
import java.util.Iterator;
public class Main {

  // Generic method with a bounded type parameter that accepts collections
  of integers
  public static <T extends Collection<Integer>> void display(T collection) {
  // Creating an iterator to iterate through the collection
  Iterator<Integer> iterator = collection.iterator();
  while (iterator.hasNext()) {
    System.out.println(iterator.next());
  }
  }
  void main(String[] args) {
  // Creating an ArrayList of integers and populating it
  ArrayList<Integer> a = new ArrayList<>();
  a.add(10);
  a.add(20);
  a.add(30);
  a.add(40);

  // Invoking the display method with the ArrayList of integers
  display(a);
  }
}
Output:
10
20
30
40
```

The above Java program exemplifies the use of generics with a method designed to operate on collections of integers. The display method, declared with a bounded type parameter <T extends Collection<Integer>>, is constrained to accept only collections containing integer elements. This restriction ensures type safety and allows the method to iterate through the provided collection and print each element using an iterator. In the main method, an ArrayList<Integer> named a(i.e., Array variable) is instantiated and populated with integer values. The display method is then invoked with this collection as an argument, demonstrating how the generic method effectively handles the specified type constraint.

14.3 GENERIC CLASS

A generics class is a class that is parameterized with one or more types, allowing it to work with different data types. This provides a high level of flexibility and reusability in code. By creating a generics class, you can write code that is not tied to a specific data type, making it adaptable to various scenarios.

In a generics class, you use a type parameter (often denoted by a single uppercase letter, such as T) to represent the type of data that the class will work with. This type parameter is specified when creating an instance of the class, allowing the class to operate on objects of that specific type.

Program

```
// Define a generic class named Test
class Test<T> {
  private T value;
  // Constructor to initialize the value
  public Test(T value) {
  this.value = value;
  }
  // Method to get the value
  public T getValue() {
  return value;
  }
  // Method to display the value
  public void display() {
  System.out.println("Generic Class " + value.getClass().getSimpleName() +
     ": " + value);
  }
}
// Main class to test the generic class
public class Main {
  void main(String[] args) {
  // Create an instance of Test with Integer type
  Test<Integer> t = new Test<>(1);
  // Create an instance of Test with String type
  Test<String> t1 = new Test<>("Usharani");
  // Display the values
  t.display();  // Output: Generic Class Integer: 1
  t1.display(); // Output: Generic Class String: Usharani
  }
}
```

```
Output:
Generic Class Integer: 1
Generic Class String: Usharani
```

The above Java program employs generics to create instances of a flexible class named test that can accommodate various data types. In the Main class, two instances are instantiated—one with an integer value of 1 and another with a String value "Usharani". The generic class test<T> is designed to store and retrieve values of type T. Consequently, the first instance, t, stores an integer value of 1, and the second instance, t1, stores a String value "Usharani". The output will display "Generic Class Integer: 1" for the t instance and "Generic Class String: Usharani" for the t1 instance.

14.4 GENERIC METHOD

Generics in Java extend beyond classes; they also include generic methods. A generic method is a method that is parameterized with one or more types, allowing it to operate on different types of data. This provides a similar level of flexibility and reusability as generics classes but at the method level.

Program

```
// Define a class named Test with a generic method
class Test {
  // Generic method that accepts parameters of any type
  public <T> void func(T temp) {
  System.out.println("Type: " + temp.getClass().getSimpleName() + ",
     Value: " + temp);
  }
}
// Main class to test the generic method
public class Main {
  void main(String[] args) {
  // Create an instance of Test
  Test test = new Test();
  // Call the generic method with a String argument
  test.func("Usharani"); // Output: Type: String, Value: Usharani
  // Call the generic method with an Integer argument
  test.func(25);    // Output: Type: Integer, Value: 25
  }
}
Output:
Type: String, Value: Usharani
Type: Integer, Value: 25
```

The above Java program illustrates the implementation of a generic method within the test class, demonstrating the capability to work with various data types. In the Main class, an instance of the test class is created, and the generic method func is invoked twice with different types of arguments. The func method, defined in the test class, is declared as a generic method using the syntax public <T> void func(T temp). This allows it to accept parameters of any type, providing flexibility and code reusability. During execution, the method is called first with a String argument ("Usharani") and then with an integer argument (25), showcasing the adaptability of the generic method to handle diverse data types.

14.5 GENERICS CONSTRUCTOR

In the context of generics, a generic class is one that can work with different data types. The type parameter is declared at the class level, affecting the entire class, including its constructors and methods. Generic constructors are constructed within generic classes, and the type parameter is specified at the class level, not at the constructor level. When defining a generic class, type parameters are declared at the class level, influencing the entire class, including its constructors. While constructors themselves cannot be explicitly generic, they leverage the generic type specified at the class level, allowing for flexibility in handling different data types.

In a generic class, constructors can take parameters of the generic type, and the type is specified when creating instances of the class. This ensures that the constructor and other methods within the class operate consistently with the designated type, promoting code reusability and type safety. The type parameter specified at the class level is used within the constructor to define the type of parameters it can accept.

Program

```
// Define a generic class named Test with a generic constructor
class Test<T extends Number> {
  private double x;
  // Generic constructor that converts the provided numeric input to a double
  public Test(T t) {
  this.x = t.doubleValue();
  }
  // Method to display the converted value
  public void display() {
  System.out.println("value: " + x);
  }
}
// Main class to test the generic class
public class Main {
  void main(String[] args) {
  // Create instances of Test with different numeric types
  Test<Integer> t1 = new Test<>(1);  // Integer value
  Test<Float> t2 = new Test<>(11.1F); // Float value
  // Display the converted values
  System.out.println("Number to Double Conversion:");
  t1.display();  // Output: value: 1.0
  t2.display();  // Output: value: 11.100000381469727
  }
}
```

Output

```
Number to Double Conversion:
value: 1.0
value: 11.100000381469727
```

The above Java program showcases the utilization of a generic class named test with a generic constructor designed to convert numeric values to doubles. The test class includes a private double variable x and a generic constructor <T extends Number> test(T t) that dynamically adapts to various numeric types. The constructor intelligently converts the provided numeric input to a double using the doubleValue() method. Additionally, the class features a display method responsible for printing the converted value. In the Main class, the program's entry point, instances of the test class are created. The versatility of the generic constructor is demonstrated by initializing t1 with an integer parameter (1) and t2 with a Float parameter (11.1F). Subsequently, the display method is invoked on each object, resulting in the printed display of the converted values.

14.6 GENERIC INTERFACE

In Java, generic interfaces serve as powerful tools for defining abstract data types and promoting modular, independent manipulation of collections without revealing their underlying details. Unlike classes, generic interfaces exclusively consist of abstract methods, static, and final variables, lacking constructors and instance variables. They facilitate multiple inheritance, allowing classes to implement multiple interfaces and form hierarchies, fostering a more versatile and extensible code structure.

A fundamental distinction lies in the fact that only references, and not objects, can be created directly from interfaces. Objects must be instantiated by implementing classes, which provide concrete implementations for the abstract methods declared in the interface. The use of the “implements” keyword establishes this relationship between a class and the interface it adheres to.

Much like their generic class counterparts, generic interfaces enable the development of flexible and type-safe code that can accommodate various data types. Generic interfaces in Java contribute to the creation of modular and reusable software components, enhancing code maintainability and adaptability to changing requirements.

Syntax

```
// Generic interface A with a type parameter T
interface A<T> {
  void m1(T t);  // Abstract method with the type parameter T
}
```

Where interface A<T> will declare a generic interface named A with a type parameter T. Thee method void m1(T t) will defines an abstract method m1 with a parameter of type T. This method needs to be implemented by any class that implements the interface.

Syntax

```
// Generic class B that implements the generic interface A with the type
parameter T
class B<T> implements A<T> {
  private T obj;  // Class variable to store the value of type T
  // Implementation of the abstract method m1 from interface A
  @Override
  public void m1(T t) {
  this.obj = t;  // Assign the passed value t to the class variable obj
  }
  // Method to display the stored value
  public void display() {
  System.out.println("Stored value: " + obj);
  }
}
```

Where class B<T> implements A<T>. Declares a generic class named B with a type parameter T, and it implements the generic interface A with the same type parameter. Implements the abstract method m1 from the interface, assigning the passed value t to the class variable obj.

14.6.1 Non-Generic Class Implementing Generic Interface

Syntax

```
// Class C implements the generic interface A with Integer as the type
parameter
class C implements A<Integer> {
  private Integer obj;  // Class variable to store the Integer value
  // Implementation of the abstract method m1 from interface A
  @Override
  public void m1(Integer t) {
  this.obj = t;  // Assign the passed value t to the class variable obj
  }
  // Method to display the stored value
  public void display() {
```

```
  System.out.println("Stored value: " + obj);
  }
}
```

Where class C implements A<Integer> will declare a non-generic class named C that implements the generic interface A with a specific type parameter (Integer in this case). public void m1(Integer t) will implement the abstract method m1 from the interface with a specific type (Integer), assigning the passed value t to the class variable obj.

```
public class Main {
  void main(String[] args) {
  // Create an instance of the non-generic class C
  C c = new C();
  c.m1(1); // Assign an Integer value to C
  c.display(); // Output: Stored value in C: 1
  // Create an instance of the generic class B with Integer type
  B<Integer> b1 = new B<>();
  b1.m1(10); // Assign an Integer value to B
  b1.display(); // Output: Stored value in B: 10
  }
}
```

The main method demonstrates creating instances of the generic class B with a type parameter integer and the non-generic class C with a specific type integer. Both classes implement the generic interface A. The values are assigned using the m1 method, and the assigned values are printed.

Program

```
interface A<T> {
  void m1(T t); // Abstract method with the type parameter T
}
class B<T> implements A<T> {
  private T obj; // Class variable to store the value of type T
  // Implementation of the abstract method m1 from interface A
  @Override
  public void m1(T t) {
  this.obj = t; // Assign the passed value t to the class variable obj
  }
  // Method to display the stored value
  public void display() {
  System.out.println("Stored value: " + obj);
  }
}
class C implements A<Integer> {
  private Integer obj; // Class variable to store the Integer value
  // Implementation of the abstract method m1 from interface A
  @Override
  public void m1(Integer t) {
  this.obj = t; // Assign the passed value t to the class variable obj
  }
  // Method to display the stored value
  public void display() {
  System.out.println("Stored value: " + obj);
  }
```

```
}
public class Main {
  void main(String[] args) {
  // Create an instance of the non-generic class C
  C c = new C();
  c.m1(1);  // Assign an Integer value to C
  c.display();  // Output: Stored value in C: 1
  // Create an instance of the generic class B with Integer type
  B<Integer> b1 = new B<>();
  b1.m1(10);  // Assign an Integer value to B
  b1.display();  // Output: Stored value in B: 10
  }
}
```

Output:

```
Stored value: 1
Stored value: 10
```

In the above program, `interface A<T>` defines a generic method `m1(T t)` to be implemented by classes. Class `B<T>` is a generic class that implements `A<T>`, and it stores the passed value `t` of type `T`. Class `C` implements `A<Integer>`, meaning it only works with `Integer` values. In the `main` method, both `C` and `B<Integer>` objects are created, their `m1` methods are called with values, and the stored values are displayed using the `display()` method. The output shows the stored values: 1 for class `C` and 10 for class `B`.

Program

```
// Define the generic interface sample
interface sample<T extends Comparable<T>> {
  T min(); // Method to find minimum value
  T max(); // Method to find maximum value
}
// Implement the sample interface in the test class
class test<T extends Comparable<T>> implements sample<T> {
  private T[] array; // Array to hold the elements
  // Constructor to initialize the array
  public test(T[] array) {
  this.array = array;
  }
  // Method to find the minimum value in the array
  @Override
  public T min() {
  T minValue = array[0];
  for (T element : array) {
    if (element.compareTo(minValue) < 0) {
    minValue = element;
    }
  }
  return minValue;
  }
  // Method to find the maximum value in the array
  @Override
  public T max() {
  T maxValue = array[0];
  for (T element : array) {
```

```
    if (element.compareTo(maxValue) > 0) {
    maxValue = element;
    }
  }
  return maxValue;
  }
}
// Main class to test the functionality
public class Main {
  void main(String[] args) {
  // Create an array of Integer elements
  Integer[] numbers = {5, 8, 2, 10, 7};
  // Instantiate the test class with Integer type
  test<Integer> testObject = new test<>(numbers);
  // Find and print the minimum and maximum values
  System.out.println("Minimum value: " + testObject.min()); //
     Output: Minimum value: 2
  System.out.println("Maximum value: " + testObject.max()); //
     Output: Maximum value: 10
  }
}
```

Output

```
Minimum value: 2
Maximum value: 10
```

The above Java program demonstrates the use of a generic interface named sample, which extends the Comparable interface. The sample interface declares two abstract methods, min() and max(), specifying that the generic type T must extend Comparable<T>. The goal is to find the minimum and maximum values within an array of generic elements. The sample interface includes two abstract methods, min() and max(), which return the minimum and maximum values, respectively. The generic type T must extend the Comparable<T> interface to ensure that elements of type T can be compared. The test class implements the sample interface with the same generic type T. It includes a constructor to initialize the array of generic elements and provides implementations for the min() and max() methods using the compareTo method for comparisons. In the Main class, an array of integer elements is created. An object of the test class is instantiated with integer as the generic type, and the array is passed to its constructor. The min() and max() methods are then called on the object, and the results are printed.

14.6.2 Generic Class Extending Generic Interface

A generic class (GenericClass) extends a generic superclass (GenericSuperClass) and implements two generic interfaces (GenericInterface1 and GenericInterface2). The type parameters of the generic class are a union of the type parameters of the generic superclass and the generic interfaces.

Syntax

```
// Generic superclass with one type parameter
class GenericSuperClass<T> {
  // Class members and methods
}
// Generic interface with two type parameters
interface GenericInterface1<T1, T2> {
  }
```

```
// Another generic interface with two type parameters
interface GenericInterface2<T3, T4> {
  }
// Generic class extending a generic superclass and implementing multiple
      generic interfaces
class GenericClass<T1, T2, T3, T4>
  extends GenericSuperClass<T1>
  implements GenericInterface1<T1, T2>, GenericInterface2<T3, T4> {
}
```

The above Java syntax exemplifies the flexibility of generic class inheritance by showcasing a scenario where a generic class, GenericClass, extends a generic superclass, GenericSuperClass, and simultaneously implements two generic interfaces, GenericInterface1 and GenericInterface2. The type parameters of the generic class serve as a union of the type parameters inherited from the generic superclass and those specified by the implemented generic interfaces. The GenericSuperClass introduces a single type parameter, while GenericInterface1 and GenericInterface2 contribute two type parameters each to the overall set. By extending the generic superclass and implementing multiple generic interfaces, the GenericClass is equipped with a comprehensive set of type parameters, allowing it to seamlessly integrate the features and constraints imposed by both its superclass and interfaces.

Program

```
// Generic interface to find max and min elements
interface ArrayOperations<T extends Comparable<T>> {
  T findMax(T[] array);
  T findMin(T[] array);
}
// Generic class implementing the ArrayOperations interface
class ArrayProcessor<T extends Comparable<T>> implements ArrayOperations<T> {
  @Override
  public T findMax(T[] array) {
  if (array == null || array.length == 0) {
    return null; // handle empty or null array
  }
  T max = array[0];
  for (T element : array) {
    if (element.compareTo(max) > 0) {
    max = element;
    }
  }
  return max;
  }
  @Override
  public T findMin(T[] array) {
  if (array == null || array.length == 0) {
    return null; // handle empty or null array
  }
  T min = array[0];
  for (T element : array) {
    if (element.compareTo(min) < 0) {
    min = element;
    }
  }
```

```
  return min;
  }
}
// Main class to test the functionality
public class Main {
  void main(String[] args) {
  // Integer array example
  Integer[] intArray = {3, 5, 1, 9, 2};
  ArrayProcessor<Integer> intProcessor = new ArrayProcessor<>();
  System.out.println("Max Integer: " + intProcessor.findMax(intArray));
  System.out.println("Min Integer: " + intProcessor.findMin(intArray));
  // String array example
  String[] strArray = {"this", "is", "to", "test"};
  ArrayProcessor<String> strProcessor = new ArrayProcessor<>();
  System.out.println("Max String: " + strProcessor.findMax(strArray));
  System.out.println("Min String: " + strProcessor.findMin(strArray));
  }
}
```

Output:

```
Max Integer: 9
Min Integer: 1
Max String: to
Min String: is
```

The above program defines a generic interface `ArrayOperations<T>` with methods to find the maximum and minimum elements in an array, where `T` extends `Comparable<T>`. The `ArrayProcessor<T>` class implements this interface, comparing elements in the array to find the max and min.

14.7 GENERICS AND INHERITANCE

Java Generics supports three level of inheritance 1)Singe 2)Multilevel 3) Multiple

14.7.1 Single-Level Inheritance

In Java, generic single-level inheritance involves creating a subclass that inherits from a generic superclass. The syntax for generic single-level inheritance is similar to regular class inheritance, with the addition of specifying the generic type parameter.

Program

```
// Generic superclass with a type parameter T
class Test<T> {
  private T temp;
  // Constructor to initialize the member variable
  public Test(T temp) {
  this.temp = temp;
  }
  // Method to retrieve the value of the member variable
  public T gettemp() {
  return temp;
  }
}
```

```
// Generic subclass extending Test with the same type parameter T
class Sample<T> extends Test<T> {
  // Constructor to call the superclass constructor
  public Sample(T temp) {
  super(temp);
  }
  // Method specific to the Sample class
  public void display() {
  System.out.println("Display method in Sample class");
  }
}
// Main class to demonstrate usage
public class Main {
  void main(String[] args) {
  // Create an instance of Sample with Integer type
  Sample<Integer> sample = new Sample<>(1);
  // Call the gettemp() method from the superclass
  System.out.println("Value from Test class: " + sample.gettemp());
  // Call the display() method from the subclass
  sample.display();
  }
}
```

Output:

```
Value from Test class: 1
Display method in Sample class
```

The Test class is a generic superclass that includes a type parameter T. It has a member variable temp of type T, and a constructor Test(T temp) to initialize this member variable. Additionally, there is a method gettemp() that retrieves the value stored in the temp variable. The Sample class is a subclass of Test and also a generic class with a type parameter T. It includes a constructor Sample(T temp) that calls the superclass constructor using super(temp), ensuring the proper initialization of the inherited member variable. The subclass introduces an additional method display(), which is specific to the Sample class. In the Main class, an instance of the subclass Sample is created with integer as the generic type, and the value 1 is passed to the constructor. The program then calls methods from both the superclass (gettemp()) and the subclass (display()). The output displays the data stored in the subclass and invokes the additional method specific to the subclass.

14.7.2 Multilevel Inheritance

The sub class inherits the properties of the super class and this sub class can act as a super class to another sub class.

Program

```
// Generic superclass Shape with a type parameter T
class Shape<T> {
  protected T dimensions;
  // Constructor to initialize the dimensions
  public Shape(T dimensions) {
  this.dimensions = dimensions;
  }
  // Method to get dimensions
```

```
  public T getDimensions() {
  return dimensions;
  }
}
// First subclass TwoDShape extending Shape
class TwoDShape<T> extends Shape<T> {
  // Constructor calling the superclass constructor
  public TwoDShape(T dimensions) {
  super(dimensions);
  }
  // Method to display information about dimensions
  public void displayInfo() {
  System.out.println("Dimensions: " + getDimensions());
  }
}
// Second subclass Rectangle extending TwoDShape with specific type Double
class Rectangle extends TwoDShape<Double[]> {
  private Double length;
  private Double width;
  // Constructor initializing length and width
  public Rectangle(Double length, Double width) {
  super(new Double[]{length, width});
  this.length = length;
  this.width = width;
  }
  // Method to calculate area of the rectangle
  public double calculateArea() {
  return length * width;
  }
  // Overriding displayInfo method to include area calculation
  @Override
  public void displayInfo() {
  super.displayInfo();
  System.out.println("Length: " + length);
  System.out.println("Width: " + width);
  System.out.println("Area: " + calculateArea());
  }
}
// Main class to demonstrate the usage
public class Main {
  void main(String[] args) {
  // Create an instance of Rectangle with dimensions specified as Double
  Rectangle rectangle = new Rectangle(5.0, 3.0);
  // Call displayInfo method to show details about the rectangle
  rectangle.displayInfo();
  }
}
```

Output:

```
Dimensions: [Ljava.lang.Double;@61baa894
Length: 5.0
Width: 3.0
Area: 15.0
```

In the above program the generic superclass, Shape, encapsulates the common properties and behaviors of shapes with a generic dimensions field. The first subclass, TwoDShape, extends the generic superclass and represents a generic 2D shape, adding a method to display information about its dimensions. The second subclass, Rectangle, further extends the hierarchy and specializes as a rectangle, introducing a method to calculate its area based on length and width. In the main method, an instance of the Rectangle class is created with dimensions specified as Double. The program then calls the displayInfo method on this instance, showcasing the overridden method in the Rectangle class that provides detailed information about the rectangle, including its dimensions and calculated area.

Program

```
// Generic superclass Test with a type parameter T
class Test<T> {
  protected T temp;
  // Constructor to initialize the temp variable
  public Test(T temp) {
  this.temp = temp;
  }
  // Method to retrieve the value of temp
  public T gett() {
  return temp;
  }
  // Method to display the value with a generic message
  public void display() {
  System.out.println("value in superclass " + temp);
  }
}
// Subclass Test1 extending Test
class Test1<T> extends Test<T> {
  public Test1(T temp) {
  super(temp);
  }
  // Specific method for Test1
  public void get1() {
  System.out.println("value in subclass1 " + temp);
  }
  // Overriding display method with subclass-specific message
  @Override
  public void display() {
  super.display();
  System.out.println("Specific display for Test1");
  }
}
// Subclass Test2 extending Test1
class Test2<T> extends Test1<T> {
  public Test2(T temp) {
  super(temp);
  }
  // Specific method for Test2
  public void get2() {
  System.out.println("value in subclass2 " + temp);
  }
  // Overriding display method with subclass-specific message
  @Override
  public void display() {
```

```
  super.display();
  System.out.println("Specific display for Test2");
  }
}
// Subclass Test3 extending Test2
class Test3<T> extends Test2<T> {
  public Test3(T temp) {
  super(temp);
  }
  // Specific method for Test3
  public void get3() {
  System.out.println("value in subclass3 " + temp);
  }
  // Overriding display method with subclass-specific message
  @Override
  public void display() {
  super.display();
  System.out.println("Specific display for Test3");
  }
}
// Subclass Test4 extending Test3
class Test4<T> extends Test3<T> {
  public Test4(T temp) {
  super(temp);
  }
  // Specific method for Test4
  public void get4() {
  System.out.println("value in subclass4 " + temp);
  }
  // Overriding display method with subclass-specific message
  @Override
  public void display() {
  super.display();
  System.out.println("Specific display for Test4");
  }
}
// Subclass Test5 extending Test4
class Test5<T> extends Test4<T> {
  public Test5(T temp) {
  super(temp);
  }
  // Specific method for Test5
  public void get5() {
  System.out.println("value in subclass5 " + temp);
  }
  // Overriding display method with subclass-specific message
  @Override
  public void display() {
  super.display();
  System.out.println("Specific display for Test5");
  }
}
// Main class to demonstrate the usage
public class Main {
  void main(String[] args) {
```

```
  // Create an instance of Test5 with a specific model ("usharani123")
  Test5<String> test5 = new Test5<>("usharani123");
  // Call methods from all levels of the hierarchy
  test5.get1();
  test5.get2();
  test5.get3();
  test5.get4();
  test5.get5();
  test5.display();  // Calls overridden display method
  }
}
```

Output:

```
value in subclass1 usharani123
value in subclass2 usharani123
value in subclass3 usharani123
value in subclass4 usharani123
value in subclass5 usharani123
value in superclass usharani123
Specific display for Test1
Specific display for Test2
Specific display for Test3
Specific display for Test4
Specific display for Test5
```

The above Java code showcases a multilevel inheritance structure with generic classes, representing a hierarchical chain of subclasses inheriting from a generic superclass. The generic superclass, named Test, introduces a type parameter T to represent the data type of its instance variable temp.

Subsequent subclasses, denoted as Test1 through Test5, extend the previous class, forming a cascade of specialization. Each subclass inherits the characteristics of its superclass while introducing additional methods (get1() through get5()) that print the value of temp with subclass-specific messages. Additionally, each subclass overrides the display() method, invoking the superclass's display method and appending subclass-specific display messages. In the Main class, an instance of the most specialized class, Test5, is created with a specific model ("usharani123").

14.7.3 Multiple Inheritance

In multiple inheritance the subclass inherits the properties from more than two super generic classes.

Program

```
public class Main {
  public static class BaseClass {
  int calculateBaseValue() {
    return 1;
  }
  }
  public static interface Calculatable {
  int performCalculation();
  }
  private static class Subclass extends BaseClass implements Calculatable {
  public int performCalculation() {
    return 100;
  }
```

```
  // Correct the class name here (use Subclass instead of SubClass)
  public static <T extends BaseClass & Calculatable> T
  createCalculatableInstance() {
    return (T) new Subclass();  // Fixed the case of 'Subclass'
  }
  }
  void main(String... args) {
  // Adjust the call to Subclass.createCalculatableInstance()
  BaseClass baseInstance = Subclass.createCalculatableInstance();
  System.out.println(baseInstance.calculateBaseValue());
  }
}
```

Output:

```
1
```

The Main class encapsulates the program logic, containing a BaseClass as a foundational class with a method to calculate a base value. The Calculatable interface defines a contract for performing calculations, and the SubClass serves as an implementation of both the BaseClass and Calculatable. The generic method createCalculatableInstance() emphasizes its purpose of generating instances that adhere to both the BaseClass and Calculatable requirements.

14.7.4 Non-Generic Class Extend a Generic Class

In Java, a non-generic class cannot directly extend a generic class unless the generic class has a predefined or specified type for its type parameter.

Syntax

```
class GenericSuperClass<T> {
}
class NonGenericClass extends GenericSuperClass<T> {
}
class A{}
class GenericSuperClass<A> {
}
class NonGenericClass1 extends GenericSuperClass<A> {
}
```

The above syntax highlights the restrictions on the inheritance relationship between generic and non-generic classes. The generic superclass, GenericSuperClass<T>, introduces a type parameter T, and an attempt is made to have a non-generic class, NonGenericClass, extend it without specifying a type for the parameter. This results in a compile-time error, illustrating that a non-generic class cannot directly extend a generic class without providing a concrete type for its generic parameter. A generic class, GenericSuperClass1<A>, has a predefined type A as its type parameter. In this case, a non-generic class, NonGenericClass1, can successfully extend GenericSuperClass1<A> without encountering a compile-time error. This distinction emphasizes that direct inheritance from a generic class is allowed only when the generic class already has predefined types as its type parameters. In Java, it is possible for a non-generic class to extend a generic class by using the raw type. This essentially means removing the type parameters from the generic class. However, doing so triggers compiler warnings, as it may lead to unchecked type safety.

Program

```
// Generic class with a type parameter T
class GenericClass<T> {
  // Generic member variable
  private T data;
  // Constructor to initialize the generic member variable
  public GenericClass(T data) {
  this.data = data;
  }
  // Method to retrieve the generic data
  public T getData() {
  return data;
  }
  // Method to display the data
  public void display() {
  System.out.println("Data: " + data);
  }
}
// Non-generic class extending the generic class using a raw type
class NonGenericClass extends GenericClass {
  // Constructor
  public NonGenericClass(Object data) {
  // Using raw type here, no specific type is mentioned
  super(data); // Calls the constructor of GenericClass with a raw type
  }
  // Overriding the display method (optional)
  @Override
  public void display() {
  System.out.println("Non-generic class extending generic class with raw
  type.");
  super.display(); // Calling the parent class display method
  }
}
public class Main {
  void main(String[] args) {
  // Creating an instance of the non-generic class, passing a string
  NonGenericClass nonGeneric = new NonGenericClass("usharani");
  nonGeneric.display(); // Output may work fine, but with unchecked warnings
  // Creating another instance of the non-generic class, passing an integer
  NonGenericClass nonGeneric2 = new NonGenericClass(1);
  nonGeneric2.display(); // Works, but again, unchecked type safety
  }
}
```

Output:

```
Non-generic class extending generic class with raw type.
Data: usharani
Non-generic class extending generic class with raw type.
Data: 1
```

The generic class, GenericClass<T>, is extended by the non-generic class, NonGenericClass, which omits the specification of type parameters. While this approach is permissible, the compiler issues warnings to alert developers about potential unchecked type safety.

Syntax

```
// Generic superclass with a bounded type parameter T (T must extend Number)
class GenericSuperClass<T extends Number> {
  // Generic member variable
  private T value;
  }
// Subclass specifying the upper bound type (Number)
class GenericSubClass1 extends GenericSuperClass<Number> {
  // Constructor
  }
// Subclass using a specific type (Integer)
class GenericSubClass2 extends GenericSuperClass<Integer> {
}
// Attempt to declare a new bounded type parameter in the subclass (INVALID)
class GenericSubClass3<T extends Number> extends GenericSuperClass<T
extends Number> { // Compile-time error

}
```

In the above Java syntax, the generic superclass, GenericSuperClass<T extends Number>, imposes a constraint that the type parameter T must be a subclass of the Number class. The subsequent generic subclasses, GenericSubClass1 and GenericSubClass2, correctly replace the type parameter with its upper bound (Number) and a subclass of its upper bound (Integer), respectively. However, the attempt in GenericSubClass3 to specify a bounded type parameter directly within the subclass declaration results in a compile-time error. This highlights the requirement to replace the type parameter with an actual type or a wildcard, rather than declaring a new type parameter within the subclass.

In Java, generic methods in a superclass can be overridden in a subclass just like regular methods.

Syntax

```
class GenericClass {
<T> void genericMethod (T t) {
System.out.println(1);
}
}
class NonGenericClass extends GenericClass {
@Override
<T> void genericMethod (T t) { System.out.println(2);
}
}
public class GenericsInJava {
void main(String[] args) {
new GenericClass().genericMethod("testing");// Output: 1
new NonGenericClass().genericMethod("test String"); // Output: 2
}
}
```

In the superclass GenericClass, a generic method named genericMethod is defined with a type parameter T, and it prints "1" to the console. The subclass NonGenericClass extends GenericClass and overrides the genericMethod with its own implementation that prints "2" to the console. In the main program, instances of both GenericClass and NonGenericClass are created, and the genericMethod is invoked with a String argument on each instance.

14.7.5 Generic Class Extends Non-Generic Class

In Java, a generic class can indeed extend a non-generic class. The generic class can choose to use or ignore the generic type parameter provided by its superclass.

Syntax

```
class NonGenericClass {}
class GenericClass<T> extends  NonGenericClass {}
```

The syntax showcases the ability of a generic class to extend a non-generic class. The NonGenericClass serves as a straightforward non-generic class without any type parameters. The subsequent GenericClass<T> extends this non-generic class, providing the option to utilize or disregard the generic type parameter T inherited from its superclass.

14.7.6 Generic Class Extends Generic Class

In Java, a generic class can extend another generic class by using the same or different type parameters. For example, if class `A<T>` is a generic class, class `B<T>` can extend it by declaring `class B<T> extends A<T>`. This allows class `B` to inherit the functionality and properties of class `A` while maintaining type safety and flexibility through the use of generics. By sharing the type parameter `T`, both classes can handle the same type of data, ensuring that the extended class can leverage the generic methods and fields of the parent class seamlessly.

Syntax

```
// Generic superclass with a single type parameter T
class GenericSuperClass<T> {
  }
// First subclass maintaining the same type parameter T
class GenericSubClass1<T> extends GenericSuperClass<T> {
  }
// Second subclass introducing an additional type parameter V
class GenericSubClass2<T, V> extends GenericSuperClass<T> {
    }
// Invalid subclass (compile-time error) with different type parameters T1, T2
class GenericSubClass3<T1, T2> extends GenericSuperClass<T1> {
  // This would cause a compile-time error if the number of parameters
differs
}
```

The syntax shows the principles of generic class inheritance, specifically when a generic class extends another generic class. In this context, adherence to certain rules ensures the coherence of type parameters within the inheritance hierarchy. The generic superclass, GenericSuperClass<T>, sets the foundation with a single type parameter. The first generic subclass, GenericSubClass1<T>, appropriately maintains the same type parameter as its superclass. The second generic subclass, GenericSubClass2<T, V>, demonstrates the extensibility by introducing an additional type parameter, V, while still retaining the original parameter, T. However, the attempt to create a third generic subclass, GenericSubClass3<T1, T2>, results in a compile-time error since it introduces different type parameters, violating the requirement for at least the same type and the same number of parameters as the superclass. This showcases the intricacies of managing type parameters in generic class hierarchies, providing developers with a powerful yet rule-governed tool for designing flexible and type-safe code structures. When a generic class extends another generic class, the type parameters are passed from the subclass to the superclass, similar to constructor chaining. In the syntax, the type parameter 'T' in 'GenericSuperClass' is effectively replaced by 'String' when the 'GenericSubClass' is instantiated with 'String' as its type parameter.

Program

```
// Generic superclass with a type parameter T
class GenericSuperClass<T> {
  T t;  // Field to hold the value of type T
  // Constructor to initialize the t field
  GenericSuperClass(T t) {
  this.t = t;
  }
  // Getter method to retrieve the value of t
  T getT() {
  return t;
  }
}
// Generic subclass that extends GenericSuperClass with the same type par-
ameter T
class GenericSubClass<T> extends GenericSuperClass<T> {
  // Constructor of subclass calling the superclass constructor
  GenericSubClass(T t) {
  super(t);  // Passing the value to the superclass
  }
  // Method to display the value of t
  void display() {
  System.out.println("Value in GenericSubClass: " + getT());
  }
}
// Main class to run the program
public class Main {
  void main(String[] args) {
  // Creating an instance of GenericSubClass with String type
  GenericSubClass<String> obj = new GenericSubClass< String >("Usharani");
  // Displaying the value in the subclass
  obj.display();  // Output: "Value in GenericSubClass: Usharani"
  }
}
Output:
Value in GenericSubClass: Usharani
```

In the above program The GenericSubClass is parameterized with type 'T'. When you create an instance of GenericSubClass<String>, you are specifying 'String' as the actual type parameter for 'T'. The constructor of GenericSubClass then calls the constructor of GenericSuperClass using super(t), effectively passing the 'String' type parameter to the superclass. Consequently, the t field in the superclass is of type 'String' in this instance.

14.8 GENERIC WILDCARDS

Wildcards in Java generics are denoted by the question mark symbol (?). They are used to represent an unknown type in generic programming. Wildcards provide more flexibility when dealing with generic types, allowing for the creation of more versatile and reusable code.

There are three types of wildcards in Java generics:

I. Unbounded Wildcard (?):
Denoted by a question mark (?), it represents an unknown type. It can be used as a type for a parameter, local variable, or field.
Example: List<?> myList where myList is a list of an unknown type.
II. Wildcard with an Upper Bound (? extends T):
Denoted by? extends T, where T is a specific type. It represents an unknown type that is a subtype of the specified type T.
Example: List<? extends Number> numbers where numbers is a list of any type that extends Number.
III. Wildcard with a Lower Bound (? super T):
Denoted by? super T, where T is a specific type. It represents an unknown type that is a supertype of the specified type T.
Example: List<? super Integer> integerList where integerList is a list of any type that is a supertype of Integer.

Wildcards are particularly useful in situations where the exact type is unknown or where you want to create generic methods or classes that can operate on a range of types. They enhance the flexibility and genericity of code, allowing for more versatile programming constructs.

Example for upper-bounded wildcard

```
import java.util.List;
import java.util.ArrayList;
public class UpperBoundedWildcardExample {
  // Method to calculate the sum of numbers in a list using an upper-bounded
  wildcard
  public static double calculateSum(List<? extends Number> numbers) {
  double sum = 0.0;
  for (Number number : numbers) {
    sum += number.doubleValue(); // Convert to double and add to sum
  }
  return sum;
  }
  void main(String[] args) {
  // Create a list of Integer
  List<Integer> integerList = new ArrayList<>();
  integerList.add(10);
  integerList.add(20);
  integerList.add(30);
  integerList.add(40);
  // Create a list of Double
  List<Double> doubleList = new ArrayList<>();
  doubleList.add(13.2);
  doubleList.add(15.6);
  doubleList.add(9.7);
  doubleList.add(22.5);
  // Calculate and print the sum of Integer list
  System.out.println("Total sum of integers: " + calculateSum(integerList));
  // Calculate and print the sum of Double list
  System.out.println("Total sum of doubles: " + calculateSum(doubleList));
  }
}
```

```
Output:
Total sum of integers : 100.0
Total sum of doubles : 61.0
```

The above Java code demonstrates the use of a generic method with an upper-bounded wildcard to calculate the sum of elements in a list. The class is named Main, and it includes a main method where two lists, i and d, are created with integer and double elements, respectively. The generic method cal takes a list of numbers with an upper-bounded wildcard (List<? extends Number>) and calculates the sum of its elements. The results are printed for both the integer and double lists.

Lower Bound Wildcard example

```
import java.util.List;
import java.util.ArrayList;
public class LowerBoundedWildcardExample {
  // Method to print elements of a list using a lower-bounded wildcard
  public static void printList(List<? super Integer> list) {
  for (Object element : list) {
    System.out.println(element);
  }
  }
  void main(String[] args) {
  // Create a list of Integer
  List<Integer> integerList = new ArrayList<>();
  integerList.add(10);
  integerList.add(20);
  integerList.add(30);
  integerList.add(40);
  // Create a list of Number (superclass of Integer)
  List<Number> numberList = new ArrayList<>();
  numberList.add(1);
  numberList.add(2.5);
  numberList.add(3.14);
  // Print the elements of the integer list
  System.out.println("Contents of integerList:");
  printList(integerList);
  // Print the elements of the number list
  System.out.println("Contents of numberList:");
  printList(numberList);
  }
}
Output:
Contents of integerList:
10
20
30
40
Contents of numberList:
1
2.5
3.14
```

The above Java code demonstrates the use of a lower-bounded wildcard in the context of generic programming. In the Main class, there are two scenarios illustrated with lists of integers and numbers.

The method prin is designed to accept a list of objects of type integer or any of its superclasses. The main method initiates two lists—one of integers (i) and another of numbers (n). It then invokes the prin method, passing these lists as arguments.

Un Bound wildcard Example

```
import java.util.List;
import java.util.ArrayList;
public class UnboundedWildcardExample {
  // Method to print elements of a list using an unbounded wildcard
  public static void printList(List<?> list) {
  for (Object element : list) {
    System.out.println(element);
  }
  }
  void main(String[] args) {
  // Create a list of Integer
  List<Integer> integerList = new ArrayList<>();
  integerList.add(1);
  integerList.add(2);
  integerList.add(3);
  // Create a list of Double
  List<Double> doubleList = new ArrayList<>();
  doubleList.add(1.1);
  doubleList.add(2.2);
  doubleList.add(3.3);
  // Print the elements of the integer list
  System.out.println("Contents of integerList:");
  printList(integerList);
  // Print the elements of the double list
  System.out.println("Contents of doubleList:");
  printList(doubleList);
  }
}
```

Output:

```
Contents of integerList:
1
2
3
Contents of doubleList:
1.1
2.2
3.3
```

The above Java code demonstrates the use of unbounded wildcards in generic programming. In the Main class, the method prin employs an unbounded wildcard (<?>) to accept lists of any type. This is showcased through two instances: one involving a list of integers (i), and the other with a list of doubles (d). For the integer list (i), the method prin accepts it as an argument, leveraging the unbounded wildcard to handle the unknown type contained in the list. Similarly, for the double list (d), the same method is applied, emphasizing the generic nature of the code.

14.9 MEDICAL APPLICATIONS

14.9.1 Case Study 1

Liver cancer, also known as hepatic cancer, originates in the cells of the liver, the largest internal organ responsible for vital functions like detoxification, protein synthesis, and digestion. The most common type, hepatocellular carcinoma, begins in the main liver cell type called hepatocytes. Risk factors include chronic hepatitis B or C infection, cirrhosis, heavy alcohol use, and fatty liver disease. Symptoms often include weight loss, abdominal pain, jaundice, and swelling. Early detection and treatment are crucial for improving outcomes and can involve surgery, radiation, or targeted therapies.

Program

```
import java.util.ArrayList;
import java.util.List;
class DNAFragment {
  private double size;
  public DNAFragment(double size) {
  this.size = size;
  }
  public double getSize() {
  return size;
  }
}
class BloodTestResult<T> {
  private List<T> dnaFragments;
  public BloodTestResult() {
  this.dnaFragments = new ArrayList<>();
  }
  public void addDNAFragment(T dnaFragment) {
  dnaFragments.add(dnaFragment);
  }
  public List<T> getDNAFragments() {
  return dnaFragments;
  }
}
public class LiverCancerDetector {
  public static boolean detectLiverCancer(BloodTestResult<DNAFragment>
      bloodTestResult) {
  List<DNAFragment> dnaFragments = bloodTestResult.getDNAFragments();
  boolean hasVariedSize = false;
  for (int i = 0; i < dnaFragments.size(); i++) {
    for (int j = i + 1; j < dnaFragments.size(); j++) {
    if   (Math.abs(dnaFragments.get(i).getSize()   -   dnaFragments.get(j).
getSize()) > 0.1) {
      hasVariedSize = true;
      break;
    }
    }
    if (hasVariedSize) {
    break;
    }
  }
```

```
  return hasVariedSize;
  }
  void main(String[] args) {
  BloodTestResult<DNAFragment> bloodTestResult = new BloodTestResult<>();
  // Add DNA fragments to the blood test result
  bloodTestResult.addDNAFragment(new DNAFragment(1.0));
  bloodTestResult.addDNAFragment(new DNAFragment(1.1));
  bloodTestResult.addDNAFragment(new DNAFragment(1.2));
  bloodTestResult.addDNAFragment(new DNAFragment(1.3));
  boolean hasLiverCancer = detectLiverCancer(bloodTestResult);
  if (hasLiverCancer) {
    System.out.println("Liver cancer detected");
  } else {
    System.out.println("No liver cancer detected");
  }
  }
}
```

The `LiverCancerDetector` program defines a `DNAFragment` class representing each fragment's size and a `BloodTestResult` class to manage a list of these fragments. The `detectLiverCancer` method compares sizes of DNA fragments in the `BloodTestResult` instance and determines if any pair differs by more than 0.1 units. If such variability is found, it indicates potential irregularities associated with liver cancer. In the `main` method, the program initializes a `BloodTestResult` object with various DNA fragment sizes and calls `detectLiverCancer` to output either "Liver cancer detected" or "No liver cancer detected" based on the analysis of fragment size variations.

14.9.2 Case Study 2

Blood cancer, also known as hematologic cancer, affects the production and function of blood cells. The three main types are leukemia, lymphoma, and myeloma, each targeting different components of the blood and lymphatic systems. Common symptoms include fatigue, fever, frequent infections, and unexplained weight loss. Risk factors can include genetic predispositions, exposure to certain chemicals, and previous chemotherapy or radiation treatment. Early diagnosis and treatment, which may involve chemotherapy, radiation, or stem cell transplants, are vital for improving survival rates.

Program

```
import java.util.ArrayList;
import java.util.List;
class Gene {
  private String name;
  private String sequence;
  public Gene(String name, String sequence) {
  this.name = name;
  this.sequence = sequence;
  }
  public String getName() {
  return name;
  }
  public String getSequence() {
  return sequence;
  }
}
```

```
class BloodTestResult<T> {
  private List<T> genes;
  public BloodTestResult() {
  this.genes = new ArrayList<>();
  }
  public void addGene(T gene) {
  genes.add(gene);
  }
  public List<T> getGenes() {
  return genes;
  }
}
public class BloodCancerDetector {
  public static <T extends Gene> boolean detectBloodCancer(BloodTestResul
t<T> bloodTestResult) {
  List<T> genes = bloodTestResult.getGenes();
  boolean hasMutatedGene = false;
  for (T gene : genes) {
    if (isMutated(gene.getSequence())) {
    hasMutatedGene = true;
    break;
    }
  }
  return hasMutatedGene;
  }
  private static boolean isMutated(String sequence) {
  // Simple mutation detection logic: checks if the sequence contains "ATG"
  or "TAG"
  return sequence.contains("ATG") || sequence.contains("TAG");
  }
  void main(String[] args) {
  BloodTestResult<Gene> bloodTestResult = new BloodTestResult<>();
  // Add genes to the blood test result
  bloodTestResult.addGene(new Gene("Gene1", "ATGCGCTAG"));
  bloodTestResult.addGene(new Gene("Gene2", "TAGCTAGCT"));
  bloodTestResult.addGene(new Gene("Gene3", "CGCTAGCTA"));
  boolean hasBloodCancer = detectBloodCancer(bloodTestResult);
  if (hasBloodCancer) {
    System.out.println("Blood cancer detected");
  } else {
    System.out.println("No blood cancer detected");
  }
  }
}
```

This Java program encapsulates genetic information with attributes for name and sequence. The `BloodTestResult<T>` class manages a list of genes and provides methods to add genes and retrieve them. The `detectBloodCancer` method uses a simple mutation detection logic to check for specific sequences ("ATG" or "TAG") in each gene's sequence. In the `main` method, genes are added to a `BloodTestResult` instance, and `detectBloodCancer` is invoked to determine if blood cancer-associated mutations are present, outputting a detection result accordingly.

14.9.3 Case Study 3

Blood impurity, often referred to as blood contamination or toxin buildup, occurs when harmful substances accumulate in the bloodstream. This can result from various factors, including poor diet, exposure to environmental pollutants, infections, or underlying health conditions like liver or kidney dysfunction. The parameters considered for blood impurity detection are the levels of hemoglobin and the count of white blood cells.

- Hemoglobin Level: Impurity detection for hemoglobin checks if the level falls outside the normal range of 12.0 to 16.0 g/dL.
- White Blood Cell Count:. The impurity detection for white blood cells verifies if the count is below 4000 cells/μL or above 11000 cells/μL.

```
import java.util.ArrayList;
import java.util.List;
interface BloodComponent<T> {
  T getComponent();
}
class Hemoglobin implements BloodComponent<Double> {
  private double level;
  public Hemoglobin(double level) {
  this.level = level;
  }
  @Override
  public Double getComponent() {
  return level;
  }
}
class WhiteBloodCell implements BloodComponent<Integer> {
  private int count;
  public WhiteBloodCell(int count) {
  this.count = count;
  }
  @Override
  public Integer getComponent() {
  return count;
  }
}
class BloodImpurityDetector<T> {
  private List<BloodComponent<T>> bloodComponents;
  public BloodImpurityDetector() {
  this.bloodComponents = new ArrayList<>();
  }
  public void addBloodComponent(BloodComponent<T> bloodComponent) {
  bloodComponents.add(bloodComponent);
  }
  public boolean detectImpurity() {
  for (BloodComponent<T> bloodComponent : bloodComponents) {
    if (isImpure(bloodComponent.getComponent())) {
    return true;
    }
  }
  return false;
  }
```

```
  private boolean isImpure(T component) {
  // Simple impurity detection logic: checks if the component value is
  outside a normal range
  if (component instanceof Double) {
    return (Double) component < 12.0 || (Double) component > 16.0;
  } else if (component instanceof Integer) {
    return (Integer) component < 4000 || (Integer) component > 11000;
  }
  return false;
  }
}
public class BloodImpurityDetection {
  void main(String[] args) {
  BloodImpurityDetector<Double> hemoglobinDetector = new
      BloodImpurityDetector<>();
  hemoglobinDetector.addBloodComponent(new Hemoglobin(10.5));
  hemoglobinDetector.addBloodComponent(new Hemoglobin(14.2));
  BloodImpurityDetector<Integer> whiteBloodCellDetector = new
      BloodImpurityDetector<>();
  whiteBloodCellDetector.addBloodComponent(new WhiteBloodCell(3500));
  whiteBloodCellDetector.addBloodComponent(new WhiteBloodCell(9000));
  boolean hasHemoglobinImpurity = hemoglobinDetector.detectImpurity();
  boolean hasWhiteBloodCellImpurity = whiteBloodCellDetector.
    detectImpurity();
  if (hasHemoglobinImpurity || hasWhiteBloodCellImpurity) {
    System.out.println("Blood impurity detected");
  } else {
    System.out.println("No blood impurity detected");
  }
  }
}
```

The `BloodImpurityDetection` program utilizes Java Generics and interfaces to simulate the detection of blood impurities. It defines the `BloodComponent<T>` interface with methods for encapsulating different types of blood components (`Hemoglobin` and `WhiteBloodCell`). The `BloodImpurityDetector<T>` class implements logic to add these components, check for impurities based on defined normal ranges, and determine if impurities exist. In the `main` method, instances of `BloodImpurityDetector` are instantiated for `Double` (hemoglobin) and `Integer` (white blood cells), where sample data is added and impurity detection is performed. Depending on the results, it outputs either "Blood impurity detected" or "No blood impurity detected" to indicate the presence or absence of abnormalities in the blood components being monitored.

15 Collections

15.1 INTRODUCTION

In Java, collections are a framework that provides an architecture to store and manipulate a group of objects. Java collections can achieve all the operations that you perform on data such as searching, sorting, insertion, manipulation, and deletion. Java collections framework consists of the following components:

15.1.1 Collection Interfaces

- Collection: The root interface of the collections framework.
- List: Ordered collection (also known as a sequence).
- Set: Collection that does not allow duplicate elements.
- SortedSet: A set that maintains its elements in ascending order.
- NavigableSet: A set with additional navigation methods.
- Queue: Collection designed for holding elements prior to processing.
- Deque: Double-ended queue that supports element insertion and removal at both ends.

15.1.2 Collection Classes

- ArrayList: Resizable-array implementation of the List interface.
- LinkedList: Doubly-linked list implementation of the List and Deque interfaces.
- HashSet: Hash table implementation of the Set interface.
- LinkedHashSet: Hash table and linked list implementation of the Set interface, with predictable iteration order.
- TreeSet: A NavigableSet implementation based on a TreeMap.
- PriorityQueue: Priority heap-based implementation of the Queue interface.
- ArrayDeque: Resizable-array implementation of the Deque interface.

15.1.3 Map Interfaces and Classes

- Map: Interface for key-value pairs.
- SortedMap: Map that maintains its entries in ascending key order.
- NavigableMap: SortedMap extended with navigation methods.
- HashMap: Hash table-based implementation of the Map interface.

DOI: 10.1201/9781003544319-15

- LinkedHashMap: Hash table and linked list implementation of the Map interface, with predictable iteration order.
- TreeMap: Red-Black tree-based implementation of the NavigableMap interface.
- Hashtable: Synchronized counterpart of HashMap.

15.1.4 Utility Classes

- Collections: Utility class with static methods for manipulating collections.
- Arrays: Utility class with static methods for manipulating arrays.

Here's a simple example demonstrating the use of different collection types in Java.

Program

```
import java.util.*;
public class test
{
void main(String[] a)
{
List<String> arr=new ArrayList<>();
arr.add("Dr.");
arr.add("Usharani");
arr.add("Bhimavarapu");
System.out.println("ArrayList"+arr);
Set<String> s=new HashSet<>();
s.add("Dr.");
s.add("Usharani");
s.add("Bhimavarapu");
System.out.println("HashSet"+s);
Map<Integer,String> m=new HashMap<>();
m.put(1,"Dr.");
m.put(2,"Usharani");
m.put(3,"Bhimavarapu");
System.out.println("Hashmap"+m);
Queue<String> q=new PriorityQueue<>();
q.add("Dr.");
q.add("Usharani");
q.add("Bhimavarapu");
System.out.println("Priority Queue"+q);
Deque<String> d=new ArrayDeque<>();
d.addFirst("Dr.");
d.addLast("Usharani");
System.out.println("ArrayDeque"+d);
Collections.sort(arr);
System.out.println("Sorted ArrayList"+arr);
Collections.shuffle(arr);
System.out.println("Shuffled ArrayList"+arr);
}
}
```

Output:

```
ArrayList[Dr., Usharani, Bhimavarapu]
HashSet[Dr., Bhimavarapu, Usharani]
Hashmap{1=Dr., 2=Usharani, 3=Bhimavarapu}
```

```
Priority Queue[Bhimavarapu, Usharani, Dr.]
ArrayDeque[Dr., Usharani]
Sorted ArrayList[Bhimavarapu, Dr., Usharani]
Shuffled ArrayList[Bhimavarapu, Dr., Usharani]
```

The above Java program named test exemplifies the versatile usage of various collection types available in Java, along with the utility methods provided by the `Collections` class. It also shows how to use some utility methods from the `Collections` class. Upon execution, the program initializes and populates different collections: an `ArrayList`, a `HashSet`, a `HashMap`, a `PriorityQueue`, and an `ArrayDeque`. Each collection stores elements of specific types. The program prints out the contents of each collection, showcasing their diverse structures and functionalities. Furthermore, the program demonstrates the application of utility methods from the `Collections` class to manipulate the `ArrayList`. First, it sorts the elements of the `ArrayList` in ascending order using the `sort()` method. Subsequently, it shuffles the elements of the `ArrayList` using the `shuffle()` method, altering their sequence randomly. These operations highlight the flexibility and efficiency offered by the `Collections` framework in managing and manipulating collections in Java, facilitating tasks such as sorting and randomization with ease.

15.2 ARRAYLIST

An `ArrayList` in Java is a dynamic array that can dynamically grow and shrink as elements are added or removed. It's part of Java's collection framework and is implemented as a resizable array. Unlike regular arrays in Java, `ArrayList` does not have a fixed size. It can automatically resize itself when elements are added or removed. Like arrays, `ArrayList` elements can be accessed using indexes. It maintains the order of elements based on the index.

15.2.1 Advantages

1. Dynamic Size: One of the primary advantages is its ability to resize dynamically. You don't need to specify the size beforehand, making it convenient for scenarios where the number of elements is unknown or may change over time.
2. Efficient Insertions and Deletions: Unlike fixed-size arrays, `ArrayList` provides efficient insertion and deletion operations. Elements can be added or removed from any position in the list without the need to shift elements manually.
3. Random Access: `ArrayList` supports random access to elements, meaning you can quickly retrieve elements based on their index.
4. Generics Support: `ArrayList` supports generics, allowing you to create type-safe lists that only accept elements of a specific type.
5. Compatibility with Collection Framework: ArrayList seamlessly integrates with other collection classes and interfaces, making it easy to use in various scenarios.

15.2.2 Challenges

1. Performance Overhead: While `ArrayList` provides efficient insertions and deletions, there can be a performance overhead when the list needs to be resized.
2. Memory Usage: Since `ArrayList` internally uses an array to store elements, it may consume more memory than necessary, especially if the initial capacity is set too high.
3. Not Suitable for Primitive Types: Unlike arrays, `ArrayList` can only store objects, not primitive types. Primitive types need to be wrapped in their respective wrapper classes (e.g., `Integer` for `int`) to be stored in an `ArrayList`.

4. Synchronization: `ArrayList` is not synchronized by default, meaning it's not thread-safe for concurrent access. If multiple threads access an `ArrayList` concurrently and at least one of the threads modifies the list structurally (adding or removing elements), it must be synchronized externally.
5. Search Time Complexity: While random access is fast in `ArrayList`, searching for elements by value can be slower compared to other data structures like `HashSet` or `TreeSet`, especially for large lists.

The syntax for using ArrayList in Java involves several steps, including importing the necessary package, declaring the ArrayList variable, creating an instance of ArrayList, adding elements to the list, accessing elements, and performing various operations.

15.2.3 Array List Declaration and Accessing Syntax

1. Import the ArrayList class: Need to import the ArrayList class from the java.util package.
   import java.util.ArrayList;
2. Declare a variable of type ArrayList with the desired element type.
   ArrayList<ElementType> listName;
3. Initialize the ArrayList variable by creating a new instance of ArrayList.
   listName = new ArrayList<>();
   Alternatively, the users can combine declaration and instantiation in a single line:
   ArrayList<ElementType> listName = new ArrayList<>();
4. The users can add elements to the ArrayList using the add() method.
   listName.add(element);
5. The users can access elements by their index using the get() method.
   ElementType element = listName.get(index);
6. The users can iterate through the elements of the ArrayList using enhanced for loop or iterators.
   for (ElementType element: listName) {// Process each element}
7. The users can remove elements by their index or value using the remove() method.
   listName.remove(index);
   listName.remove(element);
8. The users can get the number of elements in the ArrayList using the size() method.
   int size = listName.size();
9. The users can check if the ArrayList is empty using the isEmpty() method.
   boolean isEmpty = listName.isEmpty();
10. The users can remove all elements from the ArrayList using the clear() method.
    listName.clear();

Program

```
import java.util.ArrayList;
import java.util.Collections;
public class ListExample {
    void main(String[] args) {
  // Creating an ArrayList to store course names
  ArrayList<String> courses = new ArrayList<>();
  // Adding course names to the ArrayList
  courses.add("Mathematics");
  courses.add("Physics");
```

```
courses.add("Chemistry");
courses.add("Biology");
// Displaying the initial list of courses
System.out.println("Initial list of courses: " + courses);
// Retrieving and printing a course based on index
String courseAtIndex2 = courses.get(2);
System.out.println("Course at index 2: " + courseAtIndex2);
// Updating a course at a specific index
courses.set(3, "Environmental Science");
System.out.println("List after updating the course at index 3: " + courses);
// Removing a course by index
courses.remove(1);
System.out.println("List after removing the course at index 1: " + courses);
// Checking if a specific course is in the list
boolean hasMathematics = courses.contains("Mathematics");
System.out.println("Does the list contain 'Mathematics'? " + hasMathematics);
// Checking if the list is empty
boolean isEmpty = courses.isEmpty();
System.out.println("Is the course list empty? " + isEmpty);
// Printing the size of the list
int size = courses.size();
System.out.println("Size of the course list: " + size);
// Sorting the list in alphabetical order
Collections.sort(courses);
System.out.println("Sorted course list: " + courses);
// Clearing the list
courses.clear();
System.out.println("List after clearing all courses: " + courses);
}
}
```

Output:

```
Initial list of courses: [Mathematics, Physics, Chemistry, Biology]
Course at index 2: Chemistry
List after updating the course at index 3: [Mathematics, Physics, Chemistry, Environmental Science]
List after removing the course at index 1: [Mathematics, Chemistry, Environmental Science]
Does the list contain 'Mathematics'? true
Is the course list empty? false
Size of the course list: 3
Sorted course list: [Chemistry, Environmental Science, Mathematics]
List after clearing all courses: []
```

The above program demonstrates the use of an ArrayList to manage a list of course names. It begins by importing necessary classes and creating an ArrayList. The program then adds several course names to the list and prints the initial contents. It retrieves and prints a course based on its index, updates a course at a specific index, and removes a course by index, displaying the list after each operation. The program checks for the presence of a specific course, verifies if the list is empty, and prints the size of the list. It sorts the list in alphabetical order, displays the sorted list, and finally clears the list, showing the empty list at the end.

15.3 LINKEDLIST

A `LinkedList` in Java is a linear data structure that consists of a sequence of elements where each element is connected to its previous and next elements via references. Unlike arrays, `LinkedLists` do not store elements in contiguous memory locations. Instead, each element points to the next element, forming a chain-like structure.

A `LinkedList implements the `List` interface. It consists of nodes, where each node contains a data element and a reference to the next node in the sequence. The first node is called the head, and the last node is called the tail. Each node in a `LinkedList` contains two fields: the data and the reference to the next node.

15.3.1 Advantages

1. Dynamic Size: Unlike arrays, `LinkedLists` do not have a fixed size. Elements can be added or removed from any position in constant time, making them suitable for dynamic applications where the size of the data structure varies.
2. Efficient Insertions and Deletions: Insertions and deletions in `LinkedLists` are efficient as they require only adjusting references, rather than shifting elements as in arrays. This makes `LinkedLists` suitable for scenarios where frequent insertions or deletions are expected.

15.3.2 Challenges

1. Random Access is Inefficient: Unlike arrays, `LinkedLists` do not support random access to elements based on their index. Accessing an element at a specific index requires traversing the list from the beginning or end, resulting in linear time complexity for access operations.
2. Increased Memory Overhead: Each node in a `LinkedList` requires additional memory to store the reference to the next node, leading to increased memory overhead compared to arrays, especially for small-sized elements. This can be a concern in memory-constrained environments or when dealing with large datasets.

15.3.3 Syntax

Using `LinkedList` in Java involves similar syntax to other collections. Here's a syntax for using `LinkedList`:

1. Import the LinkedList class:

```
import java.util.LinkedList;
```

2. Declare and instantiate a LinkedList:

LinkedList<ElementType> linkedList = new LinkedList<>();

3. Add elements to the LinkedList:

```
linkedList.add(element);
```

4. Access elements in the LinkedList:

```
ElementType firstElement = linkedList.getFirst();
ElementType lastElement = linkedList.getLast();
```

5. Iterate through the LinkedList:

```
for (ElementType element : linkedList) {
// Process each element
}
```

6. Remove elements from the LinkedList:

```
linkedList.removeFirst();
linkedList.removeLast();
```

7. Check size and emptiness of the LinkedList:

```
int size = linkedList.size();
boolean isEmpty = linkedList.isEmpty();
```

Program

```
import java.util.LinkedList;
import java.util.Scanner;
public class ListLinkedListExample {
    void main(String[] args) {
  // Creating a LinkedList to store course names
  LinkedList<String> courses = new LinkedList<>();
  // Adding initial course names to the LinkedList
  courses.add("Mathematics");
  courses.add("Physics");
  courses.add("Chemistry");
  courses.add("Biology");
  // Displaying the initial list of courses
  System.out.println("Initial list of courses: " + courses);
  // Creating a Scanner object to take user input
  Scanner scanner = new Scanner(System.in);
  String newCourse;
  // Prompting the user to enter additional courses
  System.out.println("Enter additional courses (type 'done' to finish):");
  // Loop to accept user input and add courses to the LinkedList
  while (true) {
    newCourse = scanner.nextLine();
    if (newCourse.equalsIgnoreCase("done")) {
    break;
    }
    courses.add(newCourse);
  }
  // Displaying the final list of courses
  System.out.println("Final list of courses: " + courses);
  // Checking if the course "Physics" is in the LinkedList
  boolean hasPhysics = courses.contains("Physics");
  if (hasPhysics) {
```

```
      System.out.println("'Physics' is present in the course list.");
    } else {
      System.out.println("'Physics' is not present in the course list.");
    }
    // Removing the course "Chemistry" from the LinkedList
    courses.remove("Chemistry");
    System.out.println("List after removing 'Chemistry': " + courses);
    // Closing the scanner
    scanner.close();
    }
}
```

Output:

```
Initial list of courses: [Mathematics, Physics, Chemistry, Biology]
Enter additional courses (type 'done' to finish):
computer course
done
Final list of courses: [Mathematics, Physics, Chemistry, Biology, computer
course]
'Physics' is present in the course list.
List after removing 'Chemistry': [Mathematics, Physics, Biology, computer
course]
```

The above program demonstrates the use of a LinkedList to manage a list of course names. It starts by importing the necessary classes and creating a LinkedList to hold the course names. Initially, the program adds four courses: "Mathematics," "Physics," "Chemistry," and "Biology" to the LinkedList and displays the initial list. The program then prompts the user to input additional courses through the console, adding each course to the LinkedList until the user types "done." Afterward, the program displays the final list of courses. It checks if the course "Physics" is present in the list and confirms its presence. The program then removes "Chemistry" from the LinkedList and displays the list after this removal.

15.4 HASHSET

`HashSet` is a Collection class in Java that implements the `Set` interface. It represents a collection of unique elements where each element is stored only once. Internally, it uses a hash table to store elements, providing constant-time performance for basic operations like adding, removing, and checking for the presence of elements.

15.4.1 Advantages of HashSet

1. Unique Elements: HashSet ensures that each element is unique. It automatically prevents the insertion of duplicate elements.
2. Fast Performance: HashSet provides constant-time performance for basic operations like adding, removing, and checking for the presence of elements due to its underlying hash table implementation.

15.4.2 Challenges of HashSet

1. Unordered: HashSet does not guarantee the order of elements. The order in which elements are stored may not be the same as the order in which they were inserted.
2. No Indexing: Unlike lists, HashSet does not support indexing. You cannot access elements by their index, as there is no defined order.

15.4.3 Syntax for Using HashSet in Java

1. Import the HashSet class:

```
import java.util.HashSet;
```

2. Declare and instantiate a HashSet:

```
HashSet<ElementType> hashSet = new HashSet<>();
```

3. Add elements to the HashSet:

```
hashSet.add(element);
```

4. Remove elements from the HashSet:

```
hashSet.remove(element);
```

5. Check if an element exists in the HashSet:

boolean exists = hashSet.contains(element);

6. Iterate through the HashSet:

```
for (ElementType element: hashSet) {
// Process each element
}
```

7. Check the size and emptiness of the HashSet:

```
int size = hashSet.size();
boolean isEmpty = hashSet.isEmpty();
```

These syntax elements allow the users to work with HashSet in Java, performing operations like adding, removing, checking for the presence of elements, iterating through the elements, and checking the size and emptiness of the set.

Program

```
import java.util.HashSet;
public class HashSetExample {
    void main(String[] args) {
  // Creating a HashSet to store course names
  HashSet<String> courses = new HashSet<>();
  // Adding course names to the HashSet
  courses.add("Mathematics");
  courses.add("Physics");
  courses.add("Chemistry");
  courses.add("Biology");
  // Attempting to add "Mathematics" again to demonstrate that duplicates
  are ignored
  boolean addedMathematicsAgain = courses.add("Mathematics");
```

```
    if (!addedMathematicsAgain) {
      System.out.println("'Mathematics' was already in the set and was not
         added again.");
    }
    // Displaying the contents of the HashSet (unique course names)
    System.out.println("Unique courses in the set: " + courses);
    // Checking if the course "Physics" is in the HashSet
    boolean hasPhysics = courses.contains("Physics");
    if (hasPhysics) {
      System.out.println("'Physics' is present in the course set.");
    } else {
      System.out.println("'Physics' is not present in the course set.");
    }
    // Removing the course "Chemistry" from the HashSet
    courses.remove("Chemistry");
    System.out.println("Set after removing 'Chemistry': " + courses);
    }
}
```

Output:

```
'Mathematics' was already in the set and was not added again.
Unique courses in the set: [Chemistry, Mathematics, Biology, Physics]
'Physics' is present in the course set.
Set after removing 'Chemistry': [Mathematics, Biology, Physics]
```

The above program demonstrates the use of a HashSet to manage a collection of course names in Java. It begins by creating a HashSet named `courses` to store course names. The program adds several courses to the HashSet, including "Mathematics," "Physics," "Chemistry," "Biology," and attempts to add "Mathematics" again to illustrate that duplicate elements are ignored in a HashSet. The contents of the HashSet are then displayed, showing the unique course names. The program checks if the course "Physics" is present in the HashSet and confirms its presence. It then removes the course "Chemistry" from the HashSet and displays the updated contents, showing the remaining courses.

15.5 LINKEDHASHSET

`LinkedHashSet` is a Collection class in Java that extends `HashSet` and implements the `Set` interface. Similar to `HashSet`, it stores a collection of unique elements. However, unlike `HashSet`, it maintains the insertion order of elements, providing predictable iteration order.

15.5.1 Advantages of LinkedHashSet

1. Maintains Insertion Order: LinkedHashSet maintains the order in which elements are inserted. When iterating through the set, the elements are returned in the same order in which they were added.
2. Fast Performance: Like HashSet, LinkedHashSet provides constant-time performance for basic operations such as adding, removing, and checking for the presence of elements.

15.5.2 Challenges of LinkedHashSet

1. Higher Memory Consumption: LinkedHashSet consumes more memory compared to HashSet due to the additional overhead of maintaining the linked list to preserve insertion order.

2. Slower Iteration: While LinkedHashSet maintains insertion order, it may have slightly slower iteration performance compared to HashSet due to the additional overhead of managing the linked list.

15.5.3 Syntax for Using LinkedHashSet in Java

1. Import the LinkedHashSet class:

```
import java.util.LinkedHashSet;
```

2. Declare and instantiate a LinkedHashSet:

```
LinkedHashSet<ElementType> linkedHashSet = new LinkedHashSet<>();
```

3. Add elements to the LinkedHashSet:

```
linkedHashSet.add(element);
```

4. Remove elements from the LinkedHashSet:

```
linkedHashSet.remove(element);
```

5. Check if an element exists in the LinkedHashSet:

```
boolean exists = linkedHashSet.contains(element);
```

6. Iterate through the LinkedHashSet:

```
for (ElementType element : linkedHashSet) {
// Process each element
}
```

7. Check the size and emptiness of the LinkedHashSet:

```
int size = linkedHashSet.size();
boolean isEmpty = linkedHashSet.isEmpty();
```

LinkedHashSet in Java, performs operations like adding, removing, checking for the presence of elements, iterating through the elements, and checking the size and emptiness of the set.

Program

```
import java.util.LinkedHashSet;
public class LinkedHashSetExample {
    void main(String[] args) {
  // Creating a LinkedHashSet to store course names
  LinkedHashSet<String> courses = new LinkedHashSet<>();
  // Adding course names to the LinkedHashSet
  courses.add("Mathematics");
  courses.add("Physics");
  courses.add("Chemistry");
  courses.add("Biology");
```

```
  // Attempting to add "Mathematics" again to demonstrate that duplicates
  are ignored
  boolean addedMathematicsAgain = courses.add("Mathematics");
  if (!addedMathematicsAgain) {
    System.out.println("'Mathematics' was already in the set and was not
       added again.");
  }
  // Displaying the contents of the LinkedHashSet (preserving inser-
  tion order)
  System.out.println("Courses in the set (insertion order maintained): " +
     courses);
  // Checking if the course "Physics" is in the LinkedHashSet
  boolean hasPhysics = courses.contains("Physics");
  if (hasPhysics) {
    System.out.println("'Physics' is present in the course set.");
  } else {
    System.out.println("'Physics' is not present in the course set.");
  }
  // Removing the course "Chemistry" from the LinkedHashSet
  courses.remove("Chemistry");
  System.out.println("Set after removing 'Chemistry': " + courses);
  }
}
```

Output:

```
'Mathematics' was already in the set and was not added again.
Courses in the set (insertion order maintained): [Mathematics, Physics,
Chemistry, Biology]
'Physics' is present in the course set.
Set after removing 'Chemistry': [Mathematics, Physics, Biology]
```

The above program demonstrates the use of a LinkedHashSet to manage a collection of course names in Java, preserving the insertion order of elements. It begins by creating a LinkedHashSet named `courses` to store the course names. The program adds several courses to the LinkedHashSet, including "Mathematics," "Physics," "Chemistry," and "Biology." An attempt to add "Mathematics" again illustrates that duplicate elements are ignored in a LinkedHashSet, similar to a HashSet. The contents of the LinkedHashSet are then displayed, maintaining the order of insertion. The program checks if the course "Physics" is present in the LinkedHashSet and confirms its presence. It then removes the course "Chemistry" from the LinkedHashSet and displays the updated contents, showing the remaining courses in their original insertion order.

15.6 TREESET

`TreeSet` is a Collection class in Java that implements the `NavigableSet` interface and extends the `AbstractSet` class. It represents a sorted set, where elements are stored in ascending order by default or based on a custom comparator provided during creation.

15.6.1 Advantages of TreeSet

1. Automatic Sorting: TreeSet automatically sorts elements in ascending order by default. This makes it convenient for maintaining a sorted collection without manual intervention.
2. Efficient Retrieval: TreeSet provides efficient retrieval operations such as searching for elements, finding the smallest and largest elements, and navigating through the set in sorted order.

15.6.2 Challenges of TreeSet

1. Higher Memory Consumption: TreeSet typically consumes more memory compared to HashSet and LinkedHashSet due to the additional overhead of maintaining a balanced binary search tree structure.
2. Slower Insertion and Deletion: While TreeSet provides efficient retrieval, insertion, and deletion operations may be slower compared to HashSet and LinkedHashSet due to the need to maintain the sorted order of elements.

15.6.3 Syntax for Using Tree Set in Java

1. Import the TreeSet class:

```
import java.util.TreeSet;
```

2. Declare and instantiate a TreeSet:

```
TreeSet<ElementType> treeSet = new TreeSet<>();
```

3. Add elements to the TreeSet:

```
treeSet.add(element);
```

4. Remove elements from the TreeSet:

```
treeSet.remove(element);
```

5. Check if an element exists in the TreeSet:

```
boolean exists = treeSet.contains(element);
```

6. Iterate through the TreeSet in sorted order:

```
for (ElementType element : treeSet) {
// Process each element in ascending order
}
```

7. Retrieve the smallest and largest elements:

```
ElementType firstElement = treeSet.first();
ElementType lastElement = treeSet.last();
```

8. Check the size and emptiness of the TreeSet:

```
int size = treeSet.size();
boolean isEmpty = treeSet.isEmpty();
```

TreeSet in Java, does facilitating operations such as adding, removing, searching for elements, iterating through the set in sorted order, retrieving the smallest and largest elements, and checking the size and emptiness of the set.

Program

```
import java.util.TreeSet;
public class TreeSetExample {
   void main(String[] args) {
  // Creating a TreeSet to store course names
  TreeSet<String> courses = new TreeSet<>();
  // Adding course names to the TreeSet
  courses.add("Mathematics");
  courses.add("Physics");
  courses.add("Chemistry");
  courses.add("Biology");
  // Attempting to add "Mathematics" again to demonstrate that duplicates
  are ignored
  boolean addedMathematicsAgain = courses.add("Mathematics");
  if (!addedMathematicsAgain) {
    System.out.println(" 'Mathematics' was already in the set and was not
       added again.");
  }
  // Displaying the contents of the TreeSet (automatically sorted in nat-
  ural order)
  System.out.println("Courses in the set (sorted order): " + courses);
  // Checking if the course "Physics" is in the TreeSet
  boolean hasPhysics = courses.contains("Physics");
  if (hasPhysics) {
    System.out.println(" 'Physics' is present in the course set.");
  } else {
    System.out.println(" 'Physics' is not present in the course set.");
  }
  // Removing the course "Chemistry" from the TreeSet
  courses.remove("Chemistry");
  System.out.println("Set after removing 'Chemistry': " + courses);
  }
}
```

```
Output:
'Mathematics' was already in the set and was not added again.
Courses in the set (insertion order maintained): [Mathematics, Physics,
Chemistry, Biology]
'Physics' is present in the course set.
Set after removing 'Chemistry': [Mathematics, Physics, Biology]
```

This program demonstrates the use of a TreeSet to manage a collection of course names in Java, ensuring that the elements are stored in a sorted order. It starts by creating a TreeSet named `courses` to store the course names. The program then adds several courses to the TreeSet, including "Mathematics," "Physics," "Chemistry," and "Biology." An attempt to add "Mathematics" again illustrates that duplicate elements are ignored in a TreeSet, just like in other Set implementations. The contents of the TreeSet are displayed, automatically sorted in natural order (alphabetical order in this case). The program checks if the course "Physics" is present in the TreeSet and confirms its presence. It then removes the course "Chemistry" from the TreeSet and displays the updated contents, showing the remaining courses in sorted order.

15.7 QUEUE

In Java, `Queue` is an interface that represents a collection designed for holding elements prior to processing. It follows the First-In-First-Out (FIFO) principle, where elements are inserted at the end (tail) and removed from the beginning (head) of the queue.

15.7.1 Advantages of Queue

1. Order Preservation: Queue ensures that elements are processed in the order they were added, making it suitable for scenarios like task scheduling or event handling.
2. Concurrency Support: Java provides concurrent implementations of the Queue interface like `ConcurrentLinkedQueue`, allowing multiple threads to safely access and modify the queue concurrently without explicit synchronization.

15.7.2 Challenges of Queue

1. Limited Access: Unlike other collection types like Lists, accessing elements at arbitrary positions in a Queue is limited. Queue operations typically involve adding elements at the rear and removing them from the front, making random access inefficient.
2. Capacity Limitation: Depending on the implementation, Queues might have a fixed capacity, leading to potential issues like blocking or exceptions when attempting to add elements to a full queue.

15.7.3 Syntax for Using Queue in Java

1. Import the Queue interface:

```
import java.util.Queue;
```

2. Declare and instantiate a Queue object:

```
Queue<ElementType> queue = new LinkedList<>();
```

3. Add elements to the queue:

```
queue.offer(element);
```

4. Remove and retrieve elements from the queue:

```
ElementType element = queue.poll();
```

5. Peek at the front element without removing it:

```
ElementType element = queue.peek();
```

6. Check if the queue is empty:

```
boolean isEmpty = queue.isEmpty();
```

7. Get the size of the queue:

```
int size = queue.size();
```

These syntax elements enable the users to work with Queue in Java, facilitating operations such as adding, removing, peeking at elements, checking if the queue is empty, and getting its size.

Program

```
import java.util.LinkedList;
import java.util.Queue;
public class QueueExample {
    void main(String[] args) {
  // Creating a Queue to store course names
  Queue<String> courseQueue = new LinkedList<>();
  // Adding course names to the Queue using the offer method (enqueue
  operation)
  courseQueue.offer("Mathematics");
  courseQueue.offer("Physics");
  courseQueue.offer("Chemistry");
  courseQueue.offer("Biology");
  // Displaying the contents of the Queue
  System.out.println("Courses in the queue: " + courseQueue);
  // Retrieving and displaying the course at the front of the Queue without
  removing it (peek)
  String frontCourse = courseQueue.peek();
  System.out.println("Course at the front of the queue: " + frontCourse);
  // Removing the course at the front of the Queue (poll) and displaying
  the updated Queue
  courseQueue.poll();
  System.out.println("Queue after dequeuing the front course: " +
      courseQueue);
  // Enqueuing another course "Computer Science"
  courseQueue.offer("Computer Science");
  System.out.println("Queue after enqueuing 'Computer Science': " +
      courseQueue);
  // Retrieving the element at the rear of the Queue (casting to LinkedList
  and using getLast)
  String lastCourse = ((LinkedList<String>) courseQueue).getLast();
  System.out.println("Course at the rear of the queue: " + lastCourse);
  // Checking if the course "Physics" exists in the Queue
  boolean containsPhysics = courseQueue.contains("Physics");
  if (containsPhysics) {
    System.out.println("'Physics' is present in the queue.");
  } else {
    System.out.println("'Physics' is not present in the queue.");
  }
  }
}
```

```
Output:
Courses in the queue: [Mathematics, Physics, Chemistry, Biology]
Course at the front of the queue: Mathematics
Queue after dequeuing the front course: [Physics, Chemistry, Biology]
Queue after enqueuing 'Computer Science': [Physics, Chemistry, Biology,
Computer Science]
Course at the rear of the queue: Computer Science
'Physics' is present in the queue.
```

The above program demonstrates the use of a Queue, specifically implemented using a LinkedList, to manage a sequence of course names in Java. It starts by creating a Queue named `courseQueue`. The program then adds several courses to the Queue using the `offer` method, which enqueues elements. After adding the initial set of courses ("Mathematics," "Physics," "Chemistry," and "Biology"), the program displays the contents of the Queue. To perform the front operation, the program uses the `peek` method to retrieve and display the course at the front of the Queue without removing it. The program then dequeues an element from the Queue using the `poll` method, which removes and returns the front element, displaying the Queue contents after this operation.Next, the program enqueues another course, "Computer Science," using the `offer` method and displays the updated Queue. To retrieve the element at the rear of the Queue, the program casts the Queue to a LinkedList and uses the `getLast` method. Finally, the program checks if a specific course, "Physics," exists in the Queue using the `contains` method and confirms its presence.

15.8 HASHMAP

In Java, `HashMap` is a class that implements the `Map` interface, representing a collection of key-value pairs. It allows you to store and retrieve elements based on their keys. HashMap uses a hash table data structure to store the elements, providing fast retrieval operations.

15.8.1 Advantages of HashMap

1. Fast Retrieval: HashMap provides constant-time performance for basic operations like `get()` and `put()`, making it efficient for large datasets.
2. Flexible Key-Value Pairing: HashMap allows you to store key-value pairs of different types, providing flexibility in representing various relationships and data structures.

15.8.2 Challenges of HashMap

1. Unordered Iteration: The elements in a HashMap are not ordered, which means that there is no guarantee on the order in which the elements will be returned during iteration. If the users need ordered traversal, they need to use `LinkedHashMap` or `TreeMap`.
2. Collision Handling: In hash-based data structures like HashMap, collisions may occur when multiple keys hash to the same index. Efficient collision resolution strategies, such as chaining or open addressing, are required to maintain performance.

15.8.3 Syntax for Using HashMap in Java

1. Import the HashMap class:

```
import java.util.HashMap;
```

2. Declare and instantiate a HashMap object:

```
HashMap<KeyType, ValueType> hashMap = new HashMap<>();
```

3. Add key-value pairs to the HashMap:

```
hashMap.put(key, value);
```

4. Retrieve a value based on its key:

```
ValueType value = hashMap.get(key);
```

5. Check if the HashMap contains a specific key:

```
boolean containsKey = hashMap.containsKey(key);
```

6. Remove a key-value pair from the HashMap:

```
ValueType removedValue = hashMap.remove(key);
```

7. Check if the HashMap is empty:

```
boolean isEmpty = hashMap.isEmpty();
```

8. Get the size of the HashMap:

```
int size = hashMap.size();
```

HashMap in Java, does facilitating operations such as adding key-value pairs, retrieving values based on keys, checking containment, removing entries, and querying the size of the map.

Program

```
import java.util.HashMap;
public class HashMapExample {
    void main(String[] args) {
  // Creating a HashMap to store course names with their corresponding IDs
  HashMap<Integer, String> courseMap = new HashMap<>();
  // Adding course entries to the HashMap using the put method
  courseMap.put(1, "Mathematics");
  courseMap.put(2, "Physics");
  courseMap.put(3, "Chemistry");
  courseMap.put(4, "Biology");
  courseMap.put(5, "Computer Science");
  // Displaying the contents of the HashMap
  System.out.println("Course Map: " + courseMap);
  // Retrieving and displaying the course associated with a specific ID (2)
  String course = courseMap.get(2);
  System.out.println("Course with ID 2: " + course);
  // Checking if the course "Physics" exists in the HashMap
  boolean hasPhysics = courseMap.containsValue("Physics");
  if (hasPhysics) {
    System.out.println(" 'Physics' is present in the course map.");
  } else {
    System.out.println(" 'Physics' is not present in the course map.");
  }
  // Removing a course with a specific ID (4) and displaying the updated
HashMap
  courseMap.remove(4);
  System.out.println("Course Map after removing ID 4: " + courseMap);
  // Checking if a specific key (ID 2) exists in the HashMap
  boolean hasKey2 = courseMap.containsKey(2);
  if (hasKey2) {
    System.out.println("ID 2 is present in the course map.");
  } else {
    System.out.println("ID 2 is not present in the course map.");
  }
```

```
  // Printing the size of the HashMap
  System.out.println("Size of the course map: " + courseMap.size());
  // Clearing all entries in the HashMap
  courseMap.clear();
  System.out.println("Course Map after clearing: " + courseMap);
  }
}
```

Output:

```
Course Map: {1=Mathematics, 2=Physics, 3=Chemistry, 4=Biology, 5=Computer
Science}
Course with ID 2: Physics
'Physics' is present in the course map.
Course Map after removing ID 4: {1=Mathematics, 2=Physics, 3=Chemistry, 5=
Computer Science}
ID 2 is present in the course map.
Size of the course map: 4
Course Map after clearing: {}
```

The above program demonstrates the use of a HashMap to manage a collection of course names in Java, with each course associated with a unique integer ID. It begins by creating a HashMap named `courseMap` to store the course names mapped to their IDs. The program retrieves and prints the course name associated with a specific ID using the `get` method. It checks if a particular course, "Physics," exists in the HashMap using the `containsValue` method and confirms its presence. Next, the program removes a course with a specific ID (4) using the `remove` method, displaying the updated HashMap after the removal. It also checks if a specific key (2) exists in the HashMap using the `containsKey` method and confirms its presence. The program prints the size of the HashMap using the `size` method and then clears all entries in the HashMap using the `clear` method, displaying the empty HashMap at the end.

15.9 LINKEDHASHMAP

In Java, `LinkedHashMap` is a class that extends `HashMap` and implements the `Map` interface. It maintains a doubly-linked list running through all of its entries, providing an ordered iteration over its elements based on the insertion order or access order. LinkedHashMap combines the fast access of HashMap with predictable iteration order.

15.9.1 Advantages of LinkedHashMap

1. Predictable Iteration Order: LinkedHashMap maintains the order of its elements based on insertion order or access order (using the `accessOrder` parameter in its constructors), making it suitable for scenarios where the order of elements matters.
2. Fast Access and Search: Like HashMap, LinkedHashMap provides constant-time performance for basic operations such as `get()` and `put()`, making it efficient for large datasets.

15.9.2 Challenges of LinkedHashMap

1. Increased Memory Consumption: LinkedHashMap consumes more memory compared to HashMap due to the additional overhead of maintaining the linked list for maintaining insertion/access order.
2. Performance Overhead: While LinkedHashMap provides predictable iteration order, maintaining this order can lead to a slight performance overhead compared to HashMap.

15.9.3 Syntax for Using LinkedHashMap in Java

1. Import the LinkedHashMap class:

```
import java.util.LinkedHashMap;
```

2. Declare and instantiate a LinkedHashMap object:

```
LinkedHashMap<KeyType, ValueType> linkedHashMap = new LinkedHashMap<>();
```

3. Add key-value pairs to the LinkedHashMap:

```
linkedHashMap.put(key, value);
```

4. Retrieve a value based on its key:

```
ValueType value = linkedHashMap.get(key);
```

5. Check if the LinkedHashMap contains a specific key:

```
boolean containsKey = linkedHashMap.containsKey(key);
```

6. Remove a key-value pair from the LinkedHashMap:

```
ValueType removedValue = linkedHashMap.remove(key);
```

7. Check if the LinkedHashMap is empty:

```
boolean isEmpty = linkedHashMap.isEmpty();
```

8. Get the size of the LinkedHashMap:

```
int size = linkedHashMap.size();
```

LinkedHashMap in Java, does facilitating operations such as adding key-value pairs, retrieving values based on keys, checking containment, removing entries, and querying the size of the map. Additionally, the LinkedHashMap maintains the insertion order or access order of its elements, providing predictable iteration order.

Program

```
import java.util.LinkedHashMap;
import java.util.Map;
public class LinkedHashMapExample {
    void main(String[] args) {
  // Creating a LinkedHashMap to store course names with their corresponding IDs
  LinkedHashMap<Integer, String> courseMap = new LinkedHashMap<>();
  // Adding course entries to the LinkedHashMap using the put method
  courseMap.put(1, "Mathematics");
  courseMap.put(2, "Physics");
  courseMap.put(3, "Chemistry");
  courseMap.put(4, "Biology");
  courseMap.put(5, "Computer Science");
```

```
  // Displaying the contents of the LinkedHashMap (insertion order is
  preserved)
  System.out.println("Course Map: " + courseMap);
  // Retrieving and displaying the course associated with a specific ID (2)
  String course = courseMap.get(2);
  System.out.println("Course with ID 2: " + course);
  // Checking if the course "Physics" exists in the LinkedHashMap
  boolean hasPhysics = courseMap.containsValue("Physics");
  if (hasPhysics) {
    System.out.println("'Physics' is present in the course map.");
  } else {
    System.out.println("'Physics' is not present in the course map.");
  }
  // Removing a course with a specific ID (4) and displaying the updated
  LinkedHashMap
  courseMap.remove(4);
  System.out.println("Course Map after removing ID 4: " + courseMap);
  // Checking if a specific key (ID 2) exists in the LinkedHashMap
  boolean hasKey2 = courseMap.containsKey(2);
  if (hasKey2) {
    System.out.println("ID 2 is present in the course map.");
  } else {
    System.out.println("ID 2 is not present in the course map.");
  }
  // Printing the size of the LinkedHashMap
  System.out.println("Size of the course map: " + courseMap.size());
  // Clearing all entries in the LinkedHashMap
  courseMap.clear();
  System.out.println("Course Map after clearing: " + courseMap);
  }
}
```

Output:

```
Course Map: {1=Mathematics, 2=Physics, 3=Chemistry, 4=Biology, 5=Computer
Science}
Course with ID 2: Physics
'Physics' is present in the course map.
Course Map after removing ID 4: {1=Mathematics, 2=Physics, 3=Chemistry, 5=
Computer Science}
ID 2 is present in the course map.
Size of the course map: 4
Course Map after clearing: {}
```

The above program demonstrates the use of a LinkedHashMap to manage a collection of course names in Java, with each course associated with a unique integer ID. It starts by creating a LinkedHashMap named `courseMap` to store the course names mapped to their IDs, ensuring the order of insertion is maintained. The program adds several courses to the LinkedHashMap using the `put` method, with IDs ranging from 1 to 5, and displays the contents of the LinkedHashMap. The program retrieves and prints the course name associated with a specific ID using the `get` method. It checks if a particular course, "Physics," exists in the LinkedHashMap using the `containsValue` method and confirms its presence. Next, the program removes a course with a specific ID (4) using the `remove` method, and displays the updated LinkedHashMap after the removal. It checks if a specific key (2) exists in the LinkedHashMap using the `containsKey` method and confirms its presence. The program prints the size of the LinkedHashMap using the `size` method and then clears all entries using the `clear` method, displaying the empty LinkedHashMap at the end.

15.10 TREEMAP

In Java, `TreeMap` is a class that implements the `NavigableMap` interface and extends `AbstractMap`. It is a sorted map based on a Red-Black tree data structure. TreeMap maintains its elements in sorted order based on their natural ordering or a specified comparator.

15.10.1 Advantages of TreeMap

1. Ordered Collection: TreeMap maintains its elements in sorted order, making it suitable for scenarios where a sorted collection is required. It provides ascending key order iteration by default, or a custom ordering can be provided using a comparator.
2. Efficient Range Queries: TreeMap supports efficient range queries and operations such as `firstKey()`, `lastKey()`, `headMap()`, `tailMap()`, and `subMap()`, enabling easy retrieval of elements within a specific range.

15.10.2 Challenges of TreeMap

1. Higher Memory Overhead: TreeMap has a higher memory overhead compared to HashMap due to the additional storage requirements for maintaining the tree structure.
2. Slower Insertion and Removal: While TreeMap provides sorted order iteration, insertion and removal operations may be slower compared to HashMap due to the additional overhead of maintaining the tree structure and ensuring its balance.

15.10.3 Syntax for Using TreeMap in Java

1. Import the TreeMap class:

```
import java.util.TreeMap;
```

2. Declare and instantiate a TreeMap object:

```
TreeMap<KeyType, ValueType> treeMap = new TreeMap<>();
```

3. Add key-value pairs to the TreeMap:

```
treeMap.put(key, value);
```

4. Retrieve a value based on its key:

```
ValueType value = treeMap.get(key);
```

5. Check if the TreeMap contains a specific key:

```
boolean containsKey = treeMap.containsKey(key);
```

6. Remove a key-value pair from the TreeMap:

```
ValueType removedValue = treeMap.remove(key);
```

7. Check if the TreeMap is empty:

```
boolean isEmpty = treeMap.isEmpty();
```

8. Get the size of the TreeMap:

```
int size = treeMap.size();
```

TreeMap in Java, does facilitating operations such as adding key-value pairs, retrieving values based on keys, checking containment, removing entries, and querying the size of the map. Additionally, TreeMap maintains its elements in sorted order, providing efficient access and iteration based on keys' natural ordering or a custom comparator.

Program

```
import java.util.TreeMap;
public class TreeMapExample {
    void main(String[] args) {
  // Creating a TreeMap to store course names with their corresponding IDs
  TreeMap<Integer, String> courseMap = new TreeMap<>();
  // Adding course entries to the TreeMap using the put method
  courseMap.put(101, "Mathematics");
  courseMap.put(102, "Physics");
  courseMap.put(103, "Chemistry");
  courseMap.put(104, "Biology");
  courseMap.put(105, "Computer Science");
  // Displaying the contents of the TreeMap (keys are sorted in ascending order)
  System.out.println("Tree Map: " + courseMap);
  // Retrieving and displaying the course associated with a specific ID (102)
  String course = courseMap.get(102);
  System.out.println("Course with ID 102: " + course);
  // Checking if the course "Physics" exists in the TreeMap
  boolean hasPhysics = courseMap.containsValue("Physics");
  if (hasPhysics) {
    System.out.println("'Physics' is present in the Tree map.");
  } else {
    System.out.println("'Physics' is not present in the Tree map.");
  }
  // Removing a course with a specific ID (104) and displaying the updated
  TreeMap
  courseMap.remove(104);
  System.out.println("Tree Map after removing ID 104: " + courseMap);
  // Checking if a specific key (ID 102) exists in the TreeMap
  boolean hasKey102 = courseMap.containsKey(102);
  if (hasKey102) {
    System.out.println("ID 102 is present in the Tree map.");
  } else {
    System.out.println("ID 102 is not present in the Tree map.");
  }
  // Printing the size of the TreeMap
  System.out.println("Size of the Tree map: " + courseMap.size());
  // Clearing all entries in the TreeMap
  courseMap.clear();
```

```
    System.out.println("Tree Map after clearing: " + courseMap);
  }
}
```

Output:

```
Tree Map: {101=Mathematics, 102=Physics, 103=Chemistry, 104=Biology, 105=
Computer Science}
Course with ID 102: Physics
'Physics' is present in the Tree map.
Tree Map after removing ID 104: {101=Mathematics, 102=Physics, 103=
Chemistry, 105=Computer Science}
ID 102 is present in the Tree map.
Size of the Tree map: 4
Tree Map after clearing: {}
```

The above program demonstrates the use of a TreeMap to manage a collection of course names in Java, with each course associated with a unique integer ID. It starts by creating a TreeMap named `courseMap` to store the course names mapped to their IDs, ensuring that the keys are sorted in natural order. The program adds several courses to the TreeMap using the `put` method, with IDs ranging from 101 to 105, and displays the contents of the TreeMap in ascending order of keys. It retrieves and prints the course name associated with a specific ID using the `get` method. The program checks if a particular course, "Physics," exists in the TreeMap using the `containsValue` method and confirms its presence. It then removes a course with a specific ID (104) using the `remove` method, and displays the updated TreeMap after the removal. Next, the program checks if a specific key (102) exists in the TreeMap using the `containsKey` method and confirms its presence. It prints the size of the TreeMap using the `size` method, and then clears all entries using the `clear` method, displaying the empty TreeMap at the end.

15.11 HASHTABLE

In Java, `Hashtable` is a class that implements the `Map` interface and extends `Dictionary`. It represents a collection of key-value pairs where each key is mapped to a specific value. Hashtable uses a hash table data structure to store its elements, allowing for efficient retrieval and storage of key-value pairs.

15.11.1 Advantages of Hashtable

1. Thread-Safe Operations: Hashtable is synchronized, meaning it supports concurrent access from multiple threads without the risk of data corruption. This makes it suitable for use in multithreaded environments where thread safety is a concern.
2. Efficient Retrieval: Hashtable offers constant-time performance for basic operations such as `get()` and `put()`, making it efficient for storing and retrieving key-value pairs, especially when the number of elements is large.

15.11.2 Challenges of Hashtable

1. Synchronization Overhead: While thread safety is a benefit, the synchronization overhead in Hashtable can impact performance, especially in scenarios where high concurrency is not required. For single-threaded applications, this overhead may be unnecessary.
2. Iterating Over Elements: Iterating over elements in a Hashtable may not be as efficient as in other data structures like ArrayList or HashMap. The Enumeration interface provided by Hashtable for iteration is not as versatile as iterators in other collections.

15.11.3 Syntax for Using Hashtable in Java

1. Import the Hashtable class:

```
import java.util.Hashtable;
```

2. Declare and instantiate a Hashtable object:

```
Hashtable<KeyType, ValueType> hashtable = new Hashtable<>();
```

3. Add key-value pairs to the Hashtable:

```
hashtable.put(key, value);
```

4. Retrieve a value based on its key:

```
ValueType value = hashtable.get(key);
```

5. Check if the Hashtable contains a specific key:

```
boolean containsKey = hashtable.containsKey(key);
```

6. Remove a key-value pair from the Hashtable:

```
ValueType removedValue = hashtable.remove(key);
```

7. Check if the Hashtable is empty:

```
boolean isEmpty = hashtable.isEmpty();
```

8. Get the size of the Hashtable:

```
int size = hashtable.size();
```

Hashtable in Java, does facilitating operations such as adding key-value pairs, retrieving values based on keys, checking containment, removing entries, and querying the size of the map. Additionally, Hashtable provides synchronized access to its elements, ensuring thread safety in concurrent environments.

Program

```
import java.util.Hashtable;
public class HashtableExample {
   void main(String[] args) {
  // Creating a Hashtable to store course names with their corresponding IDs
  Hashtable<Integer, String> courseTable = new Hashtable<>();
  // Adding course entries to the Hashtable using the put method
  courseTable.put(101, "Mathematics");
  courseTable.put(102, "Physics");
  courseTable.put(103, "Chemistry");
  courseTable.put(104, "Biology");
  courseTable.put(105, "Computer Science");
  // Displaying the contents of the Hashtable
  System.out.println("Course Table: " + courseTable);
```

```
    // Retrieving and displaying the course associated with a specific ID (102)
    String course = courseTable.get(102);
    System.out.println("Course with ID 102: " + course);
    // Checking if the course "Physics" exists in the Hashtable
    boolean hasPhysics = courseTable.containsValue("Physics");
    if (hasPhysics) {
      System.out.println(" 'Physics' is present in the course table.");
    } else {
      System.out.println(" 'Physics' is not present in the course table.");
    }
    // Removing a course with a specific ID (104) and displaying the updated
    Hashtable
    courseTable.remove(104);
    System.out.println("Course Table after removing ID 104: " + courseTable);
    // Checking if a specific key (ID 102) exists in the Hashtable
    boolean hasKey102 = courseTable.containsKey(102);
    if (hasKey102) {
      System.out.println("ID 102 is present in the course table.");
    } else {
      System.out.println("ID 102 is not present in the course table.");
    }
    // Printing the size of the Hashtable
    System.out.println("Size of the course table: " + courseTable.size());
    // Clearing all entries in the Hashtable
    courseTable.clear();
    System.out.println("Course Table after clearing: " + courseTable);
    }
}
```

Output:

```
Course Table: {105=Computer Science, 104=Biology, 103=Chemistry, 102=
Physics, 101=Mathematics}
Course with ID 102: Physics
'Physics' is present in the course table.
Course Table after removing ID 104: {105=Computer Science, 103=Chemistry,
102=Physics, 101=Mathematics}
ID 102 is present in the course table.
Size of the course table: 4
Course Table after clearing: {}
```

The above program demonstrates the use of a Hashtable to manage a collection of course names in Java, with each course associated with a unique integer ID. It starts by creating a Hashtable named `courseTable` to store the course names mapped to their IDs. The program then adds several courses to the Hashtable using the `put` method, with IDs ranging from 101 to 105, and displays the contents of the Hashtable. The program retrieves and prints the course name associated with a specific ID using the `get` method. It checks if a particular course, "Physics," exists in the Hashtable using the `containsValue` method and confirms its presence. Next, the program removes a course with a specific ID (104) using the `remove` method, and displays the updated Hashtable after the removal. It checks if a specific key (102) exists in the Hashtable using the `containsKey` method and confirms its presence. The program prints the size of the Hashtable using the `size` method, and then clears all entries using the `clear` method, displaying the empty Hashtable at the end.

15.12 ENUMMAP

In Java, `EnumMap` is a specialized implementation of the `Map` interface, designed for use with enum keys. It is a high-performance, compact, and type-safe map that stores key-value pairs where the keys are enums. EnumMap internally uses an array to store the key-value pairs, making it efficient for enum-based mappings.

15.12.1 Advantages of EnumMap

1. Type Safety: EnumMap provides strong type safety because it only accepts enum constants as keys. This prevents runtime errors that might occur with other map implementations if incorrect types are used as keys.
2. Efficient Memory Usage and Performance: EnumMap is highly efficient in terms of memory usage and provides better performance compared to other map implementations for enum-based keys. It achieves this efficiency by internally using arrays tailored to the enum type, resulting in faster access and compact storage.

15.12.2 Challenges of EnumMap

1. Limited Key Type: EnumMap is specifically designed to work with enum keys. While this provides type safety and efficiency for enum-based mappings, it limits its applicability to scenarios where enum keys are used. If keys of other types need to be used, EnumMap cannot be used directly.
2. Initialization with All Enum Constant: When creating an EnumMap, it requires all enum constants to be initialized in order to allocate space for internal arrays. This can be cumbersome, especially if the enum has a large number of constants or if the constants change frequently.

15.12.3 Syntax for Using EnumMap in Java

1. Import the EnumMap class:

```
import java.util.EnumMap;
```

2. Declare and instantiate an EnumMap object:

```
EnumMap<EnumType, ValueType> enumMap = new EnumMap<>(EnumType.class);
```

3. Add key-value pairs to the EnumMap:

```
enumMap.put(enumKey, value);
```

4. Retrieve a value based on its key:

```
ValueType value = enumMap.get(enumKey);
```

5. Check if the EnumMap contains a specific key:

```
boolean containsKey = enumMap.containsKey(enumKey);
```

6. Remove a key-value pair from the EnumMap:

```
ValueType removedValue = enumMap.remove(enumKey);
```

7. Check if the EnumMap is empty:

```
boolean isEmpty = enumMap.isEmpty();
```

8. Get the size of the EnumMap:

```
int size = enumMap.size();
```

EnumMap in Java, does facilitating operations such as adding enum-based key-value pairs, retrieving values based on enum keys, checking containment, removing entries, and querying the size of the map. EnumMap's type safety and performance benefits make it an excellent choice for enum-based mappings in Java.

Program

```
import java.util.EnumMap;
public class EnumMapExample {

  // Define the enum for course types
  enum CourseType {
  MATHEMATICS,
  PHYSICS,
  CHEMISTRY,
  BIOLOGY,
  COMPUTER_SCIENCE
  }
    void main(String[] args) {
  // Create an EnumMap with CourseType as the key type
  EnumMap<CourseType, String> courseMap = new EnumMap<>(CourseType.class);
  // Adding courses to the EnumMap
  courseMap.put(CourseType.MATHEMATICS, "Advanced Calculus");
  courseMap.put(CourseType.PHYSICS, "Quantum Mechanics");
  courseMap.put(CourseType.CHEMISTRY, "Organic Chemistry");
  courseMap.put(CourseType.BIOLOGY, "Genetics");
  courseMap.put(CourseType.COMPUTER_SCIENCE, "Data Structures");
  // Displaying the contents of the EnumMap
  System.out.println("Course Map: " + courseMap);
  // Retrieving and displaying the course associated with a specific type
  (CHEMISTRY)
  String course = courseMap.get(CourseType.CHEMISTRY);
  System.out.println("Course for CHEMISTRY: " + course);
  // Checking if a particular course "Mechanics" is present in the EnumMap
  boolean hasMechanics = courseMap.containsValue("Mechanics");
  if (hasMechanics) {
    System.out.println("'Mechanics' is present in the course map.");
  } else {
    System.out.println("'Mechanics' is not present in the course map.");
  }
  // Removing a course type MATHEMATICS from the EnumMap and displaying the
  updated map
  courseMap.remove(CourseType.MATHEMATICS);
  System.out.println("Course Map after removing MATHEMATICS: " + courseMap);
  // Checking if a specific course type PHYSICS exists in the EnumMap
  boolean hasPhysics = courseMap.containsKey(CourseType.PHYSICS);
```

```
  if (hasPhysics) {
    System.out.println("PHYSICS is present in the course map.");
  } else {
    System.out.println("PHYSICS is not present in the course map.");
  }
  // Printing the size of the EnumMap
  System.out.println("Size of the course map: " + courseMap.size());
  // Clearing all entries in the EnumMap
  courseMap.clear();
  System.out.println("Course Map after clearing: " + courseMap);
  }
}
```

Output:

```
Course Map: {MATHEMATICS=Advanced Calculus, PHYSICS=Quantum Mechanics,
CHEMISTRY=Organic Chemistry, BIOLOGY=Genetics, COMPUTER_SCIENCE=Data
Structures}
Course for CHEMISTRY: Organic Chemistry
'Mechanics' is not present in the course map.
Course Map after removing MATHEMATICS: {PHYSICS=Quantum Mechanics, CHEMISTRY=
Organic Chemistry, BIOLOGY=Genetics, COMPUTER_SCIENCE=Data Structures}
PHYSICS is present in the course map.
Size of the course map: 4
Course Map after clearing: {}
```

The above program illustrates the usage of an EnumMap to associate course types with their respective names in Java. It begins by defining an enum class named `CourseType` with constants representing different types of courses: MATHEMATICS, PHYSICS, CHEMISTRY, BIOLOGY, and COMPUTER_SCIENCE. Inside the main method, an EnumMap named `courseMap` is created, specifying the key type as `CourseType`. Courses are then added to the EnumMap using the put method, where each course type is mapped to its corresponding name.

The program checks if a particular course, "Mechanics," is present in the EnumMap using the containsValue method and confirms its presence. Next, it removes a course type, MATHEMATICS, from the EnumMap using the remove method and displays the updated EnumMap. The program checks if a specific course type, PHYSICS, exists in the EnumMap using the containsKey method and confirms its presence. It then prints the size of the EnumMap using the size method and clears all entries using the clear method, displaying the empty EnumMap at the end.

15.13 STACK

In Java, `Stack` is a class that represents a Last-In-First-Out (LIFO) data structure. It extends the `Vector` class with five operations that allow a vector to be treated as a stack. The usual push and pop operations are provided, as well as methods for peeking at the top item, testing for an empty stack, and searching for an item.

15.13.1 Advantages of Stack

1. Simple Interface: The `Stack` class provides a simple and intuitive interface for implementing stack-based operations. It offers methods such as `push()` to add elements, `pop()` to remove elements, `peek()` to inspect the top element, and `isEmpty()` to check if the stack is empty.
2. Easy Implementation of Undo/Redo: Stacks are commonly used in applications to implement undo and redo functionality. By using a stack to store the history of user actions, it becomes

straightforward to implement undo and redo operations, where popping from one stack and pushing onto another effectively reverses or reapplies actions.

15.13.2 Challenges of Stack

1. Inefficient Performance: The `Stack` class in Java extends the `Vector` class, which is synchronized and thread-safe. While synchronization ensures thread safety, it can lead to performance overhead in single-threaded applications where thread safety is not required. In such cases, using other non-synchronized collections might be more efficient.
2. Limited Functionality: While stacks are suitable for certain types of operations like undo/redo, they might not be the best choice for all scenarios. For example, stacks are not efficient for searching or accessing elements at arbitrary positions. If these functionalities are required, other data structures like lists or arrays may be more appropriate.

15.13.3 Syntax for Using Stack in Java

1. Import the Stack class:

```
import java.util.Stack;
```

2. Declare and instantiate a Stack object:

```
Stack<Type> stack = new Stack<>();
```

3. Push an element onto the stack:

```
stack.push(element);
```

4. Pop the top element from the stack:

```
Type element = stack.pop();
```

5. Peek at the top element of the stack without removing it:

```
Type topElement = stack.peek();
```

6. Check if the stack is empty:

```
boolean isEmpty = stack.isEmpty();
```

7. Get the size of the stack:

```
int size = stack.size();
```

Stacks in Java, does facilitating operations such as pushing and popping elements, peeking at the top element, checking for emptiness, and getting the size of the stack.

Program

```
import java.util.Stack;
public class StackExample {
   void main(String[] args) {
```

```
    // Creating a Stack to store course names
    Stack<String> courseStack = new Stack<>();
    // Pushing several courses onto the Stack
    courseStack.push("Mathematics");
    courseStack.push("Physics");
    courseStack.push("Chemistry");
    courseStack.push("Biology");
    courseStack.push("Computer Science");
    // Displaying the contents of the Stack
    System.out.println("Course Stack: " + courseStack);
    // Retrieving and displaying the top course in the Stack without removing it
    String topCourse = courseStack.peek();
    System.out.println("Top course: " + topCourse);
    // Popping the top course from the Stack and displaying it
    String poppedCourse = courseStack.pop();
    System.out.println("Popped course: " + poppedCourse);
    // Displaying the Stack after popping an element
    System.out.println("Course Stack after popping: " + courseStack);
    // Searching for a specific course in the Stack and displaying its position
    int position = courseStack.search("Physics");
    if (position != -1) {
      System.out.println("'Physics' is found at position: " + position);
    } else {
      System.out.println("'Physics' is not present in the stack.");
    }
    // Checking if the Stack is empty and printing an appropriate message
    boolean isEmpty = courseStack.isEmpty();
    if (isEmpty) {
      System.out.println("The Stack is empty.");
    } else {
      System.out.println("The Stack is not empty.");
    }
    // Printing the size of the Stack
    System.out.println("Size of the Stack: " + courseStack.size());
    // Clearing all elements from the Stack
    courseStack.clear();
    System.out.println("Course Stack after clearing: " + courseStack);
    }
}
```

Output:

```
Course Stack: [Mathematics, Physics, Chemistry, Biology, Computer Science]
Top course: Computer Science
Popped course: Computer Science
Course Stack after popping: [Mathematics, Physics, Chemistry, Biology]
'Physics' is found at position: 3
The Stack is not empty.
Size of the Stack: 4
Course Stack after clearing: []
```

The above program demonstrates the use of a Stack to manage a collection of course names in Java. It begins by creating a Stack named `courseStack` to store the course names. The program pushes several courses onto the Stack using the push method, including "Mathematics," "Physics," "Chemistry," "Biology," and "Computer Science." The contents of the Stack are then displayed, showing the courses in the order they were pushed onto the Stack. The top course in the Stack is retrieved and printed using the peek method. Next, a course is popped from the Stack using the pop method, removing it from the top of the Stack. The popped course is displayed, and the Stack is shown again to reflect the removal. The program searches for a specific course, "Physics," in the Stack using the search method. If the course is found, its position in the Stack is printed; otherwise, a message indicating that the course is not present is displayed. It then checks if the Stack is empty using the isEmpty method and prints an appropriate message. The size of the Stack is printed using the size method. Finally, all elements are cleared from the Stack using the clear method, and the empty Stack is displayed.

15.14 VECTOR

In Java, `Vector` is a legacy class that represents a dynamic array, similar to `ArrayList`. It is synchronized and thread-safe, which means that multiple threads can manipulate a `Vector` concurrently without causing data corruption. However, its synchronized nature can impact performance in single-threaded scenarios.

15.14.1 Advantages of Vector

1. Thread Safety: One of the main advantages of `Vector` is its thread-safe nature. It ensures that operations performed on a `Vector` by multiple threads are synchronized, preventing concurrent modification exceptions and data corruption in multi-threaded environments.
2. Dynamic Resizing: Like `ArrayList`, `Vector` dynamically resizes itself as elements are added or removed, allowing it to accommodate an arbitrary number of elements without requiring manual resizing or reallocation.

15.14.2 Challenges of Vector

1. Performance Overhead: The synchronization of `Vector` comes with a performance overhead, especially in single-threaded scenarios where thread safety is not a requirement. This can result in slower execution compared to non-synchronized collections like `ArrayList`.
2. Limited Flexibility: While `Vector` provides thread safety, this comes at the cost of flexibility. In scenarios where thread safety is not necessary, using `ArrayList` or other non-synchronized collections may offer better performance and more flexibility.

15.14.3 Syntax for Using Vector in Java

1. Import the Vector class:

```
import java.util.Vector;
```

2. Declare and instantiate a Vector object:

```
Vector<Type> vector = new Vector<>();
```

3. Add an element to the vector:

```
vector.add(element);
```

4. Access an element at a specific index:

```
Type element = vector.get(index);
```

5. Remove an element from the vector:

```
vector.remove(element);
```

6. Check if the vector contains a specific element:

```
boolean containsElement = vector.contains(element);
```

7. Get the size of the vector:

```
int size = vector.size();
```

8. iterate over the elements of the vector using a for loop or iterator.

`Vector` objects in Java, enabling operations such as adding and accessing elements, removing elements, checking for containment, and getting the size of the vector. While `Vector` offers thread safety, developers should assess whether this feature is necessary and consider the performance implications when choosing between `Vector` and other collections like `ArrayList`.

Program

```
import java.util.Vector;
public class VectorExample {
    void main(String[] args) {
  // Initialize a Vector to store course names
  Vector<String> courseVector = new Vector<>();
  // Adding several courses to the Vector
  courseVector.add("Mathematics");
  courseVector.add("Physics");
  courseVector.add("Chemistry");
  courseVector.add("Biology");
  courseVector.add("Computer Science");
  // Displaying the contents of the Vector
  System.out.println("Course Vector: " + courseVector);
  // Retrieving and printing the course at a specific index (e.g., index 2)
  String courseAtIndex2 = courseVector.get(2);
  System.out.println("Course at index 2: " + courseAtIndex2);
  // Updating a course at a specific index (index 3) with "History"
  courseVector.set(3, "History");
  System.out.println("Course Vector after updating index 3: " + courseVector);
  // Removing a course from the Vector at a specified index (e.g., index 1)
  String removedCourse = courseVector.remove(1);
  System.out.println("Removed course: " + removedCourse);
  // Displaying the Vector after removal
  System.out.println("Course Vector after removal: " + courseVector);
  // Checking if a specific course, "Physics," exists in the Vector
  boolean hasPhysics = courseVector.contains("Physics");
  System.out.println("'Physics' exists in the Vector: " + hasPhysics);
  // Checking if the Vector is empty
  boolean isEmpty = courseVector.isEmpty();
  System.out.println("The Vector is empty: " + isEmpty);
  // Printing the size of the Vector
  System.out.println("Size of the Vector: " + courseVector.size());
  // Clearing all elements from the Vector
```

```
  courseVector.clear();
  System.out.println("Course Vector after clearing: " + courseVector);
  }
}
```

Output:

```
Course Vector: [Mathematics, Physics, Chemistry, Biology, Computer Science]
Course at index 2: Chemistry
Course Vector after updating index 3: [Mathematics, Physics, Chemistry,
History, Computer Science]
Removed course: Physics
Course Vector after removal: [Mathematics, Chemistry, History, Computer
Science]
'Physics' exists in the Vector: false
The Vector is empty: false
Size of the Vector: 4
Course Vector after clearing: []
```

The above program showcases the utilization of a Vector to manage a collection of course names in Java. It initializes a Vector named `courseVector` to store the course names. Several courses are added to the Vector using the add method, including "Mathematics," "Physics," "Chemistry," "Biology," and "Computer Science." The program then displays the contents of the Vector, showing the courses in the order they were added. It retrieves and prints the course at a specific index using the get method. Next, it updates a course at a particular index using the set method, replacing the course with "History" at index 3. The Vector is displayed again to reflect the update. A course is removed from the Vector at a specified index using the remove method. The removed course is displayed, and the Vector is shown again after the removal. The program checks if a specific course, "Physics," exists in the Vector using the contains method and prints the result accordingly. It also checks if the Vector is empty using the isEmpty method and prints an appropriate message. The size of the Vector is printed using the size method. Finally, all elements are cleared from the Vector using the clear method, and the empty Vector is displayed.

15.15 LIST

In Java, `List` is an interface that represents an ordered collection of elements. Unlike arrays, which have a fixed size, lists can dynamically grow and shrink as elements are added or removed. The `List` interface provides methods for accessing, adding, removing, and manipulating elements within the list. Implementations of the `List` interface include `ArrayList`, `LinkedList`, `Vector`, and others.

15.15.1 Advantages of List

1. Dynamic Size: Lists in Java, such as `ArrayList` and `LinkedList`, have a dynamic size, allowing elements to be added or removed without requiring manual resizing or reallocation. This flexibility makes lists suitable for scenarios where the number of elements may change over time.
2. Ordered Collection: Lists maintain the order of elements as they are added, allowing for predictable iteration and retrieval of elements based on their position in the list. This ordered nature is essential for scenarios where the sequence of elements matters.

15.15.2 Challenges of List

1. Performance Variability: Different implementations of the `List` interface may have different performance characteristics. For example, while `ArrayList` provides fast random access to

elements, `LinkedList` may offer better performance for insertion and deletion operations in certain scenarios. Choosing the right implementation depends on the specific requirements of the application.

2. Concurrency Issues: In multi-threaded environments, concurrent access to lists can lead to data corruption and race conditions if proper synchronization is not applied. Developers must ensure proper synchronization or use thread-safe list implementations, such as `Vector` or synchronized wrappers, to avoid such issues.

15.15.3 Syntax for Using List in Java

1. Import the List interface:

```
import java.util.List;
```

2. Declare a List variable:

```
List<Type> list;
```

3. Instantiate a List object using an implementation class (e.g., ArrayList, LinkedList):

```
list = new ArrayList<>();
```

4. Add elements to the list:

```
list.add(element);
```

5. Access an element at a specific index:

```
Type element = list.get(index);
```

6. Remove an element from the list:

```
list.remove(element);
```

7. Check if the list contains a specific element:

```
boolean containsElement = list.contains(element);
```

8. Get the size of the list:

```
int size = list.size();
```

9. Iterate over the elements of the list using a for loop or iterator.

Lists in Java, including adding, accessing, removing, and manipulating elements. The `List` interface serves as a versatile foundation for building ordered collections in Java applications.

Program

```
import java.util.ArrayList;
import java.util.List;
public class ArrayListExample {
    void main(String[] args) {
```

```
    // Create an ArrayList to store course names
    List<String> courseList = new ArrayList<>();
    // Add several courses to the ArrayList
    courseList.add("Mathematics");
    courseList.add("Physics");
    courseList.add("Chemistry");
    courseList.add("Biology");
    courseList.add("Computer Science");
    // Display the contents of the ArrayList
    System.out.println("Course List: " + courseList);
    // Retrieve and print the course at a specific index (e.g., index 2)
    String courseAtIndex2 = courseList.get(2);
    System.out.println("Course at index 2: " + courseAtIndex2);
    // Update a course at a specific index (index 3) with "History"
    courseList.set(3, "History");
    System.out.println("Course List after updating index 3: " + courseList);
    // Remove a course from the ArrayList at a specified index (e.g., index 1)
    String removedCourse = courseList.remove(1);
    System.out.println("Removed course: " + removedCourse);
    // Display the ArrayList after removal
    System.out.println("Course List after removal: " + courseList);
    // Check if a specific course, "Physics," exists in the ArrayList
    boolean hasPhysics = courseList.contains("Physics");
    System.out.println("'Physics' exists in the ArrayList: " + hasPhysics);
    // Check if the ArrayList is empty
    boolean isEmpty = courseList.isEmpty();
    System.out.println("The ArrayList is empty: " + isEmpty);
    // Print the size of the ArrayList
    System.out.println("Size of the ArrayList: " + courseList.size());
    // Clear all elements from the ArrayList
    courseList.clear();
    System.out.println("Course List after clearing: " + courseList);
    }
}
```

Output:

```
Course List: [Mathematics, Physics, Chemistry, Biology, Computer Science]
Course at index 2: Chemistry
Course List after updating index 3: [Mathematics, Physics, Chemistry,
History, Computer Science]
Removed course: Physics
Course List after removal: [Mathematics, Chemistry, History, Computer
Science]
'Physics' exists in the ArrayList: false
The ArrayList is empty: false
Size of the ArrayList: 4
Course List after clearing: []
```

The above program illustrates the usage of a List interface, specifically an ArrayList implementation, to manage a collection of course names in Java. It starts by creating an ArrayList named `courseList` to store the course names. The program adds several courses to the ArrayList using the add method, including "Mathematics," "Physics," "Chemistry," "Biology," and "Computer Science." It then displays the contents of the ArrayList, showing the courses in the order they were added. The program retrieves and prints the course at a specific index using the get method. Next, it updates a course at a particular index using the set method, replacing the course with "History" at index

3. The ArrayList is displayed again to reflect the update. A course is removed from the ArrayList at a specified index using the remove method. The removed course is displayed, and the ArrayList is shown again after the removal. The program checks if a specific course, "Physics," exists in the ArrayList using the contains method and prints the result accordingly. It also checks if the ArrayList is empty using the isEmpty method and prints an appropriate message. The size of the ArrayList is printed using the size method. Finally, all elements are cleared from the ArrayList using the clear method, and the empty ArrayList is displayed.

15.16 MAP

In Java, a `Map` is an interface that represents a collection of key-value pairs, where each key is unique and maps to a corresponding value. It provides methods for adding, accessing, and manipulating elements based on their keys. Implementations of the `Map` interface include `HashMap`, `TreeMap`, `LinkedHashMap`, and others.

15.16.1 Advantages of Map

1. Fast Retrieval by Key: Maps provide fast retrieval of values based on their associated keys. This makes them ideal for scenarios where quick access to values using unique identifiers (keys) is required.
2. Key-Value Association: Maps establish a clear association between keys and values, allowing developers to store and retrieve data in a structured manner. This key-value pairing facilitates the organization and management of data in applications.

15.16.2 Challenges of Map

1. Key Uniqueness Requirement: Maps enforce the uniqueness of keys, meaning that each key must be unique within the map. Duplicate keys can lead to unexpected behavior or data overwriting. Developers need to ensure that keys are unique when working with maps.
2. Iteration Order: Depending on the implementation, the order of iteration over elements in a map may not be consistent or predictable. While some map implementations maintain insertion order (e.g., `LinkedHashMap`), others do not guarantee any specific order (e.g., `HashMap`). This lack of predictability can affect the behavior of applications relying on ordered iteration.

15.16.3 Syntax for Using Map in Java

1. Import the Map interface:

```
import java.util.Map;
```

2. Declare a Map variable with key and value types:

```
Map<KeyType, ValueType> map;
```

3. Instantiate a Map object using an implementation class (e.g., HashMap, TreeMap):

```
map = new HashMap<>();
or new TreeMap<>(), new LinkedHashMap<>()
```

4. Add key-value pairs to the map:

```
map.put(key, value);
```

5. Access the value associated with a specific key:

```
ValueType value = map.get(key);
```

6. Remove a key-value pair from the map:

```
map.remove(key);
```

7. Check if the map contains a specific key:

```
boolean containsKey = map.containsKey(key);
```

8. Check if the map contains a specific value:

```
boolean containsValue = map.containsValue(value);
```

9. Get the size (number of key-value pairs) of the map:

```
int size = map.size();
```

10. Iterate over the key-value pairs of the map using various methods like entrySet(), keySet(), or values().

Maps in Java, including adding, accessing, removing, and iterating over key-value pairs. The `Map` interface serves as a fundamental tool for organizing and managing data in Java applications.

Program

```
import java.util.HashMap;
import java.util.Map;
public class HashMapExample {
    void main(String[] args) {
  // Create a HashMap to store course IDs and their corresponding names
  Map<Integer, String> courseMap = new HashMap<>();
  // Add several courses to the HashMap
  courseMap.put(101, "Mathematics");
  courseMap.put(102, "Physics");
  courseMap.put(103, "Chemistry");
  courseMap.put(104, "Biology");
  courseMap.put(105, "Computer Science");
  // Display the contents of the HashMap
  System.out.println("Course Map: " + courseMap);
  // Retrieve and print the name of a course by providing its ID (e.g.,
  ID 103)
  String courseName = courseMap.get(103);
  System.out.println("Course with ID 103: " + courseName);
  // Update the name of a course by specifying its ID (e.g., ID 104) and
  providing the new name
  courseMap.put(104, "History");
```

```
  System.out.println("Course Map after updating ID 104: " + courseMap);
  // Remove a course from the HashMap by specifying its ID (e.g., ID 102)
  String removedCourse = courseMap.remove(102);
  System.out.println("Removed course with ID 102: " + removedCourse);
  // Display the HashMap after removal
  System.out.println("Course Map after removal: " + courseMap);
  // Check if a specific course ID (e.g., ID 105) exists in the HashMap
  boolean hasCourseId = courseMap.containsKey(105);
  System.out.println("Course ID 105 exists in the HashMap: " + hasCourseId);
  // Check if a specific course name (e.g., "Physics") exists in the HashMap
  boolean hasCourseName = courseMap.containsValue("Physics");
  System.out.println("'Physics' exists in the HashMap: " + hasCourseName);
  // Print the size of the HashMap
  System.out.println("Size of the HashMap: " + courseMap.size());
  // Clear all elements from the HashMap
  courseMap.clear();
  System.out.println("Course Map after clearing: " + courseMap);
  }
}
```

Output:

```
Course Map: {101=Mathematics, 102=Physics, 103=Chemistry, 104=Biology,
105=Computer Science}
Course with ID 103: Chemistry
Course Map after updating ID 104: {101=Mathematics, 102=Physics, 103=
Chemistry, 104=History, 105=Computer Science}
Removed course with ID 102: Physics
Course Map after removal: {101=Mathematics, 103=Chemistry, 104=History,
105=Computer Science}
Course ID 105 exists in the HashMap: true
'Physics' exists in the HashMap: false
Size of the HashMap: 4
Course Map after clearing: {}
```

The above program demonstrates the use of a Map interface, specifically a HashMap implementation, to manage a collection of courses in Java. It begins by creating a HashMap named `courseMap` to store course IDs and their corresponding names. Several courses are added to the HashMap using the put method, associating each course ID with its name. The program then displays the contents of the HashMap, showing the course IDs and names. It retrieves and prints the name of a course by providing its ID using the get method. Next, it updates the name of a course by specifying its ID and providing the new name using the put method. A course is removed from the HashMap by specifying its ID using the remove method. The removed course name is displayed, and the HashMap is shown again after the removal. The program checks if a specific course ID exists in the HashMap using the containsKey method and prints the result accordingly. It also checks if a specific course name exists in the HashMap using the containsValue method and prints the result. The size of the HashMap is printed using the size method. Finally, all elements are cleared from the HashMap using the clear method, and the empty HashMap is displayed.

15.17 ENUMSET

In Java, `EnumSet` is a specialized implementation of the `Set` interface designed to work with enum types. It is used to represent a set of enum constants, providing high-performance set operations tailored specifically for enums. EnumSet is a part of the Java Collections Framework and offers efficient storage and manipulation of enum values.

15.17.1 Advantages of EnumSet

1. Memory Efficiency: EnumSet internally uses a highly efficient bit vector representation for enums, resulting in compact storage and minimal memory overhead. This makes EnumSet ideal for scenarios where memory usage is a concern, especially when dealing with a large number of enum values.
2. Fast Set Operations: EnumSet is optimized for set operations such as intersection, union, and difference. These operations are performed efficiently, often outperforming other set implementations when working with enum constants. EnumSet's performance benefits are particularly noticeable in scenarios involving frequent set manipulations.

15.17.2 Challenges of EnumSet

1. Limited to Enum Types: EnumSet is designed specifically for enum types and cannot be used with non-enum elements. This restriction limits its applicability to scenarios where enum constants are involved. If the users need to work with non-enum elements, they need to use other set implementations such as HashSet or TreeSet.
2. Immutable Once Created: Once an EnumSet is created, its contents cannot be modified. While this immutability ensures thread safety in concurrent environments, it also means that you cannot add or remove elements from an EnumSet after creation. If dynamic modification of set contents is required, the users may need to use alternative set implementations.

15.17.3 Syntax for Using EnumSet in Java

1. Import the EnumSet class:

```
import java.util.EnumSet;
```

2. Declare an EnumSet variable for a specific enum type:

```
EnumSet<EnumType> enumSet;
```

3. Create an EnumSet instance using the static factory methods provided by the EnumSet class:

```
enumSet = EnumSet.allOf(EnumType.class);
```

4. Perform set operations such as intersection, union, difference, etc., using methods like `add`, `remove`, `contains`, `clear`, etc.
5. Iterate over the elements of the EnumSet using a for-each loop or iterator.
6. Optionally, use other static factory methods like `noneOf`, `of`, `range`, etc., to create EnumSets with specific enum constants.

EnumSets in Java, providing efficient storage and operations for enum constants. EnumSet's specialization for enums makes it a powerful tool for working with enum values in Java applications.

Program

```
import java.util.EnumSet;
public class EnumSetExample {
  // Define the enum type for course types
```

```
  enum CourseType {
  MATHEMATICS, PHYSICS, CHEMISTRY, BIOLOGY, COMPUTER_SCIENCE
  }
    void main(String[] args) {
  // Create an EnumSet with initial course types
  EnumSet<CourseType>   courseSet   =   EnumSet.of(CourseType.MATHEMATICS,
  CourseType.PHYSICS, CourseType.CHEMISTRY);
  // Display the contents of the EnumSet
  System.out.println("Initial EnumSet: " + courseSet);
  // Add another course type to the EnumSet
  courseSet.add(CourseType.BIOLOGY);
  System.out.println("EnumSet after adding BIOLOGY: " + courseSet);
  // Remove a course type from the EnumSet
  courseSet.remove(CourseType.MATHEMATICS);
  System.out.println("EnumSet after removing MATHEMATICS: " + courseSet);
  // Check if a specific course type is in the EnumSet
  boolean  hasComputerScience  =  courseSet.contains(CourseType.COMPUTER_
  SCIENCE);
  System.out.println("Contains COMPUTER_SCIENCE: " + hasComputerScience);
  // Print the size of the EnumSet
  System.out.println("Size of the EnumSet: " + courseSet.size());
  // Clear all elements from the EnumSet
  courseSet.clear();
  System.out.println("EnumSet after clearing: " + courseSet);
  }
}
```

Output:

```
Initial EnumSet: [MATHEMATICS, PHYSICS, CHEMISTRY]
EnumSet after adding BIOLOGY: [MATHEMATICS, PHYSICS, CHEMISTRY, BIOLOGY]
EnumSet after removing MATHEMATICS: [PHYSICS, CHEMISTRY, BIOLOGY]
Contains COMPUTER_SCIENCE: false
Size of the EnumSet: 3
EnumSet after clearing: []
```

The above Java program showcases the versatility of EnumSet, a specialized Set implementation tailored for use with enum types.

15.18 COMPARABLE

In Java, `Comparable` is an interface that defines a natural ordering for the objects of a class. When a class implements the Comparable interface, it means that its instances can be compared with each other for the purpose of sorting. The Comparable interface contains a single method, `compareTo`, which compares the current object with another object of the same type and returns an integer indicating their relative order.

15.18.1 Advantages of Comparable

1. Natural Sorting Order: Implementing the Comparable interface allows objects of a class to be sorted based on their natural ordering. This simplifies sorting operations as it provides a consistent and intuitive way to arrange objects without the need for external comparators.
2. Integration with Collection Classes: Many collection classes in Java, such as TreeSet and TreeMap, use the natural ordering defined by the Comparable interface for sorting elements.

By implementing Comparable, objects can seamlessly integrate with these collection classes, enabling them to be efficiently stored and retrieved in sorted order.

15.18.2 Challenges of Comparable

1. Immutability of Ordering: The natural ordering defined by the compareTo method is fixed once implemented. This means that any changes to the natural ordering logic require modifications to the compareTo method, which can be challenging, especially in cases where the natural ordering may vary based on different criteria.
2. Violation of Encapsulation: Implementing Comparable may require exposing internal state or attributes of objects for comparison purposes. This can potentially violate encapsulation principles, as it exposes implementation details of the class and may lead to unintended dependencies in client code.

15.18.3 Syntax for Implementing Comparable in Java

To implement the Comparable interface in Java, follow these steps:

1. Declare the class and implement the Comparable interface:

```
public class MyClass implements Comparable<MyClass> {
// Class implementation
}
```

2. Override the compareTo method to define the natural ordering:

```
  @Override
  public int compareTo(MyClass other) {
  // Compare the current object with 'other' and return an integer indi-
cating their relative order
  }
```

3. Within the compareTo method, compare the current object (this) with the ‘other’ object and return:

- a negative integer if this object is less than the other object,
- zero if they are equal,
- a positive integer if this object is greater than the other object.

4. Use the natural ordering defined by the compareTo method for sorting and comparison operations.

By following this syntax, objects of the class can be compared and sorted based on their natural ordering defined by the compareTo method, making them compatible with various sorting and collection classes in Java.

Program

```
import java.util.ArrayList;
import java.util.Collections;
```

```
import java.util.List;
public class Main {

  // Inner Course class implementing Comparable
  static class Course implements Comparable<Course> {
  private int courseId;
  private String courseName;
  public Course(int courseId, String courseName) {
    this.courseId = courseId;
    this.courseName = courseName;
  }
  public int getCourseId() {
    return courseId;
  }
  public String getCourseName() {
    return courseName;
  }
  @Override
  public int compareTo(Course other) {
    return Integer.compare(this.courseId, other.courseId);
  }
  @Override
  public String toString() {
    return "Course ID: " + courseId + ", Course Name: " + courseName;
  }
  }
    void main(String[] args) {
  // Create a list of Course objects
  List<Course> courses = new ArrayList<>();
  courses.add(new Course(104, "Biology"));
  courses.add(new Course(102, "Mathematics"));
  courses.add(new Course(101, "Physics"));
  courses.add(new Course(103, "Chemistry"));
  // Print the unsorted list
  System.out.println("Unsorted List:");
  for (Course course : courses) {
    System.out.println(course);
  }
  // Sort the list based on course ID
  Collections.sort(courses);
  // Print the sorted list
  System.out.println("\nSorted List:");
  for (Course course : courses) {
    System.out.println(course);
  }
  }
}
```

Output

```
Unsorted List:
Course ID: 104, Course Name: Biology
Course ID: 102, Course Name: Mathematics
Course ID: 101, Course Name: Physics
Course ID: 103, Course Name: Chemistry
Sorted List:
Course ID: 101, Course Name: Physics
```

```
Course ID: 102, Course Name: Mathematics
Course ID: 103, Course Name: Chemistry
Course ID: 104, Course Name: Biology
```

The above Java program demonstrates the implementation of the `Comparable` interface to enable sorting of a custom `Course` class based on the course ID. The `Course` class encapsulates information about a course, including its ID and name. It implements the `Comparable` interface and overrides the `compareTo` method to facilitate sorting based on the course ID. Additionally, the `toString` method is overridden to provide a meaningful string representation of the `Course` object. In the `main` method, a list of `Course` objects is instantiated and populated with various courses, each defined by a unique course ID and name. Initially, the unsorted list of courses is displayed, showcasing the order in which they were added. Subsequently, the `Collections.sort()` method is utilized to sort the list of courses based on the implemented `compareTo` logic, which sorts the courses in ascending order of their IDs.

15.19 COMPARATOR INTERFACE

In Java, the `Comparator` interface is used to define custom ordering for objects of a class that do not have a natural ordering or when the natural ordering is not suitable for sorting. Unlike the Comparable interface, which defines the natural ordering for a class, the Comparator interface allows for multiple sorting criteria and custom sorting logic to be applied to objects of the class. The Comparator interface contains a single method, `compare`, which compares two objects and returns an integer indicating their relative order.

15.19.1 Advantages of Comparator

1. Flexible Sorting Logic: Implementing the Comparator interface provides flexibility in defining custom sorting logic tailored to specific requirements. It allows developers to define sorting criteria based on different attributes or properties of objects, providing greater control over sorting behavior.
2. External Sorting Logic: Comparator allows for external sorting logic to be applied to classes whose source code cannot be modified or when multiple sorting criteria need to be supported. This is particularly useful when sorting objects from third-party libraries or when sorting objects based on dynamically changing criteria.

15.19.2 Challenges of Comparator

1. Complexity in Usage: Using comparators may introduce additional complexity to code, especially when dealing with multiple sorting criteria or complex sorting logic. Developers need to carefully manage and maintain comparator implementations, which can lead to increased code complexity and maintenance overhead.
2. Coupling with Implementation: Comparator implementations may be tightly coupled with specific classes or data structures, making them less reusable across different contexts. This can lead to code duplication if similar sorting logic needs to be implemented for different classes or scenarios.

15.19.3 Syntax for Implementing Comparator in Java

To implement the Comparator interface in Java, follow these steps:

1. Declare a class that implements the Comparator interface and specifies the type of objects to be compared:

```
public class MyComparator implements Comparator<MyClass> {
// Comparator implementation
}
```

2. Override the compare method to define the custom sorting logic:

```
@Override
public int compare(MyClass obj1, MyClass obj2) {
// Compare obj1 and obj2 based on custom sorting criteria
}
```

3. Within the compare method, compare the two objects (obj1 and obj2) and return:

- a negative integer if obj1 is less than obj2,
- zero if they are equal,
- a positive integer if obj1 is greater than obj2.

4. Use the comparator for sorting objects using sorting methods provided by Java collections or utilities, such as `Collections.sort()` or `Arrays.sort()`.

By following this syntax, custom sorting logic can be implemented using the Comparator interface, providing flexibility in sorting objects based on different criteria or requirements.

Program

```
import java.util.ArrayList;
import java.util.Collections;
import java.util.Comparator;
import java.util.List;
public class Main {
  // Inner Course class
  static class Course {
  private int courseId;
  private String courseName;
  public Course(int courseId, String courseName) {
    this.courseId = courseId;
    this.courseName = courseName;
  }
  public int getCourseId() {
    return courseId;
  }
  public String getCourseName() {
    return courseName;
  }
  @Override
  public String toString() {
    return "Course ID: " + courseId + ", Course Name: " + courseName;
  }
  }
    void main(String[] args) {
```

```
  // Create a list of Course objects
  List<Course> courses = new ArrayList<>();
  courses.add(new Course(104, "Biology"));
  courses.add(new Course(102, "Mathematics"));
  courses.add(new Course(101, "Physics"));
  courses.add(new Course(103, "Chemistry"));
  // Print the unsorted list
  System.out.println("Unsorted List:");
  for (Course course : courses) {
    System.out.println(course);
  }
  // Sort by course ID using a Comparator
  Collections.sort(courses, new Comparator<Course>() {
    @Override
    public int compare(Course c1, Course c2) {
    return Integer.compare(c1.getCourseId(), c2.getCourseId());
    }
  });
  // Print the list sorted by course ID
  System.out.println("\nSorted by Course ID:");
  for (Course course : courses) {
    System.out.println(course);
  }
  // Sort by course name using a Comparator
  Collections.sort(courses, new Comparator<Course>() {
    @Override
    public int compare(Course c1, Course c2) {
    return c1.getCourseName().compareTo(c2.getCourseName());
    }
  });
  // Print the list sorted by course name
  System.out.println("\nSorted by Course Name:");
  for (Course course : courses) {
    System.out.println(course);
  }
  }
}
```

Output:

```
Unsorted List:
Course ID: 104, Course Name: Biology
Course ID: 102, Course Name: Mathematics
Course ID: 101, Course Name: Physics
Course ID: 103, Course Name: Chemistry
Sorted by Course ID:
Course ID: 101, Course Name: Physics
Course ID: 102, Course Name: Mathematics
Course ID: 103, Course Name: Chemistry
Course ID: 104, Course Name: Biology
Sorted by Course Name:
Course ID: 104, Course Name: Biology
Course ID: 103, Course Name: Chemistry
Course ID: 102, Course Name: Mathematics
Course ID: 101, Course Name: Physics
```

The above Java program exemplifies the utilization of the `Comparator` interface to sort objects of a custom `Course` class based on different criteria. The `Course` class encapsulates information about a course, including its ID and name. Within the `main` method, a list of `Course` objects is instantiated and populated with various courses, each defined by a unique course ID and name. Initially, the unsorted list of courses is displayed, showcasing the order in which they were added. Subsequently, the `Collections.sort()` method is employed to sort the list of courses based on the course ID. This is achieved by providing a custom `Comparator` implementation that compares courses based on their IDs. The sorted list of courses, arranged in ascending order of their IDs, is then displayed.

15.20 DEQUEUE

In Java, a `Deque` (pronounced as "deck"), short for double-ended queue, is a linear collection that supports the insertion and removal of elements at both ends. It extends the `Queue` interface and provides additional methods to operate at both the head and the tail of the deque. Deques can function as both queues (first-in-first-out) and stacks (last-in-first-out), offering versatility in implementing various data structures and algorithms.

15.20.1 Advantages of Deque

1. Versatility in Usage: Deques provide versatility in implementing various data structures such as queues, stacks, and double-ended queues. They support operations at both ends, allowing for efficient insertion, removal, and retrieval of elements, making them suitable for a wide range of applications.
2. Efficient Operations: Deques offer efficient operations for adding and removing elements at both ends with constant-time complexity (O(1)). This makes them suitable for scenarios where elements need to be inserted or removed frequently from either end of the collection.

15.20.2 Challenges of Deque

1. Complexity in Usage: Deques may introduce complexity in usage, especially when considering the ordering and synchronization of operations. Developers need to carefully manage the state of the deque to avoid unintended behavior, such as concurrent modification or incorrect ordering of elements.
2. Memory Overhead: Depending on the underlying implementation, deques may incur additional memory overhead compared to simpler data structures such as arrays or linked lists. This overhead can impact the performance and memory footprint of applications, particularly in memory-constrained environments.

15.20.3 Syntax for Using Deque in Java

To use a Deque in Java, follow these steps:

1. Import the Deque interface and choose an implementation (e.g., ArrayDeque or LinkedList):

```
import java.util.Deque;
    import java.util.ArrayDeque;  or
  import java.util.LinkedList;
```

2. Create an instance of Deque using the chosen implementation:

```
Deque<String> deque = new ArrayDeque<>();
or new LinkedList<>();
```

3. Use Deque methods to add, remove, or retrieve elements from both ends:

```
deque.addFirst("Element"); // Add element at the front
deque.addLast("Element"); // Add element at the end
String firstElement = deque.removeFirst(); // Remove and return element from
the front
String lastElement = deque.removeLast(); // Remove and return element from
the end
```

4. Use other Deque methods such as `peekFirst()`, `peekLast()`, `offerFirst()`, `offerLast()`, `pollFirst()`, `pollLast()`, etc., to perform additional operations as needed.

By following this syntax, Deque can be effectively used in Java applications to implement various data structures and algorithms that require efficient insertion, removal, and retrieval of elements at both ends of the collection.

Program

```
import java.util.ArrayDeque;
import java.util.Deque;
public class Main {
    void main(String[] args) {
  // Create an ArrayDeque to store course names
  Deque<String> courseDeque = new ArrayDeque<>();
  // Add courses to the deque
  courseDeque.offerFirst("Biology");  // Add to the front
  courseDeque.offerLast("Mathematics"); // Add to the end
  courseDeque.offerLast("Physics"); // Add to the end
  courseDeque.offerFirst("Chemistry"); // Add to the front
  // Display the current contents of the deque
  System.out.println("Deque contents: " + courseDeque);
  // Retrieve and print the first and last courses without removing them
  System.out.println("First course: " + courseDeque.peekFirst());
  System.out.println("Last course: " + courseDeque.peekLast());
  // Remove and print the first and last courses
  String removedFirst = courseDeque.pollFirst();
  String removedLast = courseDeque.pollLast();
  System.out.println("Removed first course: " + removedFirst);
  System.out.println("Removed last course: " + removedLast);
  // Display the updated contents of the deque
  System.out.println("Updated deque contents: " + courseDeque);
  // Check if a specific course is present
  boolean hasPhysics = courseDeque.contains("Physics");
  System.out.println("Deque contains 'Physics': " + hasPhysics);
  // Check if the deque is empty and display its size
  System.out.println("Deque is empty: " + courseDeque.isEmpty());
  System.out.println("Size of deque: " + courseDeque.size());
  // Clear the deque and display it again
  courseDeque.clear();
  System.out.println("Deque contents after clearing: " + courseDeque);
  }
}
```

Output:

```
Deque contents: [Chemistry, Biology, Mathematics, Physics]
First course: Chemistry
```

```
Last course: Physics
Removed first course: Chemistry
Removed last course: Physics
Updated deque contents: [Biology, Mathematics]
Deque contains 'Physics': false
Deque is empty: false
Size of deque: 2
Deque contents after clearing: []
```

The above program demonstrates the usage of the `Deque` interface through an `ArrayDeque` implementation. The program starts by creating an `ArrayDeque` named `courseDeque` to store strings representing various courses. The program then proceeds to add courses to both ends of the deque using the `offerFirst()` and `offerLast()` methods, simulating the addition of courses to the front and back of a queue, respectively. After populating the deque, it displays the current contents, showcasing the sequence of courses. Later retrieves and prints the first and last courses in the deque using the `peekFirst()` and `peekLast()` methods without removing them.

15.21 SET

In Java, a `Set` is a collection that stores unique elements. It does not allow duplicate elements, ensuring that each element appears only once in the collection. The `Set` interface is part of the Java Collections Framework and provides methods for adding, removing, and checking the presence of elements. Implementations of the `Set` interface include `HashSet`, `TreeSet`, `LinkedHashSet`, and others, each with its own characteristics and performance considerations.

15.21.1 Advantages of Set

1. Uniqueness of Elements: Sets enforce uniqueness by not allowing duplicate elements. This property is beneficial when dealing with collections where each element must occur only once, such as storing unique identifiers or removing duplicates from a collection.
2. Efficient Element Lookup: Set implementations offer efficient element lookup operations. They typically use hashing or tree-based data structures to achieve fast access times, making them suitable for scenarios where rapid retrieval of elements is required, such as searching for specific values in a large dataset.

15.21.2 Challenges of Set

1. Unordered Elements: Sets do not guarantee the order in which elements are stored. While this property is useful for many applications, it can be challenging when a specific ordering of elements is required. Developers may need to use a different collection type, such as `List`, if element ordering is important.
2. Overhead for Custom Objects: When using custom objects as elements in a set, developers need to ensure that the objects correctly implement the `equals()` and `hashCode()` methods. Failure to do so may result in unexpected behavior, such as incorrect identification of duplicate elements or inefficient performance due to hash collisions.

15.21.3 Syntax for Using Set in Java

To use a Set in Java, follow these steps:

1. Import the Set interface and choose an implementation (e.g., HashSet, TreeSet, LinkedHashSet):

```
import java.util.Set;
import java.util.HashSet;  or
import java.util.TreeSet;
or import java.util.LinkedHashSet;
```

2. Create an instance of Set using the chosen implementation:**

```
Set<String> set = new HashSet<>(); // or
new TreeSet<>(); or new LinkedHashSet<>();
```

3. Use Set methods to add, remove, or check the presence of elements:

```
set.add("Element"); // Add an element to the set
set.remove("Element"); // Remove an element from the set
boolean containsElement = set.contains("Element");
```

4. Use other Set methods such as `isEmpty()`, `size()`, `clear()`, etc., to perform additional operations as needed.

Sets can be effectively used in Java applications to store unique elements and perform operations such as adding, removing, and checking the presence of elements efficiently.

Program

```
import java.util.HashSet;
import java.util.Set;
public class Main {
    void main(String[] args) {
  // Create a HashSet to store course names
  Set<String> courseSet = new HashSet<>();
  // Add courses to the set
  courseSet.add("Mathematics");
  courseSet.add("Physics");
  courseSet.add("Chemistry");
  courseSet.add("Biology");
  // Try to add a duplicate course
  boolean added = courseSet.add("Physics"); //  Should  return  false  as
                                             "Physics" is already in the set
  System.out.println("Adding 'Physics' again: " + added);
  // Remove a course
  boolean removed = courseSet.remove("Biology"); // Should return true if
                                                   "Biology" was present
  System.out.println("Removing 'Biology': " + removed);
  // Display the updated set contents
  System.out.println("Updated set contents: " + courseSet);
  // Check if a specific course exists in the set
  boolean hasChemistry = courseSet.contains("Chemistry");
  System.out.println("Set contains 'Chemistry': " + hasChemistry);
  // Check if the set is empty and display its size
  System.out.println("Set is empty: " + courseSet.isEmpty());
  System.out.println("Size of set: " + courseSet.size());
```

```
  // Clear the set and display it again
  courseSet.clear();
  System.out.println("Set contents after clearing: " + courseSet);
  }
}
```

Output:

```
Adding 'Physics' again: false
Removing 'Biology': true
Updated set contents: [Chemistry, Mathematics, Physics]
Set contains 'Chemistry': true
Set is empty: false
Size of set: 3
Set contents after clearing: []
```

The above Java program demonstrates the usage of the `Set` interface with a `HashSet` implementation. Program begins by creating a `HashSet` named `courseSet` to store strings representing various courses. Then adds several courses to the set using the `add()` method. Since sets do not allow duplicate elements, it attempts to add a duplicate course, "Physics," to the set and prints whether the addition was successful, which should return `false`.

15.22 SORTEDSET

In Java, a `SortedSet` is a subinterface of the `Set` interface that maintains its elements in sorted order. Unlike a regular `Set`, which does not guarantee any particular order of its elements, a `SortedSet` ensures that its elements are sorted according to their natural ordering or a specified comparator. Implementations of `SortedSet` include `TreeSet`, which stores elements in a sorted tree structure.

15.22.1 Advantages of SortedSet

1. Ordered Elements: Unlike regular sets, elements in a `SortedSet` are always maintained in sorted order. This property is advantageous when iteration over the set or retrieving elements in sorted order is required, as it eliminates the need for explicit sorting operations.
2. Efficient Retrieval: SortedSet implementations use efficient data structures, such as balanced trees, to maintain the sorted order of elements. As a result, operations like finding the first or last element, or retrieving elements within a specific range, can be performed efficiently.

15.22.2 Challenges of SortedSet

1. Overhead for Custom Comparators: While `SortedSet` allows elements to be sorted according to a custom comparator, specifying and implementing a comparator can introduce additional complexity. Developers need to ensure that the comparator correctly defines the sorting order and handles all edge cases to avoid unexpected behavior.
2. Limited Flexibility in Ordering: The sorted nature of `SortedSet` restricts the ordering of elements to a single predefined order, either natural or defined by a comparator. This limitation may not be suitable for scenarios where dynamic or changing sorting criteria are required, as it necessitates recreating the `SortedSet` with a new comparator.

15.22.3 Syntax for Using SortedSet in Java

To use a `SortedSet` in Java with the `TreeSet` implementation, follow these steps:

1. Import the SortedSet interface and TreeSet class:

```
import java.util.SortedSet;
import java.util.TreeSet;
```

2. Create an instance of SortedSet using the TreeSet implementation:

```
SortedSet<String> sortedSet = new TreeSet<>();
```

3. Use SortedSet methods to add, remove, or retrieve elements:

```
sortedSet.add("Element"); // Add an element to the sorted set
sortedSet.remove("Element"); // Remove an element from the sorted set
String firstElement = sortedSet.first(); // Retrieve the first (lowest) element
String lastElement = sortedSet.last(); // Retrieve the last (highest)
element
```

4. Optionally, use methods like `headSet()`, `tailSet()`, or `subSet()` to retrieve subsets of the sorted set based on specified ranges.

Developers can effectively use `SortedSet` in Java applications to store elements in sorted order and perform operations such as adding, removing, and retrieving elements efficiently.

Program

```
import java.util.SortedSet;
import java.util.TreeSet;
public class Main {
    void main(String[] args) {
  // Create a TreeSet to store course names
  SortedSet<String> courseSet = new TreeSet<>();
  // Add courses to the set
  courseSet.add("Mathematics");
  courseSet.add("Physics");
  courseSet.add("Chemistry");
  courseSet.add("Biology");
  // Print the set contents after adding elements
  System.out.println("Set contents after adding elements: " + courseSet);
  // Try to add a duplicate course
  boolean added = courseSet.add("Physics"); // Should return false as
                                  "Physics" is already in the set
  System.out.println("Adding 'Physics' again: " + added);
  // Remove a course
  boolean removed = courseSet.remove("Biology"); // Should return true if
                                     "Biology" was present
  System.out.println("Removing 'Biology': " + removed);
  // Display the updated set contents
  System.out.println("Updated set contents: " + courseSet);
  // Check if a specific course exists in the set
  boolean hasChemistry = courseSet.contains("Chemistry");
  System.out.println("Set contains 'Chemistry': " + hasChemistry);
  // Retrieve and print the first and last elements of the sorted set
  String firstCourse = courseSet.first();
  String lastCourse = courseSet.last();
```

```
    System.out.println("First course: " + firstCourse);
    System.out.println("Last course: " + lastCourse);
    // Display the size of the sorted set
    System.out.println("Size of set: " + courseSet.size());
    // Clear the set and display it again
    courseSet.clear();
    System.out.println("Set contents after clearing: " + courseSet);
    }
}
```

Output:

```
Set contents after adding elements: [Biology, Chemistry, Mathematics, Physics]
Adding 'Physics' again: false
Removing 'Biology': true
Updated set contents: [Chemistry, Mathematics, Physics]
Set contains 'Chemistry': true
First course: Chemistry
Last course: Physics
Size of set: 3
Set contents after clearing: []
```

The above program provided showcases the usage of the `SortedSet` interface, implemented through the `TreeSet` class. Program begins by creating a `TreeSet` named `courseSet` to store strings representing various courses. Since sets do not allow duplicate elements, it attempts to add a duplicate course, "Physics," to the set and prints whether the addition was successful, which should return `false`.

15.23 SORTEDMAP

In Java, a `SortedMap` is an interface that extends the `Map` interface to maintain its key-value pairs in sorted order based on the keys. Unlike a regular `Map`, which does not guarantee any particular order of its elements, a `SortedMap` ensures that its keys are sorted according to their natural ordering or a specified comparator. Implementations of `SortedMap` include `TreeMap`, which stores elements in a sorted tree structure.

15.23.1 Advantages of SortedMap

1. Ordered Key-Value Pairs: The primary advantage of a `SortedMap` is that it maintains its entries in sorted order based on the keys. This allows for efficient retrieval of entries in sorted key order, eliminating the need for additional sorting operations.
2. Efficient Range Operations: SortedMap implementations use efficient data structures, such as balanced trees, to maintain the sorted order of keys. This makes operations like finding entries within a specific key range or retrieving the first or last entry efficient and straightforward.

15.23.2 Challenges of SortedMap

1. Overhead for Custom Comparators: While `SortedMap` allows keys to be sorted according to a custom comparator, specifying and implementing a comparator can introduce additional complexity. Developers need to ensure that the comparator correctly defines the sorting order and handles all edge cases to avoid unexpected behavior.

2. Limited Flexibility in Key Ordering: The sorted nature of `SortedMap` restricts the ordering of keys to a single predefined order, either natural or defined by a comparator. This limitation may not be suitable for scenarios where dynamic or changing sorting criteria are required, as it necessitates recreating the `SortedMap` with a new comparator.

15.23.3 Syntax for Using SortedMap in Java

To use a `SortedMap` in Java with the `TreeMap` implementation, follow these steps:

1. Import the SortedMap interface and TreeMap class:

```
import java.util.SortedMap;
import java.util.TreeMap;
```

2. Create an instance of SortedMap using the TreeMap implementation:

```
SortedMap<Integer, String> sortedMap = new TreeMap<>();
```

3. Use SortedMap methods to add, remove, or retrieve key-value pairs:

```
sortedMap.put(1, "Value1"); // Add a key-value pair to the sorted map
sortedMap.remove(1); // Remove a key-value pair from the sorted map
Integer firstKey = sortedMap.firstKey(); // Retrieve the first (lowest) key
Integer lastKey = sortedMap.lastKey(); // Retrieve the last (highest) key
```

4. Optionally, use methods like `headMap()`, `tailMap()`, or `subMap()` to retrieve subsets of the sorted map based on specified key ranges.

Developers can effectively use `SortedMap` in Java applications to store key-value pairs in sorted order and perform operations such as adding, removing, and retrieving entries efficiently.

Program

```
import java.util.SortedMap;
import java.util.TreeMap;
public class Main {
    void main(String[] args) {
  // Initialize a TreeMap to store course IDs and names
  SortedMap<Integer, String> courseMap = new TreeMap<>();
  // Add key-value pairs to the map
  courseMap.put(101, "Mathematics");
  courseMap.put(102, "Physics");
  courseMap.put(103, "Chemistry");
  courseMap.put(104, "Biology");
  // Print the map contents after adding elements
  System.out.println("Map contents after adding elements: " + courseMap);
  // Add a duplicate key with a different value
  String oldValue = courseMap.put(102, "Geology"); // Should replace the
old value "Physics" with "Geology"
  System.out.println("Replaced value for key 102: " + oldValue);
  // Print the updated map contents to show the effect of duplicate key
  insertion
```

```
  System.out.println("Updated map contents after replacing value for key
  102: " + courseMap);
  // Remove an entry with a specific key
  String removedValue = courseMap.remove(104); // Should return the value
                                                  "Biology"
  System.out.println("Removed entry with key 104: " + removedValue);
  // Print the updated map contents
  System.out.println("Updated map contents after removal of key 104: " +
     courseMap);
  // Check if a specific key exists in the map
  boolean hasKey103 = courseMap.containsKey(103);
  System.out.println("Map contains key 103: " + hasKey103);
  // Retrieve and print the first and last keys of the sorted map
  Integer firstKey = courseMap.firstKey();
  Integer lastKey = courseMap.lastKey();
  System.out.println("First key: " + firstKey);
  System.out.println("Last key: " + lastKey);
  // Display the size of the sorted map
  System.out.println("Size of map: " + courseMap.size());
  // Clear the map and display it again
  courseMap.clear();
  System.out.println("Map contents after clearing: " + courseMap);
  }
}
```

Output:

```
Map contents after adding elements: {101=Mathematics, 102=Physics, 103=
Chemistry, 104=Biology}
Replaced value for key 102: Physics
Updated map contents after replacing value for key 102: {101=Mathematics,
102=Geology, 103=Chemistry, 104=Biology}
Removed entry with key 104: Biology
Updated map contents after removal of key 104: {101=Mathematics, 102=
Geology, 103=Chemistry}
Map contains key 103: true
First key: 101
Last key: 103
Size of map: 3
Map contents after clearing: {}
```

The above Java program demonstrates the utilization of the `SortedMap` interface, implemented through the `TreeMap` class. Program starts by initializing a `TreeMap` named `courseMap` to store mappings of integer keys to string values, representing various courses.

Since `TreeMap` maintains elements in ascending order of keys, the courses are automatically sorted by their corresponding keys.

15.24 MEDICAL APPLICATIONS

15.24.1 Case Study 1

Leg disorders encompass a range of conditions affecting the bones, muscles, and joints of the leg, causing pain, weakness, or limited mobility. Common disorders include varicose veins, shin splints, and conditions like Osgood-Schlatter disease, each requiring specific medical evaluation and treatment. The parameters considered in this program are disorder (e.g., "Pain below the kneecap" for Osgood-Schlatter Disease).

Program

```
import java.util.HashMap;
import java.util.HashSet;
import java.util.Map;
import java.util.Set;
public class LegDisorderDetection {
  private static final Map<String, Disorder> disorders;
  // Map of disorder names to Disorder objects
  static {
  disorders = new HashMap<>();
  // Sample disorders and symptoms
  Disorder osgoodSchlatter = new Disorder("Osgood-Schlatter Disease");
  osgoodSchlatter.addSymptom("Pain below the kneecap");
  osgoodSchlatter.addSymptom("Tenderness to the touch");
  osgoodSchlatter.addSymptom("Pain during activity");
  disorders.put(osgoodSchlatter.getName(), osgoodSchlatter);
  Disorder patellarTendinitis = new Disorder("Patellar Tendinitis (Jumper's
     Knee)");
  patellarTendinitis.addSymptom("Pain just below the kneecap");
  patellarTendinitis.addSymptom("Pain that worsens with activity");
  patellarTendinitis.addSymptom("Stiffness in the morning");
  disorders.put(patellarTendinitis.getName(), patellarTendinitis);
  // More disorders...
  Disorder shinSplints = new Disorder("Shin Splints");
  shinSplints.addSymptom("Pain along the shinbone");
  shinSplints.addSymptom("Pain that worsens with activity");
  shinSplints.addSymptom("Tenderness to the touch");
  disorders.put(shinSplints.getName(), shinSplints);
  Disorder plantarFasciitis = new Disorder("Plantar Fasciitis");
  plantarFasciitis.addSymptom("Pain in the heel or arch of the foot");
  plantarFasciitis.addSymptom("Pain that is worse in the morning or after
     long periods of standing");
  plantarFasciitis.addSymptom("Sharp pain with the first steps in the
     morning");
  disorders.put(plantarFasciitis.getName(), plantarFasciitis);
  Disorder varicoseVeins = new Disorder("Varicose Veins");
  varicoseVeins.addSymptom("Twisted, enlarged veins");
  varicoseVeins.addSymptom("Aching or cramping in the legs");
  varicoseVeins.addSymptom("Swelling in the ankles");
  disorders.put(varicoseVeins.getName(), varicoseVeins);
}
  void main(String[] args) {
  UserInput input = new UserInput();
  // Collect user data
  String name = input.getStringInput("Enter your name");
  Set<String> symptoms = input.getSymptomsInput("Enter your leg-related
     symptoms");
  // Analyze symptoms
  Set<String> potentialDisorders = new HashSet<>();
  for (Disorder disorder : disorders.values()) {
    Set<String> disorderSymptoms = disorder.getSymptoms();
    if (symptoms.containsAll(disorderSymptoms)) {
      // Check for all symptoms present
```

```
potentialDisorders.add(disorder.getName());
    }
  }
  // Display results
  if (potentialDisorders.isEmpty()) {
    System.out.println("Based on your symptoms, no leg-related disorders
       were identified.");
  } else {
    System.out.println("Potential leg-related disorders based on your
       symptoms:");
    for (String disorder : potentialDisorders) {
  System.out.println("- " + disorder);
    }
    System.out.println("Please consult a healthcare professional for a
       proper diagnosis.");
  }
  input.closeScanner();
  }
}
```

In the `LegDisorderDetection` program, a map `disorders` is initialized to store various leg-related disorders along with their associated symptoms using `HashMap<String, Disorder>`. Each disorder (`Disorder` object) is created with a name and a set of symptoms. Users input their name and specific leg-related symptoms via the `UserInput` class. The program then compares the user-provided symptoms against each disorder's symptoms in the `disorders` map. If a user's symptoms match all symptoms of a particular disorder, that disorder is added to `potentialDisorders`. Finally, based on the presence or absence of potential disorders, the program prints out either a list of potential leg-related disorders or a message indicating no disorders were identified.

15.24.2 Case Study 2

Rickets, primarily affecting children, is a condition caused by vitamin D deficiency leading to weak and soft bones. The risk includes bone pain, delayed growth, and skeletal deformities such as bowed legs or thickened wrists and ankles. The parameters considered in this program are "Bone pain or tenderness," "Muscle weakness," "Delayed growth," "Soft skull in infants (fontanelle)," "Bowed legs or knock-knees," and "Seizures (rare)."

Program

```
public class RicketsSymptoms {
  private String symptom;
  private int severity; // 1 (low) to 5 (high)
  public RicketsSymptoms(String symptom, int severity) {
  this.symptom = symptom;
  this.severity = severity;
  }
  public String getSymptom() {
  return symptom;
  }
  public int getSeverity() {
  return severity;
  }
```

```
  @Override
  public String toString() {
  return symptom + " (Severity: " + severity + ")";
  }
}
import java.util.Scanner;
import java.util.Stack;
public class RicketsDetection {
  private static final RicketsSymptoms[] SYMPTOMS = {
  new RicketsSymptoms("Bone pain or tenderness", 5),
  new RicketsSymptoms("Muscle weakness", 4),
  new RicketsSymptoms("Delayed growth", 5),
  new RicketsSymptoms("Soft skull in infants (fontanelle)", 4),
  new RicketsSymptoms("Bowed legs or knock-knees", 4),
  new RicketsSymptoms("Seizures (rare)", 5),
  };
  void main(String[] args) {
  Scanner scanner = new Scanner(System.in);
  Stack<RicketsSymptoms> symptomStack = new Stack<>();
  System.out.println("Rickets Symptom Analysis");
  // Get user input for symptoms (can be modified for loop or other input
  methods)
  System.out.println("Enter symptoms (or 'done' to finish):");
  String symptom;
  do {
    symptom = scanner.nextLine();
    if (!symptom.equalsIgnoreCase("done") && !symptom.isEmpty()) {
  int severity = getSymptomSeverity(symptom);
  if (severity > 0) {
    symptomStack.push(new RicketsSymptoms(symptom, severity));
  } else {
    System.out.println("Invalid symptom. Please enter a valid symptom or
       'done'.");
  }
    }
  } while (!symptom.equalsIgnoreCase("done"));
  // Analyze symptoms
  int totalSeverity = 0;
  if (symptomStack.isEmpty()) {
    System.out.println("No symptoms entered.");
  } else {
    System.out.println("Entered Symptoms:");
    while (!symptomStack.isEmpty()) {
  RicketsSymptoms currentSymptom = symptomStack.pop();
  System.out.println(currentSymptom);
  totalSeverity += currentSymptom.getSeverity();
    }
    String assessment = assessRicketsRisk(totalSeverity);
    System.out.println("\nAssessment:");
    System.out.println(assessment);
    System.out.println("**Disclaimer:** This is a simplified example and
       does not constitute medical advice. Please consult a healthcare pro-
       fessional for diagnosis and treatment.");
  }
```

```
  scanner.close();
  }
  private static int getSymptomSeverity(String symptom) {
  for (RicketsSymptoms ricketsSymptom : SYMPTOMS) {
    if (ricketsSymptom.getSymptom().equalsIgnoreCase(symptom)) {
  return ricketsSymptom.getSeverity();
    }
  }
  return 0; // Invalid symptom
  }
  private static String assessRicketsRisk(int totalSeverity) {
  if (totalSeverity == 0) {
    return "Based on the entered symptoms, rickets is unlikely.";
  } else if (totalSeverity <= 10) {
    return "There is a low possibility of rickets.";
  } else if (totalSeverity <= 15) {
    return "There is a moderate possibility of rickets. Please consult a
       healthcare professional for a proper diagnosis.";
  } else {
    return "The entered symptoms suggest a high possibility of rickets..";
  }
  }
}
}
```

The `RicketsDetection` program allows users to input symptoms associated with rickets, a disorder caused by vitamin D deficiency. It begins by defining various symptoms of rickets along with their severity levels using the `RicketsSymptoms` class. Users input their symptoms via a command-line interface, and each symptom's severity is validated against predefined symptoms. The program calculates the total severity based on entered symptoms and provides an assessment of rickets risk, ranging from unlikely to high, along with a disclaimer emphasizing that it's a simplified tool and not a substitute for professional medical advice.

16 Case Studies

16.1 INTRODUCTION

This chapter delves into the application of Java in the medical field, presenting several case studies that highlight how Java can be utilized to develop systems for detecting various medical conditions. The case studies encompass a range of diseases, demonstrating the versatility and effectiveness of Java in medical diagnostics.

One of the case studies focuses on diabetes detection, showcasing how Java algorithms can analyze patient data to identify the presence of diabetes. Another study explores the detection of diabetic retinopathy, a complication of diabetes that affects the eyes, using image processing and analysis techniques implemented in Java.

The chapter also includes a case study on COVID-19 detection, illustrating how Java can be employed to develop software for diagnosing this highly infectious disease. By processing and analyzing medical data, Java-based systems can assist in early detection and management of COVID-19 cases.

Depression detection is another critical area covered in this chapter. The case study demonstrates how Java can be used to analyze behavioral data and symptoms to identify signs of depression, providing a valuable tool for mental health professionals.

Additionally, the chapter addresses Alzheimer's detection, showcasing how Java can aid in the early diagnosis of this neurodegenerative disease. Through data analysis and machine learning techniques, Java-based applications can help in identifying patterns and symptoms associated with Alzheimer's.

Lastly, the chapter presents a case study on skin cancer detection. Using image processing capabilities in Java, the system can analyze skin lesions and identify potential cancerous growths, facilitating early intervention and treatment.

Overall, this chapter illustrates the significant role Java plays in developing advanced diagnostic tools for a variety of medical conditions, highlighting its impact on improving healthcare outcomes through innovative technological solutions.

16.2 DIABETES DETECTION

The dataset comprises several critical attributes that are commonly associated with diabetes risk factors and symptoms. The attributes in the dataset include:

1. Age: The patient's age, as age is a significant risk factor for diabetes.
2. Gender: The patient's gender, which can influence the risk and prevalence of diabetes.
3. BMI (Body Mass Index): A measure of body fat based on height and weight, which is a crucial indicator of diabetes risk.

DOI: 10.1201/9781003544319-16

4. Blood Pressure: The patient's blood pressure levels, as hypertension is often linked with diabetes.
5. Fasting Blood Sugar: The blood sugar level after a period of fasting, an essential metric for diagnosing diabetes.
6. Postprandial Blood Sugar: The blood sugar level after eating, which helps in understanding how the body manages sugar intake.
7. Family History: Information about diabetes in the patient's family, indicating genetic predisposition.
8. Physical Activity: The patient's level of physical activity, which affects overall health and diabetes risk.
9. Smoker: Whether the patient smokes, as smoking is a risk factor for many chronic diseases, including diabetes.
10. Diabetic: A binary indicator of whether the patient has been diagnosed with diabetes.

16.2.1 Sample Dataset

age, gender, bmi, bloodPressure, fastingBloodSugar, postPrandialBloodSugar, familyHistory, physicalActivity, smoker, diabetic
45, Male, 29.5, 140/90, 120, 210, true, Low, false, true
50, Female, 28.0, 130/85, 110, 190, true, Moderate, false, true
30, Male, 25.0, 120/80, 95, 140, false, High, false, false
55, Female, 32.0, 145/95, 130, 220, true, Low, true, true
40, Male, 27.0, 135/85, 105, 180, false, Moderate, true, false

Program

```
import java.io.BufferedReader;
import java.io.FileReader;
import java.io.IOException;
import java.util.ArrayList;
import java.util.List;
```

Imports the `ArrayList` and `List` classes from the `java.util` package, which are used to create a dynamic array to store the data read from the file. This setup is typically used for reading a text file line by line, storing each line into a list for further processing or analysis. Using `BufferedReader` wrapped around `FileReader`, ensures efficient reading of the file contents, while `ArrayList` provides a flexible container to hold the data, allowing for dynamic resizing as new lines are read and added.

```
class Patient {
  int age;
  String gender;
  double bmi;
  String bloodPressure;
  int fastingBloodSugar;
  int postPrandialBloodSugar;
  boolean familyHistory;
  String physicalActivity;
  boolean smoker;
  boolean diabetic;
```

The `Patient` class is designed to represent the detailed medical profile of an individual with respect to diabetes. It contains several fields that capture key health metrics and lifestyle information. These fields include `age`, which records the patient's age in years, and `gender`, which stores the patient's gender as a string. The `bmi` field captures the Body Mass Index, a critical measure of body fat based on height and weight. The `bloodPressure` field stores the patient's blood pressure readings as a string, allowing for the recording of complex values like systolic/diastolic pressure.

Further, the class includes `fastingBloodSugar` and `postPrandialBloodSugar`, both of which are integers that measure blood sugar levels before and after eating, respectively. The `familyHistory` boolean field indicates whether the patient has a family history of diabetes, which is an important risk factor. The `physicalActivity` field is a string that describes the patient's level of physical activity, providing context for other health metrics.

The class also includes a `smoker` boolean field to record whether the patient is a smoker, given the significant health risks associated with smoking. Finally, the `diabetic` boolean field indicates whether the patient has been diagnosed with diabetes.

```
// Constructor to initialize the patient data
    public Patient(int age, String gender, double bmi, String
    bloodPressure, int fastingBloodSugar, int postPrandialBloodSugar,
    boolean familyHistory, String physicalActivity, boolean smoker,
    boolean diabetic) {
```

The constructor `public Patient(int age, String gender, double bmi, String bloodPressure, int fastingBloodSugar, int postPrandialBloodSugar, booleanfamilyHistory, String physicalActivity, boolean smoker, boolean diabetic)` initializes a `Patient` object with the specified parameters. It accepts several arguments that represent various aspects of a patient's health profile.

The `age` parameter is an integer representing the patient's age in years, while `gender` is a string indicating the patient's gender. The `bmi` parameter is a double value representing the Body Mass Index, a measure of body fat based on height and weight. `bloodPressure` is a string parameter capturing the patient's blood pressure readings, typically in systolic/diastolic format.

Further parameters include `fastingBloodSugar` and `postPrandialBloodSugar`, both integers representing blood sugar levels before and after eating, respectively. The `familyHistory` parameter is a boolean indicating whether the patient has a family history of diabetes, while `physicalActivity` is a string describing the patient's level of physical activity.

The `smoker` parameter is a boolean indicating whether the patient is a smoker, and `diabetic` is a boolean indicating whether the patient has been diagnosed with diabetes. Together, these parameters provide comprehensive information about the patient's health status, lifestyle factors, and potential risk factors for diabetes. This constructor facilitates the creation of `Patient` objects with initialized attributes, enabling efficient management and analysis of patient data in medical applications.

```
    this.age = age;
    this.gender = gender;
    this.bmi = bmi;
    this.bloodPressure = bloodPressure;
    this.fastingBloodSugar = fastingBloodSugar;
    this.postPrandialBloodSugar = postPrandialBloodSugar;
    this.familyHistory = familyHistory;
    this.physicalActivity = physicalActivity;
    this.smoker = smoker;
    this.diabetic = diabetic;
    }
}
```

The constructor is defined for the `Patient` class, which initializes the fields of a `Patient` object with the values passed as arguments. Each field of the `Patient` class, including `age`, `gender`, `bmi`, `bloodPressure`, `fastingBloodSugar`, `postPrandialBloodSugar`, `familyHistory`, `physicalActivity`, `smoker`, and `diabetic`, is assigned a value based on the corresponding parameter passed to the constructor.

The `this` keyword is used to refer to the current instance of the `Patient` class, allowing for the distinction between the constructor parameters and the class fields with the same names. By assigning the parameter values to the class fields, the constructor initializes the state of a `Patient` object with specific attributes representing age, gender, BMI, blood pressure, blood sugar levels, family history of diabetes, physical activity level, smoking status, and diabetic condition.

This initialization process ensures that each instance of the `Patient` class created using this constructor starts with predefined values for its attributes, enabling the accurate representation of patient data and facilitating further processing or analysis within medical applications.

```
public class Main {
  // Method to load dataset from file
  public static List<Patient> loadDataset(String fileName) {
  List<Patient> patients = new ArrayList<>();
  try (BufferedReader br = new BufferedReader(new FileReader(fileName))) {
    String line;
```

The `Main` class contains a static method named `loadDataset` that takes a `fileName` parameter representing the name of the file containing patient data. This method returns a list of `Patient` objects. Inside the method, a new `ArrayList` called `patients` is created to store the `Patient` objects read from the file. Additionally, a `BufferedReader` named `br` is instantiated to read the contents of the file specified by `fileName`. The method then enters a loop to read each line of the file using the `readLine()` method of the `BufferedReader`. Each line of the file is stored in the `line` variable.

```
    while ((line = br.readLine()) != null) {
    if (line.startsWith("#")) {
      continue; // Skip comments
    }
    String[] data = line.split(", ");
    // Parse data and create a Patient object
    int age = Integer.parseInt(data[0]);
    String gender = data[1];
    double bmi = Double.parseDouble(data[2]);
    String bloodPressure = data[3];
    int fastingBloodSugar = Integer.parseInt(data[4]);
    int postPrandialBloodSugar = Integer.parseInt(data[5]);
    boolean familyHistory = Boolean.parseBoolean(data[6]);
    String physicalActivity = data[7];
    boolean smoker = Boolean.parseBoolean(data[8]);
    boolean diabetic = Boolean.parseBoolean(data[9]);
    Patient patient = new Patient(age, gender, bmi, bloodPressure,
    fastingBloodSugar, postPrandialBloodSugar, familyHistory,
    physicalActivity, smoker, diabetic); patients.add(patient);
    }
  } catch (IOException e) {
    System.err.println("Error reading dataset: " + e.getMessage());
  }
  return patients;
  }
```

The loadDataset method utilizes a while loop to iterate through each line of the file read by the `BufferedReader`. Subsequently, the parsed data elements are extracted from the `data` array and assigned to local variables representing different attributes of a patient, such as `age`, `gender`, `bmi`, `bloodPressure`, `fastingBloodSugar`, `postPrandialBloodSugar`, `familyHistory`, `physicalActivity`, `smoker`, and `diabetic`. Using these extracted values, a new `Patient` object is instantiated, and it is added to the `patients` list using the `add` method.

Finally, after processing all lines, the `BufferedReader` is closed to release any system resources, and the list of `Patient` objects is returned.

```
  // Main method to load data and assess diabetes likelihood
  public static void main(String[] args) {
  try {
    List<Patient> patients = loadDataset("test.txt");
    if (!patients.isEmpty()) {
    Patient firstPatient = patients.get(0);
    boolean diabeticStatus = isDiabetic(patients, firstPatient);
    if (diabeticStatus) {
      System.out.println("The first patient is likely to have diabetes.");
    } else {
      System.out.println("The first patient is unlikely to have diabetes.");
    }
    }
  } catch (Exception e) {
    e.printStackTrace();
  }
  }
}
```

Firstly, within a try block, the `loadDataset` method is invoked to read the dataset from the specified file. If successful, the first patient entry is extracted from the list of patients retrieved from the dataset. Next, the `isDiabetic` method is called, passing the list of patients and the extracted patient entry as arguments. This method evaluates the likelihood of the patient having diabetes based on the dataset's information and returns a boolean value representing the assessment. Depending on the boolean result obtained from `isDiabetic`, a corresponding message is printed to the console indicating whether the patient is deemed likely or unlikely to have diabetes. In case an `IOException` occurs during the dataset loading process, the catch block is triggered. It prints an error message to the console indicating the occurrence of an error while reading the dataset and prints the stack trace to provide additional context for debugging purposes.

```
// Method to determine if a patient is diabetic based on the dataset
  public static boolean isDiabetic(List<Patient> patients, Patient
  inputPatient) {
  for (Patient p : patients) {
    if (p.fastingBloodSugar == inputPatient.fastingBloodSugar &&
    p.postPrandialBloodSugar == inputPatient.postPrandialBloodSugar &&
    p.familyHistory == inputPatient.familyHistory &&
    p.physicalActivity.equals(inputPatient.physicalActivity) &&
    p.smoker == inputPatient.smoker) {
    return p.diabetic;
    }
  }
  return false;
  }
```

The `isDiabetic` method iterates through a list of patient records to assess whether a specific patient, denoted by `inputPatient`, is likely to have diabetes based on certain criteria. Within a loop that iterates over each patient in the `patients` list, the method compares the attributes of each patient with those of the `inputPatient` to determine a match. Specifically, it checks if the fasting blood sugar level, post-prandial blood sugar level, family history of diabetes, physical activity level, and smoking status of the current patient match those of the input patient. If a match is found, the method returns the diabetic status of the current patient, indicating whether they are deemed to have diabetes. If no matching patient is found after iterating through all records in the dataset, the method returns false, indicating that the input patient is assessed as unlikely to have diabetes based on the provided criteria. This method provides a simple yet effective approach to assessing the likelihood of a patient having diabetes by comparing their attributes with those of other patients in a dataset.

16.3 DIABETIC RETINOPATHY DETECTION

Collected images form publicly available sources such as STARE, DIARETDB0, and Kaggle. These datasets contain a wide range of fundus images, annotated with information about the presence and severity of diabetic retinopathy.

```
import org.bytedeco.opencv.opencv_core.Mat;
import org.bytedeco.opencv.opencv_imgcodecs.Imgcodecs;
import org.bytedeco.opencv.opencv_imgproc.Imgproc;
import weka.classifiers.Classifier;
import weka.classifiers.functions.SMO;
import weka.core.Attribute;
import weka.core.DenseInstance;
import weka.core.Instance;
import weka.core.Instances;
import java.io.File;
import java.io.IOException;
import java.util.ArrayList;
import java.util.List;
```

The `IOException` class, also from `java.io`, is employed to handle exceptions that may occur during input-output operations. On the other hand, `ArrayList` from `java.util` facilitates the creation of dynamic arrays that can grow or shrink as needed, offering methods for adding, removing, and accessing elements efficiently.

```
public class DiabeticRetinopathyDetection {
  public static void main(String[] args) {
  try {
    // Extract features from the directory "C://dr"
    List<Instance> instances = extractFeatures("C://dr");
    // Create a dataset from the extracted features
    Instances dataset = createDataset(instances);
    // Train the classifier using the dataset
    Classifier classifier = trainClassifier(dataset);
    // Extract features from the directory "C://dr//new" for new images
    List<Instance> newInstances = extractFeatures("C://dr//new");
    // Classify new instances and output the predictions
    for (Instance newInstance : newInstances) {
    double prediction = classifyInstance(newInstance, classifier);
    System.out.println("Diabetic retinopathy prediction: " + prediction);
    }
```

```
  } catch (Exception e) {
    e.printStackTrace();
  }
  }
```

Initially, an attempt is made to extract features from images located in the directory "C://dr" using the `extractFeatures` method. These features are then used to create an `Instances` dataset through the `createDataset` function. Subsequently, a classifier is trained on this dataset via the `trainClassifier` method. Following the training, another set of instances is extracted from the directory "C://dr //new" using the same `extractFeatures` function. For each new instance, a prediction is made utilizing the trained classifier through the `classifyInstance` method. Any encountered exceptions during this process are caught and handled, with details printed for debugging purposes through the `printStackTrace` method.

```
// Method to extract features from images in a directory
  private static List<Instance> extractFeatures(String directoryPath)
throws IOException {
  List<Instance> instances = new ArrayList<>();
  File[] files = new File(directoryPath).listFiles();
  if (files != null) {
    for (File file : files) {
    if (file.isFile() && (file.getName().endsWith(".jpg") || file.getName().
       endsWith(".png"))) {
      // Load the image using OpenCV
      Mat image = Imgcodecs.imread(file.getAbsolutePath());
      // Resize the image to 100x100 pixels
      Imgproc.resize(image, image, new org.bytedeco.opencv.opencv_core.
      Size(100, 100));
      // Convert the image to grayscale
      Imgproc.cvtColor(image, image, Imgproc.COLOR_BGR2GRAY);
      // Extract features from the image
      double[] features = extractFeaturesFromImage(image);
      // Create a Weka instance from the extracted features
      Instance instance = createInstance(features);
      instances.add(instance);
    }
    }
  }
  return instances;
  }
```

This Java method, `extractFeatures`, is designed to extract features from images stored in a specified directory path. It starts by initializing an empty list of `Instance` objects to store the extracted features. Then, it retrieves the list of files from the specified directory using the `listFiles` method. If the list of files is not null, it iterates through each file. For each file that is a valid image file, it reads the image using the OpenCV library's `imread` method. The image is then resized to a standard size of 100x100 pixels and converted to grayscale using the `resize` and `cvtColor` methods from the OpenCV library, respectively. After preprocessing, the method calls `extractFeaturesFromImage` to compute the features of the image. These features are encapsulated into an `Instance` object using the `createInstance` method. Finally, the `Instance` object is added to the list of instances. The method returns the list of instances containing the extracted features from all the images in the specified directory.

```
// Method to extract features from a single image
  private static double[] extractFeaturesFromImage(Mat image) {
  // Perform Shi-Tomasi corner detection
  Mat corners = new Mat();
  Imgproc.goodFeaturesToTrack(image, corners, 100, 0.01, 10);
  // Apply Canny edge detection
  Mat edges = new Mat();
  Imgproc.Canny(image, edges, 100, 200);
  Imgcodecs.imwrite("edges.jpg", edges);  // Save the detected edges
  // Calculate histogram of pixel intensities
  Mat hist = new Mat();
  Imgproc.calcHist(new Mat[]{image}, new int[]{0}, new Mat(), hist, new
     int[]{256}, new float[]{0, 256});
  // Generate Gabor kernel and apply it to the image
  Mat gaborKernel = Imgproc.getGaborKernel(new org.bytedeco.opencv.
      opencv_core.Size(21, 21), 5, Math.PI / 4, 10, 0.5);
  Mat filteredImage = new Mat();
  Imgproc.filter2D(image, filteredImage, -1, gaborKernel);
  Imgcodecs.imwrite("filtered_image.jpg", filteredImage);
  // Save the filtered image
  // Calculate Hu moments for shape descriptors
  Mat moments = Imgproc.moments(image);
  Mat huMoments = new Mat();
  Imgproc.HuMoments(moments, huMoments);
  // Combine features into a single array (corners count, histogram, Hu
  moments, etc.)
  double[] features = new double[1 + hist.cols() + 7];
  features[0] = corners.total();  // Number of corners detected
  for (int i = 0; i < hist.cols(); i++) {
    features[i + 1] = hist.get(i, 0)[0];  // Histogram values
  }
  for (int i = 0; i < 7; i++) {
    features[hist.cols() + 1 + i] = huMoments.get(i, 0)[0];
    // Hu moments
  }
  return features;
  }
```

The `extractfeaturesFromImage` method takes a `Mat` object representing an image as input. Within the method, the image is read from a file named "image.jpg" using OpenCV's `Imgcodecs.imread` function. Next, corner detection is performed using the Shi-Tomasi corner detector through the `Imgproc.goodFeaturesToTrack` method. Then, Canny edge detection is applied to the grayscale version of the image using `Imgproc.Canny`, and the resulting edges are saved to a file named "edges.jpg" using `Imgcodecs.imwrite`. Following that, a histogram of pixel intensities is calculated using `Imgproc.calcHist` and stored in a `Mat` object named `hist`. A Gabor kernel is generated using `Imgproc.getGaborKernel` to perform texture feature extraction. The kernel is applied to the grayscale image using `Imgproc.filter2D`, and the filtered image is saved to "filtered_image.jpg".

Finally, Hu moments are computed using `Imgproc.moments` and `Imgproc.HuMoments` to extract shape descriptors.

```
  // Method to create a Weka instance from extracted features
  private static Instance createInstance(double[] features) {
  // Define the attributes of the dataset (you can add more attributes as
  needed)
```

```
ArrayList<Attribute> attributes = new ArrayList<>();
for (int i = 0; i < features.length; i++) {
  attributes.add(new Attribute("feature" + (i + 1)));
}
attributes.add(new Attribute("class"));  // The class attribute
// Create a new Weka instance
Instances dataset = new Instances("TestInstances", attributes, 1);
dataset.setClassIndex(attributes.size()                    -                   1);
// Set the class attribute as the last one
Instance instance = new DenseInstance(features.length + 1);
for (int i = 0; i < features.length; i++) {
  instance.setValue(i, features[i]);
}
instance.setDataset(dataset);  // Set the instance's dataset context
return instance;
}
```

The `createInstance`, method is responsible for creating an `Instance` object encapsulating the extracted features passed as an array. It begins by initializing an `ArrayList` called `attributeList` to store attributes representing the features. A loop iterates over each feature, and for each feature, a new `Attribute` object is created with a name based on the feature index. Subsequently, a new `Instances` object named "TestInstances" is instantiated, defining the dataset with the `attributeList` and specifying a capacity of 1 for the dataset. The class index of the dataset is set to the last attribute using `setClassIndex`.

Next, a new `DenseInstance` object is created with a size equal to the number of features plus one to accommodate the class attribute. Another loop iterates over the features, setting the value of each attribute in the instance using the `setValue` method. Finally, the instance is added to the dataset using the `add` method, and the method returns the first instance in the dataset using `firstInstance`. This method effectively creates an `Instance` object containing the extracted features, ready to be used for classification or further analysis.

```
// Method to create a dataset from a list of instances
private static Instances createDataset(List<Instance> instances) {
ArrayList<Attribute> attributes = new ArrayList<>();
for (int i = 0; i < instances.get(0).numAttributes(); i++) {
  attributes.add(new Attribute("feature" + (i + 1)));
}
attributes.add(new Attribute("class"));  // The class attribute
Instances   dataset   =   new   Instances("TrainingInstances",   attributes,
   instances.size());
dataset.setClassIndex(dataset.numAttributes() - 1);  // Set the class index
for (Instance instance : instances) {
  dataset.add(instance);
}
return dataset;
}
```

In the, `createDataset`, method dataset of instances is created from a list of instances. It begins by initializing an `Instances` object named "TrainingInstances" to represent the dataset. The constructor is called with parameters including the dataset name, `null` indicating no attribute information, and the size of the list of instances.

A loop then iterates over each instance in the input list. For each instance, it is added to the dataset using the `add` method. Once all instances are added, the method returns the populated dataset, containing all instances ready for training or further processing. This method effectively constructs a dataset encapsulating the instances extracted from the images, enabling the training of machine learning models or other analyses.

```
// Method to train a classifier (Support Vector Machine - SMO)
private static Classifier trainClassifier(Instances dataset) throws
   Exception {
Classifier classifier = new SMO();
classifier.buildClassifier(dataset);
return classifier;
}
```

The `trainClassifier` method is responsible for training a classifier using a provided dataset of instances. It starts by instantiating a SMO (Sequential Minimal Optimization) classifier object. SMO is a popular algorithm for training support vector machines (SVMs), a type of supervised learning model used for classification tasks.

After creating the classifier, the `buildClassifier` method is called, which takes the dataset as input and trains the classifier using the instances in the dataset. This step involves the optimization of the classifier's parameters based on the training data. Finally, the trained classifier object is returned, ready for use in making predictions on new instances.

This method encapsulates the training process, abstracting away the complexities of model training and allowing for the straightforward training of classifiers using provided datasets.

```
  // Method to classify a new instance using the trained classifier
  private static double classifyInstance(Instance instance, Classifier clas-
sifier) throws Exception {
  return classifier.classifyInstance(instance);
  // Returns the predicted class label
  }
}
```

The `classifyInstance` method is a crucial component of the classification. Given an instance of data and a trained classifier model, it predicts the class label or outcome associated with the provided instance. This process involves applying the trained classifier to the input instance and determining which class it belongs to based on the model's learned decision boundaries.

Inside the method, the `classifyInstance` function of the classifier object is invoked, passing the instance to be classified as an argument. This function returns the predicted class label or value for the given instance. If successful, the predicted value is returned by the method.

16.4 COVID-19 DETECTION

The attributes included in the dataset are Age, Gender, Fever, Cough, Difficulty Breathing, Fatigue, Body Aches, Loss of Taste or Smell, Sore Throat, and Test Result. Each of these attributes plays a crucial role in understanding the health status of an individual, particularly in relation to COVID-19.

1. Age: This attribute captures the patient's age, which is important because COVID-19 can affect different age groups in varying ways. Understanding the age distribution can help tailor the diagnostic process and anticipate risk levels.
2. Gender: Gender information is collected as it can influence the severity and symptoms of COVID-19. Research has shown that there can be differences in how the disease manifests and affects individuals based on gender.

3. Fever: Fever is a common symptom of COVID-19, and this attribute records whether the patient has experienced an elevated body temperature, which is a key indicator of infection.
4. Cough: This attribute captures the presence of a cough, another prevalent symptom of COVID-19. Persistent coughing is often associated with respiratory infections, including COVID-19.
5. Difficulty Breathing: Difficulty breathing or shortness of breath is a serious symptom often associated with severe cases of COVID-19. This attribute helps in identifying patients who may require immediate medical attention.
6. Fatigue: Fatigue is recorded to assess whether the patient is experiencing unusual tiredness, which can be a symptom of COVID-19, particularly in conjunction with other indicators.
7. Body Aches: This attribute notes any reported body aches or muscle pain, which are common symptoms experienced by individuals infected with COVID-19.
8. Loss of Taste or Smell: The loss of taste or smell is a distinctive symptom of COVID-19, and its presence can significantly aid in diagnosing the disease.
9. Sore Throat: A sore throat is another symptom that can accompany COVID-19, particularly in its early stages. This attribute helps in building a comprehensive profile of the patient's symptoms.
10. Test Result: The test result attribute records whether the patient has tested positive or negative for COVID-19, providing a definitive outcome for the diagnostic process.

16.4.1 Sample Dataset

Age,Gender,Fever,Cough,DifficultyBreathing,Fatigue,BodyAches,LossOfTasteOrSmell,SoreThroa
t,TestResult
45,Male,true,true,false,false,false,false,false,true
32,Female,false,true,true,true,false,true,false,false
56,Male,true,true,true,true,true,true,false,false

```
import java.io.BufferedReader;
import java.io.FileReader;
import java.io.IOException;
import java.util.ArrayList;
import java.util.List;
```

The `BufferedReader` class is utilized for efficient reading of text from a character-input stream, while `FileReader` is used to read characters from a file. The `IOException` class is included to handle any potential exceptions that may arise during file reading operations. Finally, `ArrayList` and `List` are imported to enable the storage and manipulation of data in the form of a list.

```
class Patient {
  private int age;
  private String gender;
  private boolean fever;
  private boolean cough;
  private boolean difficultyBreathing;
  private boolean fatigue;
  private boolean bodyAches;
  private boolean lossOfTasteOrSmell;
  private boolean soreThroat;
  private boolean testResult;
```

The attributes include `age`, denoting the patient's age, and `gender`, specifying their gender. These demographic details serve as fundamental identifiers. Additionally, boolean flags such as `fever`, `cough`, `difficultyBreathing`, `fatigue`, `bodyAches`, `lossOfTasteOrSmell`, and `soreThroat` capture common symptoms associated with COVID-19. These symptoms are crucial indicators in the diagnosis process.

Furthermore, the `testResult` attribute provides binary information about the outcome of a COVID-19 test, distinguishing between positive (`true`) and negative (`false`) results. This attribute is pivotal in determining the patient's infection status.

```
// Constructor
public Patient(int age, String gender, boolean fever, boolean cough,
    boolean difficultyBreathing, boolean fatigue,
    boolean bodyAches, boolean lossOfTasteOrSmell,
    boolean soreThroat, boolean testResult) {
this.age = age;
this.gender = gender;
this.fever = fever;
this.cough = cough;
this.difficultyBreathing = difficultyBreathing;
this.fatigue = fatigue;
this.bodyAches = bodyAches;
this.lossOfTasteOrSmell = lossOfTasteOrSmell;
this.soreThroat = soreThroat;
this.testResult = testResult;
}
```

The constructor method `public Patient(...)` initializes instances of the `Patient` class for COVID-19 detection. This constructor takes several parameters that represent essential attributes of a patient's condition. These parameters include `age`, representing the patient's age, and `gender`, indicating their gender identity.

Furthermore, boolean parameters such as `fever`, `cough`, `difficultyBreathing`, `fatigue`, `bodyAches`, `lossOfTasteOrSmell`, and `soreThroat` correspond to common symptoms associated with COVID-19. The `testResult` parameter is a boolean value that denotes the outcome of a COVID-19 test performed on the patient. It holds crucial information regarding the patient's infection status, with `true` indicating a positive test result and `false` indicating a negative result.

The constructor method initializes the attributes of a `Patient` instance based on the parameters provided during object creation. Each attribute of the `Patient` class, including `age`, `gender`, and various symptoms such as `fever`, `cough`, `difficultyBreathing`, `fatigue`, `bodyAches`, `lossOfTasteOrSmell`, and `soreThroat`, is assigned a value corresponding to the parameters passed into the constructor. For instance, `this.age = age;` assigns the value of the `age` parameter to the `age` attribute of the `Patient` instance being created. Similarly, the `gender`, `fever`, `cough`, `difficultyBreathing`, `fatigue`, `bodyAches`, `lossOfTasteOrSmell`, and `soreThroat` attributes are initialized with the values provided as parameters.

Lastly, the `testResult` attribute is set based on the `testResult` parameter passed to the constructor. This boolean attribute reflects the outcome of a COVID-19 test performed on the patient, where `true` indicates a positive result and `false` indicates a negative result.

```
public class Main {
  public static List<Patient> readDataset(String fileName) {
  List<Patient> patients = new ArrayList<>();
  try (BufferedReader br = new BufferedReader(new FileReader(fileName))) {
    string line;
  int lineNumber=0
```

The `Main`, class contains a static method `readDataset` responsible for reading a dataset from a file and converting it into a list of `Patient` objects. Within the method, an `ArrayList` named `patients` is initialized to store the patient data read from the file. It utilizes a `BufferedReader` to read the contents of the file specified by the `fileName` parameter.

A `String` variable named `line` is used to store each line of the file as it is read. Additionally, an `int` variable named `lineNumber` is initialized to keep track of the line number for potential error reporting purposes. This variable is useful for identifying the specific line in the file that may be causing issues during data processing.

```
while ((line = br.readLine()) != null) {
lineNumber++;
if (line.startsWith("#")) continue; // Skip comments
String[] data = line.split(",");
// Ensure we have the correct number of fields
if (data.length != 10) {
  System.err.println("Error on line " + lineNumber + ": Expected 10
     fields, got " + data.length);
  continue;
}
public int getAge() {
return age;
}
public boolean getTestResult() {
return testResult;
}
}
```

The try-catch block encapsulating the logic for reading each line of the dataset file. Within the try block, the BufferedReader reads each line of the file until reaching the end (null). During each iteration, the lineNumber variable is incremented to track the current line being processed.

Another check is implemented to ensure that each line contains exactly 10 fields of data. If the length of the data array is not equal to 10, an error message is printed to the standard error stream indicating the line number and the mismatch in the number of fields. This check helps identify and handle any discrepancies or inconsistencies in the dataset format.

```
try {
  int age = Integer.parseInt(data[0]);
  String gender = data[1];
  boolean fever = Boolean.parseBoolean(data[2]);
  boolean cough = Boolean.parseBoolean(data[3]);
  boolean difficultyBreathing = Boolean.parseBoolean(data[4]);
  boolean fatigue = Boolean.parseBoolean(data[5]);
  boolean bodyAches = Boolean.parseBoolean(data[6]);
  boolean lossOfTasteOrSmell = Boolean.parseBoolean(data[7]);
  boolean soreThroat = Boolean.parseBoolean(data[8]);
  boolean testResult = Boolean.parseBoolean(data[9]);
  // Create a new Patient object and add it to the list
  patients.add(new Patient(age, gender, fever, cough, difficultyBreathing,
  fatigue, bodyAches, lossOfTasteOrSmell,
  soreThroat, testResult));
} catch (NumberFormatException e) {
  System.err.println("Error on line " + lineNumber + ": " + e.getMessage());
}
```

```
    }
  } catch (IOException e) {
    System.err.println("Error reading dataset: " + e.getMessage());
  }
  return patients;
  }
```

The try-finally block encapsulating the logic for parsing and initializing patient data from each line of the dataset file. For each line, the String values are parsed and converted to their respective data types using methods like parseInt() for age and parseBoolean() for boolean attributes. These parsed values are then used to initialize a new Patient object, which is added to the list of patients.

A catch block is implemented to handle potential exceptions that may occur during parsing, such as NumberFormatException or ArrayIndexOutOfBoundsException. If any exception occurs, an error message is printed to the standard error stream, indicating the line number and the specific error message. Finally, in the finally block, the BufferedReader is closed to release system resources after reading the entire dataset file.

```
public static void main(String[] args) {
  List<Patient> patients = readDataset("test.txt");
  System.out.println("COVID-19 Detection Results:");
  for (Patient patient : patients) {
    boolean isPositive = patient.isPositiveForCovid();
    String testResult = patient.getTestResult() ? "Positive" : "Negative";
    System.out.println("Age: " + patient.getAge() + ", Test Result: " +
        testResult +
          ", Likely Positive for COVID-19: " + isPositive);
  }
  }
}
```

Within the try block, the readDataset method is called to load patient data from the "test.txt" file into a list of Patient objects. If the dataset is successfully loaded, a message indicating that the dataset has been loaded successfully is printed to the console. For each patient, the isPositiveForCovid method is called to determine whether the patient is likely to have COVID-19 based on their symptoms and test results. The patient's age, COVID-19 test result (positive or negative), and the likelihood of having COVID-19 are then printed to the console.

Finally, in the catch block, any IOException that occurs during the dataset loading process is caught and handled. An error message indicating that an error occurred while reading the dataset is printed to the console, followed by the stack trace of the exception.

```
  public boolean isPositiveForCovid() {
  // A simple rule: if the patient has a fever or cough, they may be posi-
tive for COVID-19
  return fever || cough;
  }
```

The `isPositiveForCovid` method is designed to determine whether a patient is likely to test positive for Covid-19 based on their symptoms. This method takes a `Patient` object as input and returns a boolean value indicating whether the patient is likely to test positive for Covid-19. Inside the method, a logical OR operation is performed on two key symptoms: fever and cough. If the patient experiences either fever or cough, the method returns true, suggesting that the patient is likely to test positive for Covid-19.

```
Patient Age: 45
Covid-19 Test Result: Positive
Is likely to have Covid-19: Yes
------------------------------------------
Patient Age: 32
Covid-19 Test Result: Negative
Is likely to have Covid-19: Yes
------------------------------------------
Patient Age: 56
Covid-19 Test Result: Negative
Is likely to have Covid-19: Yes
------------------------------------------
```

16.5 COVID-19 DETECTION USING X-RAYS

The dataset from Cohen's collection and Kaggle includes a vast array of chest X-ray images, each annotated with information about the patient's COVID-19 status.

```
import org.opencv.core.*;
import org.opencv.imgcodecs.Imgcodecs;
import org.opencv.imgproc.Imgproc;
import weka.classifiers.functions.SMO;
import weka.core.*;
import java.io.File;
import java.io.IOException;
import java.util.ArrayList;
import java.util.List;
```

The `ArrayList` class from the `java.util` package provides a resizable array implementation for dynamic lists, and the `List` interface defines an ordered collection that can contain duplicate elements.

```
public class Covid19Detection {
  static {
  System.loadLibrary(Core.NATIVE_LIBRARY_NAME); // Load OpenCV library
  }
  private String trainingDirectory = "c:/xray";
  // Directory containing training images
  private String newImagesDirectory = "c:/xray/new";
  // Directory containing new images for prediction
  private Instances dataset; // Weka dataset for classification
  public static void main(String[] args) {
  Covid19Detection detector = new Covid19Detection();
  try {
   List<Instance> instances = detector.extractFeaturesFromImages(detec
      tor.trainingDirectory);
   detector.dataset = detector.createDataset(instances);
   Classifier classifier = detector.trainClassifier(detector.dataset);
   detector.predictNewImages(classifier, detector.newImagesDirectory);
  } catch (Exception e) {
   e.printStackTrace();
  }
  }
```

The `Covid19Detection` is designed to detect COVID-19 from X-ray images using machine learning techniques. It begins by extracting features from a set of X-ray images located in the specified directory (`c:/xray`) and creating a dataset from these extracted features. A machine learning classifier is then trained using this dataset. For each new instance, the trained classifier is used to make predictions regarding the presence of COVID-19.

```
// Extract features from images in the specified directory
public List<Instance> extractFeaturesFromImages(String directoryPath) {
List<Instance> instances = new ArrayList<>();
File directory = new File(directoryPath);
File[] files = directory.listFiles((dir, name) -> name.endsWith(".jpg") ||
   name.endsWith(".png"));
if (files != null) {
  for (File file : files) {
  Mat image = Imgcodecs.imread(file.getAbsolutePath());
  double[] features = extractFeatures(image);
  Instance instance = createInstance(features);
  instances.add(instance);
  }
}
return instances;
}
```

The method `extractFeaturesFromImages` is designed to process all image files in a specified directory and extract relevant features from each image. It begins by initializing an empty list of `Instance` objects. It then retrieves all files from the given directory path. For each file, if it is an image file (either `.jpg` or `.png`), the method reads the image using the `opencv_imgcodecs.imread` function. The image is then processed by the `extractFeatures` method to obtain an array of feature values. These features are used to create an `Instance` object, which is added to the list of instances.

```
// Extract features from a given image
  public double[] extractFeatures(Mat image) {
  // Convert to grayscale
  Mat grayImage = new Mat();
  Imgproc.cvtColor(image, grayImage, Imgproc.COLOR_BGR2GRAY);
  // Corner detection
  Mat corners = new Mat();
  Imgproc.goodFeaturesToTrack(grayImage, corners, 100, 0.01, 10);
  // Edge detection
  Mat edges = new Mat();
  Imgproc.Canny(grayImage, edges, 100, 200);
  // Histogram of pixel intensities
  Mat hist = new Mat();
  Imgproc.calcHist(List.of(grayImage), new MatOfInt(0), new Mat(), hist,
     new MatOfInt(256), new MatOfFloat(0, 256));
  // Placeholder for feature values
  double[] featureValues = new double[10]; // Change size based on actual
     feature extraction
  // Populate featureValues with actual features (this is a simplified
  example)
  for (int i = 0; i < featureValues.length; i++) {
    featureValues[i] = Math.random();
    // Replace with actual feature extraction logic
  }
```

```
  return featureValues;
  }
```

The `extractFeatures` method processes an image to extract various local and global features. It begins by reading the image using `Imgcodecs.imread`. Next, it detects corners in the grayscale version of the image with the `Imgproc.goodFeaturesToTrack` method. It then performs edge detection using the `Imgproc.Canny` method and saves the resulting edge-detected image. For global features, it calculates the histogram of pixel intensities using `Imgproc.calcHist`. The method also applies a Gabor filter to the image, creating a filtered version that is saved for further analysis. Additionally, it computes the image moments with `Imgproc.moments` and derives Hu moments from these. The method concludes by returning a placeholder array of feature values, which represents a simplified example of the diverse features that could be extracted from an image. This comprehensive approach captures essential characteristics of the image for further processing or classification tasks.

```
// Create a Weka Instance from feature array
  public Instance createInstance(double[] features) {
  ArrayList<Attribute> attributes = new ArrayList<>();
  for (int i = 0; i < features.length; i++) {
    attributes.add(new Attribute("feature" + i));
  }
  // Adding the class attribute (binary classification)
  attributes.add(new Attribute("class", List.of("COVID", "Normal")));
  Instances instances = new Instances("TestInstances", attributes, 0);
  instances.setClassIndex(attributes.size() - 1);
  DenseInstance instance = new DenseInstance(instances.numAttributes());
  for (int i = 0; i < features.length; i++) {
    instance.setValue(attributes.get(i), features[i]);
  }
  instance.setClassValue("Normal"); // Placeholder for class value
  instances.add(instance);
  return instance;
  }
```

The `createInstance` method constructs a Weka `Instance` object from a given array of features. It starts by creating an `ArrayList` of `Attribute` objects, where each attribute corresponds to an element in the features array, named "feature0", "feature1", and so on. This list of attributes is then used to create an `Instances` object named "TestInstances", which serves as a container for the dataset. The class index for this dataset is set to the last attribute. A new `DenseInstance` object is created with a size equal to the number of features plus one (for the class attribute). The method populates this instance with the feature values from the array. Finally, the instance is added to the dataset, and the method returns the first instance from the dataset.

```
  // Create Weka dataset from a list of Instances
  public Instances createDataset(List<Instance> instances) {
  ArrayList<Attribute>  attributes  =  new  ArrayList<>(instances.get(0).
     numAttributes());
  for (int i = 0; i < instances.get(0).numAttributes(); i++) {
    attributes.add(instances.get(0).attribute(i));
  }
  Instances  dataset  =  new  Instances("TrainingInstances",  attributes,
     instances.size());
  for (Instance instance : instances) {
    dataset.add(instance);
```

```
}
return dataset;
}
```

The `createDataset` method is designed to generate `Instances` dataset from a given list of `Instance` objects. It begins by initializing a new `Instances` object named "TrainingInstances" with a null attribute list and a capacity set to the size of the provided list of instances.

```
// Train the classifier using SVM
public Classifier trainClassifier(Instances dataset) throws Exception {
SMO smo = new SMO();
smo.buildClassifier(dataset);
return smo;
}
```

The `trainClassifier` method is responsible for training a Support Vector Machine (SVM) classifier using the Sequential Minimal Optimization (SMO) algorithm on a given dataset of instances. It begins by creating an instance of the `SMO` classifier, which is a widely used algorithm for training SVMs. The method then calls the `buildClassifier` method on the SMO instance, passing in the provided `Instances` dataset. This method trains the SMO classifier using the data contained in the dataset. Once the classifier is trained, the method returns the trained `SMO` classifier.

```
// Method to classify an instance using a trained classifier
public double classifyInstance(Instance instance, Classifier classifier)
throws Exception {
  // Use the classifier to predict the class label for the given instance
  double predictedClassLabel = classifier.classifyInstance(instance);
  return predictedClassLabel;
}
```

The `classifyInstance` method is designed to predict the class label of a given instance using a trained classifier. It takes two parameters: an `Instance` object representing the instance to be classified and a `Classifier` object representing the trained classifier model. Inside the method, the `classifyInstance` function of the classifier is invoked, passing the instance as an argument. This function returns the predicted class label for the provided instance. If the classification process encounters any exceptions, they are propagated upward.

16.6 VITAMIN DEFICIENCY

The attributes included in the Vitamin Deficiency dataset are Age, Gender, Sun Exposure, Dietary Vitamin D Intake, Serum Vitamin D Level, Bone Pain, Muscle Weakness, Fatigue, Depression, and Hair Loss. Each attribute provides valuable insights into the patient's health status and potential vitamin deficiencies.

1. Age: This attribute captures the patient's age, which is significant as vitamin needs can vary with age. For instance, older adults are more prone to vitamin D deficiency due to reduced skin synthesis.
2. Gender: Gender information is collected as it can influence the risk of vitamin deficiencies. For example, women may have different dietary requirements and absorption rates compared to men.
3. Sun Exposure: This attribute records the amount of time the patient spends in sunlight, which is crucial for the synthesis of vitamin D in the skin. Limited sun exposure can lead to vitamin D deficiency.

4. Dietary Vitamin D Intake: This captures the amount of vitamin D consumed through the diet, which is an essential factor in maintaining adequate vitamin D levels. Foods rich in vitamin D include fatty fish, fortified dairy products, and supplements.
5. Serum Vitamin D Level: This is a direct measure of the vitamin D concentration in the blood, providing a clear indicator of whether a deficiency exists.
6. Bone Pain: Bone pain can be a symptom of vitamin D deficiency, as this vitamin is critical for bone health. This attribute helps in identifying patients who might be suffering from deficiency-related bone issues.
7. Muscle Weakness: Muscle weakness is another symptom associated with vitamin D deficiency. Recording this symptom helps in the comprehensive assessment of the patient's condition.
8. Fatigue: Chronic fatigue can be linked to various vitamin deficiencies, including vitamin D. This attribute assists in evaluating the overall health and energy levels of the patient.
9. Depression: Vitamin D deficiency has been linked to mood disorders such as depression. Including this attribute helps in understanding the broader health impacts of vitamin deficiencies.
10. Hair Loss: Hair loss can be a symptom of multiple vitamin deficiencies, including vitamin D. This attribute adds another dimension to the health profile of the patient.

16.6.1 Sample Dataset

Age, Gender, Sun Exposure, Dietary Vitamin D Intake, Serum Vitamin D Level, Bone Pain, Muscle Weakness, Fatigue, Depression, Hair Loss
35, Male, 2, 800, 10, Yes, No, Yes, No, No
45, Female, 1, 600, 8, Yes, Yes, Yes, Yes, No
28, Male, 3, 1000, 12, No, No, No, No, Yes
50, Female, 1.5, 400, 6, Yes, Yes, Yes, No, Yes
60, Male, 2.5, 1200, 15, No, Yes, No, Yes, No

```
import java.io.BufferedReader;
import java.io.FileReader;
import java.io.IOException;
import java.util.ArrayList;
import java.util.List;
```

Imports `BufferedReader`, `FileReader`, `IOException`, and `ArrayList` and `List` from the `java.util` package.

```
class Patient {
  private int age;
  private String gender;
  private double sunExposure;
  private double dietaryVitaminDIntake;
  private double serumVitaminDLevel;
  private boolean bonePain;
  private boolean muscleWeakness;
  private boolean fatigue;
  private boolean depression;
  private boolean hairLoss;
```

The `Patient` class encapsulates key attributes used in detecting vitamin deficiencies. It comprises fields to store essential patient information, including age, gender, sun exposure level, dietary vitamin D intake, serum vitamin D level, and boolean indicators for symptoms like bone pain, muscle weakness, fatigue, depression, and hair loss. Each instance of this class represents a unique patient profile, offering a comprehensive overview of their health status. By storing these attributes, the `Patient` class facilitates the analysis and detection of potential vitamin deficiencies based on the presence or absence of specific symptoms and other relevant factors.

```
// Parameterized constructor
  public Patient(int age, String gender, double sunExposure, double
     dietaryVitaminDIntake,
     double serumVitaminDLevel, boolean bonePain, boolean muscleWeakness,
     boolean fatigue, boolean depression, boolean hairLoss) {
```

The parameterized constructor in the `Patient` class facilitates the instantiation of patient objects with specific attributes related to vitamin deficiency detection. It accepts various parameters representing essential information about a patient's health status. The `age` parameter denotes the patient's age, while the `gender` parameter indicates their gender. The `sunExposure` parameter captures the level of exposure to sunlight, a factor influencing vitamin D synthesis in the body. Additionally, the `dietaryVitaminDIntake` parameter represents the amount of vitamin D consumed through the diet.

Furthermore, the `serumVitaminDLevel` parameter holds the measured serum level of vitamin D, providing insights into the patient's current vitamin D status. Boolean parameters such as `bonePain`, `muscleWeakness`, `fatigue`, `depression`, and `hairLoss` serve as indicators for various symptoms associated with vitamin deficiencies. Each parameter, when appropriately set, reflects the presence or absence of specific symptoms in the patient.

```
  this.age = age;
  this.gender = gender;
  this.sunExposure = sunExposure;
  this.dietaryVitaminDIntake = dietaryVitaminDIntake;
  this.serumVitaminDLevel = serumVitaminDLevel;
  this.bonePain = bonePain;
  this.muscleWeakness = muscleWeakness;
  this.fatigue = fatigue;
  this.depression = depression;
  this.hairLoss = hairLoss;
  }
  // Getters
  public int getAge() { return age; }
  public String getGender() { return gender; }
  public double getSunExposure() { return sunExposure; }
  public double getDietaryVitaminDIntake() { return dietaryVitaminDIntake; }
  public double getSerumVitaminDLevel() { return serumVitaminDLevel; }
  public boolean hasBonePain() { return bonePain; }
  public boolean hasMuscleWeakness() { return muscleWeakness; }
  public boolean hasFatigue() { return fatigue; }
  public boolean hasDepression() { return depression; }
  public boolean hasHairLoss() { return hairLoss; }
  @Override
  public String toString() {
  return "Patient [age=" + age + ", gender=" + gender + ", sunExposure=" +
     sunExposure +
     ", dietaryVitaminDIntake=" + dietaryVitaminDIntake + ",
          serumVitaminDLevel=" + serumVitaminDLevel +
```

```
        ", bonePain=" + bonePain + ", muscleWeakness=" + muscleWeakness + ",
            fatigue=" + fatigue +
        ", depression=" + depression + ", hairLoss=" + hairLoss + "]";
    }
}
```

The constructor method of the `Patient` class initializes the attributes of a patient object with the values passed as parameters. Each attribute of the patient object is assigned the corresponding value provided in the constructor parameters. The `age` attribute is set to the value of the `age` parameter, representing the patient's age. Similarly, the `gender` attribute is assigned the value of the `gender` parameter, indicating the patient's gender.

Additionally, boolean attributes such as `bonePain`, `muscleWeakness`, `fatigue`, `depression`, and `hairLoss` are initialized based on the respective parameters provided in the constructor. These attributes indicate the presence or absence of symptoms associated with vitamin deficiencies in the patient. By setting these attributes during object instantiation, the constructor ensures that each patient object is initialized with comprehensive health information, facilitating further analysis and detection of vitamin deficiencies.

```
public class VitaminDeficiencyDetector {
  // Method to read dataset from a file
  public static List<Patient> readDataset(String fileName) {
  List<Patient> patients = new ArrayList<>();
  String line;
  int lineNumber = 0;
```

The `readDataset` method is responsible for reading a dataset from a specified file and converting its contents into a list of `Patient` objects. Initially, an empty list called `patients` is created to store the patient data. The method opens a file specified by the `fileName` parameter for reading using a `BufferedReader`. It then initializes a variable `lineNumber` to keep track of the line number being processed in case of errors or exceptions.

Subsequently, within a try-catch block, the method reads each line of the file using the `readLine` method of the `BufferedReader`. For each line, it increments the `lineNumber` variable to track its position within the file. Any encountered exceptions or errors during this process are caught and handled, with appropriate error messages printed to the console.

Finally, after processing all lines in the file, the `BufferedReader` is closed to release system resources, and the method returns the list of `Patient` objects containing the dataset's information.

```
  try (BufferedReader br = new BufferedReader(new FileReader(fileName))) {
    while ((line = br.readLine()) != null) {
    lineNumber++;
    if (line.startsWith("#")) continue; // Skip comments
    String[] data = line.split(",");
    if (data.length != 10) {
      System.err.println("Error on line " + lineNumber + ": Expected 10
         fields, found " + data.length);
      continue;
    }
```

The try block within the `readDataset` method is responsible for iterating over each line of the dataset file, processing its contents, and populating the `Patient` objects. Following this, the code checks if the length of the `data` array is not equal to 10, which indicates an incorrect number of fields for a `Patient` object. If the length is incorrect, an error message is printed to the standard error stream indicating the line number and the number of fields found. The `continue` statement then skips further processing for that line and proceeds to the next one.

```
try {
    int age = Integer.parseInt(data[0].trim());
    String gender = data[1].trim();
    double sunExposure = Double.parseDouble(data[2].trim());
    double dietaryVitaminDIntake = Double.parseDouble(data[3].trim());
    double serumVitaminDLevel = Double.parseDouble(data[4].trim());
    boolean bonePain = data[5].trim().equalsIgnoreCase("Yes");
    boolean muscleWeakness = data[6].trim().equalsIgnoreCase("Yes");
    boolean fatigue = data[7].trim().equalsIgnoreCase("Yes");
    boolean depression = data[8].trim().equalsIgnoreCase("Yes");
    boolean hairLoss = data[9].trim().equalsIgnoreCase("Yes");
    Patient patient = new Patient(age, gender, sunExposure,
       dietaryVitaminDIntake,
      serumVitaminDLevel, bonePain, muscleWeakness,
    fatigue, depression, hairLoss);
    patients.add(patient);
  } catch (NumberFormatException e) {
    System.err.println("Error parsing line " + lineNumber + ": " +
       e.getMessage());
  } catch (ArrayIndexOutOfBoundsException e) {
    System.err.println("Error on line " + lineNumber + ": " + e.getMessage());
  }
  }
} catch (IOException e) {
  System.err.println("IOException while reading the dataset: " +
     e.getMessage());
}
return patients;
}
```

The try block within the readDataset method, focusing on the parsing of data from each line of the dataset and the creation of Patient objects. Inside the try block, each field of the data array is parsed and assigned to the corresponding attributes of a Patient object. The parseInt and parseDouble methods are used to convert string representations of numerical values into their respective integer and double data types, while the parseBoolean method converts string representations of boolean values. If any parsing errors occur, such as invalid number formats or missing fields, the catch block catches NumberFormatException and ArrayIndexOutOfBoundsException, prints an error message indicating the line number and the specific error encountered, and continues to the next line.

Finally, the BufferedReader is closed within the finally block to ensure proper resource management, and the list of patients is returned.

```
public static void main(String[] args) {
  List<Patient> patients = readDataset("test.txt");
  System.out.println("Loaded " + patients.size() + " patients from
     dataset.");
  // Perform vitamin deficiency detection (placeholder for model predic-
  tion logic)
  for (Patient patient : patients) {
    System.out.println(patient); // Display patient information
    // Here you would typically call your machine learning model to predict
    deficiency.
```

```
      // e.g., String prediction = model.predict(patient);
      System.out.println("Predicted Vitamin D Deficiency: [Insert Prediction
         Logic Here]");
      System.out.println("----------");
    }
    }
}
```

The main method begins with a try block, where it attempts to read the dataset file named "test.txt" using the readDataset method. If successful, it prints messages confirming the successful loading of the dataset and proceeds to perform the vitamin deficiency detection. In the catch block, it handles IOException, which may occur if there is an error while reading the dataset file.

16.7 DEPRESSION DETECTION

Each attribute contributes valuable information that can be analyzed to understand an individual's mental health status, particularly concerning depression.

1. Age: This attribute captures the patient's age, which is significant because depression can manifest differently across various age groups. Understanding the age distribution helps in tailoring the diagnostic process and anticipating risk levels.
2. Gender: Gender information is collected as it can influence the prevalence and symptoms of depression. Research indicates that depression can affect men and women differently, with variations in symptom presentation and severity.
3. Marital Status: This attribute records the patient's marital status, as relationship dynamics and social support systems can significantly impact mental health. Being married, single, divorced, or widowed can correlate with different levels of depression risk.
4. Employment Status: Employment status provides insight into the patient's socioeconomic stability and stress levels. Unemployment or job insecurity can be major stressors contributing to depression.
5. Education Level: This captures the highest level of education attained by the patient. Education can influence mental health through factors like job opportunities, social status, and coping mechanisms.
6. Family History of Depression: This attribute notes whether there is a history of depression in the patient's family, which is a significant risk factor. Genetic predisposition and family dynamics can play a crucial role in the development of depression.
7. Sleep Disturbances: Sleep problems are common in depression, and this attribute records issues like insomnia or hypersomnia. Sleep disturbances are both symptoms and potential exacerbators of depression.
8. Appetite Changes: This attribute captures changes in appetite, which are often seen in depressive episodes. Significant weight loss or gain can be indicative of depression.
9. Loss of Interest or Pleasure: This records whether the patient has lost interest or pleasure in activities they once enjoyed, a core symptom of depression known as anhedonia.
10. Fatigue or Loss of Energy: Persistent fatigue or a noticeable decrease in energy levels is another common symptom of depression. This attribute helps in identifying patients who may be experiencing this aspect of the disorder.
11. Feelings of Worthlessness or Guilt: These feelings are significant indicators of depression and can severely impact a person's mental health and daily functioning.
12. Difficulty Concentrating: This attribute notes any reported difficulties in concentrating or making decisions, which are common cognitive symptoms of depression.

13. Suicidal Thoughts: The presence of suicidal thoughts is a critical symptom of severe depression that requires immediate attention and intervention.
14. Depression Diagnosis: This is the outcome variable indicating whether the patient has been diagnosed with depression. This attribute is used to train and validate the predictive model.

16.7.1 Sample Dataset

Age,Gender,MaritalStatus,EmploymentStatus,EducationLevel,Family History of Depression,Sleep Disturbances,AppetiteChanges,Loss of Interest or Pleasure,Fatigue or Loss of Energy,Feelings of Worthlessness or Guilt,DifficultyConcentrating,SuicidalThoughts,Depression Diagnosis
35,Male,Married,Employed,Bachelor's degree,Yes,Yes,Yes,Yes,Yes,Yes,Yes,No,No,No
28,Female,Single,Employed,High school diploma,No,No,No,Yes,No,Yes,No,No,Yes,No
45,Female,Married,Unemployed,Master's degree,Yes,Yes,Yes,Yes,Yes,Yes,Yes,Yes,Yes,No
50,Male,Divorced,Employed,Doctorate degree,No,Yes,No,Yes,Yes,Yes,Yes,Yes,No,No

```
import java.io.BufferedReader;
import java.io.FileReader;
import java.io.IOException;
import java.util.ArrayList;
import java.util.List;
```

These classes and interfaces are essential for reading data from a file and storing it in memory for further processing or analysis.

```
// Patient class representing an individual's mental health attributes
class Patient {
  private int age;
  private String gender;
  private String maritalStatus;
  private String employmentStatus;
  private String educationLevel;
  private boolean familyHistoryOfDepression;
  private boolean sleepDisturbances;
  private boolean appetiteChanges;
  private boolean lossOfInterestOrPleasure;
  private boolean fatigueOrLossOfEnergy;
  private boolean feelingsOfWorthlessnessOrGuilt;
  private boolean difficultyConcentrating;
  private boolean suicidalThoughts;
  private boolean depressionDiagnosis;
```

The class "Patient" represents an individual's characteristics and potential indicators related to depression. It includes fields such as age, gender, marital status, employment status, and education level to capture demographic information. Additionally, there are boolean fields indicating various symptoms and factors associated with depression, such as family history of depression, sleep disturbances, appetite changes, loss of interest or pleasure, fatigue or loss of energy, feelings of worthlessness or guilt, difficulty concentrating, suicidal thoughts, and depression diagnosis. These fields aim to encapsulate a comprehensive set of attributes that may contribute to identifying or assessing depression in an individual.

```
  // Constructor to initialize Patient object
  public Patient(int age, String gender, String maritalStatus, String
     employmentStatus,
```

```
    String educationLevel, boolean familyHistoryOfDepression, boolean
       sleepDisturbances,
    boolean appetiteChanges, boolean lossOfInterestOrPleasure, boolean
       fatigueOrLossOfEnergy,
    boolean feelingsOfWorthlessnessOrGuilt, boolean difficultyConcentrating,
       boolean suicidalThoughts,
    boolean depressionDiagnosis) {
```

The constructor of the "Patient" class initializes its attributes. It takes in various demographic and behavioral indicators related to depression. These parameters include age, gender, marital status, employment status, and education level, which provide insights into the individual's background and socioeconomic context. By encapsulating these attributes within the constructor, the "Patient" object can be instantiated with comprehensive information relevant to assessing depression in an individual.

```
  this.age = age;
  this.gender = gender;
  this.maritalStatus = maritalStatus;
  this.employmentStatus = employmentStatus;
  this.educationLevel = educationLevel;
  this.familyHistoryOfDepression = familyHistoryOfDepression;
  this.sleepDisturbances = sleepDisturbances;
  this.appetiteChanges = appetiteChanges;
  this.lossOfInterestOrPleasure = lossOfInterestOrPleasure;
  this.fatigueOrLossOfEnergy = fatigueOrLossOfEnergy;
  this.feelingsOfWorthlessnessOrGuilt = feelingsOfWorthlessnessOrGuilt;
  this.difficultyConcentrating = difficultyConcentrating;
  this.suicidalThoughts = suicidalThoughts;
  this.depressionDiagnosis = depressionDiagnosis;
  }
  // Getters for the Patient attributes
  public int getAge() {
  return age;
  }
  public String getGender() {
  return gender;
  }
  public boolean isDepressionDiagnosis() {
  return depressionDiagnosis;
  }
}
```

In the "Patient" class, the constructor initializes the attributes of a patient object with the values provided as arguments. Each attribute corresponds to a specific aspect of the patient's condition or history relevant to depression. The constructor assigns the provided values to these attributes, ensuring that each patient object holds accurate information. The attributes include age, gender, marital status, employment status, and education level, providing demographic context. Additionally, boolean attributes such as family history of depression, sleep disturbances, changes in appetite, loss of interest or pleasure, fatigue or loss of energy, feelings of worthlessness or guilt, difficulty concentrating, suicidal thoughts, and depression diagnosis capture various symptoms and risk factors associated with depression. By setting these attributes within the constructor, the "Patient" class encapsulates essential patient information, facilitating the assessment and analysis of depression-related factors.

```
// Main class containing the dataset reading method and execution logic
public class Main {
  // Method to read the dataset from a file and return a list of Patient
objects
  public static List<Patient> readDataset(String fileName) {
  List<Patient> patients = new ArrayList<>();
  try (BufferedReader br = new BufferedReader(new FileReader(fileName))) {
    String line;
    int lineNumber = 0;
```

The “Main” class contains a method named “readDataset,” responsible for reading a dataset file and creating a list of patient objects based on the information provided in the file. The method takes the file name as input and returns a list of patients. Inside the method, it initializes an empty list to store patient objects and creates a BufferedReader to read the contents of the file. Parses the data from the array into the appropriate data types (e.g., integers, strings, booleans) and creates a new “Patient” object using the parsed values. Any parsing errors or array index out-of-bounds exceptions are caught and handled, printing an error message with the line number where the issue occurred. After processing all lines, the BufferedReader is closed, and the list of patients is returned.

```
    // Skip the header line
    br.readLine();
    // Read each line of the dataset
    while ((line = br.readLine()) != null) {
    lineNumber++;
    // Skip comment lines
    if (line.startsWith("#")) continue;
    String[] data = line.split(",");
    // Check for valid data length
    if (data.length != 15) {
      System.err.println("Error at line " + lineNumber + ": Expected 15
         fields but found " + data.length);
      continue;
    }
```

Verifies that the length of the array is exactly 15, as expected for a valid dataset entry. If the length differs, indicating an invalid data format, it prints an error message specifying the line number and the number of fields found. Finally, if the length matches the expected number of fields, the code proceeds to parse the data into appropriate types and create a new “Patient” object using the parsed values.

```
    try {
      // Parsing the patient attributes
      int age = Integer.parseInt(data[0].trim());
      String gender = data[1].trim();
      String maritalStatus = data[2].trim();
      String employmentStatus = data[3].trim();
      String educationLevel = data[4].trim();
      boolean familyHistoryOfDepression = Boolean.parseBoolean(data[5].
         trim());
      boolean sleepDisturbances = Boolean.parseBoolean(data[6].trim());
      boolean appetiteChanges = Boolean.parseBoolean(data[7].trim());
      boolean lossOfInterestOrPleasure = Boolean.parseBoolean(data[8].
         trim());
```

```
    boolean fatigueOrLossOfEnergy = Boolean.parseBoolean(data[9].trim());
    booleanfeelingsOfWorthlessnessOrGuilt=Boolean.parseBoolean(data[10].
       trim());
    boolean  difficultyConcentrating  =  Boolean.parseBoolean(data[11].
       trim());
    boolean suicidalThoughts = Boolean.parseBoolean(data[12].trim());
    boolean depressionDiagnosis = Boolean.parseBoolean(data[13].trim());
    // Creating a new Patient object and adding it to the list
    Patient  patient  =  new  Patient(age,  gender,  maritalStatus,
       employmentStatus, educationLevel,
      familyHistoryOfDepression, sleepDisturbances, appetiteChanges,
      lossOfInterestOrPleasure, fatigueOrLossOfEnergy, feelingsOfWorthle
         ssnessOrGuilt,
      difficultyConcentrating, suicidalThoughts, depressionDiagnosis);
    patients.add(patient);
  } catch (NumberFormatException | ArrayIndexOutOfBoundsException e) {
    System.err.println("Error at line " + lineNumber + ": " + e.getMessage());
  }
  }
} catch (IOException e) {
  System.err.println("Error reading dataset: " + e.getMessage());
}
return patients;
}
```

Inside the "try" block of the "readDataset" method, each line of the dataset is parsed to extract the relevant information for creating a new "Patient" object. The age, gender, marital status, employment status, and education level are extracted as strings from the corresponding indices in the "data" array after trimming any leading or trailing whitespace. The boolean values for family history of depression, sleep disturbances, appetite changes, loss of interest or pleasure, fatigue or loss of energy, feelings of worthlessness or guilt, difficulty concentrating, suicidal thoughts, and depression diagnosis are parsed from the respective string values using the "Boolean.parseBoolean" method after trimming.

Subsequently, a new "Patient" object is instantiated with the parsed values. If any parsing errors occur, such as encountering a non-integer value when parsing the age or any other data type mismatch, a "NumberFormatException" or "ArrayIndexOutOfBoundsException" is caught. In such cases, an error message is printed specifying the line number where the error occurred along with the exception message. Finally, in the "finally" block, the BufferedReader is closed to release the associated resources, ensuring proper cleanup, and the list of patients is returned.

```
public static void main(String[] args) {
List<Patient> patients = readDataset("test.txt");
// Print patient information
if (!patients.isEmpty()) {
  System.out.println("Dataset loaded successfully. Patient Information:");
  for (Patient patient : patients) {
  System.out.println("Age: " + patient.getAge() + ", Gender: " + patient.
     getGender() +
    ", Depression Diagnosis: " + (patient.isDepressionDiagnosis() ? "Yes"
: "No"));
  System.out.println("------------------------------------");
  }
} else {
```

```
    System.out.println("No patient data available.");
  }
  }
}
```

For each patient in the list, the age, gender, and depression diagnosis status are printed to the console. The age and gender of the patient are retrieved directly from the patient object, while the depression diagnosis status is determined by accessing the "depressionDiagnosis" boolean attribute of the patient object. If the value is true, it indicates that the patient has been diagnosed with depression; otherwise, it indicates that the patient does not have a diagnosis of depression.

After printing the patient's information, a separator line consisting of dashes is printed to visually separate the information for each patient.If an IOException occurs while reading the dataset, an error message is printed to the console indicating that an error occurred while reading the dataset, and the stack trace of the exception is also printed for further debugging purposes.

16.8 DEPRESSION DETECTION USING BRAIN IMAGES

These studies utilize features derived from magnetic resonance imaging (MRI) data, highlighting the significance of neuroimaging techniques in understanding the neural correlates of depression.

```
import org.opencv.core.*;
import org.opencv.imgcodecs.Imgcodecs;
import org.opencv.imgproc.Imgproc;
import weka.classifiers.Classifier;
import weka.classifiers.functions.SMO;
import weka.core.Instance;
import weka.core.Instances;
import weka.core.DenseInstance;
import weka.core.SerializationHelper;
```

Imports necessary OpenCV and Weka libraries for image processing and machine learning tasks. It includes classes for core functionalities like loading images, resizing, and applying image processing techniques such as histogram equalization.

```
public class DepressionDetection {
  static {
  System.loadLibrary(Core.NATIVE_LIBRARY_NAME);
  }
  public static void main(String[] args) {
  String imagePath = "brain_image"; // Path to the input image
  Mat preprocessedImage = preprocessImage(imagePath);
  double[] features = extractFeatures(preprocessedImage);

  // Assuming the features are being used to train a model
  trainModel(features);
  }
```

The `DepressionDetection` class serves as the entry point for detecting depression using brain images. Upon execution, it first loads the necessary native libraries required for OpenCV functionality by calling `System.loadLibrary(Core.NATIVE_LIBRARY_NAME)`.

After preprocessing, the `extractFeatures` method is invoked to extract relevant features from the preprocessed image. This typically involves techniques such as Histogram of Oriented Gradients

(HOG) or Gray-Level Co-occurrence Matrix (GLCM) feature extraction, which analyze texture and structural patterns in the image associated with depression.

Once the features are extracted, the `trainModel` method is called to train a model using the extracted features. This model aims to classify whether the input brain image exhibits signs of depression based on the extracted features.

```
public static Mat preprocessImage(String imagePath) {
  // Read the image and convert to grayscale
  Mat image = Imgcodecs.imread(imagePath, Imgcodecs.IMREAD_GRAYSCALE);
  Mat resizedImage = new Mat();
  Imgproc.resize(image, resizedImage, new Size(256, 256));
  // Normalize the image
  Mat normalizedImage = new Mat();
  Core.normalize(resizedImage, normalizedImage, 0, 255, Core.NORM_MINMAX);
  // Apply histogram equalization
  Mat equalizedImage = new Mat();
  Imgproc.equalizeHist(normalizedImage, equalizedImage);

  return equalizedImage; // Return the preprocessed image
  }
```

Initially, the method reads the image file specified by the `imagePath` parameter using the OpenCV `Imgcodecs.imread` function, converting it into a grayscale image using the `IMREAD_GRAYSCALE` flag. After loading the image, it resizes the image to a new size of 256x256 pixels using the `Imgproc.resize` function, ensuring uniformity in image dimensions for subsequent processing steps. Next, it normalizes the pixel intensities of the resized image to a range of 0 to 255 using the `Core.normalize` function with the `NORM_MINMAX` normalization method. This step helps in improving the contrast and dynamic range of pixel values in the image. Finally, it enhances the contrast of the normalized image using histogram equalization performed by the `Imgproc.equalizeHist` function. This process redistributes the intensity values in the image histogram to improve the overall contrast and visibility of image features. The method returns the preprocessed and enhanced image, ready for further analysis or feature extraction tasks.

```
public static double[] extractFeatures(Mat image) {
  // Placeholder for feature extraction using HOG and GLCM
  double[] features = new double[10]; // Adjust size based on actual fea-
     ture extraction

  // HOG Feature Extraction (Placeholder)
  // Implement HOG extraction logic here and populate features array
  // GLCM Feature Extraction (Placeholder)
  // Implement GLCM extraction logic here and populate features array
  return features; // Return the extracted features
  }
```

The Java method `extractFeatures` extracts features from a given input image using two different techniques: Histogram of Oriented Gradients (HOG) and Gray-Level Co-occurrence Matrix (GLCM). For HOG feature extraction, initializes parameters such as window size, block size, block stride, cell size, and number of bins. Next, it calculates four statistical features from the normalized GLCM: mean, standard deviation, minimum value, and maximum value. These features provide information about the texture and spatial relationships present in the image. Finally, returns an empty array as it currently does not return the computed features.

```
public static void trainModel(double[] features) {
  try {
    // Load or create your dataset for training (Weka Instances)
    Instances dataSet = createDataset(features);
    // Set class index (the last attribute in your dataset)
    dataSet.setClassIndex(dataSet.numAttributes() - 1);
    // Initialize and build the classifier
    Classifier classifier = new SMO(); // Support Vector Machine
    classifier.buildClassifier(dataSet);
    // Create an instance for prediction
    Instance instance = new DenseInstance(1.0, features);
    instance.setDataset(dataSet); // Set dataset for the instance
    // Perform classification
    double predictedClass = classifier.classifyInstance(instance);
    System.out.println("Predicted class: " + predictedClass);

    // Save the model if needed
    SerializationHelper.write("DepressionModel.model", classifier);
  } catch (Exception e) {
    e.printStackTrace(); // Print any exceptions for debugging
  }
  }
```

The Java method `trainModel` is designed to train a machine learning model using a given set of featuresInside the method, sets the class index of the dataset and initializes a classifier, in this case, a Support Vector Machine (SVM) classifier. Then, builds the classifier using the provided dataset.

```
public static Instances createDataset(double[] features) {
  // Placeholder for creating a Weka Instances object
  // You should replace this with actual dataset creation logic
  // Example:
  // 1. Create an Attribute List
  // 2. Create Instances object
  // 3. Add features to the Instances object
  return new Instances("DepressionDataset", /* attributes */, 0); // Adjust
attributes
  }
}
```

Next, is prepared an instance using the input features; and set the dataset for this instance. This instance is then evaluated using the trained SVM model to predict the class label. Finally, the predicted class label is printed to the console. If any exception occurs during the process, it is caught and printed to the console for debugging purposes.

16.9 ALZEIHMER'S DETECTION

Employed brain images sourced from publicly accessible datasets such as OASIS and Kaggle.

```
import java.io.File;
import org.opencv.core.Core;
import org.opencv.core.Mat;
import org.opencv.core.MatOfFloat;
import org.opencv.core.MatOfKeyPoint;
import org.opencv.core.Size;
```

```
import org.opencv.imgcodecs.Imgcodecs;
import org.opencv.imgproc.Imgproc;
import org.opencv.objdetect.HOGDescriptor;
import weka.classifiers.Classifier;
import weka.classifiers.functions.SMO;
import weka.core.DenseInstance;
import weka.core.Instance;
import weka.core.Instances;
import weka.core.converters.ConverterUtils.DataSource;
import weka.classifiers.Evaluation;
```

The `Core` class from OpenCV is crucial for accessing fundamental functionalities such as loading the native OpenCV library using `Core.NATIVE_LIBRARY_NAME`. This statement ensures that the OpenCV library is properly loaded before any image processing operations take place. The `Mat` class represents matrices, which are the primary data structures used in OpenCV for storing image data. It allows for various image manipulations such as resizing, transformation, and feature extraction. The `MatOfFloat`, `MatOfInt`, and `MatOfKeyPoint` classes are specialized data structures used to store specific types of data, such as arrays of floating-point values, integers, and key points (used in feature detection algorithms like SIFT and SURF), respectively.

The `Size` class represents the size of an image or a region of interest within an image. It is commonly used for specifying dimensions during image resizing operations.

```
public class AlzheimerDetection {
  public static void main(String[] args) throws Exception {
  // Load OpenCV native library
  System.loadLibrary(Core.NATIVE_LIBRARY_NAME);
  // Preprocess brain image
  Mat preprocessedImage = preprocessImage("brain_image");
  // Extract features
  double[] features = extractFeatures(preprocessedImage);
  // Train and evaluate the model
  trainModel(features);
  }
```

First, the `System.loadLibrary(Core.NATIVE_LIBRARY_NAME)` statement loads the OpenCV native library required for image processing tasks. Next, the `preprocessImage` method is called to preprocess the input brain image. This method performs preprocessing steps such as converting the image to grayscale, resizing it to a standard size, and applying histogram equalization to enhance its contrast and brightness.

After preprocessing, the `extractFeatures` method is invoked to extract relevant features from the preprocessed image. In this case, the method utilizes the Histogram of Oriented Gradients (HOG) technique to compute feature descriptors that capture the image's texture and shape characteristics. Once the features are extracted, the `trainModel` method is called to train a machine-learning model using the extracted features. The trained model is expected to learn patterns indicative of Alzheimer's disease from the provided brain images.

```
  public static Mat preprocessImage(String imagePath) {
  // Load the input image as grayscale
  Mat image = Imgcodecs.imread(imagePath, Imgcodecs.IMREAD_GRAYSCALE);
  // Resize the image to 256x256 pixels
  Mat resizedImage = new Mat();
  Imgproc.resize(image, resizedImage, new Size(256, 256));
```

```
// Apply histogram equalization for contrast enhancement
Mat equalizedImage = new Mat();
Imgproc.equalizeHist(resizedImage, equalizedImage);
return equalizedImage;
}
```

The `preprocessImage` method is designed to preprocess an input image before further analysis or feature extraction. It is specifically tailored for processing grayscale images using the OpenCV library.

First, the method loads the input image located at the specified `imagePath` using the `Imgcodecs.imread` function, ensuring that it is read as a grayscale image (`Imgcodecs.IMREAD_GRAYSCALE` flag). This grayscale conversion simplifies subsequent processing steps as it reduces the complexity of the image data.Next, the method resizes the image to a new size of 256x256 pixels using the `Imgproc.resize` function. Resizing the image to a standardized size ensures consistency in the input data and facilitates subsequent feature extraction steps. After resizing, the image is further resized to a smaller size of 225X225 pixels. This additional resizing step may be performed to further reduce computational complexity or to match the input size requirements of downstream algorithms or models.

Finally, the method applies histogram equalization to enhance the contrast and brightness of the image using the `Imgproc.equalizeHist` function. The preprocessed image, after undergoing these series of transformations, is then returned by the method for further analysis or processing.

```
// Method to extract features using HOG and histogram of pixel intensities
public static double[] extractFeatures(String imagePath) {
// Load the image from the provided path
Mat image = Imgcodecs.imread(imagePath, Imgcodecs.IMREAD_GRAYSCALE);
if (image.empty()) {
  System.out.println("Error: Cannot load image");
  return null;
}
// Resize the image to a standard size for HOG descriptor
Size imageSize = new Size(256, 256);
Imgproc.resize(image, image, imageSize);
// Initialize HOGDescriptor with parameters
HOGDescriptor hog = new HOGDescriptor(
  new Size(256, 256),  // Window size
  new Size(16, 16),    // Block size
  new Size(8, 8),     // Block stride
  new Size(8, 8),     // Cell size
  9        // Number of bins
);
// Compute the HOG features
MatOfFloat descriptors = new MatOfFloat();
hog.compute(image, descriptors);
// Compute histogram of pixel intensities
ArrayList<Mat> imagesList = new ArrayList<>();
imagesList.add(image);
Mat histogram = new Mat();
Imgproc.calcHist(imagesList, new MatOfInt(0), new Mat(), histogram, new
   MatOfInt(256), new MatOfFloat(0, 256));
// Combine both HOG features and histogram values into a single fea-
     ture vector
double[] hogArray = descriptors.toArray();
```

```
double[] histArray = new double[(int) histogram.total()];
for (int i = 0; i < histogram.total(); i++) {
  histArray[i] = histogram.get(i, 0)[0];
}
// Concatenate HOG and histogram arrays into one feature vector
double[] featureVector = new double[hogArray.length + histArray.length];
System.arraycopy(hogArray, 0, featureVector, 0, hogArray.length);
System.arraycopy(histArray, 0, featureVector, hogArray.length, histArray.
   length);
return featureVector;
}
```

The `extractFeatures` method is designed to extract features from a given image using the Histogram of Oriented Gradients (HOG) technique. It utilizes the OpenCV library to perform feature extraction. First, an instance of the `HOGDescriptor` class is created, which is responsible for computing the HOG features. Parameters such as window size, block size, block stride, cell size, and the number of bins are set to configure the HOG descriptor. Additionally, a Support Vector Machine (SVM) detector is set using the `setSVMDetector` method, although it's not directly used for feature extraction in this context. The `compute` method of the `HOGDescriptor` class is then invoked to compute the HOG descriptors for the input image. These descriptors represent the distribution of gradients within localized regions of the image and serve as features for subsequent analysis. Additionally, the `calcHist` method from OpenCV is used to compute the histogram of pixel intensity values in the image. This histogram provides additional information about the distribution of pixel intensities across the image. Finally, the descriptors computed by both HOG and the histogram are converted into a double array and returned by the method, representing the extracted features from the input image.

```
public static void trainModel(double[] features) throws Exception {
  // Load dataset (replace with actual path)
  DataSource source = new DataSource("brain_data.arff");
  Instances dataset = source.getDataSet();
  // Set class index to the last attribute
  dataset.setClassIndex(dataset.numAttributes() - 1);
  // Convert features to Weka Instance
  Instance instance = new DenseInstance(features.length);
  for (int i = 0; i < features.length; i++) {
    instance.setValue(i, features[i]);
  }
  instance.setDataset(dataset);
  // Initialize SVM classifier
  Classifier svm = new SMO();
  svm.buildClassifier(dataset);
  // Evaluate model
  Evaluation evaluation = new Evaluation(dataset);
  double predictedClass = evaluation.evaluateModelOnce(svm, instance);
  // Print the predicted class
  System.out.println("Predicted class: " + predictedClass);
  }
}
```

The `trainModel` method takes an array of features as input, representing the extracted features from brain images. Inside the method, the features are converted into a Weka `Instance` using the

`DenseInstance` class. Then, the class index of the dataset is set, and a Support Vector Machine (SVM) classifier is initialized using the `SMO` class.

The SVM classifier is trained on the dataset using the `buildClassifier` method. After training, an evaluation is performed using the `evaluateModelOnce` method of the `Evaluation` class, which predicts the class of the input features. Finally, the predicted class is printed to the console.

16.10 SKIN CANCER DETECTION

Skin images from publicly available datasets such as ISIC (International Skin Imaging Collaboration) and HAM10000 (Human Against Machine with 10000 training images) have been collected.

```
import org.opencv.core.*;
import org.opencv.imgcodecs.Imgcodecs;
import org.opencv.imgproc.Imgproc;
import weka.classifiers.functions.SMO;
import weka.core.*;
import weka.classifiers.Evaluation;
import java.io.File;
import java.util.ArrayList;
import java.util.List;
Imports various classes from both libraries, including those for image
processing (e.g., `Mat`, `FeatureDetector`) and machine learning (e.g.,
`Classifier`, `Evaluation`).
public class SkinCancerDetection {
  static { System.loadLibrary(Core.NATIVE_LIBRARY_NAME); }
  public static void main(String[] args) throws Exception {
  // Step 1: Load and Preprocess Images
  String imageDir = "path_to_dataset";
  List<Mat> preprocessedImages = preprocessImages(imageDir);

  // Step 2: Extract Features from Images
  List<double[]> featureVectors = extractFeatures(preprocessedImages);
  // Step 3: Train Machine Learning Model
  trainModel(featureVectors);
  }
```

Initially, the OpenCV library is loaded to leverage its image processing capabilities. Following this, the program proceeds with preprocessing the skin lesion images, which involves tasks like resizing, noise reduction, and contrast enhancement. Then, features are extracted from the preprocessed images, utilizing techniques such as texture analysis, color histogram computation, and shape descriptors. These features are represented as numerical vectors and stored in a list. Subsequently, the extracted features are used to train a machine-learning model for classifying skin lesions as benign or malignant. The training process involves feeding the feature vectors into a classification algorithm, such as support vector machines (SVM), to learn the underlying patterns in the data. Optionally, the trained model can be evaluated for its performance using metrics like accuracy, precision, and recall.

```
  // Preprocessing images: resizing, grayscale conversion
  public static List<Mat> preprocessImages(String directoryPath) {
  List<Mat> preprocessedImages = new ArrayList<>();
  File folder = new File(directoryPath);
  File[] imageFiles = folder.listFiles();
  if (imageFiles != null) {
```

```
    for (File file : imageFiles) {
    Mat image = Imgcodecs.imread(file.getAbsolutePath());
    if (!image.empty()) {
      // Resize image to 225x225 pixels
      Imgproc.resize(image, image, new Size(225, 225));
      // Convert image to grayscale
      Imgproc.cvtColor(image, image, Imgproc.COLOR_BGR2GRAY);
      preprocessedImages.add(image);
    }
    }
  }
  return preprocessedImages;
  }
```

The `preprocessImages` method is responsible for preparing the skin lesion images for further analysis and feature extraction. It accepts a directory path containing the images as input and returns a list of OpenCV `Mat` objects, each representing a preprocessed image. Initially, the method initializes an empty list to store the preprocessed images. It then iterates through the files in the specified directory, loading each image using the OpenCV `Imgcodecs.imread` function. If the image loading is successful and the image is not empty, the method proceeds with preprocessing steps. These steps include resizing the image to a standard size of 225X225 pixels using `Imgproc.resize`, and converting the image to grayscale using `Imgproc.cvtColor` to simplify subsequent feature extraction. Finally, the preprocessed image is added to the list of images. After processing all the images in the directory, the method returns the list of preprocessed images. This preprocessing step is crucial for ensuring uniformity and reducing the complexity of the input data before feature extraction and model training.

```
// Extracting features: Histogram of Gradients (HOG) as an example
public static List<double[]> extractFeatures(List<Mat> images) {
List<double[]> featureVectors = new ArrayList<>();
for (Mat image : images) {
  MatOfFloat hogDescriptor = new MatOfFloat();
  // Compute HOG features for each image
  Imgproc.calcHist(List.of(image), new MatOfInt(0), new Mat(),
     hogDescriptor, new MatOfInt(256), new MatOfFloat(0, 256));
  // Convert MatOfFloat to double array
  double[] featureVector = new double[(int) hogDescriptor.total()];
  hogDescriptor.get(0, 0, featureVector);
  featureVectors.add(featureVector);
}
return featureVectors;
}
```

The `extractFeatures` method is tasked with extracting relevant features from the preprocessed skin lesion images. It takes a list of preprocessed images represented as OpenCV `Mat` objects as input and returns a list of feature vectors, where each vector contains the extracted features for a corresponding image. Within the method, a loop iterates over each preprocessed image in the input list. Initially, the method initializes an empty list to store the extracted features. It then utilizes the OpenCV library to detect keypoints in the image using the `FeatureDetector` class. Subsequently, the `calcHist` function calculates the histogram of gradients for the image, providing a quantitative representation of its texture and shape features. The resulting descriptors are converted into a double array format and added to the list of features. This process is repeated for each image in the input list. Ultimately, the method returns a list containing feature vectors, where each vector encapsulates the extracted features for a corresponding preprocessed image. These extracted features serve as valuable input for subsequent stages, such as model training and classification, in the skin cancer detection pipeline.

```
// Train the SVM model using Weka
  public static void trainModel(List<double[]> featureVectors) throws
Exception {
  // Prepare data for Weka
  ArrayList<Attribute> attributes = new ArrayList<>();
  for (int i = 0; i < featureVectors.get(0).length; i++) {
    attributes.add(new Attribute("feature_" + i));
  }
  ArrayList<String> classValues = new ArrayList<>();
  classValues.add("benign");
  classValues.add("malignant");
  attributes.add(new Attribute("class", classValues));
  Instances dataset = new Instances("SkinCancerData", attributes,
     featureVectors.size());
  dataset.setClassIndex(attributes.size() - 1);
  // Add instances to dataset
  for (double[] featureVector : featureVectors) {
    Instance instance = new DenseInstance(featureVector.length + 1);
    instance.setDataset(dataset);
    for (int i = 0; i < featureVector.length; i++) {
    instance.setValue(i, featureVector[i]);
    }
    // Here you can set the class value manually (0 = benign, 1 = malignant)
    instance.setClassValue(Math.random() > 0.5 ? "benign" : "malig-
       nant"); // Example random classification
    dataset.add(instance);
  }
  // Train SVM model
  SMO svm = new SMO();
  svm.buildClassifier(dataset);
  // Evaluate the model (Optional: Perform cross-validation)
  Evaluation eval = new Evaluation(dataset);
  eval.crossValidateModel(svm, dataset, 10, new java.util.Random(1));
  // Print evaluation metrics
  System.out.println(eval.toSummaryString());
  }
}
```

The `trainModel` method is responsible for training a machine learning model using the extracted features from skin lesion images. The dataset is then prepared for training by setting the class index to the last attribute. Subsequently, a classifier, specifically a Support Vector Machine (SVM), is instantiated using the `SMO` class. The `buildClassifier` method is invoked on the SVM instance, which trains the model using the provided dataset. Optionally, model evaluation can be performed using cross-validation to assess its performance.

Index

For Product Safety Concerns and Information please contact our EU representative GPSR@taylorandfrancis.com
Taylor & Francis Verlag GmbH, Kaufingerstraße 24, 80331 München, Germany

www.ingramcontent.com/pod-product-compliance
Lightning Source LLC
Chambersburg PA
CBHW072005230326
41598CB00082B/6719

* 9 7 8 1 0 3 2 8 9 7 1 9 6 *